A tailored education experience —
Sherpath book-organized collections

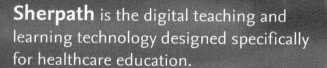

Sherpath is the digital teaching and learning technology designed specifically for healthcare education.

ELSEVIER

Sherpath book-organized collections offer:

Objective-based, digital lessons, mapped chapter-by-chapter to the textbook, that make it easy to find applicable digital assignment content.

Adaptive quizzing with personalized questions that correlate directly to textbook content.

Teaching materials that align to the text and are organized by chapter for quick and easy access to invaluable class activities and resources.

Elsevier ebooks that provide convenient access to textbook content, even offline.

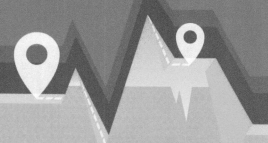

VISIT
myevolve.us/sherpath
today to learn more!

CONTENTS

Understanding Nursing Research

Building an Evidence-Based Practice

8th EDITION

SUSAN K. GROVE, PhD, RN, ANP-BC, GNP-BC

Professor Emeritus
College of Nursing and Health Innovation
The University of Texas at Arlington
Arlington, Texas;
Adult Nurse Practitioner
Arlington, Texas

JENNIFER R. GRAY, PhD, RN, FAAN

Dean
College of Professional Studies
Oklahoma Christian University
Edmond, Oklahoma;
Professor Emeritus
College of Nursing and Health Innovation
The University of Texas at Arlington
Arlington, Texas

ELSEVIER

Elsevier
3251 Riverport Lane
St. Louis, Missouri 63043

UNDERSTANDING NURSING RESEARCH: BUILDING AN
EVIDENCE-BASED PRACTICE, EIGHTH EDITION

ISBN: 978-0-323-82641-9

Notice

Practitioners and researchers must always rely on their own experience and knowledge in evaluating and
using any information, methods, compounds or experiments described herein. Because of rapid advances
in the medical sciences, in particular, independent verification of diagnoses and drug dosages should
be made. To the fullest extent of the law, no responsibility is assumed by Elsevier, authors, editors or
contributors for any injury and/or damage to persons or property as a matter of products liability,
negligence or otherwise, or from any use or operation of any methods, products, instructions, or ideas
contained in the material herein.

Previous editions copyrighted 2019, 2015, 2011, 2007, 2003, 1999, and 1995.

Executive Content Strategist: Lee Henderson
Senior Content Development Manager: Luke Held
Senior Content Development Specialist: Maria Broeker
Publishing Services Manager: Shereen Jameel
Project Manager: Karthikeyan Murthy/Beula Christopher
Design Direction: Renee Duenow

Printed in the United States of America.

Last digit is the print number: 9   8   7   6   5   4   3   2   1

Working together
to grow libraries in
developing countries

www.elsevier.com • www.bookaid.org

To all the nursing students and registered nurses
who are using the best research evidence in their practice.
Susan and Jennifer

To my grandchildren, Jack, Boone, and Cole Appleton,
who have added so much joy to my life.
Susan

To my husband Randy Gray, our children, and our grandchildren,
who make me laugh and remember the importance of memories.
Jennifer

CONTRIBUTOR AND REVIEWERS

CONTRIBUTOR

Polly A. Hulme, PhD, APRN-NP, RN
Emeritus Associate Professor
College of Nursing
University of Nebraska Medical Center
Omaha, Nebraska

REVIEWERS

Maritsa Cholmondeley, BA, ADN, RN
RN Graduate Fellow, Adolescent Psychiatry
Inova Fairfax Hospital/University of Virginia
Falls Church, Virginia

Jaime Lyn Crabb, DNP, RN, FNP-BC
Associate Professor
Practical Nursing Program Coordinator
Northern Michigan University
Marquette, Michigan

Katherine Marie Hagerott, MSN, BA, RN
Registered Nurse, Professor of Pre-Licensure
    Nursing Programs
AdventHealth
Hendersonville, North Carolina

Kathleen B. Heacock, EdD, RN, MSN
Nursing Retention Instructor
Delaware Technical Community College
Georgetown, Delaware

Briana Modes, BSN, RN
Registered Nurse
St Mary Mercy Hospital
Livonia, Michigan

Alicia M. Morrish, BS, BSN, RN
Registered Nurse, Medical Intensive Care Unit
Hurley Medical Center
Flint, Michigan

Patricia O'Malley, PhD, APRN-CNS
Nurse Researcher/Scientist Faculty
Premier Health
Dayton, Ohio

Xuzhe Zhang, PhD
Research Assistant
Division of Human Genetics, Center for Prevention
    of Preterm Birth, Perinatal Institute
Cincinnati Children's Hospital Medical Center
Cincinnati, Ohio

The delivery of evidence-based care is a major goal of professional nursing and health care. By making nursing research an integral part of baccalaureate education, we hope to prepare graduates who can read, critically appraise, and synthesize research. In this way, BSN-prepared nurses can make evidence-based changes in practice. Our aim in writing this research text, *Understanding Nursing Research: Building an Evidence-Based Practice*, is to create excitement about research in undergraduate students. We want students like you to be aware of the relevant knowledge that has been generated through nursing research. Only through research can nursing truly be recognized as a profession with documented effective outcomes for the patient, family, nurse provider, and healthcare system.

Developing the eighth edition of *Understanding Nursing Research* has provided us with an opportunity to update, clarify, and refine the essential content of this undergraduate research text. In addition, a new feature, ***Research/EBP Tip,*** was included throughout each chapter to increase your understanding of providing an evidence-based practice (EBP) in nursing. The revisions in this edition are based on our own experiences with the text and input from dedicated reviewers, inquisitive students, and supportive faculty from across the country who provided us with many helpful suggestions.

Chapter 1, Introduction to Nursing Research and Its Importance in Building an Evidence-Based Practice, introduces you to nursing research, the history of research, and the significance of research evidence for nursing practice. We introduce the types of research synthesis being conducted in nursing—systematic review, meta-analysis, meta-synthesis, and mixed methods research synthesis. The definition of EBP has been updated based on current literature and EBP activities of nurses. The research methodologies of quantitative, qualitative, mixed methods, and outcomes research are explained with the use of examples from published articles. We describe each methodology's contribution to evidence-based practice.

Chapter 2, Introduction to Quantitative Research, presents the steps of the quantitative research process in a clear, concise manner. Extensive, current examples of descriptive, correlational, quasi-experimental, and experimental studies are provided, which reflect the quality of research being conducted in nursing and health care.

For Chapter 3, Introduction to Qualitative Research, we selected four approaches to qualitative research that are frequently reported in the literature. These approaches include phenomenology, grounded theory, ethnography, and exploratory-descriptive qualitative research. Data collection and analysis methods specific to qualitative research are discussed. Guidelines for reading and critically appraising qualitative studies are explained using examples of published studies.

Chapter 4, Examining Ethics in Nursing Research, provides an extensive discussion of the use of ethics in research and the Common Rule, the federal regulations that govern the protection of human subjects. Guidelines are provided to assist students in critically appraising the ethical discussions in published studies and to participate in the ethical review of research in clinical agencies.

In Chapter 5, Examining Research Problems, Purposes, and Hypotheses, we clarify the difference between a study problem and purpose. Examples of problems and purposes are included from current quantitative, qualitative, mixed methods, and outcomes studies. Detailed appraisal guidelines are provided for critically appraising the problems and purposes in studies; the objectives, questions, or hypotheses that may be included; and the variables or concepts that are manipulated or measured.

Chapter 6, Understanding and Critically Appraising the Literature Review, begins by describing different types of publications that might be included in a review, with attention to their quality. The steps for finding relevant sources, reading studies, and synthesizing information into a logical, cohesive review are presented. We provide guidelines for critically appraising literature reviews, distinguishing between the purpose and timing of the literature review in quantitative and qualitative studies.

Chapter 7, Understanding Theory and Research Frameworks, presents the components of theory, different types of theories, and using theories or parts of theories as research frameworks. The purpose of a research framework is discussed, recognizing that researchers may not include the framework in the publication. Guidelines for critically appraising the research framework are presented as well. The guidelines are applied to studies with frameworks derived from research findings and from different types of theories.

Chapter 8, Clarifying Quantitative Research Designs, addresses descriptive, correlational, quasi-experimental, and experimental designs. Because design validity is a key part of a study's quality, we summarize the strengths and threats to design validity in a table and discuss them in relation to current studies. Guidelines are provided for critically appraising the designs of quantitative studies and their validity.

Chapter 9, Examining Populations and Samples in Research, provides a detailed discussion of the concepts of sampling in research. Different types of sampling methods for quantitative, qualitative, mixed methods, and outcomes research are discussed. Guidelines are included for critically appraising the sampling criteria, sampling method, and sample size of nursing studies.

Chapter 10, Clarifying Measurement and Data Collection in Quantitative Research, has been updated to reflect current knowledge about measurement methods used in nursing research. Content has been expanded and uniquely organized to assist students in critically appraising the reliability and validity of scales; precision and accuracy of physiological measures; and the sensitivity, specificity, and likelihood ratios of diagnostic and screening tests.

Chapter 11, Understanding Statistics in Research, focuses on the principles and concepts of the statistical analysis process. We presented the analyses used for describing variables, examining relationships, predicting outcomes, and examining group differences in studies. Excerpts from studies are used as examples of data analyses and results. Guidelines are provided for critically appraising the Results and Discussion sections of nursing studies.

Chapter 12, Critical Appraisal of Quantitative and Qualitative Research for Nursing Practice, was revised to present the three major criteria for critically appraising quantitative and qualitative studies. These criteria are (1) to identify the steps or components of studies; (2) to determine the strengths and weaknesses of studies; and (3) to evaluate the credibility, trustworthiness, and meaning of studies. Within each criterion are specific questions to ask in critically appraising quantitative and qualitative studies. We provide detailed examples of critical appraisals of a current quantitative study and qualitative study using the guidelines provided in the chapter. The studies we use are available in the online Research Article Library for this text.

Chapter 13, Building an Evidence-Based Nursing Practice, has been significantly updated to reflect the current trends in providing evidence-based nursing practice. Detailed guidelines are provided for critically appraising the four common types of research synthesis conducted in nursing (systematic review, meta-analysis, meta-synthesis, and mixed methods research synthesis). These guidelines were used to assist students in examining the quality of published research syntheses and the potential use of research evidence in practice. The chapter includes models to assist nurses and agencies in moving toward EBP. Translational research is introduced as a method for promoting the use of research evidence in practice.

Chapter 14, Introduction to Additional Research Methodologies in Nursing: Mixed Methods and Outcomes Research, includes current information about mixed methods and outcomes studies. Mixed methods studies are making significant contributions to what we know about chronic illness and new infections, such as COVID-19. Outcomes studies are important as they examine patient and financial outcomes using large databases. Because both types of studies are important to healthcare, we wanted you to be able to read and critically appraise these studies to determine their contribution to your EBP.

The eighth edition is written and organized to facilitate ease in reading, understanding, and critically appraising studies. The major strengths of the text are as follows:
- State-of-the art coverage of EBP—a topic of vital importance in nursing.
- **Research/EBP Tips** to increase students' understanding and use of research evidence in practice.
- Balanced coverage of qualitative and quantitative research methodologies.
- Inclusion of mixed methods and outcomes research methodologies throughout the book, with Chapter 14 focused on these two types of research.
- Rich and frequent illustration of major points and concepts from the most current nursing research literature from a variety of clinical practice areas.
- A clear, concise writing style that is consistent among the chapters to facilitate student learning.
- Electronic references and websites that direct the student to an extensive array of information that is important in reading, critically appraising, synthesizing, and using research knowledge in practice.

This text provides a background for understanding quantitative, qualitative, mixed methods, and outcomes research methodologies, making it appropriate for use in research courses for both RN and pre-licensure students. In addition, the text can serve as a valuable resource for practicing nurses in critically appraising studies and implementing research evidence in their clinical settings.

LEARNING RESOURCES TO ACCOMPANY *UNDERSTANDING NURSING RESEARCH*, 8th EDITION

The teaching and learning resources to accompany *Understanding Nursing Research* have been revised for both the instructor and student to reflect content updates to the eighth edition and to promote a maximum level of flexibility in course design and student review.

Evolve Instructor Resources

A comprehensive suite of Instructor Resources is available online at http://evolve.elsevier.com/Grove/understanding/ and consists of a Test Bank, PowerPoint slides, Image Collection, Answer Guidelines for the Appraisal Exercises provided for students, and TEACH for Nurses, which include teaching strategies and other educator resources for research and EBP courses.

Test Bank

The Test Bank consists of approximately 550 NCLEX® Examination–style questions, including approximately 10% of questions in alternate item formats. Each question is coded with the correct answer, a rationale from the textbook, and the cognitive level in the new Bloom's Taxonomy. The Test Bank is provided in ExamView and Evolve LMS formats.

PowerPoint Slides

The PowerPoint slide collection contains approximately 550 slides, including seamlessly integrated Audience Response System Questions, images, and Unfolding Case Studies. The PowerPoints have been simplified, with the Notes area of the slides featuring additional content details. Unfolding Case Studies focus on practical EBP/PICO or PICOS questions, such as a nurse on a unit needing to perform a literature search or to identify a systematic review or meta-analysis to address a practice problem. PowerPoint presentations are fully customizable.

Image Collection

The electronic Image Collection consists of all images from the text. This collection can be used in classroom or online presentations to reinforce student learning.

TEACH for Nurses

TEACH for Nurses is a robust, customizable, ready-to-use collection of chapter-by-chapter teaching strategies and educational resources that provide everything you need to create an engaging and effective course. Each chapter includes the following:
- Chapter Objectives
- Student Resources
- Instructor Resources
- Teaching Strategies
- In-Class/Online Case Study
- Nursing Curriculum Standards

Evolve Student Resources

The Evolve Student Resources include interactive Review Questions, a Research Article Library consisting of 10 full-text research articles, and Appraisal Exercises based on the articles in the Research Article Library.
- The interactive Review Questions (approximately 25 per chapter) aid the student in reviewing and focusing on the chapter material.
- The Research Article Library is an updated collection of 10 research articles taken from leading nursing journals.
- The Appraisal Exercises are a collection of application exercises, based on the articles in the Research Article Library, that help students learn to critically appraise and apply research findings. Answer Guidelines are provided for the instructor.

Study Guide

The companion Study Guide, written by the authors of the main text, provides both time-tested and innovative exercises for each chapter in *Understanding Nursing Research*, 8th Edition. Included for each chapter are a brief Introduction, Terms and Definitions exercises, Linking Ideas exercises, Web-Based Information and Resources exercises, and Conducting Critical Appraisals to Build an Evidence-Based Practice exercises. An integral part of the Study Guide are the appendices, which feature three published research studies that are referenced throughout the critical appraisal exercises. These three recently published nursing studies (a quantitative study, a qualitative study, and a mixed methods study) can be used in classroom or online discussions, as well as to address the Study Guide questions. Key features of the eighth edition Study Guide include the following:
- Increased emphasis on EBP: This edition of the Study Guide continues the EBP emphasis of the revised textbook and reinforces the value of understanding the research process and critical appraisal.

- Web-Based Activities: This section promotes the appropriate use of the Internet for scholarly research and EBP learning experiences.
- Back matter has been updated for quick reference: An "Answer Key" is provided for the exercises developed for each chapter. Each published study is in a separate appendix (three appendices total), which simplifies cross referencing in the body of the Study Guide. Also included is a Critical Appraisal Guidelines appendix that details critical appraisal guidelines for quantitative and qualitative research.
- Quick-reference printed tabs: Quick-reference printed tabs have been added to differentiate the Answer Key and each of the book's three published studies (four tabs total), for improved navigation and usability.

ACKNOWLEDGMENTS

Developing the eighth edition of *Understanding Nursing Research* was a 2-year project, and there are many people we would like to thank. We want to extend a very special thank you to Dr. Polly Hulme for her revision of Chapter 2, Introduction to Quantitative Research, and Chapter 6, Understanding and Critically Appraising the Literature Review. We are very fortunate that Polly was willing to share her expertise and time in developing the eighth edition of this text.

We want to express our appreciation to our universities, The University of Texas at Arlington College of Nursing and Health Innovation and Oklahoma Christian University, which continue to support our writing. We would like to thank nursing faculty members across the world who are using our book to teach research, especially those who take time to send us information on errors. Special thanks to the students who have read our book and provided honest feedback on its clarity and usefulness to them. We would also like to recognize the excellent reviews of the colleagues, listed on the previous pages, who helped us make important revisions in the text.

In conclusion, we would like to thank the people at Elsevier who helped produce this book. We thank those who have devoted extensive time to the development of this eighth edition, the instructor's ancillary materials, the student study guide, and all of the web-based components. These individuals include Lee Henderson, Luke Held, Maria Broeker, Beula Christopher, Karthikeyan Murthy, Aparna Venkatachalam, and Ramkumar Bashyam. Maria Broeker and Beula Christopher have been in constant communication with us to promote the quality and consistency of the formatting and content in this text. It has been such a pleasure working with you.

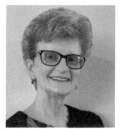

Susan K. Grove,
PhD, RN, ANP-BC, GNP-BC

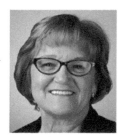

Jennifer R. Gray,
PhD, RN, FAAN

CONTENTS

Introduction to Nursing Research and Its Importance in Building an Evidence-Based Practice

Jennifer R. Gray

CHAPTER OVERVIEW

LEARNING OUTCOMES

After completing this chapter, you should be able to:

1. Define research, nursing research, and evidence-based practice (EBP).
2. Discuss the past and present activities influencing research in nursing.
3. Examine ways of informally and formally acquiring nursing knowledge.
4. Describe the common types of research—quantitative, qualitative, mixed methods, and outcomes—conducted to generate evidence for nursing practice.
5. Describe the purposes of research in implementing an evidence-based nursing practice.
6. Discuss your role in research as a professional nurse.
7. Describe the following strategies for synthesizing healthcare research: systematic review, meta-analysis, meta-synthesis, and mixed methods research synthesis.
8. Examine the levels of research evidence available to nurses for practice.

Welcome to nursing research! Learning about nursing research is similar to moving to a new country. What would you need to do if you moved to a new country? You might need to learn a new language, understand new laws and social customs, and become integrated into the culture of the country. Your experiences in the new country might change your way of evaluating situations and gathering new information. Throughout the process of becoming part of the new country, you may become more observant and ask relevant questions. You may refer to a book about the country as a guide. We developed this book to be a trusted resource, a guide to the world of research.

Research has its own language. This chapter will clarify the meaning of nursing research and its significance in developing an evidence-based practice (EBP) for nursing. Key terms and definitions are introduced throughout the book. You also have a glossary at the back of the book in which each term that appears in the main text in bold font is listed with its definition. Knowing the history of a country may provide a new resident insight into the country. For that reason, this chapter also will include a short description of the history of nursing research. The research accomplishments in the profession since the 1850s are discussed. Research has standard scientific processes that are followed to produce credible, reliable evidence. We will describe these processes and provide examples to help you understand research.

We believe understanding research is necessary for you to be an effective nurse in practice. In this chapter, we will compare ways nurses acquire the knowledge they use in practice, including acquiring knowledge through research. The research methodologies that are commonly used to generate evidence for practice are introduced. We also want you to understand how your role in nursing research will change as you increase the level of your nursing education. Nurses with graduate degrees have additional ways by which they can contribute to ensuring EBP. Your knowledge of research will allow you to contribute to EBP by providing quality, safe, cost-effective care for patients and families. The chapter will conclude with the critical elements of evidence-based nursing practice, such as strategies for synthesizing research evidence, levels of research evidence, and evidence-based guidelines.

WHAT IS NURSING RESEARCH?

The word *research* means "to search again" or "to examine carefully." More specifically, research is a diligent systematic inquiry or study that validates and refines existing knowledge and develops new knowledge. Diligent systematic study indicates planning, organization, and persistence. The ultimate goal of research is to develop an empirical body of knowledge for a discipline or profession, such as nursing.

> **📄 RESEARCH/EBP TIP**
>
> Nursing research is validating existing knowledge and developing new knowledge in a systematic way.

Understanding nursing research requires determining the relevant knowledge needed by nurses. Because nursing is a practice profession, research is essential to develop and refine knowledge that nurses can implement to improve clinical practice and promote quality outcomes (McMenamin et al., 2019; Moorhead et al., 2018; Powers, 2020). Expert researchers have studied many interventions, and nurses have synthesized these studies to provide guidelines and protocols for use in practice. Implementation of practice guidelines in clinical settings, however, has been challenging. Several clinical practice guidelines have been developed for confirming placement of feeding tubes (FTs) in adults. The guidelines recommend using gastric acidity and radiographic confirmation as safe and appropriate methods for confirming placement of a FT in adults (Bourgault et al., 2020).

A national agency in the United Kingdom has banned the use of auscultation and observation of gastric aspirate to determine FT placement (National Patient Safety Agency, 2011). Bourgault et al. (2020) conducted a survey of 408 critical care nurses in the United States and found that 80% used auscultation at least sometimes to verify initial placement of a FT. The most frequently used method was observing for signs of respiratory distress (96%). Most nurses used auscultation in conjunction with other methods, although 35% of their institutions had policies against using auscultation to determine FT placement. The study conducted by Bourgault et al. (2020) confirms the challenges of implementing appropriate methods based on evidence and de-implementing methods not supported by evidence (Makic & Granger, 2019).

Nursing research is also needed to generate knowledge about nursing education. Nursing education research is essential to provide quality learning experiences for nursing students using the most up-to-date methods. For example, Bayram and Caliskan (2019) found that a virtual reality phone learning application improved the tracheostomy care provided by nursing students. With a continuing nursing shortage, it is critical that nursing education finds innovative and effective ways to prepare additional nurses to address relevant health issues, such as opioid abuse and chronic illnesses. In a small study, nursing faculty collaborated with a local health department to provide naloxone education for their students (Carter & Caudill, 2020). The students' knowledge and self-efficacy related to naloxone administration increased and their naloxone stigma decreased after the educational intervention.

Nursing administration and health services researchers examine nurse characteristics, staffing levels, work environment, nurses' intent to leave, cost of care, quality concerns, and patient outcomes. Studies on these topics influence national and state health policy and institutional decisions. Persons with burns are an example of a patient population with risk factors for mortality and complex care needs. A payment claims database was used to extract care outcomes of 14,064 patients with thermal burns who received care in 653 hospitals across the United States (Bettencourt et al., 2020). Nurses in these hospitals provided data on staffing levels and work environment. The researchers found that, in low-volume burn units, nursing staffing and work environment did not have a significant effect on patient mortality. However, in high-volume burn units, each patient that was added to a nurse's workload increased the risk for mortality by 30%. They also found that quality work environments in high-volume burn units were associated with lower patient mortality (Bettencourt et al., 2020). Studies such as these have lifesaving implications. In summary, nursing research is a scientific process that validates and refines existing knowledge and generates new knowledge that directly and indirectly influences nursing practice. Nursing research is the key to building an EBP for our profession.

WHAT IS EVIDENCE-BASED PRACTICE?

The ultimate goal of nursing is an EBP that promotes quality, safe, and cost-effective outcomes for patients, families, healthcare providers, and the healthcare system (Melnyk & Fineout-Overholt, 2019; Melnyk et al., 2018). EBP in nursing evolves from the integration of the best research evidence with our clinical expertise and our patients' circumstances and values to produce quality health outcomes (Melnyk & Fineout-Overholt, 2019; Straus et al., 2019). Fig. 1.1 identifies the elements of EBP and demonstrates the major contribution of best research evidence to the delivery of this practice. The best research evidence is the empirical knowledge generated from the synthesis of quality health studies to address a clinical problem.

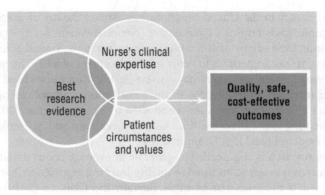

FIG. 1.1 Model of Evidence-Based Practice.

Teams of expert researchers, healthcare professionals, and sometimes policymakers and consumers synthesize the best research evidence in different areas to develop national clinical guidelines or standards of practice for patient and family care (Grinspun & Bajnok, 2018). For example, a professional organization devoted to infusion therapy, the Infusion Nurses Society, published the standards of care for peripheral intravenous (PIV) therapy. The standards of care were developed by a team of clinical nurse experts who identified, critically appraised, and synthesized research to develop EBP standards of care that are discussed later in this section (Gorski et al., 2016; Nickel, 2019).

Clinical expertise is the knowledge and skills of the healthcare professional providing care. The clinical expertise of a nurse depends on his or her years of clinical experience, current knowledge of the research and clinical literature, and educational preparation. The stronger the nurse's clinical expertise, the better is her or his clinical judgment in implementing the best research evidence in practice.

EBP also incorporates the circumstances and values of a patient. Patient circumstances include the individual's physical condition, disease trajectory, family structure, economic resources, and educational level. In addition, a patient brings values or unique preferences, expectations, concerns, and cultural beliefs to each clinical encounter that need to be integrated by the nurse into the care delivered. Within the nurse–patient relationship, the nurse learns about the unique characteristics of the patient that affect the care that is needed (Feo et al., 2018). Thus EBP is the unique combination of the best research evidence being implemented by expert nurse clinicians in providing care to patients and families with specific health circumstances and values to promote quality, safe, cost-effective outcomes (Melnyk & Fineout-Overholt, 2019; Straus et al., 2019; see Fig. 1.1).

📄 **RESEARCH/EBP TIP**

Combining best research evidence, clinical expertise, and patients' preferences and values results in EBP, which promotes quality, safety, and cost-effectiveness.

Evidence-Based Standards of Care for Peripheral Intravenous Access

Research findings from multiple studies are synthesized to develop guidelines, standards, protocols, algorithms (clinical decision trees), and/or policies to direct the implementation of a variety of nursing interventions. Inserting a PIV catheter is the most common invasive procedure in hospitals worldwide (Nickel, 2019). The members of the Infusion Nurses Society used evidence from many studies to develop standards of care for every aspect of PIV therapy. The standards of care for PIV therapy, more than 150 pages long, provides detail about every aspect of PIV therapy (Gorski et al., 2016). As an example of applying evidence in practice, we are going to apply the evidence-based standards of care for initial PIV placement to an older patient (Nickel, 2019). As a nursing student or practicing nurse, you must apply the EBP recommendations for PIV therapy to ensure safety of the patient. Table 1.1 provides guidance for determining the site for PIV, selecting an appropriate catheter, preparing the site, inserting the catheter, and documenting the insertion.

Delivery of Evidence-Based Care to a Selected Patient Needing Peripheral Intravenous Therapy

Fig. 1.2 provides an example of the delivery of evidence-based nursing care to an adult female patient, Evelyn Jackson, who is 79 years old. She is dehydrated and may have a kidney infection. By assessing Mrs. Jackson, the nurse notes that she has fragile skin with skin tears on her nondominant hand from a recent fall. The best research evidence identifies:

1. Selecting a 22-gauge catheter or smaller because of the patient's age
2. Using vascular visualization technology, if needed, to identify an appropriate site for PIV placement
3. Preparing the site aseptically
4. Inserting the catheter at a reduced angle (5–15 degrees) to accommodate less subcutaneous tissue often found in older adults

TABLE 1.1	EVIDENCED-BASED STANDARDS OF CARE FOR PERIPHERAL INTRAVENOUS DEVICE PLACEMENT	
ACTION	**STANDARDS OF CARE**
Selection of device	• For older adults, use the smallest gauge (22–24 gauge) device for the therapy that has been prescribed (p.S51; Std 26.I.B.2[a]). • Catheters greater than 20 gauge are associated with an increased incidence of phlebitis (p.S51; Std 26.I. B.1).
Selection of site	• The forearm is the preferred site to increase dwell time, decrease pain, promote self-care, prevent occlusion, and avoid accidental removal (p.S54; Std 27.I.A.1). • Use the nondominant hand or arm when possible (p.S54; Std 27.I.C.1). • Avoid compromised areas and distal to this area, such as site of prior infiltration (p.S54; Std 27.I.C.3). • Promote vascular distention using a tourniquet or blood pressure cuff so that venous flow is impeded but arterial circulation is not (p. S64; Std 33.II.C.1). • If patient has compromised circulation, bruises easily, or fragile veins, use another method, such as warmth or gravity, to promote vascular distention (p. S64; Std 33.II.C.1). • Palpate the veins in the limb at the planned insertion site, maintaining the integrity of the glove (p. S64; Std 33.II.E.1). • Use visible light devices or near infrared light technology to aid in visualization of appropriate veins (p.S44; Std 22.I.B.1–4 and 22.I.C.1–2).

Continued

TABLE 1.1	EVIDENCED-BASED STANDARDS OF CARE FOR PERIPHERAL INTRAVENOUS DEVICE PLACEMENT—cont'd
ACTION	**STANDARDS OF CARE**
Preparation of the site	• Use a new pair of disposable, nonsterile gloves (p. S64; Std 33.II.E.1). • Clean the skin at the intended site with 5% or more chlorohexidine in alcohol solution. Use an approved alternate solution if chlorhexidine is contraindicated (p. S64; Std 33.II.D). • Allow adequate time after cleaning of the site for the skin to dry (p. S64; Std 33.II.D). • Do not palpate the vein after the skin is cleaned to avoid contamination (p. S64; Std 33.II.E.1).
Insertion of catheter	• Use a new sterile device (catheter) for each attempt (p. S64; Std 33.1). • Insert the catheter. Adjust the catheter insertion angle based on the thickness of the skin and subcutaneous tissue (Coulter, 2016). With blood return or perceived entrance into the vein, reduce the angle further to almost parallel to the skin (Coulter, 2016).
Securing the PIV catheter	• Use an adhesive "engineered stabilization device (ESD)" or "bordered polyurethane securement dressing" to maintain the PIV and visualize the insertion site (p. S72–S73; Std 37.D.1–3). • Do not use rolled bandages of any type to secure a PIV catheter because they may impair visualization of the site and infusion of solution (p. S72–S73; Std 37.H).
Documentation of insertion	• Document in the electronic healthcare record the patient or family member's understanding of the need for the PIV and subsequent therapy; site preparation; type, length, and gauge of PIV device; date and time; number of insertions; patient teaching of signs and symptoms to report; and other elements based on facility policies (p. S29; Std 10.A.1–7).
Ongoing assessment of PIV insertion site	• Assess signs of infiltration such as pain, edema, changes in color, and fluid leakage at the insertion site (p. S99; Std 46.F.1–4). • Immediately stop the infusion if any signs of infiltration exist (p. S99; Std 46.G). • Recognize that subsequent PIVs are at higher risk for infiltration (p. S98; Std 46.C.4). • In case of infiltration, outline the area of infiltration with a skin marker to allow assessment of subsequent changes (p. S99; Std 46.G.7). • Assess insertion site for signs of infection, such as erythema, edema, pain, and changes in body temperature (p. S106; Std 49.A). • Remove PIV if patient develops any signs of infection (p. S106; Std 49.C).

[a]All page numbers in the table are from Gorski et al. (2016). The page numbers are in a supplemental issue; therefore pages are preceded with capital S. The numbers after the page number refer to the Standard number and subpart, such as 33.3. For some standards, the subsequent numbers refer to the Practice Criteria sections, subsections, and numbered Statements. Page numbers are included, although not direct quotations, to facilitate finding specific standard in the 160-page standard document.

PIV, Peripheral intravenous.

Adapted from Coulter, K. (2016). Successful infusion in older adults. *Journal of Infusion Nursing, 39*(6), 352–358. https://doi.org/10.1097/NAN.0000000000000196; Gorski et al. (2016). Infusion therapy standards of practice. *Journal of Infusion Nursing, 39*(1S), S1-S159; Nickel, B. (2019). Peripheral intravenous access: Applying infusion therapy standards of practice to improve patient safety. *Critical Care Nurse, 39*(1), 61–71. https://doi.org/10.4037/ccn2019790.

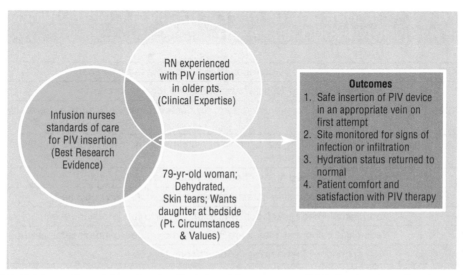

FIG. 1.2 Evidence-Based Practice for Peripheral Intravenous (PIV) Device Insertion in an Older Adult Woman. *Pt.,* Patient; *pts.,* patients; *RN,* registered nurse.

5. Securing the PIV catheter in a way that allows visualization and assessment of the site
6. Monitoring the infusion and the PIV site routinely (see Table 1.1; Gorski et al., 2016; Nickel, 2019).

EBP goes beyond knowing and applying standards of care or clinical guidelines, however. As shown in Fig. 1.2, the evidence must be integrated with the nurse's clinical expertise and the patient's preferences. The nurse asks Mrs. Jackson about previous PIV insertions and learns that she has not had one recently. Although the standards of care indicate using the nondominant forearm for PIV devices, the nondominant side is ruled out because of the skin injury. The assessment of Mrs. Jackson's skin and experiences with PIV therapy in older adults are indicators of the nurse's clinical expertise. Mrs. Jackson does not like needles and asks that her daughter be able to hold her other hand during the procedure. These standards of care, developed from the best research evidence, are translated by registered nurses (RNs) and nursing students to address the characteristics, circumstances, and values of adult patients being hospitalized for dehydration and possible infection.

HISTORICAL DEVELOPMENT OF RESEARCH IN NURSING

Initially, nursing research evolved slowly following the investigations of Florence Nightingale in the 19th century. During the 1930s and 1940s, nurse researchers studied nursing education. Their focus moved to exploring and describing nurses and nursing roles in the 1950s and 1960s. From the 1970s to the present, nurse researchers have focused their research on clinical problems, nursing interventions, and the outcomes of the interventions. These topics were important because of their growing commitment to providing EBP for patients. Reviewing the history of nursing research enables us to identify the accomplishments of nurses earlier in our profession. It also helps us understand the need for further research to determine the best research evidence for use in practice. Table 1.2 outlines the key historical events that have influenced the development of research in nursing.

TABLE 1.2	CHRONOLOGY OF KEY EVENTS IN THE DEVELOPMENT OF NURSING RESEARCH
YEAR	**EVENT**
1850	Florence Nightingale was recognized as first nurse researcher.
1900	*American Journal of Nursing* was published for the first time.
1923–1929	First graduate educational program for nurses began at Columbia University and Yale University.
1932	Association of Collegiate Schools of Nursing was formed to develop standards for education and practice.
1950	ANA commissioned study of nursing functions and activities.
1952	First research journal in nursing, *Nursing Research*, was published.
1955	American Nurses Foundation was established to fund nursing research.
1957	Regional nursing societies were developed to support and disseminate nursing research.
1965	ANA sponsored first nursing research conferences.
1970	ANA Commission on Nursing Research was established.
1972	Cochrane published *Effectiveness and Efficiency,* introducing concepts relevant to EBP.
1973	First Nursing Diagnosis Conference held and became the NANDA.
1976	*Stetler-Marram Model for Application of Research Findings to Practice* was published.
1980s–1990s	Methodologies were developed to determine *best evidence* for practice by Sackett and colleagues.
1982–1983	The report of the *Conduct and Utilization of Research in Nursing Project* was published.
1983	*Annual Review of Nursing Research* was published for the first time.
1985	NCNR was established at the National Institutes of Health.
1989	AHCPR was established.
1990	American Nurses Credentialing Center implemented the Magnet Hospital Designation Program for Excellence in Nursing Services.
1992	*Healthy People* was initiated by the federal government; the Cochrane Center was established.
1993	NCNR renamed the National Institute of Nursing Research (NINR); The Cochrane Collaboration initiated providing systematic reviews and EBP guidelines.
1999	AHCPR renamed Agency for Healthcare Research and Quality (AHRQ).
2001	Stetler revised the model, *Steps of Research Utilization to Facilitate EBP;* Institute of Medicine published report *Crossing the Quality Chasm: A New Health System for the 21st Century.*
2002	The Joint Commission revised accreditation policies for hospitals supporting EBP; NANDA became international—NANDA-I.
2005	Quality and Safety Education for Nurses program was initiated with one competency being EBP.
2006	AACN published statement on nursing research.

TABLE 1.2	CHRONOLOGY OF KEY EVENTS IN THE DEVELOPMENT OF NURSING RESEARCH—cont'd	
YEAR	**EVENT**
2016	NINR mission statement and strategic plan updated.
2017	AACN leading initiatives of research and data management; AHRQ current mission and funding priorities; *Healthy People 2020* topics and objectives; NINR current research funding and other activities to promote research in nursing.
2020	*Healthy People 2030* was published. Nursing professional organizations responded to the coronavirus disease 2019 (COVID-19) pandemic by providing continuing education about the disease and stress management.

AACN, American Association of Colleges of Nursing; *AHCPR*, Agency for Health Care Policy and Research; *ANA*, American Nurses Association; *EBP*, evidence-based practice; *NANDA*, North American Nursing Diagnosis Association; *NCNR*, National Center for Nursing Research; *NINR*, National Institute of Nursing Research.

Florence Nightingale

Florence Nightingale (1840–1910) was a British nurse who is viewed as the Mother of Modern Nursing because of her work during the Crimean War, research activities, and involvement in the education of nurses. Nightingale (1859) is also recognized as the first nurse researcher for her studies focused on the influence of a healthy environment, such as ventilation, cleanliness, and purity of water, on patients' health (Herbert, 1981). She investigated maternal mortality related to puerperal fever and found that the deaths of many mothers were preventable (McDonald, 2001). She also became involved in training nurses and began moving nursing from an uneducated, poorly respected group to a profession that is among the most respected (Pickler, 2020).

Nightingale became well-known because of her work during the Crimean War and the reports of her work in the *London Times*. In addition to leading trained nurses who provided care, she collected data and conducted statistical analyses. She studied soldiers' mortality rates and the conditions related to mortality. By presenting her results in tables, bar graphs, and pie charts, she was able to present a clear argument for clean conditions and trained nursing care (McDonald, 2001). She advocated for systematic collection of data in hospitals. Nightingale was the first woman elected to the Royal Statistical Society based on her research and statistical expertise (Oakley, 2010).

🗎 RESEARCH/EBP TIP

Nightingale, often called the Lady of the Lamp, was a researcher and statistician.

Nightingale's research enabled her to instigate attitudinal, organizational, and social changes. She changed the attitudes of the military and society about the care of the sick. The military began to view the sick as individuals who require adequate food, suitable quarters, and appropriate medical treatment. This realization greatly reduced the mortality rate (Cook, 1913). Because of Nightingale's research evidence and influence, society began to slowly accept responsibility for testing public water, improving sanitation, preventing starvation, and decreasing morbidity and mortality rates (Palmer, 1977).

Nursing Research in the 1900s Through the 1970s

The *American Journal of Nursing* was first published in 1900, with the first research, case studies, appearing in this journal in the late 1920s. A case study involves an in-depth analysis and systematic description of one patient or group of similar patients to promote the understanding of healthcare interventions, problems, and/or situations (Yin, 2018). Case studies are one example of the practice-related research that has been conducted in nursing over the last century. Research capacity grew among nurses as graduate education programs were developed for nurses. The first doctoral program for nurses was offered at Columbia University, and the first master's degree in nursing was offered by Yale University.

The American Nurses Association (ANA) initiated a 5-year study on nursing functions and activities, which was published in 1959. The findings from this study were used to develop statements on functions, standards, and qualifications for professional nurses. Some new nursing specialty organizations included in their missions to develop standards of care for their specialties. The research conducted by the ANA and specialty groups provided the basis for the first nursing practice standards that have been revised over time and continue to guide professional practice (Fitzpatrick, 1978; McMenamin et al., 2019).

📄 RESEARCH/EBP TIP

As more nurses completed graduate degrees, nurses developed more studies on clinical topics. Graduate nursing education increased nurses' ability to provide evidence-based care and conduct research.

Research became part of the curricula of baccalaureate and master's in nursing programs in the 1950s and 1960s. The increase in research activities prompted the publication of the first research journal, *Nursing Research*, in 1952 (Fitzpatrick, 1978). *Nursing Research* is still one of the most respected nursing research journals today. The American Nurses Foundation was established in 1955 to fund nursing research projects. The Southern Regional Educational Board, Western Interstate Commission on Higher Education, Midwestern Nursing Research Society, and New England Board of Higher Education were formed in 1957 and have important roles today in supporting and disseminating nursing research across the United States.

In the 1960s, an increasing number of clinical studies focused on quality care and the development of criteria to measure patient outcomes. Intensive care units were developed, which promoted the investigation of nursing interventions, staffing patterns, and cost-effectiveness of care for a new setting (Gortner & Nahm, 1977). Nurses also began developing models, conceptual frameworks, and theories to guide nursing practice. These nursing theorists generated propositions that required testing, which provided direction for nursing research. In 1970 the ANA Commission on Nursing Research was formed to expand the conduct of research. The commission influenced the development of federal guidelines for research with human subjects (See, 1977).

Despite these accomplishments, nurses were not recognized for their intelligence and expertise. However, in a nursing school in Indiana, six nursing students decided to start an honor society for nurses. They would be surprised to see that the honor society they started, Sigma Theta Tau International, has grown to include chapters around the world. Sigma, the current name of the society, advocates for the dissemination of research findings. Sigma leaders recognize that clinical nurses cannot use research findings in practice when they do not know about the findings. Over time, Sigma has sponsored national and international research conferences, and chapters of this organization sponsor many local conferences to communicate research findings.

Moving from knowing research findings to using them in practice is not an easy process. Archie Cochrane, a medical professor, recognized that fact. To facilitate the use of research evidence in practice, the Cochrane Center was established in 1992 and the Cochrane Collaboration in 1993. The Cochrane Collaboration and Library house numerous resources to promote EBP, such as systematic reviews of research, evidence-based guidelines, and other quality evidence to use in practice (see the Cochrane website, http://www.cochrane.org).

Researchers who wanted to study nursing care and its influence on patient outcomes found that work very difficult. Nurses in different hospitals and different parts of the country used a variety of terms for aspects of the nursing process. To work toward consistency, the first Nursing Diagnosis Conference was held in 1973. From the conference, the North American Nursing Diagnosis Association (NANDA) was formed and expanded internationally to be known as NANDA International (NANDA-I). The organization started a journal to publish research related to nursing diagnoses and interventions (see Table 1.2). Details on NANDA-I can be found on their website (http://www.nanda.org). The standardization of nursing diagnoses and interventions allowed researchers to extract data from electronic health records and laid the groundwork for outcomes research.

Nursing Research in the 1980s and 1990s

The conduct of clinical research received increased focus in the 1980s, and clinical journals began publishing more research reports. New nursing journals were also published specifically to report studies and the application of theory to practice. Although the body of empirical knowledge generated through clinical research increased rapidly in the 1980s, little of this knowledge was used in practice. During 1982 and 1983, a project called the Conduct and Utilization of Research in Nursing was funded by the federal government. The project published a guide on how to use research to improve clinical practice (Horsley et al., 1983).

Qualitative research was introduced in nursing in the late 1970s; the first studies appeared in nursing journals in the 1980s. Qualitative research used text, instead of numbers, to explore the holistic nature of people and phenomena, discovering meaning and gaining new insights into issues relevant to nursing. The number of qualitative researchers and studies expanded greatly in the 1990s, with qualitative studies appearing in most of the nursing research and clinical journals.

Another priority of the 1980s was to obtain increased funding for nursing research. Most of the federal funds in the 1980s were designated for medical studies involving the diagnosis and treatment of diseases. However, the ANA achieved a major political victory for nursing research with the creation of the National Center for Nursing Research in 1985. The purpose of this center was to support the conduct and dissemination of knowledge developed through basic and clinical nursing research, training, and other programs in patient care research (Bauknecht, 1985). The National Center for Nursing Research became the National Institute of Nursing Research (NINR) in 1993 to increase the status of nursing research and to obtain more funding for studies (NINR, n.d.).

Outcomes research emerged in the late 1980s and 1990s as an important methodology for documenting the effectiveness of healthcare services. Outcomes research, sometimes called effectiveness research, evolved when the federal government raised concerns about the quality and appropriateness of care that patients received. The government was especially concerned about the outcomes of patients for whom government programs, such as Medicare, were the insurers. Dr. Linda Aiken led a group of nurse researchers, statisticians, and other scientists to study the outcomes of nursing care in hospitals. Aiken et al. (2002) reported that for every additional patient assigned to nurses, the likelihood that a patient would die within 30 days of discharge increased by 7%. Dr. Aiken has continued this program of research and expanded it to work with researchers in other countries. Dr. Aiken has continued to affect health policy by reporting that patient mortality decreased when the percentage of nurses in the hospital with a BSN or higher degree increased (Cheung & Aiken, 2006) and demonstrating the effect of nurses on patient outcomes in numerous countries (Aiken et al., 2011).

📄 RESEARCH/EBP TIP

Research has shown that nurses' workload and education influence patient outcomes.

Other agencies and centers were established within the US Department of Health and Human Services to promote positive health outcomes, such as the Agency for Health Care Policy and Research (AHCPR) (Rettig, 1991). AHCPR was responsible for publishing the first clinical practice guidelines, which were syntheses of the best research evidence. In 1999 AHCPR's name was changed to the Agency for Healthcare Research and Quality (AHRQ), which signaled an increased focus on improving the quality and safety of patient care. Also within the US Department of Health and Human Services, the Centers for Disease Control and Prevention (CDC) was established with its name being a statement of its mission. The CDC was viewed as an authority on public health when the pandemic caused by coronavirus 19 (COVID-19) affected the United States in 2020. The Centers for Medicare and Medicaid Services oversee Medicare for older adults and some aspects of state-administered care for the uninsured, children, and families in poverty. Although the primary functions of the CDC and the Centers for Medicare and Medicaid Services do not include research, they employ many scientists who analyze data and conduct research to improve health. Some of these scientists are nurses who study the effects of Medicare decisions, and others are deployed around the world to work with communities in low-income countries and to provide surveillance of emerging infections.

EBP became more refined in the 1990s. A research group led by Dr. David Sackett developed explicit research methodologies to determine the *best evidence* for practice. EBP grew in importance for nursing in 1990 when the American Nurses Credentialing Center implemented the Magnet Hospital Designation Program for Excellence in Nursing Services. The criteria for Magnet designation have evolved but continue to include demonstrating that (1) nurses are delivering evidence-based care to patients and (2) nurses at the bedside are leading studies to improve the outcomes of their patients.

Nursing Research in the 21st Century

The vision for nursing research in the 21st century includes conducting quality studies using a variety of methodologies, synthesizing the study findings into the best research evidence, and using this research evidence to guide practice (Melnyk & Fineout-Overholt, 2019; Melnyk et al., 2018). To expand EBP in clinical agencies, Stetler (2010) revised the Research Utilization to Facilitate EBP Model, and it continues to be used as a model to integrate research into practice in some healthcare systems (Karl & Mion, 2020; see Chapter 13 for a description of this model). In 2004 Sigma began publishing a journal related to EBP titled *Worldviews on Evidence-Based Nursing* that contains research syntheses and systematic reviews of research for clinical practice.

The focus of healthcare research and funding has expanded from the treatment of illness to include health promotion and illness prevention. The *Healthy People 2000, 2010,* and *2020* plans increased the visibility of health promotion goals and the motivation to study interventions to improve health (see Table 1.1). *Healthy People 2030* (USDHHS, n.d.) topics and objectives can be reviewed on the *Healthy People* website (https://health.gov/healthypeople). The topics cover all ages and a wide range of topics related to living healthy and using available technologies that facilitate health-promoting behaviors. In the coming decade, nurse researchers will have a major role in the development of interventions to promote health and prevent illness in individuals and families.

Nurse researchers also have a critical role in promoting safe and quality health care. *To Err Is Human: Building a Safer Health System* (Kohn et al., 2000) was published by the Institute of Medicine (IOM) to report the high incidence of errors in health care. The IOM followed the next year with *Crossing the Quality Chasm: A New Health System for the 21st Century* (IOM, 2001). The second report identified the characteristics of a high-quality health system and the competencies needed by healthcare professionals to create that environment. Based on this report, six competency areas were identified as essential for nursing education to ensure that students were able to deliver quality, safe care. Specific competencies were identified in six areas (Box 1.1). The Quality and Safety Education for Nurses (QSEN) initiative (2017) identified the requisite knowledge, skills, and attitude statements for each of the competencies for nurses and recommended strategies for incorporating the competencies into nursing education (http://qsen.org). The competency most relevant for this book is the EBP competency, which is defined as "integrating the best current evidence with clinical expertise and patient/family preferences and values for delivery of optimal health care" (QSEN, 2020). You, as an undergraduate nursing student, need to be skilled in the critical appraisal of studies. A critical appraisal of research involves the careful examination of all aspects of a study to judge its strengths, limitations, meaning, and significance. Undergraduate nursing students also need to be skilled in the use of appropriate research evidence in practice, adherence to institutional review board guidelines, and appropriate data collection. Your expanded knowledge of research is necessary to attain EBP and the QSEN competencies.

The AHRQ (2018) continues to be the lead agency for studies designed to improve health and safety while reducing cost and medical errors within healthcare facilities. AHRQ conducts and sponsors research that provides evidence-based information on healthcare outcomes, quality, cost, use, and access. This research information is needed to promote effective healthcare decision making by patients, clinicians, health system executives, and policymakers.

In the past few years, the NINR has focused its research awards in the areas of symptom science and palliative care. For example, one nurse researcher, Dr. A. M. McCarthy, has developed a website for pediatric nurses and parents to assess a hospitalized child's risk for distress from medical procedures. The website also includes ways to minimize the child's distress. Other stories of discovery can be found at NINR (n.d.). The NINR continues to advocate for increased funding to support nursing research and encourage innovative technologies and methodologies to generate essential knowledge for nursing practice. The NINR website (http://ninr.nih.gov) provides current information on the Institute's research funding opportunities and supported studies. In this chapter, we

---

BOX 1.1   COMPETENCIES REQUIRED FOR HEALTHCARE PROFESSIONALS TO PROVIDE HIGH-QUALITY CARE

- Patient-centered care
- Teamwork and collaboration
- Evidence-based practice
- Quality improvement
- Safety
- Informatics

have focused on research as a way to build knowledge. The next section of this chapter is about other ways that nurses acquire knowledge and make decisions, in addition to research.

ACQUIRING KNOWLEDGE IN NURSING

Knowledge is essential information that is acquired in a variety of ways, is expected to be an accurate reflection of reality, and can potentially be used to direct a person's actions (Kaplan, 1964). Because you are in a nursing education program, you are in a time of rapid acquisition of an extensive amount of knowledge. You are learning to synthesize, incorporate, and apply this knowledge so that you can practice as a nurse. Nursing has historically acquired knowledge informally and formally. The informal ways we acquire knowledge is through traditions, authority, borrowing, trial and error, personal experience, intuition, and professional practice. More formally, we learn through role modeling and mentoring, logical reasoning, education, and research. This section introduces these different ways of acquiring knowledge and how you will use knowledge at different stages of professional development.

Informal Acquisition of Knowledge

"We have always done it that way." The statement exemplifies how traditions shape our knowledge. Traditions include "truths" or beliefs based on customs and habits. Traditions influence the nursing practice today, sometimes in positive ways, because they maintain structures that are effective in guiding care. However, traditions can narrow and limit our knowledge. Nurses may cling to traditions when the context or situation has changed significantly, making their actions ineffective.

Tradition is often linked to authority. An authority is a person with expertise and power who is able to influence opinion and behavior. A person is given authority because it is thought that she or he is more knowledgeable in a given area. Knowledge acquired from an authority is illustrated when one person credits another as the source of information. You may view your instructors as authorities. During clinical experiences, experienced nurses may be seen as authorities. Nurses with authority must be careful to teach and practice based on evidence and standards of care because they are influencing the actions of others.

As nurses, we use information from other disciplines to guide some areas of practice. Borrowing in nursing involves appropriating and using knowledge from other fields or disciplines to guide nursing practice. At times that knowledge has not been integrated with a nursing focus. For example, the medical model and its focus on diagnosis and treatment of illness is often used to guide nursing practice. A more useful way of borrowing is to identify information from other disciplines that can be used within nursing's focus on the whole person. For example, knowledge from other disciplines such as psychology and sociology can guide nurses as they therapeutically communicate with patients and families.

Trial and error is an approach to acquiring knowledge that has unknown outcomes. Patients respond uniquely to nursing interventions, so nursing practice includes many situations of uncertainty. In these situations, nurses frequently scan their minds for applicable information and use that knowledge to inform their actions. They collect information about the outcomes of an initial action to guide subsequent actions. Even when using interventions supported by research, you will encounter some degree of uncertainty because you do not know how the patient will respond. Unfortunately, trial and error frequently involves no formal documentation of which actions worked and which did not. The individual nurse gains knowledge through these personal experiences but may not share it with others.

Personal experience involves gaining knowledge by being involved in an event, situation, or circumstance. Personal experience enables you to gain skills and expertise through life experience. For example, a nurse who has had surgery may be able to empathize more easily with the anxiety experienced by patients scheduled for a surgery. As a student, you may have had a job that provided experience in setting priorities and working as part of a team. Such experiences may have given you additional skills related to flexibility and teamwork. Learning through personal experience enables you to cluster ideas into a meaningful whole. As you practice as a nurse, you may be able to apply the knowledge you previously acquired through your personal experiences.

Intuition is an insight into or understanding of a situation or event as a whole that a person usually cannot explain logically (Benner & Tanner, 1987). Because intuition is a type of knowing that seems to come unbidden, you may describe it as a gut feeling or a hunch. Experienced nurses may take initial actions based on intuition but continue to assess and integrate details in the situation to refine their initial impression. Some describe intuition as deep knowledge that is incorporated so completely into the subconscious that intuitive people cannot explain how they knew what to do. Using intuitive knowledge, nurses can assess the patient's condition, intervene, and contact the provider as needed for medical intervention.

Acquiring knowledge informally occurs in professional practice and overlaps with the other informal ways of learning. Professional practice is providing knowledgeable, skillful, and holistic care to patients, families, and communities as part of a healthcare team. During professional practice, nurses develop relationships with recipients of their interventions and select interventions consistent with available research evidence and ethical standards. Benner (1984) was curious about the process by which nurses became experts in their professional practice. She conducted a phenomenological qualitative study to identify the development of expertise in nursing practice. She identified the following levels of expertise: (1) novice, (2) advanced beginner, (3) competent, (4) proficient, and (5) expert. Novice nurses have no personal experience in the work they are to perform. They may have some preconceptions and expectations from their educational experiences but will often rely on tradition and authority in the development of their clinical knowledge. A preceptor or clinical mentor may guide new nurses as they develop knowledge. Advanced beginner nurses have limited experience but can recognize and intervene in recurrent situations. For example, the advanced beginner recognizes a patient's pain and will select from familiar interventions to manage the pain. As they develop professionally, they may begin integrating interventions that are evidence based (Benner, 1984).

Competent nurses are able to generate plans of care based on additional years of clinical experience (Benner, 1984). Competent nurses have developed personal knowledge that they will use to take conscious and deliberate actions that are efficient and organized. Proficient nurses will incorporate interventions from experience, evidence-based guidelines, and standards of care. Proficient nurses recognize that patients and families respond differently to illness and health and can make adjustments based on those responses. The expert nurse has extensive experience and can supplement the facts in a situation with intuition. Their clinical expertise increases their ability to seamlessly incorporate EBP with accuracy and speed. In other words, expert nurses can skillfully and seamlessly integrate personal experience and research evidence in their responses to patients' changing circumstances (Benner, 1984).

Formal Acquisition of Knowledge

Role modeling is acquiring knowledge by imitating the behaviors of an expert. In nursing, role modeling enables the novice nurse to learn through observing and interacting with highly competent, expert nurses. Role models include admired teachers, expert clinicians, researchers, and those who inspire others through their example. An intense form of role modeling is mentorship, in which the expert nurse serves as a teacher, sponsor, guide, and counselor for a less experienced nurse. The knowledge gained through personal experience is greatly enhanced by a quality relationship with a role model or mentor. Mentoring relationships may be formalized through internships and residencies that help new nurses transition into practice. In addition, mentoring relationships are essential for cultivating EBP (Schuler et al., 2020).

Reasoning is the processing and organizing of ideas to reach conclusions. There are many types of reasoning; we are focusing on logical reasoning and making inferences (Hayes et al., 2018). Logical reasoning is using a defined process of thinking to draw conclusions. The science of logic includes inductive and deductive reasoning. Inductive reasoning moves from the specific to the general; particular instances are observed and then combined into a larger whole or a general statement (Gravetter & Forzano, 2018). An example of inductive reasoning is provided in Table 1.3. Inductive reasoning is involved in synthesizing the findings of multiple studies to draw conclusions about best practices. Later in this chapter, you will find formal ways that inductive reasoning is applied in the development of EBP.

Deductive reasoning moves from the general to the specific or from a general premise to a particular situation or conclusion (Gravetter & Forzano, 2018). A general premise is an abstract statement that may be based on a theory, beliefs, or facts. An example of deductive reasoning is provided in Table 1.3. Conclusions are reached as abstract statements are applied to specific situations. However, the conclusions generated from deductive reasoning are valid only if they are based on valid statements. Research is a means to test and confirm or refute a statement. Once shown to be valid, the statement can be used as a basis for reasoning in nursing practice (Gray & Grove, 2021).

The learning that is the goal of education is another formal means of acquiring knowledge. Education is a structured presentation of information, usually by a person identified to be the expert (teacher). Education includes nursing programs that prepare students to deliver quality nursing care and for the licensing examination to become an RN. Education may also include a program for RNs with a diploma or an associate's degree in nursing to move to a baccalaureate degree. In the future, you may enter a graduate-level education program to prepare yourself for an advanced practice or leadership role. As a nurse in practice, you will have the opportunity to participate in continuing professional education to keep up to date with clinical advances and technology improvements.

TABLE 1.3   LOGICAL REASONING: INDUCTIVE AND DEDUCTIVE

Example of Inductive Reasoning	
Particular instances	• A headache is an altered level of health that is stressful. • An acute viral infection is an altered level of health that is stressful. • A terminal illness is an altered level of health that is stressful.
General statement	• Therefore it can be induced that all altered levels of health are stressful.
Example of Deductive Reasoning	
Propositions	• All humans experience loss. • All adolescents are humans.
Conclusion	• Therefore it can be deduced that all adolescents experience loss.

Research is a means of acquiring information through systematic investigation, as defined earlier in the chapter. The purpose of research is to develop new knowledge or validate existing knowledge. Research knowledge needed for practice should be specific and holistic, as well as process oriented and outcomes focused. Because of the breadth of knowledge needed, a variety of research methods are implemented to generate this knowledge. One of the important skills you will learn through this book is to critically appraise research findings to determine whether the findings are reliable and valid. The following sections will describe the types of evidence needed for developing an EBP.

TYPES OF NEEDED EVIDENCE

Nurses need a solid research base as a foundation for implementing selected nursing interventions and documenting their effectiveness in treating patient health problems. Effective interventions promote positive patient and family outcomes. The research evidence needed in clinical practice includes studies focused on the description, explanation, prediction, and control of phenomena (Gray & Grove, 2021).

Description

Description involves identifying and understanding the nature of nursing phenomena and, sometimes, the relationships among them (Chinn & Kramer, 2018). Through research, nurses describe what exists in nursing practice and discover new information. Descriptive research is also used to promote understanding of situations and classify information for use in the discipline. Studies conducted for the broad purpose of description might include:

- Describing the resilience of nurses who are caring for patients with COVID-19 infection
- Determining the incidence of burnout among health professionals
- Exploring the experience of being hopeful after being diagnosed with cancer
- Identification and classification of nursing interventions
- Description of the responses of individuals to a variety of health conditions and aging
- Determination of the incidence of a disease in a geographical area, such as Ebola infection in West Africa or diagnosed hypertension in the United States.

An example of research conducted for the purpose of description was a qualitative study of fatigue management among acute care nurses in the United States (Groves et al., 2020). "The purpose of this study phase was to describe how hospital nurses manage fatigue in order to inform future regulation and organizational fatigue risk management programs" (Groves et al., 2020, p. 36). This study involved data collected from interviews with 120 nurses from eight hospitals. Barriers to fatigue management at work were "workload," "schedules and shifts," and "slowing down," and at home were "not enough sleep" and "competing time demands" (Groves et al., p. 39). The participants also provided insight into how they managed their fatigue. Studies that identify concerns and describe important characteristics provide essential knowledge. Studies that provide explanations, predictions, and control of nursing phenomena in practice are built on the essential knowledge provided by descriptive studies.

Explanation

An explanation clarifies the relationships among phenomena and identifies possible reasons why certain events occur. Research focused on explanation provides the following types of evidence essential for practice:

- Understanding which factors are related to caring for an older relative at home
- Examining the relationships among the patient's preadmission functional status, hospital complications, and length of stay in the hospital

- Determining the relationships among the physical environment, community socioeconomic characteristics, and health status
- Exploring relationships among nursing students' hours worked per week, family responsibilities, coping strategies, and academic performance.

Studying the relationships among characteristics of research participants allows researchers to explain situations and factors that may interact in these situations. For example, when faculty better understand factors that may explain nursing students' academic performance, the faculty may be able to identify possible strategies to improve students' outcomes.

Deetz et al. (2020) conducted a study with nurse managers to be able to better explain the managers' perceptions of their work and the work engagement of their employees after a union-led strike. The researchers had employment engagement data that had been collected routinely as part of the Press Ganey survey of patient satisfaction and the hospital's work environment. Deetz et al. (2020) collected data from 32 managers using a validated, but relatively new, instrument that was designed to measure meaning and joy in their work. No significant correlations were found among mangers' meaning and joy in their work and their employees' work engagement. However, Deetz et al. (2020) did find a strong, significant correlation between work engagement and the employees' perception of the manager. This significant finding was found anecdotally and was not a hypothesis proposed by the researchers. The researchers recommended that the study be repeated with larger samples of nurse managers.

Studies designed to explain characteristics of events, situations, and people typically report correlations as an indicator of relationships among a study's variables. Although the study conducted by Deetz et al. (2020) was a quantitative study using numerical data, some studies may use qualitative methods to collect and analyze data. When the explanatory aspects are well understood of a specific phenomenon, researchers may design a study with the aim of predicting one or more variables based on the characteristics of other variables.

Prediction

Through prediction, one can estimate the probability of a specific outcome in a given situation (Chinn & Kramer, 2018). However, predicting an outcome does not necessarily enable one to modify or control the outcome. It is through prediction that the risk for illness or injury is identified and linked to possible screening methods to identify and prevent health problems. Knowledge generated from research focused on prediction is essential for EBP and includes:

- Prediction of the risk for a disease or injury in different populations
- Prediction of behaviors that promote health and prevent illness
- Prediction of nursing student outcomes in programs using innovative teaching strategies
- Prediction of the nursing care required based on a patient's circumstances and values.

Kähkönen et al. (2020) collected data from a large sample of patients ($n = 416$) who had had a percutaneous coronary intervention (PCI) in 2013. The researchers wanted to identify the predictive factors, such as emotional and family support, that facilitated their adherence to medications and to lifestyle modifications. Six years later, Kähkönen et al. (2020) collected data again from 169 of the original participants. They "investigated and identified the level of adherence and the predictive factors of adherence to treatment six years after PCI" (Kähkönen et al., 2020, p. 340). The follow-up participants were more adherent than they were 4 months after PCI. Long-term adherence to treatment was predicted by several factors: close family support, relationships with nurses and physicians, sense of responsibility, fears about complications, continuity of care, and outcomes of care (Kähkönen et al., 2020). Based on these findings, nurses working with patients with a history of PCI could assess the presence and strength of the predictive factors and respond by supplementing absent or weak factors that promote adherence.

Control

If one can predict the outcome of a situation, the next step is to control or manipulate the situation to produce the desired outcome. In health care, control is the ability to write a prescription to produce the desired results. Using the best research evidence, nurses could prescribe specific interventions to meet the needs of patients and their families (Melnyk & Fineout-Overholt, 2019). The results of multiple studies in the following areas have enabled nurses to deliver care that increases control over the outcomes desired for practice:

- Testing the effectiveness of interventions to improve the health status of individuals and families
- Synthesis of research for development into EBP guidelines
- Determining the effectiveness of EBP guidelines in your clinical agency.

As discussed earlier, extensive studies have been conducted related to techniques of inserting a PIV device into older patients and the findings integrated into standards for practice (Gorski et al., 2016). In later chapters, you will also learn about randomized control trials (RCTs) conducted by nurse researchers to test the effects of specific interventions on the outcomes of care. Evidence-based guidelines and standards of care have been developed based on the findings of many studies.

Broadly, the nursing profession is accountable to society for providing quality, safe, and cost-effective care for patients and families (Powers, 2020; Sherwood & Barnsteiner, 2017). The extensive number of clinical studies conducted since 1970 has greatly expanded the scientific knowledge available to you for describing, explaining, predicting, and controlling phenomena within your nursing practice.

📄 RESEARCH/EBP TIP

Nurses need research evidence on which to base their practice because they are accountable for providing quality, safe, and cost-effective care.

DIFFERENT TYPES OF RESEARCH

This section introduces studies that are conducted using quantitative, qualitative, mixed methods, and outcomes research methods. These types of research are distinct approaches to generating empirical knowledge for nursing practice (Box 1.2).

Quantitative Research

Many of the studies conducted in nursing included quantitative research methods, which are considered the traditional scientific method. Quantitative research is a formal, objective, systematic process in which numerical data are used to obtain information about the world. The quantitative approach toward scientific inquiry emerged from a branch of philosophy called logical positivism. Logical positivism is the philosophy that knowledge is developed based on strict rules of logic, objective truth, and laws (Table 1.4). Quantitative researchers hold the position that "truth" is absolute, and that a single reality can be defined by careful measurement. To find truth, the researcher must be objective, which means that values, feelings, and personal perceptions should not enter into the measurement of reality. Quantitative research is conducted to test theory by describing variables (descriptive research), examining relationships among variables (correlational research), and determining cause-and-effect interactions between variables (quasi-experimental and experimental research). The methods of measurement commonly used in quantitative research include scales, questionnaires, and physiological measures (see Table 1.4).

BOX 1.2   RESEARCH METHODS FOR THIS TEXT

Types of Quantitative Research
Descriptive research
Correlational research
Quasi-experimental research
Experimental research

Types of Qualitative Research
Phenomenological research
Grounded theory research
Ethnographic research
Exploratory-descriptive qualitative research

Mixed Methods Research

Outcomes Research

TABLE 1.4   CHARACTERISTICS OF QUANTITATIVE AND QUALITATIVE RESEARCH METHODS

CHARACTERISTICS	QUANTITATIVE RESEARCH	QUALITATIVE RESEARCH
Philosophical origin	Logical positivism	Naturalistic, interpretive, humanistic
Basis of knowing	Cause-and-effect relationships	Meaning, discovery, understanding
Theoretical focus	Tests theory	Develops theory and frameworks
Researcher involvement	Objective	Shared interpretation
Common methods of measurement	Scales, questionnaires, and physiological measures	Unstructured interviews, observations, focus groups
Data	Numbers	Words
Analysis	Statistical analysis	Text-based analysis
Findings	Description of variables, relationships among variables, and effectiveness of interventions; generalization	Unique, dynamic, focused on understanding of phenomena and facilitating theory development

---

The data collected are numbers that are analyzed with statistical techniques to determine results (Grove & Cipher, 2020). Quantitative researchers strive to extend their findings beyond the situation studied. When extensive evidence is available on a topic, the findings may be generalized to different populations and settings. Chapter 2 describes the types of quantitative research and the quantitative research process.

Types of Quantitative Research

Several types of quantitative and qualitative research have been conducted to generate nursing knowledge for practice. These types of research can be classified in a variety of ways. The classification system for this text is presented in Box 1.2 and includes the most common types of quantitative and qualitative research conducted in nursing. The quantitative research methods are classified into four categories: descriptive, correlational, quasi-experimental, and experimental (Gray & Grove, 2021).

- Descriptive research explores new areas of research and describes situations as they exist in the world.
- Correlational research examines relationships and is conducted to develop and refine explanatory knowledge for nursing practice.
- Quasi-experimental and experimental studies determine the effectiveness of nursing interventions in predicting and controlling the outcomes desired for patients and families.

Qualitative Research

Qualitative research is a systematic, subjective approach used to describe life experiences and situations and give them meaning (Creswell & Poth, 2018). The philosophical base of qualitative research is interpretive, humanistic, and naturalistic (see Table 1.4). Experiences, often referred to as phenomena (singular phenomenon), are studied in their natural environment that encompasses social, historical, and cultural influences. Phenomena are events, processes, and situations experienced by human beings during their lives. Qualitative research is concerned with understanding the meaning of social interactions and shared interpretations among those involved (see Table 1.4). Qualitative researchers believe that truth is complex and dynamic and can be found only by studying people as they interact with and in their sociohistorical settings (Creswell & Poth, 2018). Because human emotions are difficult to quantify (assign a numerical value to); qualitative research is the appropriate method for studying emotional responses and personal experiences rather than quantitative research. Data in qualitative research are in the form of words, which are collected through interviews, observations, and focus groups and analyzed for meaning. Qualitative research findings are unique, dynamic, focused on understanding, and facilitate theory development. A variety of qualitative studies are conducted to generate findings. Chapter 3 describes different types of qualitative research with example studies.

Types of Qualitative Research

The qualitative research methods included in this text are phenomenological, grounded theory, ethnographic research, and exploratory-descriptive (see Box 1.2).

- Phenomenological research is an inductive holistic approach used to describe an experience as it is lived by individuals, such as the lived experience of adopting a child.
- Grounded theory research is an inductive research technique used to formulate, test, and refine a theory about a phenomenon (Bryant & Charmaz, 2019). Grounded theory research initially was described by Glaser and Strauss (1967) in their development of a theory about grieving.
- Ethnographic research was developed by anthropologists for investigating cultures through an in-depth study among the members of the culture. Health practices vary among cultures, and these practices need to be recognized when delivering care to patients and families (Creswell & Poth, 2018).
- Exploratory-descriptive qualitative research is conducted to address an issue or problem in need of a solution and/or understanding. Qualitative nurse researchers use this methodology to explore a problem area using varied qualitative techniques, with the intent of describing the topic of interest and promoting understanding.
  Although quantitative and qualitative research share some similarities, there are clear distinctions.

Comparing Quantitative and Qualitative Research

Quantitative and qualitative research methods complement each other because they generate different types of knowledge that are useful in nursing practice. Familiarity with these two types of research will help you identify, understand, and critically appraise these studies. Quantitative and qualitative research methodologies have some similarities; both require researcher expertise, involve rigor in conducing the studies, and generate scientific knowledge for nursing practice. Some of the differences between the two methodologies are presented in Table 1.4.

Introduction to Mixed Methods Research

Mixed methods research is an approach to addressing a research question that combines quantitative and qualitative research methods in a single study. Mixed methods studies involve the collection of qualitative and quantitative data and the analysis of both forms of data (Creswell & Creswell, 2018). Researchers might have a stronger focus on either a quantitative or qualitative research method based on the purpose of their study. The data are analyzed and integrated as directed by the study design. Sometimes quantitative and qualitative research methods are implemented concurrently or consecutively based on the knowledge to be generated. For example, researchers might examine the effectiveness of an intervention using a quasi-experimental design and then conduct qualitative research to obtain an understanding of the patients' perceptions of the intervention. The different strategies for combining qualitative and quantitative research methods in mixed methods studies are described in Chapter 14.

Introduction to Outcomes Research

The results of outcomes research are used to make clinical decisions and develop effective interventions (Dodd et al., 2020). The spiraling costs of health care have generated many questions about healthcare services and patient outcomes related to these services. Insurers, patients, and families want to know what services they are purchasing and whether these services will improve the health of the recipients of care. Healthcare policymakers want to know whether the care is cost-effective and of high quality. These concerns have promoted the conduct of outcomes research, which focuses on examining the results of care and determining the changes in health status for the patient and family. Some essential areas that require investigation through outcomes research include (1) patient responses to nursing and medical interventions; (2) functional maintenance or improvement of physical, mental, and social functioning for the patient; (3) financial outcomes achieved with the provision of healthcare services; and (4) patient satisfaction with health outcomes, care received, and healthcare providers.

Nurses are actively involved in identifying nurse-sensitive outcomes and conducting outcomes studies. A nursing-sensitive outcome is a characteristic of the health of individuals or groups that are linked to the "quantity and quality of nursing care" (Barrientos-Trigo et al., 2019. p. 209). The Nursing Outcomes Classification (NOC) was developed to standardize terminology for nursing-sensitive outcomes. NOC is to be used across nursing specialties and in a variety of practice settings to capture changes in patient status after an intervention. NOC contains 540 outcomes that have been developed over the last 30 years (Moorhead et al., 2018). The National Database of Nursing Quality Indicators is another repository for information and references for outcomes research. The nursing quality indicators include decreasing patient falls, nosocomial infections, pressure ulcers, and nursing turnover (ANA, n.d.). Chapter 14 includes a discussion of outcomes research.

Different types of research methods (see Box 1.2) provide information important to nurses in implementing an EBP. To help you in comparing quantitative, qualitative, mixed methods, and outcomes studies, Table 1.5 includes examples of studying home care and cardiac care using each type of research.

TABLE 1.5	**TOPICS FOR DIFFERENT RESEARCH METHODOLOGIES**	
RESEARCH METHODOLOGY	**TOPICS RELATED TO HOME HEALTH CARE**	**TOPICS RELATED TO CARDIAC DISEASE**
Quantitative research	Characteristics of home healthcare patients 60 days after hospital discharge	Relationships among functional status, medication adherence, and social support of patient after MI
Qualitative research	The experience of caring for a spouse at home after hospital discharge	Women's concerns about living with heart failure after MI
Mixed methods research	The physical, financial, emotional, and social effects of caring for a spouse at home after hospital discharge	Developing and testing the MI-Concerns Scale: Focus groups followed by initial validation of the scale
Outcomes research	Comparison of 30-day rehospitalization rates of patients with heart failure who receive visits from a home health nurse and those who do not	Cost and effectiveness of troponin levels in treatment of possible MIs

MI, Myocardial infarction.

📄 **RESEARCH/EBP TIP**

Quantitative, qualitative, mixed methods, and outcomes research contribute to the evidence nurses need to provide quality, safe, and cost-effective care to patients and their families.

UNDERSTANDING YOUR ROLE IN NURSING RESEARCH

Generating an empirical knowledge base for implementation in practice requires the participation of all nurses in a variety of research activities. Some nurses are developers of research and conduct studies to generate and refine the knowledge needed for nursing practice. Others are consumers of research and use research evidence to improve their nursing practice. The American Association of Colleges of Nursing (AACN, 2006) and ANA (2010) have published statements about the roles of nurses in research. No matter their education or position, all nurses have roles in research; some ideas about those roles are presented in Table 1.6. The research role that a nurse assumes usually expands as his or her education advances and clinical expertise grows. Nurses with a BSN degree understand the research process and possess the skills needed to critically appraise studies. A critical appraisal of research involves the careful examination of all aspects of a study to judge its strengths, limitations, meaning, and significance. They assist with the implementation of evidence-based guidelines, protocols, algorithms, and policies in practice (Melnyk et al., 2017). In addition, these nurses might provide valuable assistance in identifying research problems and collecting data for studies. The QSEN (2020) competencies identify such knowledge and skills as being essential for prelicensure students.

In addition to being able to critically appraise studies, nurses with an MSN have undergone the educational preparation to synthesize findings from studies and revise or develop protocols,

TABLE 1.6 NURSES' PARTICIPATION IN RESEARCH AT VARIOUS LEVELS OF EDUCATION	
NURSES' EDUCATIONAL PREPARATION	**RESEARCH EXPECTATIONS AND COMPETENCIES**
Bachelor of Science in Nursing (BSN)	Read and critically appraise studies; use best research evidence in practice with guidance; assist with problem identification and data collection.
Master of Science in Nursing (MSN)	Critically appraise and synthesize studies to develop and revise protocols, algorithms, and policies for practice. Implement best research evidence in practice; collaborate in research projects and provide clinical expertise for research.
Doctor of Nursing Practice (DNP)	Participate in evidence-based guideline development; develop, implement, evaluate, and revise as needed protocols, policies, and evidence-based guidelines in practice; conduct clinical studies, usually in collaboration with other nurse researchers.
Doctor of Philosophy (PhD) in Nursing	Major role, such as primary investigator, in conducting research and contributing to the empirical knowledge generated in a selected area of study; obtain funding for research; coordinate research teams of BSN, MSN, and DNP nurses.
Postdoctorate	Implement a funded program of research; lead and/or participate in nursing and interdisciplinary research teams; identified as experts in their areas of research; mentor PhD-prepared researchers.

algorithms, or policies for use in practice. They also have the ability to identify and critically appraise the quality of evidence-based guidelines developed by national organizations. Advanced practice nurses—nurse practitioners, clinical nurse specialists, nurse anesthetists, and nurse midwives—and nurse administrators have the ability to lead healthcare teams in making essential changes in nursing practice and in the healthcare system based on current research evidence. Some MSN-prepared nurses conduct studies but usually do so in collaboration with other nurse scientists (see Table 1.6).

The doctoral degrees in nursing can have a practice focus (Doctor of Nursing Practice [DNP]) or research focus (Doctor of Philosophy [PhD]). Nurses with DNPs are educated to have the highest level of clinical expertise, which includes the ability to translate scientific knowledge for use in practice. DNP-prepared nurses have advanced research and leadership knowledge to develop, implement, evaluate, and revise evidence-based guidelines, protocols, algorithms, and policies for practice (Gray & Grove, 2021; Melnyk & Fineout-Overholt, 2019). In addition, DNP-prepared nurses have the expertise to conduct and/or collaborate with an interprofessional team to conduct clinical studies.

PhD-prepared nurses assume a major role in the conduct of research and the generation of nursing knowledge in a selected area of interest (McSweeney et al., 2020). These nurse scientists often coordinate research teams that include DNP-, MSN-, and BSN-prepared nurses to facilitate the conduct of rigorous studies in a variety of healthcare agencies and universities. Nurses with postdoctoral education have the expertise to develop highly funded programs of research. They lead interdisciplinary teams of researchers and sometimes conduct studies in multiple settings. These scientists often are identified as experts in selected areas of research and provide mentoring for new PhD-prepared researchers (see Table 1.6).

DETERMINING THE BEST RESEARCH EVIDENCE FOR PRACTICE

EBP involves the use of the best research evidence to support clinical decisions in practice. Best research evidence was previously defined as a summary of the highest-quality, current, empirical knowledge in a specific area of health care that has been developed from a synthesis of quality studies in that area. As a nurse, you make numerous clinical decisions each day that affect the health outcomes of your patients. By using the best research evidence available, you can make quality clinical decisions that will improve patients' and families' health outcomes. This section focuses on expanding your understanding of best research evidence for practice by providing (1) descriptions of the strategies used to synthesize research evidence, (2) a model of the levels of research evidence, and (3) the connection of the best research evidence to evidence-based guidelines for practice.

Strategies Used to Synthesize Research Evidence

The synthesis of study findings is a complex, highly structured process that is best conducted by at least two people and more effectively by a team of researchers and healthcare providers. Various types of research synthesis are conducted based on the quality, number, and types of research evidence available. Research evidence in nursing is usually synthesized by (1) systematic review, (2) meta-analysis, (3) meta-synthesis, and (4) mixed methods research synthesis. Depending on the quantity and strength of the research findings available, nurses and healthcare professionals use one or more of these four synthesis processes to determine the current best research evidence in an area. Table 1.7 identifies the common processes used in research synthesis, the purpose of each synthesis process, the types of research included in the synthesis, and the analytical techniques used to achieve the synthesis of research evidence (Fisher et al., 2020; Havill et al., 2014; Higgins & Thomas, 2019; Meadows-Oliver, 2019; Melnyk & Fineout-Overholt, 2019).

A systematic review is a structured, comprehensive synthesis of the research literature to determine the best research evidence available to address a healthcare question. A systematic review involves identifying, locating, appraising, and synthesizing quality research evidence for expert clinicians to use to promote an EBP (Gray & Grove, 2021; Melnyk & Fineout-Overholt, 2019). Teams of expert researchers, clinicians, and sometimes students conduct these reviews to determine the current best knowledge for use in practice. Systematic reviews are also used in the development of national and international standardized guidelines for managing health problems, such as acute pain, high BP, and depression. Standardized guidelines are made available online, published in articles and books, and presented at conferences and professional meetings. The process for critically appraising systematic reviews is discussed in Chapter 13.

A meta-analysis is conducted to combine or pool the results from previous quantitative studies into a single statistical analysis that provides strong evidence about an intervention's effectiveness (Glasofer & Townsend, 2019; Higgins & Thomas, 2019; Melnyk & Fineout-Overholt, 2019). Because qualitative studies do not produce statistical findings, they cannot be included in a meta-analysis. Some of the strongest evidence for using an intervention in practice is generated from a

TABLE 1.7 **PROCESSES USED TO SYNTHESIZE RESEARCH EVIDENCE**

CHARACTERISTICS	SYSTEMATIC REVIEW	META-ANALYSIS	META-SYNTHESIS	MIXED METHODS RESEARCH SYNTHESIS
Purpose	Identify studies on a clinical topic, critically appraise the study findings, and summarize what is known on a clinical topic; may start with a practice question	Determine strength of an intervention or correlation; combine samples and statistical results of two or more studies measuring the same variable	Understand a clinical phenomenon from participants' perspectives; analyze, compare, integrate findings	Combine and synthesize findings from studies using different methodologies to determine current knowledge in an area
Research type included	Quantitative	Quantitative	Qualitative	Quantitative, qualitative, mixed methods studies
Types of study	Comparable designs, such as RCTs or experimental	Correlational, RCTs, quasi-experimental, experimental	Phenomenological, grounded theory, ethnography, exploratory-descriptive qualitative studies	Any type of quantitative, qualitative, or mixed methods study
Analysis	Narrative and statistical	Statistical	Content analysis and narrative	Narrative and statistical
Result	Statements of what is known and not known; evaluation of level of evidence	Summary statistic of effectiveness of intervention	Unique, holistic summary or translation of findings	Statements of what is known and not known; evaluation of level of evidence; direct future research

All these processes begin with systematically searching the literature, identifying possible studies, selecting studies based on inclusion criteria, summarizing findings, and critically appraising the studies.
RCT, Randomized control trial.
Based on content from Gray, J. R., & Grove, S. K. (2021). *Burns and Grove's the practice of nursing research: Appraisal, synthesis, and generation of evidence* (9th ed.). Elsevier; Higgins, J. P. T., & Thomas, J. (2019). *Cochrane handbook for systematic reviews of interventions* (2nd ed.). Wiley-Blackwell and The Cochrane Collaboration; Meadows-Oliver, M. (2019). Critically appraising qualitative evidence for clinical decision making. In B. Melnyk & E. Fineout-Overholt (Eds.), *Evidence-based practice in nursing and healthcare: A guide to best practice* (4th ed., pp.189–218). Wolters Kluwer; Melnyk, B. M., & Fineout-Overholt, E. (2019). *Evidence-based practice in nursing and healthcare: A guide to best practice* (4th ed., pp. 189–218). Wolters Kluwer; and Straus, S. E., Glasziou, P., Richardson, W. S., & Haynes, R. B. (2019). *Evidence-based medicine: How to practice and teach EBM.* Elsevier Limited.

meta-analysis of quasi-experimental and experimental studies. In addition, a meta-analysis can be performed on correlational studies to determine the type (positive or negative) and strength of relationships among selected variables (Glasofer & Townsend, 2019; Grove & Cipher, 2020). Many systematic reviews conducted to generate evidence-based guidelines include meta-analyses (see Chapter 13).

Qualitative research synthesis is the process and product of systematically reviewing and formally integrating the findings from qualitative studies (Meadows-Oliver, 2019; Sandelowski & Barroso, 2007). In this text, the concept of meta-synthesis is used to describe the process for synthesizing qualitative research. Meta-synthesis is defined as the systematic compilation and integration of qualitative study results to expand understanding and develop a unique interpretation of study findings in a selected area. The focus is on interpretation rather than on combining study results, as with quantitative research synthesis. Chapter 13 provides more details on meta-synthesis.

Over the last 15 years, nurse researchers have conducted mixed methods studies that include quantitative and qualitative research methods (Creswell & Creswell, 2018; Higgins & Thomas, 2019). A new method was needed to synthesize the evidence produced by quality studies that used quantitative, qualitative, and mixed methods studies. Methods for reviewing multiple types of studies and combining their findings has been called integrative reviews by some researchers. We are using the term *mixed methods research synthesis* to describe this process. Mixed methods research synthesis is a review, evaluation, integration, and summation of findings of a variety of study designs. The value of these reviews depends on the standards used to conduct them (see Chapter 13).

Levels of Research Evidence

Experimental quantitative studies, such as RCTs, provide the strongest research evidence (see Chapter 8). Also, the replication or repeating of studies with a similar methodology increases the strength of the research evidence generated. The levels of research evidence are presented in a pyramid (Fig. 1.3) that shows a continuum, with the highest quality of research evidence at the apex and the weakest research evidence at the base. The systematic research reviews and meta-analyses of RCTs and high-quality quasi-experimental and experimental studies provide the strongest or best research evidence for use by clinicians in practice. Meta-analyses of correlational, quasi-experimental, experimental, and outcomes studies also provide very strong research evidence for managing practice problems. Mixed methods systematic reviews and meta-syntheses provide quality syntheses of quantitative, qualitative, and/or mixed methods studies. The evidence from individual correlational, predictive correlational, and cohort studies provides direction for future research but is not ready for use in practice. Descriptive and qualitative studies often provide initial knowledge, which serves as a basis for generating correlational, quasi-experimental, experimental, and outcomes studies (see Fig. 1.3). The weakest evidence is generated from opinions of expert committees and authorities.

When making a decision in your clinical practice, be sure to base that decision on the best research evidence available. The levels of research evidence identified in Fig. 1.3 will help you determine the quality of the evidence that is available. The best research evidence generated from systematic reviews, meta-analyses, meta-syntheses, and mixed methods systematic reviews is used to develop standardized evidence-based guidelines for use in practice.

INTRODUCTION TO EVIDENCE-BASED GUIDELINES

Evidence-based guidelines are rigorous and explicit clinical guidelines that have been developed based on the best research evidence available in that area. These guidelines are usually developed by a team or panel of expert clinicians (nurses, physicians, pharmacists); researchers; and sometimes consumers, policymakers, and economists. The expert panel works to achieve consensus on the content of the guideline to provide clinicians with the best information for making clinical

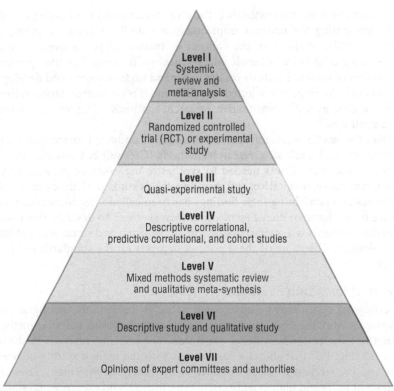

FIG. 1.3 Levels of Research Evidence. (From Gray, J. R., & Grove, S. K. [2021]. *Burns and Grove's the practice of nursing research: Appraisal, synthesis, and generation of evidence* [9th ed.]. Elsevier).

decisions in practice. There has been a dramatic growth in the production of evidence-based guidelines to assist healthcare providers in delivering an EBP and improving healthcare outcomes for patients, families, providers, and healthcare agencies.

Every year, new guidelines are developed, and some of the existing guidelines are revised based on new research evidence. These guidelines have become the gold standard (standard of excellence) for patient care, and nurses and other healthcare providers are highly encouraged to incorporate these standardized guidelines into their practice.

Many of these evidence-based guidelines have been made available online by national and international government agencies, professional organizations, and centers of excellence. AHRQ was initially a repository for clinical guidelines in the United States. After the AHRQ funding for this service was stopped, many health-related nonprofit organizations and specialty medical organizations began collaborating to support Guideline Central (https://www.guidelinecentral.com/). Guideline Central provides guideline summaries, drug information, a searchable database of clinical trials, and formula calculators for clinical indicators such as bleeding risk or appropriate medication levels for a person with decreased renal function. In addition, Guideline Central provides a downloadable application for smartphones to make the information immediately available to clinicians. Collections of clinical practice guidelines that you can trust are available from other entities as well, such as the one maintained at the National Center for Complementary and Integrative Health (2020), the American Association of Family Physicians (2020), and the American Medical Association (2019).

The purpose of this textbook is to prepare you to fulfill your research role as a BSN-prepared nurse. A key component of that role is being about to critically appraise studies. Chapters 2 through 12 were developed to expand your understanding of the quantitative and qualitative research processes so you will be able to critically appraise these types of studies. Chapter 13 provides additional information on how to build an EBP in your setting. Chapter 14 provides more information about mixed methods and outcomes research. The content of this book, when applied, prepares you to have an EBP and lays a foundation for graduate study. We hope that you will find nursing research to be an exciting adventure that holds promise for the future practice of nursing.

KEY POINTS

- Nursing research is defined as a scientific process that validates and refines existing knowledge and generates new knowledge that directly and indirectly influences nursing practice.
- EBP is the conscientious integration of best research evidence with clinical expertise and patient circumstances and values in the delivery of quality, safe, and cost-effective health care.
- Quantitative research uses numerical data to obtain information about the world. This research method is used to describe, examine relationships, and determine cause and effect.
- Qualitative research used textual data to describe life experiences and elicit their meaning from the perspective of the participants.
- Mixed methods research is an approach to inquiry that combines quantitative and qualitative research methods in a single study.
- Outcomes research focuses on examining the end results of care, determining the changes needed to improve the health of patients, and evaluating the quality of the healthcare system.
- The purposes of research in nursing include description, explanation, prediction, and control of phenomena in practice.
- Nurses with a BSN, MSN, doctoral degree (DNP, PhD), and postdoctorate education have clearly designated roles in research based on the breadth and depth of the research knowledge gained during their educational programs and their clinical and research experiences.
- Research evidence in nursing is synthesized using the following processes: (1) systematic review, (2) meta-analysis, (3) meta-synthesis, and (4) mixed methods research synthesis.
- A systematic review is a structured, comprehensive synthesis of quantitative studies in a particular healthcare area to determine the best research evidence available for clinicians to use to promote an EBP.
- Meta-analysis is a type of study that statistically combines or pools the results from previous studies into a single quantitative analysis to provide one of the highest levels of evidence for an intervention's efficacy.
- Meta-synthesis involves the systematic compilation and integration of qualitative studies in an area to expand understanding and develop a unique interpretation of the findings.
- A mixed methods research synthesis is the synthesis of findings from individual studies conducted with a variety of methods—quantitative, qualitative, and mixed methods—to determine the current knowledge in an area.
- The levels of research evidence are a continuum, with the highest quality of research evidence at the top of the pyramid and the weakest research evidence at its base (see Fig. 1.3). Systematic

research reviews and meta-analyses of quality experimental studies provide the best research evidence for practice.

- Evidence-based guidelines are rigorous and explicit statements that guide the assessment, interventions, and evaluation of patients and families' healthcare needs that have been developed based on the best research evidence available in a clinical area or specialty.

REFERENCES

Agency for Healthcare Research and Quality. (2018). *Guidelines and measures update: Information about the National Guideline Clearinghouse (NGC).* Retrieved from https://www.ahrq.gov/gam/updates/index.html

Aiken, L., Clarke, S., Sloane, D., Sochalski, J., & Silber, J. (2002). Hospital nurse staffing and patient mortality, nurse burnout, and job dissatisfaction. *Journal of the American Medical Association, 288*(16), 1987–1993. https://doi.org/10.1001.jama.288.16.1987

Aiken, L., Sloane, D., Clarke, S., Poghosyan, L., Cho, E., You, L., … Aungsuroch, Y. (2011). Importance of work environments in nine countries. *International Journal of Quality in Health Care, 23*(4), 357–364. https://doi.org/10.1093/intqhc/mzr022

American Association of Colleges of Nursing. (2006). *AACN position statement on nursing research.* Washington, DC: AACN. Retrieved from https://www.aacnnursing.org/Portals/42/News/Position-Statements/Nursing-Research.pdf

American Association of Family Physicians. (2020). *Clinical practice guidelines.* Retrieved from https://www.aafp.org/family-physician/patient-care/clinical-recommendations/clinical-practice-guidelines/clinical-practice-guidelines.html

American Medical Association. (2019). *Guidelines summary.* Retrieved from https://www.guidelinecentral.com/summaries/#_specialties/nursing/

American Nurses Association. (n.d.). *National Database of Nursing Quality Indicators (NDNQI).* Retrieved from https://nursingandndnqi.weebly.com/ndnqi-indicators.html

American Nurses Association. (2010). *Nursing: Scope and standards of practice* (2nd ed.). American Nurses Association.

Barrientos-Trigo, S., Gil-García, E., Romero-Sanchez, J., Badanta-Romero, B., & Porcel-Galvez, A. (2019). Evaluation of psychometric properties of instruments measuring nursing-sensitive outcomes: A systematic review. *International Nursing Review, 66*(2), 209–223. https://doi.org/10.1111/inr.12495

Bauknecht, V. L. (1985). Capital commentary: NIH bill passes, includes nursing research center. *American Nurse, 17*(10), 2.

Bayram, S., & Caliskan, N. (2019). Effect of a game-based virtual reality phone application on tracheostomy care education for nursing students: A randomized controlled trial. *Nurse Education Today, 79,* 25–31. https://doi.org/10.1016/j.nedt.2019.05.010

Benner, P. (1984). *From novice to expert: Excellence and power in clinical nursing practice.* Addison-Wesley.

Benner, P., & Tanner, C. (1987). How expert nurses use intuition. *American Journal of Nursing, 87*(1), 23–31.

Bettencourt, A., McHugh, M., Sloane, D., & Aiken, L. (2020). Nurse staffing, the clinical work environment, and burn patient mortality. *Journal of Burn Care & Research, 41*(4), 796–802. http://doi.org/10.1093/jbcr/iraa061

Bourgault, A., Powers, J., Aguirre, L., Hines, R., Sebastian, A., & Upvall, M. (2020). National survey of feeding tube verification practices: An urgent call for auscultation deimplementation. *Dimensions of Critical Care Nursing, 39*(6), 329–338. http://doi.org/10.1097/DCC.0000000000000440

Bryant, A., & Charmaz, K. (2019). *The Sage handbook of current developments of grounded theory.* Sage.

Carter, G., & Caudill, P. (2020). Integrating naloxone education into an undergraduate nursing course: Developing partnerships with a local department of health. *Public Health Nursing, 37*(3), 439–445. http://doi.org/10.1111/phn.12707

Cheung, R., & Aiken, L. (2006). Hospital initiative to support a better-educated workforce. *Journal of Nursing Administration, 36*(7-8), 357–362. https://doi.org.10.1097/00005110-200607000-00007

Chinn, P. L., & Kramer, M. K. (2018). *Knowledge development in nursing: Theory and process* (10th ed.). Mosby Elsevier.

Cook, E. (1913). *The life of Florence Nightingale* (Vol. 1). Macmillan.

Coulter, K. (2016). Successful infusion in older adults. *Journal of Infusion Nursing, 39*(6), 352–358. https://doi.org/10.1097/NAN.0000000000000196

Creswell, J., & Creswell, D. (2018). *Research design: Qualitative, quantitative, and mixed methods approaches* (5th ed.). Sage.

Creswell, J. W., & Poth, C. N. (2018). *Qualitative inquiry & research design: Choosing among five approaches* (4th ed.). Sage.

Deetz, J., Davidson, J., Daugherty, J., Graham, P., & Carroll, D. (2020). Exploring correlation of nurse manager meaning and joy in work with employee engagement. *Applied Nursing Research, 55,* 151297. https://doi.org/10.1016/j.apnr.2020.151297

Dodd, S., Harman, N., Taske, N., Minchin, M., Tan, T., & Williamson, P. (2020). Core outcome sets through the healthcare ecosystem: The case of type 2 diabetes mellitus. *Trials, 21,* 570. https://doi.org/10.1186/s13063-020-04403-1

Feo, R., Kitson, A., & Conroy, T. (2018). How fundamental aspects of nursing care are defined in the literature: A scoping review. *Journal of Clinical Nursing, 27,* 2189–2229. https://doi.10.1111/jocn.14313

Fisher, M., McKechnie, D., & Pryor, J. (2020). Conducting a critical review of the research literature. *Journal of the Australasian Rehabilitation Nurses' Association, 23*(1), 20–29. https://doi.org/10.33235/jarna.23.1.20-29

Fitzpatrick, M. L. (1978). *Historical studies in nursing.* Teachers College Press.

Glaser, B. G., & Strauss, A. L. (1967). *The discovery of grounded theory: Strategies for qualitative research.* Aldine.

Glasofer, A., & Townsend, A. (2019). Determining the level of evidence: Experimental research appraisal. *Nursing Critical Care, 14*(6), 22–25. https://doi.org.10.1097/01.CCN.0000580120.03118.1d

Gorski, L., Hadaway, L., Hagle, M., McGoldrick, M., Orr, M., & Doellman, D. (2016). Infusion therapy standards of practice. *Journal of Infusion Nursing, 39*(1S), S1–S159.

Gortner, S. R., & Nahm, H. (1977). An overview of nursing research in the United States. *Nursing Research, 26*(1), 10–33.

Gravetter, F., & Forzano, L. A. (2018). *Research methods for the behavioral sciences.* Cengage.

Gray, J. R., & Grove, S. K. (2021). *Burns and Grove's the practice of nursing research: Appraisal, synthesis, and generation of evidence* (9th ed.). Elsevier.

Grinspun, D., & Bajnok, I. (2018). *Transforming nursing through knowledge: Best practices for guideline development, implementation science, and evaluation.* Sigma Theta Tau International.

Grove, S. K., & Cipher, D. J. (2020). *Statistics for nursing research: A workbook for evidence-based practice* (3rd ed.). Elsevier.

Groves, P., Farag, A., & Bunch, J. (2020). Strategies for and barriers to fatigue management among acute care nurses. *Journal of Nursing Regulation, 11*(2), 36–43. http://doi.org/10.1016/S2155-8256(20)30108-3

Havill, N., Leeman, J., Shaw-Kot, J., Knafl, K., Crandell, J., & Sandelowski, M. (2014). Managing large-volume literature searches in research synthesis studies. *Nursing Outlook, 62,* 112–118. http://dx.doi.org/10.1016/j.outlook.2013.11.002

Hayes, B., Stephens, R., Ngo, J., & Dunn, J. (2018). The dimensionality of reasoning: Inductive and deductive inference can be explained by a single process. *Journal of Experimental Psychology, Learning, Memory, and Cognition, 44*(9), 1333–1351. http://dx.doi.org/10.1037/xlm0000527

Herbert, R. G. (1981). *Florence Nightingale: Saint, reformer or rebel?* Robert E. Krieger.

Higgins, J. P. T., & Thomas, J. (2019). *Cochrane handbook for systematic reviews of interventions* (2nd ed.). Wiley-Blackwell and The Cochrane Collaboration.

Horsley, J. A., Crane, J., Crabtree, M. K., & Wood, D. J. (1983). Using research to improve nursing practice: A guide. *CURN project.* Grune & Stratton

Institute of Medicine. (2001). *Crossing the quality chasm: A new health system for the 21st century.* National Academy Press. https://doi.org.10.172226/10027

Kähkönen, O., Kyngäs, H., Saaranen, T., Kankkunen, P., Miettinen, H., & Oikarinen, A. (2020). Support from next of kin and nurses are significant predictors of long-term adherence to treatment in post-PCI patients. *European Journal of Cardiovascular Nursing, 19*(4), 339–350. https://doi.org.10.1177/14745151198878

Kaplan, A. (1964). *The conduct of inquiry; Methodology for behavioral science.* Chandler. E book was published 2017. https://doi.org/10.4324/9781315131467

Karl, J., & Mion, L. (2020). Research data in hospitals and health systems. In M. McNett (Ed.), *Data for Nurses: Understanding and using data to optimize care delivery in hospitals and health systems* (pp. 31–46). Academic Press.

Kohn, L., Corrigan, L., & Donaldson, M. (Eds.). (2000). *To err is human: Building a safer health system.* National Academies Press. https://doi.org.10.17226/9728

Makic, M., & Granger, B. (2019). Deimplementation in clinical practice: What are we waiting for? *AACN Advanced Critical Care, 30*(3), 282–286. https://doi.org/10.4037/aacnacc2019607

McDonald, L. (2001). Florence Nightingale and the early origins of evidence-based nursing. *Evidence-Based*

Nursing, 4(7), 68–69. http://dx.doi.org/10.1136/ebn.4.3.68

McMenamin, A., Sun, C., Prufeta, P., & Raso, R. (2019). The evolution of evidence-based practice. *Nursing Management, 50*(9), 14–19.

McSweeney, J., Weglicki, L., Munro, C., Hickman, R., & Pickler, R. (2020). Preparing nurse scientists: Challenges and solutions. *Nursing Research, 69*(6), 414–418. https://doi.org/10.1097/NNR.0000000000000471

Meadows-Oliver, M. (2019). Critically appraising qualitative evidence for clinical decision making. In B. Melnyk & E. Fineout-Overholt (Eds.), *Evidence-based practice in nursing and healthcare: A guide to best practice* (4th ed., pp. 189–218). Wolters Kluwer.

Melnyk, B. M., & Fineout-Overholt, E. (2019). *Evidence-based practice in nursing and healthcare: A guide to best practice* (4th ed., pp. 189–218). Wolters Kluwer.

Melnyk, B. M., Gallagher-Ford, E., & Fineout-Overholt, E. (2017). *Implementing evidence-based practice competencies in healthcare: A practical guide for improving quality, safety, & outcomes.* Sigma Theta Tau International.

Melnyk, B., Gallagher-Ford, E., Zellefrow, C., Tucker, S., Thomas, B., Sinnott, L., & Tan, A. (2018). The first U.S. study on nurses' evidence-based practice competencies indicates major deficits that threaten healthcare quality, safety, and patient outcomes. *Worldviews on Evidence-Based Nursing, 15*(1), 16–25.

Moorhead, S., Johnson, M., Maas, M. L., & Swanson, E. (2018). *Nursing outcomes classification (NOC): Measurement of health outcomes* (6th ed.). Elsevier.

National Center for Complementary and Integrative Health. (2020). *Clinical practice guidelines.* Retrieved from https://www.nccih.nih.gov/health/providers/clinicalpractice

National Institute of Nursing Research. (n.d.). *Stories of discovery.* Retrieved from https://www.ninr.nih.gov/all-stories-of-discovery#8884

National Patient Safety Agency. (2011). *Patient Safety Alert NPSA/2011/PSA002: Reducing the harm caused by misplaced nasogastric feeding tubes in adults, children and infants.* National Health Service. Retrieved from http://www.gbukenteral.com/pdf/NPSA-Alert-2011.pdf

Nickel, B. (2019). Peripheral intravenous access: Applying infusion therapy standards of practice to improve patient safety. *Critical Care Nurse, 39*(1), 61–71. https://doi.org/10.4037/ccn2019790

Nightingale, F. (1859). *Notes on nursing: What it is, and what it is not.* Lippincott.

Oakley, K. (2010). Nursing by the numbers. *Occupational Health, 62*(4), 28–29.

Palmer, I. S. (1977). Florence Nightingale: Reformer, reactionary, researcher. *Nursing Research, 26*(2), 84–89.

Pickler, R. H. (2020). The year that wasn't. *Nursing Research, 29*(6), 413. https://www.doi.org/10.1097/NNR.0000000000000467

Powers, J. (2020). Increasing capacity in nursing research in magnet-designated organizations to promote nursing research [Special issue]. *Applied Nursing Research, 55,* 151286. https://doi.org/10.1016/j.apnr.2020.151286

Quality and Safety Education for Nurses. (2017). *QSEN competencies.* Retrieved from http://qsen.org/competencies/pre-licensure-ksas/

Quality and Safety Education for Nurses. (2020). *QSEN competencies: Pre-licensure knowledge, skills, and attitudes (KSAs).* Retrieved from http://qsen.org/competencies/pre-licensure-ksas/

Rettig, R. (1991). History, development, and importance to nursing of outcomes research. *Journal of Nursing Quality Assurance, 5*(2), 13–17.

Sandelowski, M., & Barroso, J. (2007). *Handbook for synthesizing qualitative research.* Springer.

Schuler, E., Paul, F., Connor, L., Doherty, D., & DeGrazia, M. (2020). Cultivating evidence-based practice through mentorship. *Applied Nursing Research, 55,* 151295. https://doi.org/10.1016/j.apnr.2020.151295

See, E. M. (1977). The ANA and research in nursing. *Nursing Research, 26*(3), 165–171.

Sherwood, G., & Barnsteiner, J. (2017). *Quality and safety in nursing: A competency approach to improving outcomes* (2nd ed.). Wiley-Blackwell.

Stetler, C. B. (2010) Stetler model. In J. Rycroft-Malone & T. Bucknall (Eds.), *Models and frameworks for implementing evidence-based practice: Linking evidence to action* (pp. 51–81). Wiley-Blackwell.

Straus, S. E., Glasziou, P., Richardson, W. S., & Haynes, R. B. (2019). *Evidence-based medicine: How to practice and teach EBM.* Elsevier Limited.

US Department of Health and Human Services. (n.d.). *Healthy People 2030: Building a health future for us all.* Retrieved from https://health.gov/healthypeople

Yin, R. (2018). *Case study research and applications: Design and methods* (6th ed.). Sage.

Introduction to Quantitative Research

Polly A. Hulme

LEARNING OUTCOMES

After completing this chapter, you should be able to:

1. Define terms relevant to the quantitative research process—basic research, applied research, rigor, and control.
2. Compare and contrast the problem-solving process, nursing process, and research process.
3. Describe the steps of the quantitative research process in descriptive, correlational, quasi-experimental, and experimental published studies.
4. Read quantitative research reports to expand your knowledge of nursing research findings.
5. Conduct initial critical appraisals of quantitative research reports.

What do you think of when you hear the word *research*? Frequently, the idea of experimentation or study comes to mind. Typical features of an experiment include randomizing participants into groups, collecting data, and conducting statistical analyses. You may think of researchers conducting a study to determine the effectiveness of an intervention, such as determining the effect of a walking program on body mass index of patients with type 2 diabetes. These ideas are associated with quantitative research, which includes specific steps that are detailed in a research report. A research report summarizes the major elements of a study and identifies the contributions of that study to nursing knowledge.

This chapter introduces the quantitative research process so that you may be able to read and understand these types of research reports and gain the skills necessary for critically appraising the strengths and weaknesses of these studies. Relevant terms are defined, and a discussion of the problem-solving process and the nursing process is presented to provide a background for understanding the quantitative research process. The steps of the quantitative research process are introduced, and a correlational study is presented as an example to promote understanding of this process. Critical thinking skills needed for reading research reports and guidelines for conducting an initial critical appraisal of these reports are also provided. The chapter concludes with the identification of the steps of the research process from a quasi-experimental study, with an initial critical appraisal of this study.

WHAT IS QUANTITATIVE RESEARCH?

Quantitative research is a formal, objective, rigorous, and systematic process for generating information about the world from numerical data. Nurses typically conduct quantitative research to (1) describe new situations, events, or concepts; (2) examine relationships among health-related variables, and (3) determine the effectiveness of interventions on health outcomes that matter to patients and society. An example of each of these types of quantitative research follows:

1. Describing the current spread of COVID-19 cases and their potential influence on local, national, and global health
2. Examining the relationships among screen time minutes per week, average number of hours of sleep per day, and body mass index of a school-age child
3. Determining the effectiveness of a fall prevention program on the fall rate of hospitalized older patients

The history of modern quantitative research begins with Sir Ronald Fisher (1935), a noted statistician and geneticist. Fisher originated classic experimental designs to test the effectiveness of interventions (also called treatments) on biological outcomes. He is noted for adding structure to the steps of the quantitative research process with ideas such as the hypothesis, research design, and statistical analysis. Fisher's studies provided the groundwork for what is now known as experimental research. Throughout the years, other types of quantitative approaches have been developed. Campbell and Stanley (1963) developed quasi-experimental research to study the effects of interventions under less controlled conditions (Shadish et al., 2002). Karl Pearson developed statistical approaches for examining relationships among variables, known as correlational research (Porter, 2004). And finally, the fields of sociology, education, and psychology are noted for their development and expansion of strategies for conducting descriptive research.

A broad range of quantitative research approaches is needed to develop the empirical knowledge for building evidence-based practice (EBP) in nursing (Melnyk & Fineout-Overholt, 2019). EBP was introduced in Chapter 1 and is discussed in detail in Chapter 13, with EBP tips provided in all chapters. EBP is essential for promoting quality, safe, cost-effective outcomes for patients and families, nursing education, and the healthcare system (Straus et al., 2019). Understanding the quantitative research process is essential for meeting the Quality and Safety Education for Nurses (QSEN, 2021) competencies for undergraduate nursing students, which are focused on patient-centered care, teamwork and collaboration, EBP, quality improvement, safety, and informatics (Sherwood & Barnsteiner, 2017). This section introduces the different types of quantitative research and provides definitions of terms relevant to the quantitative research process.

Types of Quantitative Research

The four common types of quantitative research conducted in nursing are presented in Fig. 2.1. The type of quantitative research conducted is influenced by current knowledge about a research problem. When little knowledge is available, descriptive studies are conducted that provide a basis for correlational research. Descriptive and correlational studies are conducted frequently to provide a basis for quasi-experimental and experimental studies to test nursing interventions.

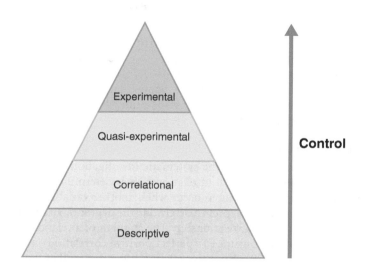

FIG. 2.1 Types of Quantitative Research Conducted in Nursing.

Descriptive Research

Descriptive research is the exploration and description of phenomena in real-life situations. Its purpose is to provide an accurate account of characteristics of particular individuals, situations, or groups using numbers (Grove & Cipher, 2020). Descriptive studies are usually conducted with large numbers of participants, in natural settings (see Chapter 9), with no manipulation of the situation. Descriptive studies are conducted to (1) determine the frequency with which a phenomenon occurs, (2) categorize the attributes of a phenomenon and measure the relative amount of each category, and (3) determine quantity when a phenomenon can be characterized by amount. In descriptive studies, researchers often compare the results across different groups and/or time. The underlying research questions in descriptive research are (1) To what extent does this variable exist? (2) What are the principal types of this variable? (3) What are the relative amounts of this variable? (4) Are there differences between existing groups, such as females and males, on this variable? (5) Do individuals change over time regarding this variable? Box 2.1 provides definitions for the following terms: constructs, concepts, and variables. You can easily refer to these definitions as you read this chapter (for further details, see Chapters 5 and 7).

Schoenfisch and colleagues (2019) conducted a descriptive study to increase understanding of the use of assistive devices by nursing staff with hospitalized patients. The results showed that only

---

BOX 2.1 DEFINITIONS OF CONSTRUCTS, CONCEPTS, AND VARIABLES

Constructs: concepts at very high levels of abstraction that have general meanings
Concepts: terms that abstractly describe and name objects or phenomena, thus providing them with a separate identity or meaning
Variables: concrete or abstract qualities, properties, or characteristics of persons, things, or situations that change or vary and are manipulated, measured, or controlled in research

Adapted from Gray, J. R., & Grove, S. K. (2021). *The practice of nursing research: Appraisal, synthesis, and generation of evidence* (9th ed.). Elsevier.

40% of participants used assistive devices for ≥50% of their lifts or transfers. These participants were compared with the remaining 60% of participants who used assistive devices for less than 50% of their lifts or transfers. Surprisingly, the two groups did not differ by age, hospital type, unit type, job title, or patient care experience. Barriers to assistive device use were multiple and consisted of a combination of patient, nurse, equipment, and situational categories. A correlational study on the relative strength of relationships among barriers and assistive device use would be a logical next step for expanding knowledge on this important nursing topic.

Correlational Research

Correlational research involves the systematic investigation of relationships between or among variables. The numerical strength of relationships is determined to discover whether a change in the value of one variable is likely to occur when another variable increases or decreases. Correlational analysis allows the researcher to determine the degree or strength of the relationship and the type (positive or negative) of relationship. The strength of a relationship varies, ranging from −1 (perfect negative correlation) to +1 (perfect positive correlation), with 0 indicating no relationship (Grove & Cipher, 2020). A positive relationship indicates that the variables vary together; that is, both variables increase or decrease together. For example, research has shown that the more minutes people exercise each week the greater their bone density. A negative relationship indicates that the variables vary in opposite directions; thus as one variable increases, the other will decrease. As an example, research has shown that as the number of smoking pack-years (number of years smoked multiplied by the number of packs smoked per day) increases, an individual's life span decreases.

The intent of correlational studies is either to explain the nature of relationships or to allow prediction, all in the context of the real world. It is important for you to remember that the relationships revealed in correlation studies are associations, not cause-and-effect relationships (Gray & Grove, 2021; Kazdin, 2017). The associations identified by correlational studies provide the basis for generating hypotheses to guide quasi-experimental and experimental studies that do focus on cause-and-effect relationships (see Fig. 2.1). Examples of underlying research questions in correlational research include the following: What is the nature of the relationship between these two variables? To what extent do these variables predict a specified outcome? Are the relationships in a model or theory supported by research?

Cho and colleagues (2021) conducted a correlational study to determine the relationship between quality of sleep and daytime fatigue in hospital nurses. They examined this relationship in participants who came back to work from time off and then worked two 12-hour consecutive day shifts. Not surprisingly, they found that a poor night's sleep was associated with increased fatigue the next day for both shifts. However, the relationships were strongest for the first shift. Based on these results, the researchers suggested that nurses find ways to psychologically disengage from work on their days off for better sleep quality the night before coming back to work. In addition, "healthcare organizations should facilitate work schedules to ensure that nurses have sufficient recovery between shifts and systematically monitor and support nurses in the management of their sleep and fatigue levels" (Cho et al., 2021, p. 133).

Quasi-Experimental Research

The purpose of quasi-experimental research is the objective, systematic study of cause-and-effect relationships. Cause-and-effect relationships are examined by using numerical means to determine whether manipulating one variable affects other variables. These studies involve implementing an intervention and examining its effects using selected measurement methods (Kazdin, 2017;

BOX 2.2 **ELEMENTS CONTROLLED IN QUANTITATIVE RESEARCH**

- Extraneous variables
- Selection of setting(s)
- Sampling process
- Assignment of study participants to groups
- Development and implementation of the study intervention

Waltz et al., 2017). For example, an intervention of a swimming exercise program might be implemented to improve balance and muscle strength of elderly women with osteoarthritis.

Quasi-experimental studies differ from experimental studies by the level of control achieved by researchers. Box 2.2 identifies the elements that are controlled in these two types of quantitative research. Quasi-experimental studies have less control over management of the setting, selection of study participants, and/or the implementation of the intervention. When studying human behavior, especially in clinical settings, researchers frequently are unable to control certain variables related to these aspects of the study. In addition, researchers sometimes are unable to randomly assign participants to intervention and control groups in clinical settings. As a result, nurse researchers conduct more quasi-experimental than experimental studies.

When reading quasi-experimental and experimental studies, you need to understand the terminology used. The manipulated variable (the intervention) is called the independent variable. The delivery of the independent variable should be highly controlled and consistently implemented, such as using a detailed protocol to direct an exercise program. The variables subjected to controlled manipulation of the independent variable are the dependent variables (also called outcomes). Returning to the example of a swimming exercise program designed to improve the balance and muscle strength of elderly women with osteoarthritis, the independent variable is the swimming exercise program, and the dependent variables are balance and muscle strength.

Karsten and colleagues (2020) conducted a quasi-experimental study on the effectiveness of peppermint aromatherapy on postoperative nausea and vomiting. The independent variable (the intervention) was a one-time dose of peppermint oil inhalation provided to patients on arrival to the postanesthesia care unit. The dependent variable (the outcome) was nausea and vomiting while in the postanesthesia care unit. The control group did not receive the intervention. Statistical analysis demonstrated no differences in nausea and vomiting between the intervention and control groups. In this study, the implementation of the intervention was highly controlled: 3 drops of peppermint oil were placed on a cotton ball and placed under the patient's nares for a one-time inhalation. However, other aspects of the study were not controlled, including type of surgery, type of anesthesia, and assignment to the intervention and control groups.

Experimental Research

Experimental research is the objective, systematic, and highly controlled investigation of cause-and-effect relationships (Gray & Grove, 2021; Kazdin, 2017). Experimental research is the most powerful quantitative method because of the rigorous control of all elements of the study (see Box 2.2). At least two separate groups must be present, one of which is a distinct control group that does not receive the intervention. In addition, participants must be randomly assigned to either the intervention or control group. Random assignment is the process of assigning participants so that each has an equal opportunity (or probability) of being in either group. Conducting an experimental study in a laboratory or a research facility provides environmental control.

Nurse educators Atthill and colleagues (2021) conducted an experimental study to test their hypothesis that virtual asynchronous debriefing is as effective as face-to-face debriefing after a clinical simulation activity. The independent variable (the intervention) was virtual asynchronous debriefing. The dependent variables (the outcomes) were the students' (1) anxiety and (2) self-confidence in engaging in clinical decision making. Students were randomly assigned to the intervention group (virtual asynchronous debriefing) or the control group (face-to-face debriefing). Through statistical analysis, the researchers found that students in the intervention group had significantly decreased anxiety and increased self-confidence after the intervention. Compared with the control group, they demonstrated similar or even better outcomes. Based on their findings, the researchers concluded that virtual asynchronous debriefing "is a reliable alternative to face-to-face debriefing" (Atthill et al., 2021, p. 10).

📄 RESEARCH/EBP TIP

Quantitative studies have varying levels of control from low in descriptive studies to high in experimental studies (see Fig. 2.1). Control can be used to improve the selection of the study setting and participants, assignment of participants to groups, and measurement of study variables, which influence the quality of findings for practice.

Defining Terms Relevant to Quantitative Research

Understanding quantitative research requires comprehension of four important terms: basic research, applied research, rigor, and control. These terms are defined in the following sections, with examples provided from quantitative studies.

Basic Research

Quantitative research can be divided into two types: basic and applied. Basic research aims to increase knowledge or understanding of the "fundamental aspects of phenomena and of observable facts without specific applications toward processes or products in mind" (Basic Research, n.d.). In the health sciences, which includes nursing, basic researchers seek new knowledge and understanding about human biology, behavior, and disease. They study these phenomena on the molecular, cellular, tissue, and/or organism levels. Basic research is conducted in a research laboratory or other artificial setting with animals, paid human volunteers, or animal or human tissue. Because basic research is often conducted in research laboratories on long tables or benches, it is sometimes referred to as bench research. Scientific principles gained from basic research require applied research to determine their use in nursing practice.

An important source of funding for nursing research is the National Institute of Nursing Research (NINR; https://www.ninr.nih.gov/). NINR is an institute of the National Institutes of Health, which functions under the US Department of Health and Human Services. An example of basic research supported by NINR is a study by Vizioli and colleagues (2021). The researchers examined subcutaneous adipose tissue (SAT) samples obtained during bariatric surgery and stored at the Human Metabolic Tissue Bank at the University of Pennsylvania. They wanted to find out how the metabolites in SAT differed between two groups: obese individuals with type 2 diabetes mellitus (T2DM) and obese individuals without T2DM. Their goal was to contribute to an "improved understanding of the complex relationship between abdominal SAT and T2DM" (Vizioli et al., 2021, p. 110). Although their results did not show significant differences in metabolites between those with and without T2DM, they laid a foundation for future studies on the topic.

Applied Research

Applied research in nursing focuses specifically on generating knowledge that will directly influence or improve nursing practice. Therefore applied research is conducted to solve real-life problems, to make decisions, and to predict or control outcomes in practice situations. Nursing practice is defined broadly to include not only direct care of patients and families in clinical and community settings but also indirect care that focuses on populations. In addition, nurse educators and administrators conduct applied research that seeks to improve nursing education and administration practices (see Chapter 1). Two studies discussed earlier, Atthill et al. (2021) and Cho et al. (2021), are applied research examples from the areas of nursing education and nursing administration, respectively. Also falling under the umbrella of applied research are studies that test and validate theories for their usefulness in nursing practice (Gray & Grove, 2021). Because the questions that applied researchers seek to answer arise from practice situations, applied research is conducted in practice settings quite similar to those where the results will be applied. Most nursing research is applied, not basic.

Hammer et al. (2021) conducted an applied study to test the feasibility of a 6-mo walking intervention designed to reduce symptoms in patients undergoing chemotherapy for cancer. This intervention was based on the premise that walking would reduce hyperglycemia, which in turn would reduce symptom severity. Basic research findings informed the researchers that hyperglycemia may increase symptom severity by way of oxidative stress induced by hyperglycemia. Oxidative stress is known to trigger inflammation, which in turn can increase symptom severity. The researchers recruited patients with cancer who were undergoing chemotherapy and did not have diabetes, and then randomly assigned them to the intervention or control group. The outcomes measured included glycosylated hemoglobin A1c and cancer-related symptoms (e.g., sleep disturbances, depression, fatigue, and pain). As a feasibility study, the sample size was not large enough to accurately determine the effect of the intervention on the outcomes. Because the feasibility data were favorable, the next step for the research team would be to conduct a study using the same methods with a large sample.

📄 RESEARCH/EBP TIP

Researchers often examine the new knowledge discovered through basic research for its usefulness in practice by conducting applied research, making these approaches complementary. The knowledge gained from applied research can benefit not only nursing practice but also policymakers addressing health and social concerns.

Rigor in Quantitative Research

Rigor is the striving for excellence in research, which requires discipline, adherence to detail, precision, and accuracy. A rigorously conducted quantitative study has precise measuring tools, a representative sample, and a tightly controlled study design. Critically appraising the rigor of a study involves examining the reasoning used in conducting the study. Logical reasoning, including deductive and inductive reasoning (see Chapter 1), is essential to the development of quantitative studies (Chinn & Kramer, 2018). The research process, discussed later in this chapter, includes specific steps that are rigorously developed with meticulous detail and are logically linked in descriptive, correlational, quasi-experimental, and experimental studies.

Another aspect of rigor is precision, which encompasses accuracy, detail, and order. Precision is evident in the concise statement of the research purpose and detailed development of the study design. However, the most explicit example of precision is the measurement or quantification of the study variables (Bandalos, 2018; Waltz et al., 2017). For example, a researcher might use a cardiac monitor to measure and record the heart rate of participants in a database during an exercise program, rather than palpating a radial pulse for 30 seconds and recording it on a data collection sheet. Precision is essential for transparency in research so that other investigators know as explicitly as possible the exact steps and elements that make up a study. Precision allows for replication and for variation, which is necessary for other researchers to validate or extend the findings.

Control in Quantitative Research

Control involves the imposing of rules by researchers to decrease the possibility of error, thereby increasing the probability that the study's findings are an accurate reflection of reality. The rules used to achieve control in research are referred to as design. Quantitative studies include various degrees of control, ranging from uncontrolled to highly controlled, depending on the type of study (see Fig. 2.1). Table 2.1 contains a list of the applied studies provided as examples in this chapter by type of quantitative research and the typical control and setting characteristics for each type. Descriptive

TABLE 2.1 LIST OF QUANTITATIVE RESEARCH EXAMPLES IN THIS CHAPTER WITH CONTROL AND SETTING CHARACTERISTICS FOR EACH TYPE OF RESEARCH

AUTHORS	TITLE	TYPE	CONTROL	TYPICAL SETTING
Schoenfisch et al. (2019)	Use of assistive devices to lift, transfer, and reposition hospital patients	Descriptive	No intervention; limited or no control of extraneous variables	Natural or partially controlled setting
Sosa et al. (2021)	The effect of demographic and self-management factors on physical activity in women	Correlational	No intervention; limited or no control of extraneous variables	Natural or partially controlled setting
Hammer et al. (2021)	Prescribed walking for glycemic control and symptom management in patients without diabetes undergoing chemotherapy	Quasi-experimental (pilot study)	Controlled intervention; rigorous control of extraneous variables	Partially controlled setting
Reaves & Angosta (2021)	The relaxation response: influence on psychological and physiological responses in patients with chronic obstructive pulmonary disease	Quasi-experimental	Controlled intervention; rigorous control of extraneous variables	Partially controlled setting
Atthill et al., (2021)	Exploring the effect of a virtual asynchronous debriefing method after a virtual simulation game to support clinical decision making	Experimental	Highly controlled intervention and extraneous variables	Research unit or laboratory setting

and correlational studies are rigorously conducted but are often designed with minimal researcher control because no intervention is implemented and study participants are examined as they exist in their natural setting, such as home, work, school, or healthcare clinic. Quasi-experimental and experimental studies have increased control with the implementation of an intervention to determine the effects on selected outcomes (see Box 2.2 for elements controlled).

Extraneous variables. Through control, the researcher can reduce the influence of extraneous variables. An extraneous variable is something that is not the focus of a study but can make the independent variable appear more powerful or less powerful than it really is. Extraneous variables exist in all studies and can interfere with obtaining a clear understanding of the relationships among the study variables (see Chapter 5). For example, Karsten et al. (2020), as discussed previously, studied aromatherapy's effect on postoperative nausea and vomiting. The researchers did not control for type of surgery or anesthesia, which might have altered the findings. Selecting only patients with abdominal incisions who received certain types of anesthesia would have helped control these two extraneous variables.

Research settings. The setting is the location in which a study is conducted. There are three common settings for conducting research: natural, partially controlled, and highly controlled (see Table 2.1). A natural (or field) setting is an uncontrolled real-life situation or environment. Conducting a study in a natural setting means that the researcher does not manipulate or change the environment for the study. Descriptive and correlational studies often are conducted in natural settings. A partially controlled setting is an environment that the researcher has manipulated or modified in some way to limit the effects of extraneous variables on the findings. A highly controlled setting is an artificially constructed environment developed for the sole purpose of conducting research. Laboratories, research centers, and test units in universities or healthcare agencies are highly controlled settings in which bench and experimental studies often are conducted (see Chapter 9).

Sampling and assignment of participants to groups. Sampling is a process of selecting participants who are representative of the population being studied. In quantitative research, random and nonrandom samples are used. Random sampling is best practice for obtaining a sample that is representative of a population because each member of the population is selected independently and has an equal chance, or probability, of being included in the study. In addition, random sampling helps prevent bias (slanting of the findings away from what is true or accurate) in selecting study participants and assigning them to the intervention or control group. A randomly selected sample, however, is difficult to obtain in nursing research, so quantitative studies often are conducted with nonrandom samples (see Chapter 9).

An example of a nonrandom sample is found in a descriptive study by Brewer and colleagues (2021). The researchers' long-term goal was to improve the outcomes of church-based weight management programs for African Americans. As an initial step to achieving their goal, they created a questionnaire to determine key characteristics of their population of interest, such as weight, social support, and motivation to change. To sample their population of interest, the researchers distributed the questionnaire electronically to the members of a predominantly African American faith-based organization. This strategy provided a nonrandom sample that consisted of 1439 individuals who completed the questionnaire.

Study interventions. Quasi-experimental and experimental research examine the effect of an intervention (the independent variable) on an outcome(s) (the dependent variable[s]). A study intervention needs to be (1) clearly and precisely developed, (2) consistently implemented, and (3) examined for effectiveness through quality measurement of the dependent variables. The detailed development of a quality intervention and the consistent implementation of this intervention are known as intervention fidelity (Bonar et al., 2020). Controlling the development and implementation of a study intervention increases the validity of the study design (see Chapter 8) and credibility of the findings.

PROBLEM-SOLVING AND NURSING PROCESSES: BASIS FOR UNDERSTANDING THE QUANTITATIVE RESEARCH PROCESS

The research process is similar in some ways to other processes. Therefore the background acquired early in nursing education in (1) problem solving and (2) the nursing process are both useful in research. A process includes a purpose, series of actions, and goal. The purpose provides direction for the implementation of a series of actions to achieve an identified goal or outcome. The specific steps of the process can be revised and reimplemented to reach the endpoint or goal. Table 2.2 links the steps of the problem-solving process, nursing process, and research process. Relating the research process to the problem-solving and nursing processes may be helpful in understanding the steps of the quantitative research process.

Comparing Problem Solving With the Nursing Process

The problem-solving process involves (1) systematic collection of data to identify a problem, difficulty, or dilemma; (2) determination of goals related to the problem; (3) identification of possible approaches or solutions to achieve those goals (plan); (4) implementation of the selected solutions;

TABLE 2.2   COMPARISON OF THE PROBLEM-SOLVING PROCESS, NURSING PROCESS, AND RESEARCH PROCESS

PROBLEM-SOLVING PROCESS	NURSING PROCESS	RESEARCH PROCESS
Data collection	Assessment	Knowledge of nursing world
	Data collection (objective and subjective data)	Clinical experiences
	Data interpretation	Literature review
Problem definition	Nursing diagnosis	Problem and purpose identification
Plan	Plan	Methodology
Setting goals	Setting goals	Design
Identifying solutions	Planning interventions	Sample
		Measurement methods
		Data collection
		Data analysis
Implementation of plan	Implementation of plan	Implementation of methodology
Evaluation and revision	Evaluation and modification	Outcomes, communication, and synthesis of study findings to promote evidence-based nursing practice

and (5) evaluation of goal achievement (Chinn & Kramer, 2018). Problem solving frequently is used in daily activities and nursing practice. For example, you use problem solving when you select your clothing, decide where to live, or turn a patient with a fractured hip.

The nursing process is a subset of the problem-solving process. The steps of the nursing process are assessment, diagnosis, plan, implementation, evaluation, and modification (see Table 2.2). Assessment involves the collection and interpretation of subjective data (health history) and objective data (physical examination) for the development of nursing diagnoses. These diagnoses guide the remaining steps of the nursing process, just as the step of identifying the problem directs the remaining steps of the problem-solving process. The planning step in the nursing process is the same as in the problem-solving process. Both processes involve implementation (putting the plan into action) and evaluation (determining the effectiveness of the process). If the process is ineffective, nurses need to review all steps and revise (modify) them as necessary to achieve quality outcomes for the patient and family. Nurses implement the nursing process until the diagnoses are resolved and the identified goals are achieved.

Comparing the Nursing Process With the Research Process

The nursing process and research process have important similarities and differences. The two processes are similar because they both involve abstract critical thinking and complex reasoning. These processes help identify new information, discover relationships, and make predictions about phenomena. In both processes, information is gathered, observations are made, problems are identified, plans are developed (methodology), and actions are taken (data collection and analysis). Both processes are reviewed for effectiveness and efficiency—the plan is evaluated in the nursing process, and outcomes are determined in the research process (see Table 2.2). Implementing the two processes expands and refines the user's knowledge. With this growth in knowledge and critical thinking, the user can implement increasingly complex nursing processes and studies.

Knowledge of the nursing process will assist you in understanding the research process. However, the research process is more complex than the nursing process and involves the rigorous application of a variety of research methods (Creswell & Creswell, 2018). The research process also has a broader focus than that of the nursing process, in which the nurse focuses on a specific patient and family. During the quantitative research process, the researcher focuses on large groups of individuals, such as a population of patients with hypertension. In addition, researchers must be knowledgeable about the world of nursing to identify problems that require study. This knowledge comes from clinical and other personal experiences and by conducting a review of relevant literature (see Chapter 6).

The theoretical underpinnings of the research process are much stronger than those of the nursing process. All steps of the research process are logically linked to each other, as well as to the theoretical foundations of the study (see Chapter 7). The conduct of research requires greater precision, rigor, and control than those that are needed in the implementation of the nursing process. The outcomes from research frequently are shared with a large number of nurses and other healthcare professionals through presentations and publications. In addition, the outcomes from several studies can be synthesized to provide sound evidence for nursing practice (Melnyk & Fineout-Overholt, 2019).

DESCRIBING THE STEPS OF THE QUANTITATIVE RESEARCH PROCESS

The quantitative research process involves conceptualizing a research project (gathering information, making observations, and identifying problems), planning and implementing that project,

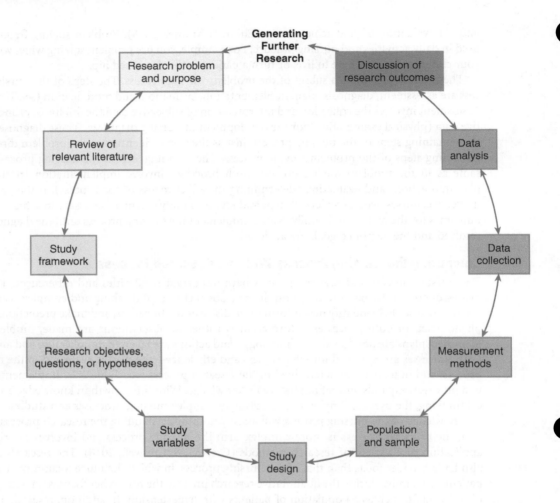

FIG. 2.2 Steps of the Quantitative Research Process.

and communicating the findings. Fig. 2.2 identifies the steps of the quantitative research process that are usually included in a research report. The figure illustrates the logical flow of the process as one step builds progressively on another. The research process is depicted in a circle because there is a flow back and forth as the different steps of a study are developed and implemented. The steps of the quantitative research process are briefly introduced here; Chapters 4 to 11 discuss them in more detail. The predictive correlational study conducted by Sosa and colleagues (2021) on factors that predict physical activity levels in women is used as an example to introduce the steps of the quantitative research process.

Research Problem and Purpose

A research problem is an area of concern in which there is a gap in the knowledge needed for nursing practice. Research is conducted to generate knowledge that addresses the practice concern, with the ultimate goal of developing sound research evidence for nursing practice (Melnyk & Fineout-Overholt, 2019). The research problem is typically broad and could provide the basis for several studies. Most research reports contain one or more paragraphs that describe the essential elements of the research problem, often as a part of the review of relevant literature. This section often concludes with the problem statement, which identifies the area of concern and a particular population on which the research will focus.

The research purpose is generated from the problem and identifies the specific focus or goal of the study. The focus of a quantitative study might be to identify, describe, or explain a situation; predict a solution to a situation; or control a situation to produce positive outcomes in practice. The purpose includes the variables, population, and often the setting for the study (see Chapter 5).

Sosa et al. (2021) noted that physical activity is a type of self-management behavior that helps reduce risk for cardiac disease. Despite its clear health benefits, women are less likely than men to engage in physical activity. This is especially true of minority women and women of lower socioeconomic status. The researchers explained that more information is needed on factors that contribute to less physical activity in women. "With this information, nurses are in a key position to develop interventions based on an understanding of factors known to relate to physical activity for self-management of disease risk" (Sosa et al., 2021, Introduction and background section). The study problem statement and purpose are presented in Research Example 2.1.

RESEARCH EXAMPLE 2.1

Problem and Purpose

Research/Study Excerpts
Research Problem Statement

Further research regarding factors influencing physical activity in the female population is necessary to increase self-management of chronic disease, particularly cardiac risk, through physical activity. (Sosa et al., 2021, Introduction and background section)

Research Purpose

To examine *demographic and self-management [factors] that impact the outcome of physical activity.* (Sosa et al., 2021, Abstract)

Review of Relevant Literature

Researchers conduct a review of relevant literature to generate a picture of what is known and not known about a particular problem and to document why a study needs to be conducted. Relevant literature refers to those sources that are highly pertinent or highly important in providing the in-depth knowledge needed to study a selected problem and purpose. Although a review of the literature includes research reports, it may also contain other nonresearch information, such as theories, clinical practice articles, clinical guidelines, and other professional sources. Often, the literature review section concludes with a summary paragraph that indicates the current knowledge of a problem area and identifies the additional research that is needed to generate essential evidence for practice (see Chapter 6).

Sosa et al.'s (2021) review of relevant literature consisted of research reports that supported their choice of which specific demographic/situational factors and external influencing factors to study. In the studies reviewed, these factors were found to be related to either lower or higher physical activity levels in women. An excerpt of this review is presented in Research Example 2.2.

RESEARCH EXAMPLE 2.2

Review of Relevant Literature

Research/Study Excerpt

Within the literature, several demographic and situational factors are associated with lack of physical activity in women. Family and societal expectations of women to prioritize the role as parent or work responsibility result in lack of time for physical activity....Modifiable external influencing...factors in the literature [include] such [factors] as knowledge and beliefs, self-efficacy, and social facilitation. Social facilitation through support from friends...and collaboration with both family...and others...has been shown to positively influence physical activity levels in women. (Sosa et al., 2021, Introduction and background section)

Study Framework

In research, a concept is a term to which abstract meaning is attached (see Box 2.1), and a framework is a combination of concepts and the connections between them. A relational statement explains the connection between two concepts. In the statement, "Fatigue can impair performance," *fatigue* and *performance* are concepts; *can impair* is the relational term that explains the connection between those concepts. A framework is an abstract version of the relationships between the study's variables. The relational statements or propositions in a study's framework are tested through research (Smith & Liehr, 2018).

A theory is similar to a framework: both are abstract, both guide the development of research, and both are tested through quantitative research. A theory consists of assumptions, an integrated set of defined concepts, and relational statements that present a view of a phenomenon and can be used to describe, explain, predict, or control the phenomenon (Chinn & Kramer, 2018). Assumptions are statements that are taken for granted or are considered true, even though they have not been scientifically tested, and they provide a basis for the phenomenon described by the theory. A theory can exist by itself and be used to explain the concepts of various studies. A framework is usually linked to a given study. Researchers conduct the study to test the relationships in the framework. Because a framework provides an idea of how the concepts in a given study are related, it should help the reader of the research report understand the connections among study variables. Sometimes a framework is represented graphically as a diagram in a research report. The diagram may be called a map, a research framework, or a model. Chapter 7 provides an explanation of frameworks, theories, and related terms.

Sosa et al. (2021) based their framework on a theory called the Individual and Family Self-Management Theory (IFSMT). The concepts are (1) Demographic/Situational Factors, (2) Influencing External Factors, and (3) Self-Management Outcome Behavior. These concepts are abstract enough to meet the definition of constructs (see Box 2.1). However, for learning purposes, we will continue to call them concepts. The relationships among the concepts were explained in the narrative as found in Research Example 2.3 and demonstrated in a diagram (Fig. 2.3). You can easily capture the relationships among the three concepts and their direction by looking at the arrows in the diagram.

RESEARCH EXAMPLE 2.3

Framework

Research/Study Excerpt

The Individual and Family Self-Management Theory (IFSMT) (Ryan & Sawin, 2009) was developed to address multiple levels of self-management in chronic disease...As a result of considering these factors, the IFSMT states that the likelihood of engagement in self-management behavior...[is] determined (Ryan & Sawin, 2009). (Sosa et al., 2021, Theoretical basis and review of literature section)

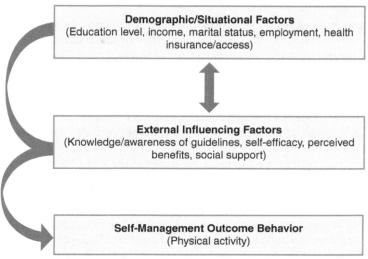

FIG. 2.3 Diagram of the Study Framework. (From Sosa, M., Sethares, K. A., & Chin, E. (2021). The impact of demographic and self-management factors on physical activity in women. *Applied Nursing Research, 57,* 151353. https://doi.org/10.1016/j.apnr.2020.151353) Theoretical basis and review of literature section.

Research Objectives, Questions, or Hypotheses

Investigators formulate research objectives (or aims), questions, or hypotheses to bridge the gap between the more abstractly stated research problem and purpose and the study design and plan for data collection and analysis. Objectives, questions, and hypotheses are narrower in focus than the purpose and often specify only one or two study variables. They also identify the relationship between the variables and indicate the population to be studied. Some descriptive studies include only a research purpose, whereas others include a purpose and objectives or questions to direct the study. Correlational studies often include a purpose and objectives or questions or occasionally hypotheses for predictive correlation studies. Hypotheses are rarely included in descriptive and correlational studies, but quasi-experimental and experimental studies need to include hypotheses to direct the conduct of the studies and the interpretation of findings (see Chapter 5; Gray & Grove, 2021). Sosa et al. (2021) posed two research questions, as identified in Research Example 2.4.

◢ RESEARCH EXAMPLE 2.4

Research/Study Excerpt
Research Questions

1. *What are the relationships of demographic/situational factors (age, race/ethnicity, educational level, income, marital status, employment, health insurance) to external influencing factors in women (awareness of the AHA [American Heart Association] physical activity guidelines, self-efficacy for physical activity, perceived benefits of exercise, and social support from family and friends)?*

2. *To what extent do demographic/situational factors (age, race/ethnicity, educational level, income, marital status, employment, health insurance) and external influencing factors (awareness of the AHA physical activity guidelines, self-efficacy for physical activity, perceived benefits of exercise, and social support from family and friends) predict participation of women in the self-management behavior of physical activity? (Sosa et al., 2021, Introduction and background section)*

Study Variables

The research purpose and objectives, questions, or hypotheses identify the variables to be examined in a study. Variables are qualities, properties, or characteristics at various levels of abstraction that are measured, manipulated, or controlled in a study (see Box 2.1). Variables with low levels of abstraction are called concrete variables. Examples of concrete variables include temperature, weight, or blood pressure. On the other end of the spectrum are abstract variables. Examples of abstract variables are creativity, empathy, and social support. Abstract variables often share the same label or name as a research concept. In other words, an abstract variable such as empathy can function in quantitative research as both a concept (as in a study framework) and a variable (that will be measured in a study).

Researchers operationalize (make measurable) the variables in a study by identifying conceptual and operational definitions. Researchers specify a conceptual definition to provide a variable with theoretical meaning (Gray & Grove, 2021; Smith & Liehr, 2018). Conceptual definitions can be based on a theorist's definition of the variable, a concept analysis, or a definition from the expert literature. Researchers develop an operational definition so that the variable can be measured, manipulated, or controlled in a study (see Chapter 5). Conceptual definitions of variables provide a link from concepts in the study framework to the study variables. The knowledge gained from studying the variables will increase understanding of the theoretical concepts from the study framework that the variables represent.

In the study by Sosa et al. (2021), the three concepts from the study framework functioned as study variables as well. Their conceptual and operational definitions are presented in Research Example 2.5. For this particular study, it is helpful to know that the term *factor* is interchangeable with variable in correlational studies that seek to predict an outcome.

RESEARCH EXAMPLE 2.5

Study Variables

Demographic/Situational Factors
Conceptual definition: factors that influence health disparities (Sosa et al., 2021)
Operational definition: (1) age, (2) race/ethnicity, (3) educational level, (4) income, (5) marital status, (6) employment, and (7) health insurance

External Influencing Factors
Conceptual definition: factors that influence self-management behavior (Sosa et al., 2021)
Operational definition: (1) awareness of American Heart Association (AHA) physical activity guidelines, (2) self-efficacy for physical activity, (3) perceived benefits of exercise, and (4) social support from family and friends

Self-Management Outcome Behavior
Conceptual definition: the process that individuals and families use to improve disease outcomes and promote health (Sosa et al., 2021)
Operational definition: self-reported physical activity in past 7 days

Study Design

Research design is a blueprint for the conduct of a study that maximizes control over factors that could interfere with the study's desired outcome. The type of design directs the selection of a population, procedures for sampling, methods of measurement, and plans for data collection and analysis. The choice of research design depends on what is known and not known about the research problem, the researcher's expertise, the purpose of the study, and the intent to generalize the findings. Sometimes the design of a study indicates that a pilot study was conducted. A pilot study is often a smaller version of a proposed study, and researchers frequently conduct these to refine the study sampling process, intervention, or measurement of variables (Gray & Grove, 2021). The feasibility study conducted by Hammer et al. (2021), discussed earlier in this chapter, is an example of a pilot study.

Designs have been developed to meet unique research needs as they emerge; thus a variety of descriptive, correlational, quasi-experimental, and experimental designs have been generated over time. In descriptive and correlational studies, no intervention is administered, so the purposes of these study designs include improving the precision of measurement, describing what exists, and clarifying relationships that provide a basis for quasi-experimental and experimental studies. Quasi-experimental and experimental study designs usually involve intervention and control groups and focus on achieving high levels of control, as well as precision in measurement (see Table 2.1 and Box 2.2). A study's design typically is in the Methods section of a research report (see Chapter 8 for details on designs). The research design used by Sosa et al. (2021) was predictive correlational.

Population and Sample

The population is all elements (individuals, objects, or situations) that meet certain criteria for inclusion in a study. A sample is a subset of the population selected for a particular study, and the members of a sample are the participants. Sampling was introduced earlier in this chapter, and Chapter 9 provides a background for critically appraising populations, samples, and settings in research reports.

For their population, Sosa et al. (2021) focused on women who have low levels of physical activity and high cardiac risk. Research Example 2.6 provides an excerpt from their sample description.

RESEARCH EXAMPLE 2.6

Population and Sample

Research/Study Excerpt

Because of background data indicating that minority, disadvantaged women, and women with children have the lowest physical activity rates, recruitment was targeted in Providence County, Rhode Island, which has the lowest rates of physical activity and highest cardiac risk in females in the study area.... To target women meeting study demographics, women were recruited at community locations such as schools and public festivals in both high and low-income areas and areas of higher diversity. (Sosa et al., 2021, Methods section)

Measurement Methods

Measurement is the process of "assigning numbers to objects (or events or situations) in accord with some rule" (Kaplan, 1964, p. 177). A component of measurement is instrumentation, which is the application of specific rules to the development of a measurement method or instrument (Waltz et al., 2017). An instrument is selected to measure a specific variable in a study. The numerical data generated with an instrument may be at the nominal, ordinal, interval, or ratio level of measurement, with nominal being the lowest form of measurement and ratio being the highest. Chapter 10 introduces the concept of measurement, describes different types of measurement methods, and provides direction to critically appraise measurement methods in studies. Research Example 2.7 provides a compilation of the instruments used by Sosa et al. (2021). The instruments are organized by the concepts that they represent. The variable or variables that were measured by each instrument are italicized in parentheses.

RESEARCH EXAMPLE 2.7

Measurement Methods

The research study instruments are from Sosa et al. (2021).

Demographic and Situational Factors
- Demographics and Situational Factors Questionnaire *(age, race/ethnicity, educational level, income, marital status, employment, and health insurance)*

External Influencing Factors
- One question on knowledge about American Heart Association (AHA) physical activity guidelines *(Awareness of AHA physical activity guidelines)*
- Self-Efficacy and Exercise Survey (Sallis et al., 1988) *(Self-efficacy for physical activity)*
- Benefits subscale of the Exercise Benefits/Barriers Scale (Sechrist et al., 1987) *(Perceived benefits of exercise)*
- Social Support for Exercise Scale (Sallis et al., 1987) *(Social support from family and friends)*

Self-Management Outcome Behavior
- 7 Day Physical Activity Recall (7 Day PAR) (Sallis et al., 1985) *(Self-reported physical activity in past 7 days)*

Data Collection

Data collection is the precise, systematic gathering of information relevant to the research purpose or the specific objectives, questions, or hypotheses of a study. To collect data, the researcher must obtain permission from the setting or agency in which the study will be conducted. Researchers must also obtain consent from all study participants to indicate their willingness to be in the study. Frequently, the researcher asks the participants to sign a consent form, which describes the study, promises them confidentiality, and indicates that they can withdraw from the study at any time. The research report should document permission from an agency to conduct a study and consent of the study participants (see Chapter 4). Research Example 2.8 provides an excerpt from Sosa et al.'s (2021) description of their data collection procedures.

RESEARCH EXAMPLE 2.8

Data Collection

Research/Study Excerpt

Each participant meeting inclusion criteria and providing consent was given a packet of [the] self-report instruments including the demographics questionnaire…and a private place to complete the instruments. The researcher remained available nearby for assistance. After completion of the self-report instruments, the participant notified the researcher and subsequently participated in an in-person interview to complete the 7 Day PAR with the researcher. (Sosa et al., 2021, Measures section)

Data Analysis

Data analysis involves organization and statistical testing of data to determine prevalence, relationship, and cause. Analysis techniques conducted in quantitative research include descriptive and inferential analyses (see Chapter 11; Grove & Cipher, 2020). Inferential analyses are conducted to examine relationships between variables and differences between groups. Investigators base their choice of analysis techniques primarily on the research objectives, questions, or hypotheses and level of measurement achieved by the measurement methods. Research reports identify the data analysis techniques conducted in the study in the last portion of the Methods section (Grove & Cipher, 2020). You can find the outcomes of the data analysis process in the Results section of the research report; this section is best organized by the research objectives, questions, or hypotheses of the study. An excerpt from Sosa et al.'s (2021) Results section is included in Research Example 2.9.

RESEARCH EXAMPLE 2.9

Data Analysis

Research/Study Excerpts

The study included 119 participants.... Moderate levels of self-efficacy through the behaviors of 'sticking to it'... and 'making time'... for exercise were found.... Awareness of the guidelines revealed that 68.1% of the sample was unaware of AHA physical activity guidelines. Awareness of the guidelines was not related to demographics/situational factors or physical activity levels.

Hierarchical regression was used...to assess prediction of levels of physical activity.... The model as a whole explained 13.8% of the variance in physical activity levels.... There were no individual independent variables significantly contributing to explanation of physical activity levels in women. (Sosa et al., 2021, Results section)

Discussion of Research Outcomes

The results obtained from data analyses require interpretation to be meaningful. Interpretation of research outcomes involves (1) examining the results of data analysis, (2) explaining what the results mean in light of current practice and previous research, (3) identifying study limitations, (4) forming conclusions, (5) deciding on the appropriate recommendation for generalization of the findings, (6) considering the implications for nursing's body of knowledge, and (7) suggesting the direction of further research. Limitations are restrictions in a study methodology and/or framework that may decrease the credibility and generalizability of the findings. A generalization is the extension of the conclusions made based on the research findings from the sample studied to a larger population. The interpretation of research outcomes is typically found in the Discussion section of research reports.

During the process of interpretation of research outcomes, the study results from data analyses are translated and interpreted to become study findings, and these study findings are synthesized to form conclusions. By necessity, study conclusions are influenced by the limitations of the study. Study conclusions provide a basis for the implications of the findings for practice and to identify areas for further research (see Chapter 11). Implications for nursing's body of knowledge include ways to incorporate the conclusions into nursing theory and practice (Gray & Grove, 2021; Melnyk & Fineout-Overholt, 2019). Suggestions for further research help close the feedback loop of the steps of the quantitative research process with wise guidance for generating further research (see Fig. 2.2).

Excerpts from Sosa et al. (2021)'s Discussion section are provided in Research Example 2.10. The excerpts include examples of findings, limitations, conclusions, implications for nursing's body of knowledge, and suggestions for future research.

RESEARCH EXAMPLE 2.10

Discussion

Research/Study Excerpts

Findings

> This attempt to again look at the operation of the theory with the chosen factors revealed that demographics as opposed to external influencing factors, were more influential on physical activity levels in this sample.... Demographic/situational factors having primary influence on physical activity deviates from previous literature. (Sosa et al., 2021, Discussion section)

Limitations

> Despite attempts to recruit a diverse sample through utilizing multiple sites, the convenience sample recruited for this inquiry was largely homogeneous, limiting the generalizability of the results.... Given that the study was a single data collection, patterns of physical activity over time, which are often iterative depending on situation, could not be elicited. (Sosa et al., 2021, Limitations section)

Conclusions

> Because cardiac risk factors are increased in many minority populations and physical activity plays an important role in decreasing cardiovascular disease, it is vital to create a body of research and intervention for all populations of women. The IFSMT has shown great value in acquiring a holistic view of a self-management behavior. (Sosa et al., 2021, Conclusions section)

Implications for Nursing's Body of Knowledge

> Based on [expanded] evidence [from future recommended studies], intervention from the healthcare provider, particularly the nurse can assist patients in self-management through physical activity. (Sosa et al., 2021, Future recommendations section)

Suggestions for Further Research

> Further research should focus on both defining relationships within the phenomenon as well as further developing theoretical relationships in order to improve understanding and care of self-management of physical activity in women. (Sosa et al., 2021, Conclusions section)

RESEARCH/EBP TIP

There are no shortcuts in the research process. Identifying the steps of the research process in a research report helps you evaluate the quality of that study's evidence. The Discussion section provides you with implications for nursing practice and areas for further study that guide the development of EBP.

READING RESEARCH REPORTS

Understanding the steps of the research process and learning new terms related to those steps will assist you in reading research reports. These reports often are difficult for nursing students and practicing nurses to read and to apply the knowledge in practice. Maybe you have had difficulty locating research articles or understanding the content of these articles. We would like to help you overcome some of these barriers and assist you in understanding the research literature by (1) identifying sources that publish research reports, (2) describing the content of a research report, and (3) providing tips for reading the research literature.

Sources of Research Reports

The most common sources for nursing research reports are professional journals. Research reports are the major focus of multiple nursing research journals, which are identified in Chapter 6. Two journals in particular, *Applied Nursing Research* and *Clinical Nursing Research*, focus on communicating research findings to practicing nurses. The journal *Worldviews on Evidence-Based Nursing* focuses on innovative ideas for using evidence to improve patient care globally. Many clinical specialty journals also place a high priority on publishing research findings, such as *Oncology Nursing Forum*, *Journal of Pediatric Nursing*, and *Heart & Lung*. More than 100 nursing journals are published in the United States, and most of them include research articles. Nursing journals can be accessed on the internet and in print through university libraries or a subscription (see Chapter 6).

Content of Research Reports

At this point, you may be overwhelmed by the seeming complexity of a research report. You will find it easier to read and comprehend these reports if you understand each of the component parts. A research report often includes six sections: (1) Abstract, (2) Introduction, (3) Methods, (4) Results, (5) Discussion, and (6) References. Box 2.3 outlines the content covered in each of these sections. A brief description of these sections follows.

Abstract Section

A research report usually begins with an abstract, which is a clear, concise summary of a study. Abstracts range from 100 to 250 words and usually include the study purpose, design, setting, sample size, major results, and conclusions. The American Psychological Association (APA, 2020) has provided guidance for critically appraising abstracts in studies. Researchers hope that their abstracts will convey the findings from their study concisely and capture your attention so that you will read the entire report. Research Example 2.11 is an abstract from the quasi-experimental study by Reaves and Angosta (2021) that is detailed later in this chapter. In this abstract, the problem's significance and a possible solution are stated in the first two sentences. The abstract lacks a clear purpose statement, and the aims expressed are really hypotheses that were tested in the study. The design, methods, results, and conclusion are clearly and concisely presented.

⚡ RESEARCH EXAMPLE 2.11

Abstract

In patients with COPD [chronic obstructive pulmonary disease], distress is significantly prevalent and can have adverse psychological and physiological effects. The Relaxation Response Meditation Technique (RRMT), a technique that elicits the relaxation response, was developed by Dr. Herbert Benson to counter the fight-or-flight response to decrease psychological and physiological effects.

Aim: (1) To assess whether implementing the RRMT decreases anxiety in patients with COPD, (2) to determine whether RRMT reduces the patients' perception of breathlessness, and (3) to investigate whether RRMT improves the physiological responses of patients with COPD.

Design: This quasi-experimental study used a pre- and posttest design. The sample (N = 25) consisted of a single group of patients diagnosed in stages 2 to 4 of COPD at an outpatient pulmonary rehabilitative clinic.

Methods: Inferential statistics were used to determine the psychological and physiological differences pre- and postintervention utilizing the State-Trait Anxiety Inventory, Modified Borg Scale, and BP [blood pressure], HR [heart rate], respiratory rate, and oxygen saturation levels.

Continued

---

⑤ RESEARCH EXAMPLE 2.11—cont'd

Results: Results indicated a significant mean change in anxiety ($p \le 0.001$), perception of dyspnea ($p \le 0.001$), and a decrease in respiratory rate ($p = 0.001$) after implementing the RRMT. There was clinical improvement in systolic and diastolic BPs and HR.

Conclusion: Findings from this study support the inclusion of the RRMT as part of the pulmonary rehabilitative program to assist patients with COPD in adapting to the negative psychological and physiological responses of distress. (Reaves & Angosta, 2021, Abstract)

Introduction Section

The introduction section of a research report identifies the nature and scope of the problem being investigated and provides a case for conducting the study. You should be able to identify the significance of conducting the study and the problem statement. Introduction sections may have a heading called Introduction or Background, or may not have any heading at all. Even without a heading, the Introduction section is identifiable as the very first part of the research report after the abstract. Depending on the type of research report, the literature review and framework may be in separate sections or part of the introduction, but both usually come before the Methods section. The literature review documents the current knowledge of the problem, including what is known and not known, and provides a basis for the study purpose.

A research report should include a framework, but only about half of published studies identify one. The relationships in the framework provide a basis for the formulation of hypotheses to be tested in quasi-experimental and experimental studies. Investigators often end the introduction by identifying the objectives, questions, or hypotheses that they used to direct the study.

Methods Section

The Methods section of a research report describes how the study was conducted and usually includes the study design, sample, setting, intervention (if appropriate), measurement methods, data collection process, and data analysis plan (see Box 2.3). This section of the report needs to be presented in enough detail so that readers can critically appraise the adequacy of the study methodology to produce credible findings.

Results Section

The Results section includes the outcomes of implementing the data analysis plan. The researchers often start this section with a description of the sample, as in their mean age, gender, and marital status. The researchers then identify the statistical analyses conducted to address the purpose or each objective, question, or hypothesis and present the results in tables, figures, and the narrative of the report (see Box 2.3; Grove & Cipher, 2020). Each statistical result is accompanied by its statistical significance, identified by the p value.

Discussion Section

The Discussion section ties together the other sections of the research report and gives them meaning. This section includes the major findings, limitations of the study, conclusions drawn from the findings, implications of the findings for nursing, and suggestions for further research (see Box 2.3).

The conclusions drawn from a research project can be useful in at least three different ways. First, you can implement the intervention tested in a study with your patients to improve their care

BOX 2.3 **MAJOR SECTIONS OF A RESEARCH REPORT**

Introduction
- Statement of the problem, with background and significance
- Statement of the purpose
- Brief literature review
- Identification of the framework
- Identification of the research objectives, questions, or hypotheses (if applicable)

Methods
- Identification of the research design
- Description of the sample and setting
- Description of the intervention (if applicable)
- Description of the methods of measurement
- Discussion of the data collection process
- Data analysis plan

Results
- Description of the data analysis procedures
- Presentation of results in tables, figures, and narrative organized by the purpose(s) and/or objectives, questions, or hypotheses

Discussion
- Discussion of major findings
- Identification of the limitations
- Presentation of conclusions
- Implications of the findings for nursing practice
- Suggestions for further research

and promote a positive health outcome. Second, reading research reports might change your view of a patient situation or provide greater insight into the situation. Finally, studies heighten your awareness of the problems experienced by patients and assist you in assessing and working toward solutions for these problems.

References Section

The Reference section or list includes the studies, theories, and methodology resources that provided a basis for the conduct of the study. The Reference section just includes sources that were cited in the article. Citations within a research report provide only the author and date of publication, with the Reference section providing the full citation (APA, 2020). The full citations allow readers to retrieve sources of interest. These sources provide an opportunity to read about the research problem in greater depth.

▤ RESEARCH/EBP TIP

Knowing the sections of a research report increases your confidence in reading studies and determining evidence for use in practice.

Tips for Reading Research Reports

When you start reading research reports, you may be confused by the new terms and complex information presented. You probably will need to read the report slowly two or three times. You can also use the glossary at the end of this book to review the definitions of unfamiliar terms. We recommend that you read the abstract first and then the Discussion section of the report. This approach will enable you to determine the relevance of the findings to you personally and to your practice. Initially, your focus should be on research reports that you believe can provide relevant information for your practice.

Reading a research report requires the use of a variety of critical thinking skills, such as skimming, comprehending, and analyzing, to facilitate an understanding of the study (Wilkinson, 2012). Skimming a research report involves quickly reviewing the source to gain a broad overview of the content. Try this approach. First, familiarize yourself with the title, and check the author's name. Next, scan the Abstract or Introduction and Discussion sections. Knowing the findings of the study will provide you with a standard for evaluating the rest of the article. Then read the major headings and perhaps one or two sentences under each heading. Finally, reexamine the conclusions and implications for practice from the study. Skimming enables you to make a preliminary judgment about the value of a source and whether to read the report in depth.

Comprehending a research report requires that the entire study be read carefully. During this reading, focus on understanding major concepts and the logical flow of ideas within the study. You may wish to highlight information about the researchers, such as their education, current positions, and any funding they received for the study. As you read the study, steps of the research process might also be highlighted. Record any notes in the margin so that you can easily identify the problem, purpose, framework, major variables, study design, sample, intervention, measurement methods, data collection process, analysis techniques, results, and study findings. Also, record any creative ideas or questions that you have in the margin of the report (see Fig. 2.2).

We encourage you to highlight the parts of the article that you do not understand, and ask your instructor or other nurse researchers for clarification. Your greatest difficulty in reading the research report probably will be in understanding the statistical analyses (see Chapter 11). Basically, you must identify the particular statistics used, results from each statistical analysis, and meaning of the results. Statistical analyses describe variables, examine relationships among variables, and/or determine differences among groups. The study purpose or specific objectives, questions, or hypotheses indicate whether the focus is on description, relationships, or differences (Grove & Cipher, 2020). Therefore you need to link each analysis technique to its results and then to the study purpose or objectives, questions, or hypotheses.

The final reading skill, analyzing a research report, involves determining the value of the report's content. Break the content of the report into parts and examine the parts in depth for accuracy, completeness, uniqueness of information, and organization. Note whether the steps of the research process build logically on each other or whether steps are missing or incomplete. Examine the Discussion section of the report to determine whether the researchers have provided a critical argument for using the study findings in practice.

📄 **RESEARCH/EBP TIP**

Using the skills of skimming, comprehending, and analyzing while reading research reports will increase your comfort with studies, allow you to become an informed consumer of research, and expand your knowledge for making changes in practice.

PRACTICE READING A QUASI-EXPERIMENTAL STUDY

Knowing the sections of the research report—Introduction, Methods, Results, and Discussion (see Box 2.3)—provides a basis for reading research reports of quantitative studies. You can apply the critical thinking skills of skimming, comprehending, and analyzing to your reading of the quasi-experimental study by Reaves and Angosta (2021). The abstract from this study was introduced earlier in Research Example 2.11. The study focused on determining the effects of the Relaxation Response Meditation Technique (RRMT) on anxiety, dyspnea, and physiological responses of patients with chronic obstructive pulmonary disease (COPD). To help enhance your thinking skills for reading research reports, the steps of the research process are illustrated with excerpts from the Reaves and Angosta (2021) study in Research Example 2.12.

Being able to read research reports and identify the steps of the research process (see Fig. 2.2) should enable you to conduct an initial critical appraisal of the report. Throughout this text, you will find boxes, entitled "Critical Appraisal Guidelines," which provide questions that you will want to consider in your appraisal of various research steps. This chapter concludes with an initial critical appraisal of Reaves and Angosta's (2021) study using the guidelines provided as follows (see last section of Research Example 2.12).

⑦ CRITICAL APPRAISAL GUIDELINES

Quantitative Research
The following questions are important in conducting an initial critical appraisal of a quantitative research report:
1. What type of quantitative study was conducted—descriptive, correlational, quasi-experimental, or experimental?
2. Can you identify the following sections in the research report—Abstract, Introduction, Methods, Results, and Discussion—as identified in Box 2.3?
3. Were the steps of the study clearly identified (see Fig. 2.2)?
4. Were any of the steps of the research process missing?

◢ RESEARCH EXAMPLE 2.12

Steps of the Research Process in a Quasi-Experimental Study with Initial Critical Appraisal

Research/Study Excerpts
1. Introduction
Research Problem Statement

> *In patients with COPD, distress is significantly prevalent and can have adverse psychological and physiological effects. (Reaves & Angosta, 2021, Abstract)*

Research Purpose
The research purpose is formulated as study aims (see Research Objectives, Questions, or Hypotheses later in this box).

Review of Relevant Literature

> *The relaxation response [describes] the body's ability to counter the fight-or-flight response to decrease physiological and psychological symptoms of distress, such as HR [heart rate], BP [blood pressure], and*

Continued

◢ RESEARCH EXAMPLE 2.12—cont'd

anxiety...One way to elicit the relaxation response is by practicing the Relaxation Response Meditation Technique [RRMT] (Benson, 2000), a variation of Transcendental Meditation, the process of repeating a mantra to guide oneself to self-awareness and relaxation. (Reaves & Angosta, 2021, Background section)

Study Framework

Reaves and Angosta (2021) did not identify a framework for their study. However, the concept of relaxation was identified as a way to reduce the concepts of physiological and psychological distress in patients with a chronic illness.

Research Objectives, Questions, or Hypotheses

The aims of this study were to: (1) assess whether implementing the RRMT decreases anxiety in patients with COPD, (2) determine whether RRMT reduces the patients' perception of dyspnea, and (3) investigate whether RRMT improves the physiological responses of patients with COPD. (Reaves & Angosta, 2021, Purpose section)

Study Variables

The independent variable (intervention) was the RRMT. The dependent variables (outcomes) were anxiety, dyspnea, and physiological responses (BP, HR, respiratory rate, and oxygen saturation).

2. Methods

Study Design

This study was quasi-experimental with a pre- and posttest design consisting of a single group of patients (N = 25). (Reaves & Angosta, 2021, Methods section)

Population and Sample

A...convenience sample [was recruited] at a single pulmonary rehabilitation clinic...in the Midwest region of the United States. (Reaves & Angosta, 2021, Methods section)

Intervention

The researcher created prerecorded audio instructions written by an Advanced Holistic Nurse Board Certified...practitioner and recorded by the researcher to guide the patient through the RRMT for 10 min. (Reaves & Angosta, 2021, Methods section)

Measurement Methods

- State-Trait Anxiety Inventory (Spielberger et al., 1983) (Anxiety)
- Modified Borg Scale (Kendrick et al., 2000) (Perception of dyspnea)
- BP, HR, respiratory rate, and oxygen saturation (Physiological responses)

Data Collection

Prior to completing the questionnaires, the patient was instructed to rest for a few minutes. The researcher obtained the patient's BP, respiratory rate, HR, and oxygen saturation. After instructions were given on what to expect during the study intervention, the researcher provided an MP4 player and headphones to the patient....After the patient listened to the prerecorded RRMT, the researcher reassessed the [dependent variables]. (Reaves & Angosta, 2021, Methods section)

3. Results

The results of the analysis indicated that implementing the RRMT significantly reduced anxiety, dyspnea, and respiratory rate. Patients scored lower on the [anxiety] questionnaire postintervention...than preintervention...The results also indicated [dyspnea] scores were significantly lower on the post-test...than on the pretest....Finally, patients' respiratory rate measurements were lower after the intervention...than before the intervention...Although there was clinical improvement in systolic BP, diastolic BP, and HR, these findings were not statistically significant (p > .05). (Reaves & Angosta, 2021, Results section)

4. Discussion

Findings

The significant reduction in anxiety after practicing the RRMT is consistent with Mahdavi et al.'s (2013) study. They reported a reduction in anxiety in hemodialysis patients after practicing the RRMT. (Reaves & Angosta, 2021, Discussion section)

Conclusions

The RRMT is a cost-effective intervention that can be used for patients with COPD. It is imperative for patients with COPD to have multiple tools they can deploy when dealing with the unwanted symptoms the disease brings. (Reaves & Angosta, 2021, Conclusion section)

Limitations

The single recruitment site...may not provide a representation of the sample population of patients with COPD. (Reaves & Angosta, 2021, Limitation section)

Implications

Nurses must expand their current plan of care by incorporating cost-effective interventions to reduce the psychological and physiological effects of COPD. (Reaves & Angosta, 2021, Implications and future research section)

Direction of Future Research

These findings cannot be solely linked to the intervention itself unless a replicated study is conducted with the inclusion of a larger sample size and control group at a different setting. (Reaves & Angosta, 2021, Implications and future research section)

Initial Critical Appraisal

Reaves and Angosta (2021) clearly identified their study as quasi-experimental research. However, the gap in the knowledge needed for nursing practice was not identified in the problem statement. All the steps of the research process were included in the research report except for the study framework. When a framework is not identified, the reader usually can figure out the researchers' proposed relationships among the concepts by carefully reading the review of literature. The aims of the study suggested the researchers' central hypothesis: RRMT as an intervention for patients with COPD induces a relaxation response that manifests as reduced anxiety, reduced perceptions of dyspnea, and improved physiological responses. The study took place in a clinical setting with a standardized data collection protocol, which qualifies the setting as partially controlled. A recorded intervention was appropriate for the aims of the study and provided a high level of control in its delivery. The pretest and posttest design with a single group was weak because there was no control group for comparison (Gray & Grove, 2021). To increase confidence in the promising results, the researchers accurately stated that further research on the topic should be conducted with a control group.

KEY POINTS

- Quantitative research is the traditional research approach in nursing; it includes descriptive, correlational, quasi-experimental, and experimental types of studies.
- Basic, or bench, research is a scientific investigation that involves the pursuit of knowledge for knowledge's sake or for the pleasure of learning and finding truth.
- Applied research is a scientific investigation conducted to generate knowledge that will directly influence or improve nursing practice.
- Conducting quantitative research requires rigor and control, which are necessary for confidence in the quality of the results.
- The quantitative research process involves conceptualizing a research project, planning and implementing that project, and communicating the findings.
- Numerous quantitative research designs have been developed, but the steps of the quantitative research process are the same for each design (see Fig. 2.2).
- Typically, the six sections of a research report are (1) Abstract, (2) Introduction, (3) Methods, (4) Results, (5) Discussion, and (6) References.
- Research reports can be read on three levels depending on the depth of the critical thinking skills involved: skimming, comprehending, and analyzing.
- The steps of a quasi-experimental study are identified, followed by an initial critical appraisal of this study.

REFERENCES

American Psychological Association. (2020). *Publication manual of the American Psychological Association* (7th ed.). American Psychological Association.

Atthill, S., Witmer, D., Luctkar-Flude, M., & Tyerman, J. (2021). Exploring the impact of a virtual asynchronous debriefing method after a virtual simulation game to support clinical decision-making. *Clinical Simulation in Nursing, 50*, 10–18. https://doi.org/10.1016/j.ecns.2020.06.008

Bandalos, D. L. (2018). *Measurement theory and applications for the social sciences.* The Guilford Press.

Basic Research. (n.d.). *In glossary of NIH terms.* Retrieved from https://grants.nih.gov/grants/glossary.htm

Benson, H. (2000). *The relaxation response.* Harper Collins Publishers.

Brewer, S. F., Gilder, C. M., & Leahey, T. M. (2021). Obesity treatment in African American churches: Current treatment targets and preferences among parishioners. *Western Journal of Nursing Research, 43*(4), 307–315. https://doi.org/10.1177/0193945920949954

Bonar, J. R. M., Wright, S., Yadrich, D. M., Werkowitch, M., Ridder, L., Spaulding, R., & Smith, C. E. (2020). Maintaining intervention fidelity when using technology delivery across studies. *CIN: Computers, Informatics, Nursing, 38*(8), 393–400. https://doi.10.1097/CIN.0000000000000625

Campbell, D. T., & Stanley, J. C. (1963). *Experimental and quasi-experimental designs for research.* Rand McNally.

Chinn, P. L., & Kramer, M. K. (2018). *Knowledge development in nursing: Theory and process* (10th ed.). Mosby.

Cho, H., Brzozowski, S., Arsenault Knudsen, É. N., & Steege, L. M. (2021). Changes in fatigue levels and sleep measures of hospital nurses during two 12-hour work shifts. *Journal of Nursing Administration, 51*(3), 128–134. https://doi.org/10.1097/NNA.0000000000000983

Creswell, J. W., & Creswell, J. D. (2018). *Research design: Qualitative, quantitative, and mixed methods approaches* (5th ed.). Sage.

Fisher, R. A. (1935). *The designs of experiments.* Hafner.

Gray, J. R., & Grove, S. K. (2021). *The practice of nursing research: Appraisal, synthesis, and generation of evidence* (9th ed.). Elsevier.

Grove, S. K., & Cipher, D. J. (2020). *Statistics for nursing research: A workbook for evidence-based practice* (3rd ed.). Elsevier.

Hammer, M. J., Eckardt, P., Cartwright, F., & Miaskowski, C. (2021). Prescribed walking for glycemic control and symptom management in patients without diabetes undergoing chemotherapy. *Nursing Research, 70*(1), 6–14. https://doi.10.1097/NNR.0000000000000468

Kaplan, A. (1964). *The conduct of inquiry: Methodology for behavioral science.* Chandler.

Karsten, M., Prince, D., Robinson, R., & Stout-Aguilar, J. (2020). Effects of peppermint aromatherapy on postoperative nausea and vomiting. *Journal of PeriAnesthesia Nursing, 35*(6), 615–618. https://doi.org/10.1016/j.jopan.2020.03.018

Kazdin, A. E. (2017). *Research design in clinical psychology* (5th ed.). Pearson.

Kendrick, K. R., Baxi, S. C., & Smith, R. M. (2000). Usefulness of the modified 0-10 Borg scale in assessing the degree of dyspnea in patients with COPD and asthma. *Journal of Emergency Nursing, 26*(3), 216–222. https://doi.10.1067/men.2000.107012

Mahdavi, A., Gorji, M. A. H., Gorji, A. M. H., Yazdani, J., & Ardebil, M. D. (2013). Implementing Benson's relaxation training in hemodialysis patients: Changes in perceived stress, anxiety, and depression. *North American Journal of Medical Sciences, 5*(9), 536–540. https://doi.org/10.4103/1947-2714.118917

Melnyk, B. M., & Fineout-Overholt, E. (2019). *Evidence-based practice in nursing and healthcare: A guide to best practice* (4th ed.). Wolters Kluwer.

Porter, T. M. (2004). *Karl Pearson: The scientific life in a statistical age.* Princeton University Press.

Quality and Safety Education for Nurses (QSEN). (2021). *Pre-licensure knowledge, skills, and attitudes (KSAs).* Retrieved from http://qsen.org/competencies/pre-licensure-ksas/

Reaves, C., & Angosta, A. D. (2021). The relaxation response: Influence on psychological and physiological responses in patients with COPD. *Applied Nursing Research, 57,* 151351. https://doi.org/10.1016/j.apnr.2020.151351

Ryan, P., & Sawin, K. J. (2009). The Individual and Family Self-Management Theory: Background and perspectives on context, process, and outcomes. *Nursing Outlook, 57*(4), 217–225. https://doi.org/10.1016/j.outlook.2008.10.004

Sallis, J. F., Grossman, R. M., Pinski, R. B., Patterson, T. L., & Nader, P. R. (1987). The development of scales to measure social support for diet and exercise behaviors. *Preventive Medicine, 16*(6), 825–836. https://doi.org/10.1016/0091-7435(87)90022-3

Sallis, J. F., Haskell, W. L., Wood, P. D., Fortmann, S. P., Rogers, T., Blair, S. N., & Paffenbarger, R. S., Jr. (1985). Physical activity assessment methodology in the Five-City Project. *American Journal of Epidemiology, 121*(1), 91–106. https://doi.10.1093/oxfordjournals.aje.a113987

Sallis, J. F., Pinski, R. B., Grossman, R. M., Patterson, T. L., & Nader, P. R. (1988). The development of self-efficacy scales for health-related diet and exercise behaviors. *Health Education Research, 3*(3), 283–292. https://doi.org/10.1093/her/3.3.283

Schoenfisch, A. L., Kucera, K. L., Lipscomb, H. J., McIlvaine, J., Becherer, L., James, T., & Avent, S. (2019). Use of assistive devices to lift, transfer, and reposition hospital patients. *Nursing Research, 68*(1), 3–12. https://doi.org/10.1097/NNR.0000000000000325

Sechrist, K. R., Walker, S. N., & Pender, N. J. (1987). Development and psychometric evaluation of the Exercise Benefits/Barriers Scale. *Research in Nursing & Health, 10*(6), 357–365. https://doi.org/10.1002/nur.4770100603

Shadish, W. R., Cook, T. D., & Campbell, D. T. (2002). *Experimental and quasi-experimental designs for generalized causal inference.* Rand McNally.

Sherwood, G., & Barnsteiner, J. (2017). *Quality and safety in nursing: A competency approach to improving outcomes* (2nd ed.). Wiley-Blackwell.

Smith, M. J., & Liehr, P. R. (2018). *Middle range theory for nursing* (4th ed.). Springer.

Sosa, M., Sethares, K. A., & Chin, E. (2021). The impact of demographic and self-management factors on physical activity in women. *Applied Nursing Research, 57,* 151353. https://doi.org/10.1016/j.apnr.2020.151353

Spielberger, C. D., Gorsuch, R. L., Lushene, R. E., Vagg, P. R., & Jacobs, G. A. (1983). *Manual for the state-trait anxiety inventory (STAI) (form Y-1: Self-evaluation questionnaire).* Consulting Psychologists Press.

Straus, S. E., Glasziou, P., Richardson, W. S., & Haynes, R. B. (2019). *Evidence-based medicine: How to practice and teach EBM* (5th ed.). Elsevier.

Vizioli, C., Jaime-Lara, R. B., Franks, A. T., Ortiz, R., & Joseph, P. V. (2021). Untargeted metabolomic approach shows no differences in subcutaneous adipose tissue of diabetic and non-diabetic subjects undergoing bariatric surgery: An exploratory study. *Biological Research for Nursing, 23*(1), 109–118. https://doi.org/10.1177/1099800420942900

Waltz, C. F., Strickland, O. L., & Lenz, E. R. (2017). *Measurement in nursing and health research* (5th ed.). Springer Publishing Company.

Wilkinson, J. M. (2012). *Nursing process and critical thinking* (5th ed.). Pearson.

CHAPTER

3

Introduction to Qualitative Research

Jennifer R. Gray

LEARNING OUTCOMES

After completing this chapter, you should be able to:

1. Identify the steps of the qualitative research process.
2. Describe four qualitative research methodologies—phenomenological research, grounded theory research, ethnography, and exploratory-descriptive qualitative research—and their intended outcomes.
3. Describe methods related to sampling, recruitment, data collection, data analysis, and data interpretation in qualitative studies.
4. Describe strategies used by qualitative researchers to increase the credibility and transferability of their findings.
5. Critically appraise qualitative studies for application to practice.

Qualitative research is a systematic approach used to describe experiences and situations from the perspective of persons in the situation. The researcher analyzes the words of the participant(s), finds meaning in the words, and provides a description of the experience that promotes deeper understanding of the experience (Creswell & Poth, 2018). Because caring about people and wanting to help them are core nursing values, you may find qualitative research valuable for the insights it provides into the lives and circumstances of your patients. Qualitative research can generate rich descriptions of the experiences of patients and families that increase nurses' understanding of the best ways to intervene and be supportive (Meadows-Oliver, 2019). As a result, qualitative findings make a distinct contribution to evidence-based practice (EBP; Gray & Grove, 2021).

This chapter includes the elements of the qualitative research process and presents an overview of four qualitative methodologies commonly conducted in nursing: phenomenological research, grounded theory research, ethnographic research, and exploratory-descriptive qualitative research. An example of a study using each design is included in this chapter. You will also be introduced to some of the more common methods used in qualitative studies, beginning with sampling and recruiting participants. The methods used to collect, analyze, and interpret qualitative data also will be described. This content provides a background for you to use in reading and comprehending published qualitative studies, critically appraising these studies, and applying study findings to your practice.

STEPS IN THE RESEARCH PROCESS FOR QUALITATIVE STUDIES

Qualitative research is conducted in natural settings to learn about a topic from the perspectives of the participants. The researcher's ability to develop rapport and build trust with the participants determines the quality of the data that are collected. The data that are collected, analyzed, and interpreted are textual and experiential data (Creswell & Poth, 2018). Other characteristics of qualitative research include multiple sources of data, emergent methods, and reflexivity. Box 3.1 displays several characteristics of qualitative research. One of the terms in the box may be unfamiliar. Reflexivity is the researcher's acknowledgment of personal biases and experiences that may influence a qualitative study.

The qualitative research process follows the same general steps as the quantitative research process. However, the underlying philosophical values and assumptions of qualitative research are different from those of quantitative research. Because of these differences, some steps of the qualitative research process are different (Table 3.1). In most quantitative studies, researchers seek information about a well-defined problem from a group (sample) to generalize to a larger group (population). Qualitative researchers seek information about a less defined research problem by obtaining multiple individual perspectives of those who are knowledgeable of the problem. By doing this, qualitative researchers strive to develop a deeper understanding of the phenomenon. The steps of the qualitative research process are interconnected, with each one being influenced by the previous step and affecting subsequent steps.

📄 RESEARCH/EBP TIP

Qualitative research explores the perspectives of those who are experiencing the phenomenon being studied. Some steps of the research process are different from the steps of the quantitative research process. The focus of qualitative research is on understanding individuals, social processes, and cultures. In contrast, the focus of quantitative research is on generalizing findings from a sample to the related population.

BOX 3.1 CHARACTERISTICS OF QUALITATIVE RESEARCH

Natural setting
Context dependent
Researcher as instrument
Multiple sources of data
Inductive and deductive analysis
Reflexivity
Focuses on participants' perspective
Emergent and evolving methods
Holistic, complex description

Adapted from Creswell, J., & Poth, C. (2018). *Qualitative inquiry and research design: Choosing among five approaches* (4th ed., p. 45). Sage.

TABLE 3.1 SIMILARITIES AND DIFFERENCES IN THE QUANTITATIVE AND QUALITATIVE RESEARCH PROCESSES

QUANTITATIVE RESEARCH PROCESS	QUALITATIVE RESEARCH PROCESS
1. Identify a Research Problem	
Building on previous knowledge, a gap in knowledge is identified.	Little may be known about the topic; qualitative approach used to explore and describe.
2. Formulate the Research Purpose	
Should be congruent with the research problem.	Should be congruent with the research problem.
3. Identify the Study Methodology	
Selected quantitative methodology should be implied in the purpose.	Selected qualitative methodology should be implied in the purpose.
4. Review the Literature	
Extensive review should be conducted to ensure that questions and/or hypotheses reflect what is known and not known.	Limited review of the literature; extent will vary depending on qualitative design; researcher does not want to be biased by the literature.
5. Describe the Theoretical Framework	
Researcher may or may not make the framework explicit.	Researcher may use a philosophy instead of a framework or may not select a framework to remain open to participants' perspectives.
6. State the Research Objectives, Questions, Hypotheses, and Procedures	
The researcher may use any of these; when possible, she or he will state hypotheses based on what is known. Questions or hypotheses are set before data collection.	Researcher will use research objectives or questions. Hypotheses are not consistent with qualitative methods. Questions may evolve over the course of the study.
7. Develop and Implement the Study Methods	
Define variables, conceptually and operationally.	No comparable step in qualitative research.
Specify procedures consistent with the study design. These may include a controlled setting and an intervention.	Specify how data will be collected (interview, observation, focus groups) in a natural setting; no intervention. Procedures may evolve.
Recruit a large sample of predetermined size.	Use purposive, network, and theoretical sampling methods, the size of which will not be predetermined. Size will depend on when saturation of the data occurs.
Collect numerical data.	Collect textual, verbal, visual, and sensory data.
Analyze data according to predetermined statistical analyses.	Analyze data using flexible and iterative steps of spending extended periods of time reading and processing the data.
Determine results and prepare tables and/or figures.	Determine results, which will vary according to qualitative methodology (e.g., ethnography—a description of a culture; grounded theory—an emerging framework).
8. Present Results	
Concisely state outcomes of statistical analyses. Tables and figures may be used with limited narrative.	Provide a narrative of patterns or themes identified. Participant quotations from interviews or focus groups to support results may be used.
9. Discuss Findings	
Compare findings with previous research findings.	Compare findings with previous research findings.
Identify limitations.	Identify limitations.
State implications of the findings, including future research needed on the topic.	State implications of the findings, including future research needed on the topic.

Research Problem

The research problem is a gap in knowledge. The patient or practice concerns that can best be addressed by qualitative research are those about which very little is known. Even for problems that have been studied, what may be missing is the perspective of those affected. The purpose of qualitative studies should be congruent with the research problem. For example, Lundquist et al. (2019) conducted a phenomenological study of living with advanced breast cancer among 12 young women, aged 25 to 39 years. The research gap was that the literature contained limited studies of the breast cancer experiences of this age group. The study's purpose was to "describe and interpret the lived experiences of young women with advanced breast cancer from their perspective" (Lundquist et al., 2019, p. 330). Three of the women had metastatic disease at the time of diagnosis. From interviews with the women, the researchers extracted the overarching theme of "wearing the mask of wellness in the presence of a life-threatening illness" (Lundquist et al., 2019, p. 332). The women appeared to be like other young women, but they experienced daily life differently, knowing their lives were likely to be cut short. Even clinicians had limited understanding of their experiences. The study demonstrated Creswell and Poth's (2018, p. 52) statement that qualitative research problems are "emotion-laden, close to people, and practical."

Methodology, Literature, and Framework

The next three steps in the qualitative research process—identifying a study's methodology, reviewing the literature, and selecting a theoretical framework—share some similarities to the initial steps of the quantitative research process, but they require modifications (see Table 3.1). Qualitative researchers make decisions about the study methodology early in the process of developing a study. Methodology as a research term can mean the general type of research, such as qualitative research (Gray & Grove, 2021). However, the term also can be applied to the different types of qualitative research, such as phenomenology. When the study purpose is written, the researcher has selected the methodology that allows the research gap to be addressed (Creswell & Creswell, 2018).

Qualitative researchers view the step of reviewing the literature cautiously because they want to remain open to the insider's perspective. As a result, qualitative researchers may review the literature to identify the research problem, but may delay further literature review until after the data are collected. The type and extent of the early literature review may vary, depending on the research design being used (see Chapter 6).

> ### 📄 RESEARCH/EBP TIP
>
> The purpose identifies the focus of the study. It also implies the methodology needed to address the research problem. The methodology of a qualitative study is a general approach within which methods, such as data collection, may evolve during the study as the researcher gains new insights.

Selecting a theoretical framework may or may not occur. For example, in grounded theory studies, the qualitative researcher is seeking to describe the social processes at work in an experience to develop a beginning theory (Kelle, 2019). Researchers using grounded theory methods usually do not select a theoretical framework. In other types of studies, such as exploratory-descriptive qualitative studies and ethnographic studies, researchers may select a theoretical framework to guide the study. Lundquist et al. (2019, p. 330) stated their qualitative study methods were based on a "hermeneutic phenomenologic approach," which indicates the philosophical foundation. They did not, however, specify a theoretical framework, which is typical for phenomenological studies. The literature review was very limited. However, what was reported in the article may not have represented all the literature that the researchers reviewed before the study. Some journals have page limits for articles, and researchers may summarize the literature to have adequate space in the article for the findings.

Research Objectives and Questions

Determining the research objectives, questions, or hypotheses is the next step in the research process. Hypotheses imply using statistical analysis to identify the strength of a relationship or effect of an intervention process, making them incongruent with qualitative research. As a result, qualitative researchers may use objectives or questions to provide direction to the collection of the data (Creswell & Poth, 2018). Lundquist et al. (2019) did not identify objectives or questions, which is common in qualitative studies. Their methods were guided by the study's purpose statement and philosophical approach.

Sampling

Qualitative and quantitative research differ a great deal in the methods, results, and discussion of the results. The sampling step in the research process occurs in both quantitative and qualitative studies, but the characteristics of a quality sample for each type of research are different. Ideally, quantitative researchers can recruit a large random sample so that the findings can be generalized to the target population. By conducting a power analysis, the researchers can determine the minimum sample size for a quantitative study (see Chapter 9). Because qualitative researchers want to understand the identified research problem from the perspective of the participants, they deliberately recruit fewer participants but ensure that each one has experience with the research topic or culture. Sample size may vary according to the study's qualitative method. Phenomenological studies may need 10 or fewer participants if the topic is narrow and the participants provide adequate data (Creswell & Poth, 2018). Grounded theory studies may require more than 30 participants to ensure that adequate detail is available to develop the emerging theory (Hennink et al., 2019).

Typically, sampling occurs until saturation is reached (Creswell & Poth, 2018), defined as when additional participants or data sources do not provide new information. Each participant provides rich data that allows the researcher to identify the participants' perspective and meaning of the phenomenon. Marcil et al. (2020) conducted 26 interviews for their grounded theory study with mothers of children who were younger than 5 years. The purpose of the study was to develop a conceptual theory of financial strain to "inform clinical care and research" (Marcil et al., 2020, p. 582). The researchers conducted interviews "until we achieved thematic saturation" (Marcil et al., 2020, p. 583).

Data Collection and Analysis

Quantitative and qualitative researchers collect different types of data. The data collected by quantitative researchers for each variable will be numerical; in contrast, qualitative researchers collect data in the form of text and images, so identifying variables and defining them are inappropriate (see Table 3.1). The data collection methods should be consistent with the research problem and study purpose. The data collection methods may evolve as the study progresses. In a supplement to the published study report, Marcil et al. (2020) provided a list of all interview questions and probes used, noting that no participant was asked all the listed questions. "We removed questions when thematic saturation was reached (i.e., interviews yielded repetitive information for multiple participants). We added questions to explore new themes that emerged" (Marcil et al., p. 583).

RESEARCH/EBP TIP

Samples for qualitative studies are usually smaller than samples for quantitative studies. The number of participants is determined by when data saturation is achieved.

Data analysis occurs in both quantitative and qualitative studies. For quantitative studies, the numerical data are analyzed using formulas and statistical equations calculated by a computer program. The analysis of qualitative data is nonstatistical, meaning that hypotheses are not tested in qualitative studies. In qualitative studies, the researcher's mind is the "program" that analyzes the data, notices patterns, identifies themes, and allows the meaning of the data to emerge. The researcher's mind inductively finds common elements and then thinks deductively, going back to the data to find more evidence to support the common element (Creswell & Poth, 2018). A software program specific to qualitative research may be used during the data analysis process to keep a record of themes that the researcher finds and the decisions made during the study. In the study conducted by Marcil et al. (2020, p. 584), the researchers inductively analyzed the "interviews using the constant comparative approach to develop a theoretical model for the effects of financial strain on women with young children." Their description of data analysis included discussing and organizing "emerging categories and themes to capture key aspects of participants' experiences with financial strain" (Marcil et al., 2020, p. 585).

Results and Interpretation

For both types of research, the results of the study are presented in the research report. The presentation of quantitative results will be numbers and statistical outcomes, often displayed in tables and figures. The qualitative results are presented as rich descriptions, themes, or an emerging theory. For qualitative studies, the results section may be very long because the researcher presents a theme and supports the theme with one or more quotations from the participants (see Table 3.1).

RESEARCH/EBP TIP

Results sections of qualitative research reports may be long because the themes or categories are supported by quotations from participants or examples of a theme found in the textual data.

During the step of interpreting the findings, the researchers compare what they found with what others have previously published (see Table 3.1). Lundquist et al. (2019, p. 334) found that young women with advanced breast cancer wore a "mask of wellness," which they compared with the "mask of aging" metaphor found in a study with older adults conducted by Rozario and Derienzis (2009). Like the older adults, the women with breast cancer experienced a "disconnection between how they feel and how they appear" (Lundquist et al., 2019, p. 334).

Limitations and Implications

Quantitative and qualitative researchers identify study limitations and then discuss whether the findings can be generalized or applied to other groups. Generalizability is a desired outcome for quantitative studies when the sample is representative of the target populations. Applicability of the findings to similar individuals or transferability is the desired outcome for qualitative studies. The researchers also make recommendations for practice, when appropriate, and for future studies. The recommendations for future studies may include studies that would be designed to overcome the current study's limitations, expand the sample to other groups, or refine the data collected. Lundquist et al. (2019, p. 335) indicated that the findings of their grounded theory study with young women with advanced breast cancer could "provide strategies for clinical and advanced practice nurses that can be implemented easily." The researchers recommended additional studies to better understand the "multidimensional coping process for this population" (Lundquist et al., 2019, p. 336). Refer to Table 3.1 to review the differences and similarities between quantitative and qualitative research.

To conclude this section and introduce the next, there are two additional qualitative research terms that may be helpful. Phenomena are the conscious awareness of experiences that comprise the lives of humans (Gray & Grove, 2021). An experience is considered unique to the individual, time, and context. Qualitative researchers seek to describe the "subjective" and "meaning making at the center of social life" (Miles et al., 2020, p. 5). Qualitative researchers recognize that we experience life from different perspectives because our thoughts, words, and actions are influenced by the past and present, as well as by the physical, psychological, and social contexts of our behaviors and experiences. The findings from a qualitative study lead to an understanding of a phenomenon in a specific situation and are not generalized in the same way as the findings of a quantitative study. The goal of qualitative researchers is to ensure and document that the identified meanings and themes represent the perspectives of the participants accurately. To achieve that goal, qualitative researchers document the processes they used to remain open to the perspectives of the participants and to reach the study's conclusions.

Each of the four qualitative methodologies included in this chapter is based on a philosophical or discipline orientation that influences the interpretation of the data. For each methodology, whether phenomenology, grounded theory, ethnography, or exploratory-descriptive qualitative research, it is critical to understand the philosophy on which the method is based. Each approach is discussed in relation to its philosophical orientation and intended outcome. Fig. 3.1 provides a display of each qualitative design with its philosophical orientation (yellow arrows), types of

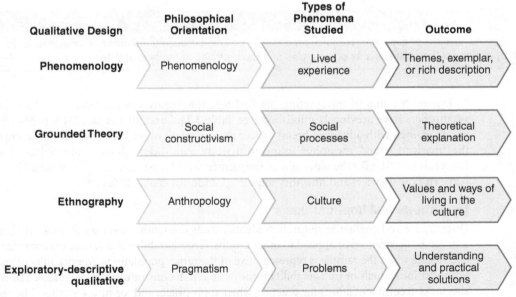

Qualitative Design	Philosophical Orientation	Types of Phenomena Studied	Outcome
Phenomenology	Phenomenology	Lived experience	Themes, exemplar, or rich description
Grounded Theory	Social constructivism	Social processes	Theoretical explanation
Ethnography	Anthropology	Culture	Values and ways of living in the culture
Exploratory-descriptive qualitative	Pragmatism	Problems	Understanding and practical solutions

FIG. 3.1 Comparing Qualitative Research Designs.

phenomena studied with this design (orange arrows), and the intended outcome (blue arrows). A study is provided to illustrate each methodology. Deciding which qualitative methodology to use depends on the research question and purpose of the study (Creswell & Poth, 2018). Each of the studies will be critically appraised using the following guidelines for identifying and understanding the qualitative methodology.

? CRITICAL APPRAISAL GUIDELINES

Qualitative Studies

1. What qualitative methodology was implemented: phenomenology, grounded theory, ethnography, or exploratory-descriptive qualitative research?
2. Was the outcome of the study as presented in the research report appropriate for the methodology?
   a. Phenomenology—rich description of lived experience
   b. Grounded theory—theoretical description of social processes
   c. Ethnography—description of a culture, whether race/ethnic or an organization
   d. Exploratory-descriptive qualitative research—problem-solving answer to the research question
3. Were the following sections clear, concise, and complete in the research report: Introduction, Methods, Results, and Discussion?
4. Were the steps of the study clearly identified? Table 3.1 identifies the steps of the qualitative research process.
5. Were any of the steps of the research process missing?
6. Did the researchers discuss the relevance of the study findings for practice?

PHENOMENOLOGICAL METHODOLOGY

Philosophical Orientation

Phenomenology refers to both a philosophy and a methodology congruent with the philosophy that guides the study of experiences or phenomena (see Fig. 3.1) (Fernandez, 2020). Phenomenologists view the person as integrated with the environment. The world shapes the person, and the person shapes the world. The broad research question that phenomenologists ask is, "What is this lived experience like?" (van Manen, 2017, p. 776). Through a phenomenological study, the researcher collects data from persons who have had the experience and seeks to create a composite of the essence of experience (Ranse et al., 2020). Two of the early phenomenologists, Husserl and Heidegger, had slightly different philosophies. Each of these philosophical perspectives supports a specific type of phenomenological research.

Husserl's focus was on the phenomenon itself. The aim of the research is to "bring into light the essence of a thing by setting aside presupposition and prejudice" (Ranse et al., 2020, p. 946). The meaning-laden statements are analyzed to discover the structure within the phenomenon. Husserl's philosophy supports descriptive phenomenological research, whose purpose is to describe experiences as they are lived or, in phenomenological terms, to capture the "lived experience" of study participants. To describe lived experiences, according to Husserl, researchers must bracket or set aside their own biases and preconceptions to describe the phenomenon as reported by the participants (Ranse et al., 2020).

Heidegger argued that it was impossible to set aside one's preconceptions and understand the world without being influenced by one's own experiences. He believed that phenomenological researchers describe how participants have interpreted or given meaning to their experiences.

Interpretative phenomenological research, consistent with Heidegger's philosophy, involves analyzing the data and presenting a rich word picture of the phenomenon, as interpreted by the participants and the researcher. The researcher's own experiences or viewpoint on the experience being studied influences the final product (Ranse et al., 2020).

📄 RESEARCH/EBP TIP

Nursing qualitative researchers use several types of phenomenological approaches to research. The main types are Husserl's descriptive approach (bracketing) and Heidegger's interpretative approach (no bracketing).

Hermeneutics is one type of interpretative phenomenological research that is congruent with Heidegger's philosophical perspective and is being used by nurse researchers (Meadows-Oliver, 2019). Hermeneutics involves textual analysis that begins with reading the texts. Texts may include journals written by participants, transcripts of interviews and focus groups, and all types of documents, such as online discussions, letters, or books. To read a text, the researcher consciously remains open to the specific participant's social, cultural, and historical position, as well as geographical location. The perspectives of hermeneutic researchers are also shaped by their unique positions in society, culture, history, and geography. Reading and analyzing texts hermeneutically requires moving from the more abstract interpretation across texts to the individual specifics of one text and then back to the overall interpretation (Ranse et al., 2020). From these readings and rereadings, the researcher identifies subthemes and themes that are examined considering the study's research questions. As the text, themes, and relevant literature are integrated, a description of the phenomenon as interpreted is produced.

Intended Outcome

The purpose of phenomenological research is to provide a thorough description of a lived experience. Some researchers write a detailed rich description or an exemplar of the experience. Other researchers who conduct phenomenological studies will describe themes that together provide a picture of the lived experience. To provide quality care, nurses need to understand the experiences of patients and how healthcare treatments and conditions may affect their well-being. Shaban et al. (2020) were concerned about the needs of persons who were isolated for suspected or confirmed infection with the novel coronavirus, commonly known as COVID-19. They initiated the research because no studies had been conducted about the experiences of the patients. The data were collected through interviews with the first 11 patients in Australia isolated for COVID-19. Excerpts of the study are provided in Research Example 3.1. Following the study excerpts, the study will be critically appraised.

🔏 RESEARCH EXAMPLE 3.1

Phenomenological Study

Research/Study Excerpt
Methods

An interpretive phenomenological approach using the core elements of Heideggerian hermeneutical perspective was employed. ... This approach enabled us to understand the totality of participants' lived experience through a blend of meanings and understandings articulated between them and the investigators.
(Shaban et al., 2020, p. 1446)

RESEARCH EXAMPLE 3.1—cont'd

Interviews were conducted at the bedside and went for between 15 and 45 minutes. ...All interviews were conducted by the lead investigator...To gain an overall understanding of the data, transcripts were read, and audio files of interviews were listened to. Summaries of each transcript were drafted. ...Identified themes and patterns in data were verified through discussion, and transcripts were re-read to link relationships and overlaps between themes. ...Generating thick descriptions of the participants' lived experience in this setting...afforded transferability to other contexts or settings. ...[T]he investigators examined the relationship between their individual conceptual lenses, assumptions, values and preconceptions, and the research. (Shaban et al., 2020, p. 1446)

Findings

There were eleven participants (4 females and 7 males) aged 27-61 years in the study....Five themes encapsulated the lived experiences and perceptions of the COVID-19 patients in the designated isolation facility in New South Wales, Australia.

Theme 1: "Knowing about COVID-19"

The participants' lived experience of COVID-19 was anchored to commercial news and other similar media forums. They had made considerable efforts to obtain up-to-date information from different sources.

Theme 2: "Planning for a response to COVID-19"

Self-isolation and home-quarantining were practiced by some participants before admission to hospital as they considered them to be effective measures to ensure the health and safety of their close contacts (e.g., family members). (Shaban et al., 2020, p. 1446–1447)

Theme 3: "Being infected"

The feeling of being diagnosed with laboratory-confirmed COVID-19 resulted in anxiety, shock, and doubt, and was described by participants as being surreal": ...[A]ll 11 participants indicated that they, for the most part, had mild and nonspecific symptoms, such as cough, low-grade fever, and body pain. (Shaban et al., 2020, p. 1448)

Theme 4: "Life in isolation, and the room"

For some of the participants, isolation and quarantine practices were positive experiences...for others, their lived experiences of being under source isolation brought a range of negative emotions and effects due to a lack of social interactions, losing the track of time, and being physically isolated with limited mobility. (Shaban et al., 2020, p. 1448–1449)

Theme 5: "Post-discharge life"

All participants anticipated making a full recovery from COVID-19 and expressed this experience as life post-discharge....Their experience resulted in them wanting to make changes to their lifestyles to boost overall health and improve the immune system. Many expressed a concern about remaining infective or re-infection in relation to post-discharge life. (Shaban et al., 2020, p. 1449)

Discussion

Source isolation and quarantine measures are instruments for outbreak management and disease control...Notwithstanding this there are negative and unintended psychological consequences of isolation such as anxiety, depression, and aggression which are well documented in the existing literature. ...Some of the practical ways to minimize the negative and unintended consequences of isolation include provision of sufficient physical space to walk around, allowing more activities, and having large windows to enable the participants to connect to spaces outside their room. (Shaban et al., 2020, p. 1449)

Continued

> **RESEARCH EXAMPLE 3.1—cont'd**
>
> *The Heideggerian hermeneutical perspective employed in this study led to a holistic understanding of the COVID-19 patients in the context of isolation...Developing and implementing models of care for COVID-19 and other high-consequence infectious diseases requires that the negative and unintended consequences of isolation be minimized. ...[T]he study study does have limitations. Interviews were conducted with participants during their hospitalization, and it was not possible to follow-up with them post discharge to conduct member-checking. ...We also acknowledge that participants' cultural background and their sociocultural context influences their experiences, and further sociocultural research should examine this. (Shaban et al., 2020, p. 1449–1450)*
>
> **Critical Appraisal**
>
> Shaban et al. (2020, p. 1446) identified their study as being "an interpretive phenomenological approach using the core elements of Heideggerian hermeneutical perspective." The outcome of the study was a robust description of the lived experience of being isolated because of COVID-19 infection early in the epidemic. The methods and outcomes were consistent with phenomenology.
>
> The first section of the research report had no heading but provided the history of the epidemic, the importance of isolation for public health, and the infectious disease precautions. The first steps of the research process, the research problem and study purpose, were clearly identified (Shaban et al., 2020). The purpose of the study included the phrase "the lived experience." This phrase implies that phenomenology is the study design. Other than the study purpose, the study had no other objectives or research questions. The cited literature supported the background and significance of the study, but was limited. A limited literature review is typical for phenomenological studies. No theoretical framework was identified, but the philosophical approach was Heideggerian phenomenology.
>
> The Methods section included interviews as the primary tool used to collect data from the isolated patients diagnosed with COVID-19 infection. Purposive sampling was used to recruit the participants: the first 11 patients isolated for COVID-19 at the researchers' hospital. Reaching saturation was not mentioned, rather the researchers recruited all isolated patients with COVID-19 during a specified time frame. The researchers used team-based analysis and described the methods used to ensure rigor of the study.
>
> Instead of Results, the next section was labeled as Findings. The identified themes were supported by quotations from the participants' interviews. The Discussion section compared the study findings with prior studies with persons in isolation for other infectious diseases. The researchers also identified possible clinical interventions to minimize the negative effects of isolation and recommendations for future studies. They ended the research report with the strength of having a multidisciplinary team and the limitations of the study. None of the steps of the research process were missing. The research conducted by Shaban et al. (2020) is an example of a quality phenomenological study on a relevant clinical topic.

GROUNDED THEORY METHODOLOGY

Philosophical Orientation

Grounded theory research is an inductive technique that emerged from the discipline of sociology. The term *grounded* means the theory was developed from the research; in other words, the theory is grounded in the real world based on data provided by participants. The philosophy of social constructivism provides a foundation for grounded theory. Social constructivism as a philosophy posits that our beliefs and actions are based on our perceived reality, a shared reality that has been constructed through our interactions with individuals and groups (Creswell & Poth, 2018) (Fig. 3.1). These interactions occur between family members, friends, coworkers, organizations, and communities in the context of our place and time in history. In social life, meanings are developed and shared by groups and are communicated to new members through socialization processes. Group life is based on consensus and shared meanings. Interaction may lead to redefining a meaning or constructing new meanings. "Social constructivism contends that knowledge is sustained by social processes" and as a result, groups act and interact based on what they know (Young & Collin, 2004, p. 376). The grounded theory researcher seeks to understand the interaction between self and group from the perspective of those involved and, from that understanding, develop a theory of interactions or social processes (Creswell & Poth, 2018).

Grounded theory has been used most frequently to study areas in which little previous research has been conducted and to gain a new viewpoint in familiar areas of research. Through their interviews to understand the perspectives of persons who were dying, Glaser and Strauss (1967) developed grounded theory research as a method and published a book describing it as a qualitative method. Nurse researchers use grounded theory methods to study a wide range of topics, such as night-shift nurses driving home drowsy (Smith et al., 2020), experiences of homeless veterans in emergency departments (Weber et al., 2020), the effect of financial strain on parenting and mental health of mothers (Marcil et al., 2020), and experiences of parents whose chronically ill children are attending school (Nieto-Eugenio et al., 2020).

Intended Outcome

Fully developed grounded theory studies result in theoretical frameworks with relational statements between concepts. Some grounded theorists provide a diagram displaying the interactions among the social processes that were identified. Others describe the concepts and relationships through a narrative description.

📄 RESEARCH/EBP TIP

Within the philosophy of social constructivism, grounded theory studies examine the interactions among individuals sharing an experience. The goal is to develop a theoretical explanation of the social processes occurring within the experience.

Southby et al. (2019, p. 1) conducted a grounded theory study of "women's experiences of expecting a baby aged 35 years or older." The researchers identified a gap in the knowledge needed by midwives and obstetrical nurses to provide care for this group of mothers. Research Example 3.2 is a description of their study. Fig. 3.2 depicts the model of the emerging theory that was provided by the researchers. After the excerpts from the article, the study will be critically appraised.

📊 RESEARCH EXAMPLE 3.2

Grounded Theory Study

Research/Study Excerpt
Introduction

The average age at which women are having their first baby is rising . . . Cooke et al. (2010) noted a lack of literature seeking to understand pregnancy at AMA [advanced maternal age] from the woman's perspective. . . . Therefore, the purpose of this study is to deepen our understanding of women's experiences of expecting a first baby aged 35 years or more. (Southby et al., 2019, pp. 1–2)

Theoretical Framework

Grounded theory was considered to be an ideal methodology to identify key processes relating to how older first-time mothers experience pregnancy and prepare for childbirth. (Southby et al., 2019, p. 2)

Continued

RESEARCH EXAMPLE 3.2—cont'd

Setting

Interviews took place in the participants' home... Women were made aware of the study by their maternity care professional and by posters displayed in clinic waiting areas.

Recruitment

Recruitment ceased when no new categories emerged and it was considered that theoretical saturation had been reached.

Data Collection and Data Analysis

Data analysis and data collection were simultaneous and data analysis commenced with first participant's interview....Each participant engaged in one in-depth interview, lasting approximately one hour....[T]he [i]nterviews were audio recorded and transcribed. ...Techniques adopted for data analysis were: summarising during the interview, listening and re-listening during transcribing, memo writing, line by line coding and focused coding. Constant comparison of the data...eventually resulted in the development of a core category and subsequent theory generation. (Southby et al., 2019, p. 2–3)

Results

The sample consisted of 15 nulliparous women, whose ages ranged from 35 to 44 years. Participants were white, generally highly educated, had diverse careers and had attended antenatal classes. The majority of women were in relationships and had a planned pregnancy.

Figure 3.2 illustrates the results of the data analysis. 'It's now or never' is the core category underpinning the interpretive theory of the experience of expecting a first baby after the age of 35 years. Three theoretical categories; 'becoming ready', 'dealing with anxieties' and 'decision making' were formulated from seven theoretical codes...

Our theory is that women's awareness that their age can limit future opportunities to have another baby can affect key aspects of the pregnancy experience, including feelings of readiness to have a baby, perception of risk and decision-making regarding care options. This concept appeared to be more apparent in the participants nearing or beyond the age of forty and for those who had undergone assisted conceptions. (Southby et al., 2019, p. 3–4)

Discussion

Analysis of the core category, "it's now or never" has generated a theoretical understanding that the journey to becoming a mother may be different for women of AMA. ...This theory can help to explain key aspects of the pregnancy experience, including feelings of readiness to have a baby, perception of risk and decision-making regarding care choices. (Southby et al., 2019, p. 6)

Strengths and Limitations

A strength of this study is the development of a theory induced from the voices of the participants. ...A limitation of the study was that it took place in one part of the UK [United Kingdom] and voices from women of diverse ethnicities were not represented. (Southby et al., 2019, p. 7)

Conclusions

Further research is now needed to test the applicability of this theory with a larger group of women of AMA in their first pregnancy prior to changes in practice being recommended. ...Health professionals can play an important role in helping women to feel supported in their pregnancy by understanding and acknowledging issues that are important to women of AMA. (Southby et al., 2019, p. 7)

Critical Appraisal

Southby et al. (2019) stated the methodology of the study was grounded theory. A theory was developed, complete with a model displaying concepts and relationships among them. This is the expected outcome of a grounded theory.

RESEARCH EXAMPLE 3.2—cont'd

The sections of the research report were clearly identified. The Introduction section included information about the significance of pregnancy among women of AMA and some of the medical complications that may occur. The literature was cited to support facts about pregnancy in mothers older than 35 years, including previous research findings about medical risks and AMA mothers' concerns. The researchers appropriately identified the limitations of the available literature to support the need for the current study. The beginning steps of the research process, identifying the research problem and formulating the study purpose, were stated clearly. The study was guided by the purpose and did not include objectives or questions.

The study's design was identified in the section titled Theoretical Framework, which is unusual but consistent with the desired outcome. The theoretical framework was identified as constructivist grounded theory, which was a specific philosophical approach to the qualitative methods the researchers used. The data were collected in participant homes of 15 women recruited from a maternity clinic. Two interviews were conducted with each woman to provide increased depth on the codes and categories that emerged from the initial data analysis. The analysis process was supported with quotations from the participants for each theoretical code. Recruitment continued until the researchers achieve theoretical saturation. Data included text from the interview transcripts, as well as answers to a demographic questionnaire. The researchers described the methods with adequate detail to allow readers to critically appraise the rigor of the study methods.

The Results section contained the typical content. Tables were used to provide a sample description and categories related to interview questions. In addition to the narrative, the researchers developed an interpretive theory (see Fig. 3.2) with the concepts of "Decision Making," "Becoming Ready," and "Dealing with Anxieties" (Southby et al., 2019, p. 4). The core category was identified as "It's Now or Never."

In a section titled Discussion, the researchers compared the findings with previous research findings. They identified a strength of the study to be the methods used to ensure and document rigor. Limitations included a sample from one region that was not diverse. The participants were also well educated and interviewed only during pregnancy.

The report's final section was Conclusions. The conclusions were consistent with the findings and recognized the need for additional research to explore the experiences of AMA mothers of other countries and ethnicities. No step of the research process was omitted.

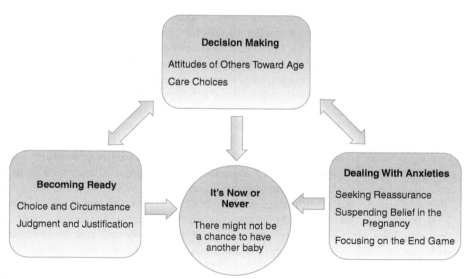

FIG. 3.2 Core category and theoretical categories with theoretical codes.(From Southby, C., Cooke, A., & Lavender, T. [2019]. 'It's now or never'—nulliparous women's experience of pregnancy at advanced maternal age: A grounded theory study. *Midwifery*, 68[1], 1–8.)

ETHNOGRAPHIC METHODOLOGY

Philosophical Orientation

Ethnographic research was developed by anthropologists as a method to study how cultures develop and are maintained over time (Newman & Newman, 2020). Through immersion in the culture, anthropologists study a group of people who share a culture and their origins, past ways of living, and ways of surviving through time (Creswell & Poth, 2018). The term *ethnography* can also be applied to the product of the investigation, the written description of the study of the culture (Erickson, 2018). Early ethnography researchers studied primitive, foreign, or remote cultures. Such studies enabled the researcher who spent a year or longer in another culture to acquire new perspectives about a specific people, including their ways of living, believing, and adapting to changing environmental circumstances. This reflects the emic approach of studying behaviors from within the culture that recognizes the uniqueness of the individual (Leininger, 1985). The emic view from inside the culture is the typical goal of ethnography but may be alternated with the etic approach. The etic approach is to view the culture as a naive outsider and analyze its elements as a researcher. Both viewpoints are helpful in conducting an ethnography. Broadly speaking, ethnography is "an approach that seeks to find meanings of cultural phenomena by getting close to the experience of these phenomena" (Markham, 2018, p. 653).

The philosophical perspective of ethnographic research is based in anthropology and recognizes that culture is material and nonmaterial (Fig. 3.1). Material culture consists of all created or constructed aspects of culture, such as buildings used for cultural events, symbols of the culture, family traditions, networks of social relations, and the beliefs reflected in social and political institutions. Symbolic meaning, social customs, and beliefs—components of the nonmaterial culture—may be apparent in a different culture only over time, but they are essential elements of cultures. Cultures also have ideals that people hold as desirable, even though they do not always live up to these standards. Anthropologists and nurse ethnographers seek to discover the multiple parts of a culture and determine how these parts are interrelated. An overall picture of the culture becomes clearer.

Nurses may not observe a culture over months or years, but may observe an organizational culture repeatedly for shorter spans of time to explore and examine the relationships, status, interactions, and symbols within a smaller social unit (Butcon & Chan, 2017). This type of study is called a focused ethnography. Observations shorter than months or years are appropriate when the research question is narrower, and the scope of the study is limited to a specific place or organization. Even a focused ethnography is a time-intensive research method.

The nurse who increased the visibility of ethnography in nursing was Madeline Leininger, a nurse who earned her doctoral degree in anthropology (Fawcett & McFarland, 2012). The 2 years of fieldwork for her degree were spent in Papua New Guinea (Miller, 2019). From this experience, she developed the Sunshine Model of Transcultural Nursing Care, which identifies aspects of culture to consider when communicating with patients and families of another culture (Leininger, 1988). Nurses use Leininger's theory of transcultural nursing (Leininger, 2002) in practice by assessing multiple aspects of the patient, family, and their environment, including religion, societal norms, economic status, country of origin, ethnic subgroup, and beliefs about illness and healing. This theory has led to an ethnographic research strategy for nursing, termed ethnonursing research. Ethnonursing research "focuses mainly on observing and documenting interactions with people [and] how these daily life conditions and patterns are influencing human care, health, and nursing care practices" (Leininger, 1985, p. 238). However, several nurse anthropologists not associated with the ethnonursing orientation are also providing important contributions to nursing's body of knowledge using ethnographic methods.

The ethnographic researcher must become a student of the culture by observing it, actively participating in it, and interviewing members of the culture. Even for focused ethnographies, the researcher must become immersed in the culture being studied. Being immersed involves being in the culture for an extended time. This allows the researcher to become increasing familiar with aspects of the culture, such as language, sociocultural norms, traditions, and other social dimensions. Social dimensions may include family relationships, communication patterns (verbal and nonverbal), religion and its role, division of work, and expressions of emotion. Through immersion, the ethnographic researcher becomes increasingly accepted into the culture. Although ethnographic researchers must be actively involved in the culture they are studying, they must avoid going native, which would interfere with data collection and analysis. In going native, the researcher becomes a part of the culture and loses her or his ability to observe clearly (Creswell & Poth, 2018).

📄 RESEARCH/EBP TIP

Ethnography began within the discipline of anthropology. The ethnographer spends time immersed in the culture being studied, either for a prolonged time or for shorter but multiple times. Ethnographers are observant and inquisitive about the values, traditions, and reasons supporting the participants' behaviors.

Intended Outcome

The ethnographer prepares a written report based on the analysis of the culture. Traditional ethnographies are often book length and exceed what can be published in a professional journal. Focused ethnographies are more likely to be published in a nursing journal. Another type of ethnography used by nurses that also has a narrower focus is critical ethnography. Critical ethnography is a method that focuses on the socioecological and political factors within a culture. Laging et al. (2018) conducted a critical ethnography of the reasons staff may not recognize deterioration of residents in nursing homes. They cited the RNs' lack of autonomy in making decisions, financial pressure to avoid unnecessary hospital transfers, and limited education of personal care assistants. Ethnographic studies may provide information to develop a health intervention that is culturally acceptable, incorporate health promotion behaviors into routine life activities, and improve the quality of care that is being delivered in an organization.

Hassankhani et al. (2020) conducted a focused ethnography of mothers being involved in painful procedures of their stable infants in a neonatal intensive care unit (NICU). The setting was in a referral hospital in Iran (Research Example 3.3). The excerpts from the research report are provided along with a critical appraisal.

🔍 RESEARCH EXAMPLE 3.3

Ethnographic Study

Background

There is still little information about the experiences of mothers and nurses in regards to maternal presence. Awareness and understanding of the experiences of mothers and nurses could help establish a protocol regarding the participation of mothers in managing infant pain during painful procedures. This study explored the experiences of Iranian mothers and nurses with regard to mothers' role during painful procedures. (Hassankhani et al., 2020, p. 340–341)

Continued

⚡ RESEARCH EXAMPLE 3.3—cont'd

Methods

Fieldwork involved field notes, informal and formal individual interviews. ... During observations, 70 cases of painful procedures were observed. To clarify ambiguities during observations, informal discussion occurred, allowing questions to be asked about observed events and interactions. ... All participants gave written informed consent. Face-to-face in-depth interviews were also conducted by the PI [primary investigator]. ... All interviews were transcribed verbatim. Roper and Shapira's (2000) framework for analyzing data was used. ... In order to increase the credibility of the study, both fieldwork and interviews were used, with analysis conducted concurrently. (Hassankhani et al., 2020, p. 341)

Results

From the data collected, three main themes emerged. . . .

Theme 1 – determining maternal presence at painful procedures, as assessed by the mother and nurses

Prior to beginning the procedure, neonatal nurses indicated that they conducted an assessment before making a decision regarding the mother's presence and possible involvement. One of the main criteria in their decision-making was the view of the procedure by mother. (Hassankhani et al., 2020, p. 341)

Theme 2 – negative impacts of the maternal role

A number of participants recalled an outpouring of maternal emotion and distress during the procedure that could affect both the mother and the nursing staff.

Theme 3 – positive impacts of a maternal role

Participants discussed this influence in three ways – positive impacts on the mother's wellbeing, positive impacts on the neonate's wellbeing, and the mother as an aide to nurses. (Hassankhani et al., 2020, p. 342)

Discussion

The likelihood of nurses supporting and promoting maternal inclusion tended towards excluding parents unless the parent was considered able to witness pain and not disturb clinical staff during the procedure. Mothers likewise varied in their need to be included during procedures and their likelihood of acquiescing to directions by clinical staff to leave. This contrasts with other research that has suggested that parent empowerment through communication, inclusion and shared decision-making are paramount. ... The results of the present study showed that the majority of mothers preferred to be present during procedures. Part of this preference was grounded in the belief that their presence was beneficial to the baby. ... Nurses have a key role to play in motivating mothers to strengthen their confidence to attend painful procedures. (Hassankhani et al., 2020, p. 342–343)

Limitations

This study is not without limitations. Whilst focused on the experiences of nurses and mothers in Iran, it did not consider the cultural context or its possible influence upon the findings. (Hassankhani et al., 2020, p. 343)

Critical Appraisal

Hassankhani et al. (2020) identified their qualitative method to be focused ethnography. The outcome of the study was a description of the culture of selected NICUs with stable infants. Because fathers were able to visit only 1 hour per day, the study focused on mothers and their interactions with nurses related to painful procedures.

The research report included a section titled Background, instead of Introduction (Hassankhani et al., 2020). The section included the importance of family-centered care, the necessity of painful procedures in the NICU,

RESEARCH EXAMPLE 3.3—cont'd

and characteristics of NICUs in Iran. The statement of the research problem was "little information about the experiences of mothers and nurses in regards to maternal presence" (Hassankhani et al., 2020, p. 340). The study purpose was stated after the research problem, but no research questions or objectives were identified. The purpose had two phrases, exploring the "experiences of Iranian mothers and nurses with regard to mothers' role during painful procedures" and "whether this role" affected "neonatal as well as parental stress" (Hassankhani et al., 2020, p. 340).

The Methods section was divided into additional headings for relevant steps of the research process. The setting was a NICU in a children's referral hospital in northwest Iran. Although the infants were in an NICU, their condition was stable. The data collection methods were fieldwork, observation, informal conversations, and formal unstructured interviews. During 200 hours of observation, 70 painful procedures were observed. The mothers and nurses who provided data were informed about the study and consented to participate. Data were analyzed following specific steps identified by Roper and Shapiro (2000). The initial work of analysis was completed by the primary researcher with ongoing discussion among team members.

The Results section was organized by the three themes identified by the researchers during data analysis. Each theme was described with ample support from mothers' and nurses' quotations. The Discussion section contained several comparisons of the findings with findings of other studies. The literature review of the study was incorporated into the discussion of the findings. The limitations of the study were presented in a separate section. The steps of the research process were identified with the exceptions of identifying the theoretical framework or philosophy and stating the implications for future research. Despite these omissions, the study conducted by Hassankhani et al. (2020) is an example of a credible focused ethnography.

EXPLORATORY-DESCRIPTIVE QUALITATIVE METHODOLOGY

Some reports of qualitative studies do not include mention of a specific design or approach, such as phenomenology or grounded theory. The researchers may have described their studies as being naturalistic inquiry, descriptive, or just qualitative. Usually, the researchers are exploring a new topic or describing a situation, so we have chosen to label these studies as exploratory-descriptive qualitative research (Gray & Grove, 2021). Studies consistent with this approach are not a specific type of research; rather, they are studies conducted for a specific purpose that do not fit into another of the qualitative research categories (Sandelowski, 2000, 2010).

Philosophical Orientation

Exploratory-descriptive qualitative studies are developed to provide information and insight into clinical or practice problems. Researchers design exploratory-descriptive qualitative studies to obtain information needed to understand patients' and families' perspectives, evaluate a program, or develop an intervention for a specific group of patients. The philosophical orientation of exploratory-descriptive qualitative research may vary, depending on the purpose of the study. A pragmatic philosophy is an approach that supports researchers in search of useful information and practical solutions (Fig. 3.1; Creswell & Poth, 2018).

Intended Outcome

A well-designed, exploratory-descriptive qualitative study answers the research question. The purpose of the study is achieved, and the researchers have the information that they need to address the situation or patient concern that was the focus of the study. The findings of the study are applied to the practice problem that instigated the inquiry.

📄 RESEARCH/EBP TIP

Exploratory-descriptive qualitative designs are appropriate when a problem or situation can be better understood and potentially resolved if the patients' perspectives are known. For example, if a clinic had a high proportion of no-shows, an exploratory-descriptive qualitative study could help clinicians understand participants' barriers to keeping appointments.

Successfully reducing hospitalizations of patients with heart failure (HF) is dependent on the patient's adherence to self-care behaviors that change the patient's diet and level of physical activity and affects multiple decisions about taking medications (Myers et al., 2020). Research Example 3.4 provides information about the study and a critical appraisal of the study's strengths and weaknesses.

⚡ RESEARCH EXAMPLE 3.4

Exploratory-Descriptive Qualitative Study

Research/Study Excerpt
Introduction

Although much work has been done to identify mechanisms and test interventions to improve self-care, HF self-care interventions are inconsistently successful...The primary guiding framework for this study was the Health Belief Model (HBM)...[W]e also used the Situation Specific Theory of HF Self-Care to guide our interpretations of the study results. ....[T]he objective of this study was to explore perceptions and motivations of individuals with HF who had transitioned from self-care non-adherence to self-care adherence. (Myers et al., 2020, p. 817–818)

Methods
Study Design and Sampling

A qualitative descriptive approach was used to explore participants' transitions from self-care non-adherence to self-care adherence. This study was approved by the center's institutional review board, and all participants gave written informed consent. A purposive sample of eight participants was recruited from the outpatient cardiology clinics of an academic medical center. (Myers et al., 2020, p. 818)

Data Collection

Individuals who provided consent participated in face-to-face, 60-minute audio-recorded interviews and provided socio-demographic data using a brief questionnaire....Follow-up questions sought participant perspectives about factors that contributed to their understanding of HF, ways to care for themselves, and their description of factors that make their HF symptoms better or worse. We also included questions about their fears, hope, control over their HF, any sense of discouragement, and the support they received. (Myers et al., 2020, p. 818)

Data Analysis

All interviews were transcribed verbatim and verified for accuracy. ....In the first round of analysis, the primary author reviewed each line of the transcripts to identify key words and phrases reflecting ways participants spoke about their transition...We documented our reactions and initial thoughts about the data in memos and referred to the memos during the following stages of analysis. ...The primary author...met with other members of the study team...to review raw data, coding practices and coding definitions/rules, and interpretations of findings. (Myers et al., 2020, p. 818)

RESEARCH EXAMPLE 3.4—cont'd

Results

During the screening process, all participants were identified by their provider as being non-adherent to most of the HF self-care recommendations and making behavior changes to become adherent. ... The findings from this study of transition from non-adherence to adherence reflect five key themes: 1) mortality, 2) optimism and hope, 3) making connections between behavior and health, 4) self-efficacy, and (5) role of the clinician.

Mortality

All participants made references to their death or thinking they were going to die.... Many participants spoke about their mortality as a motivating factor to change their health behaviors....

The Importance of Optimism and Hope

While all participants referenced their mortality, they also described feeling optimistic—an overall general positive state of mind or view of the future. ...

Making Connections Between Behaviors and Health

Three categories of connections were identified, with connections between: 1) adherence to treatment/self-care recommendations and their HF status (i.e., becoming better or worse); 2) adherence to treatment/self-care recommendations and their active symptoms; and 3) their active symptoms and their HF status.

Self-Efficacy

All participants described having some degree of control, knowledge or ability to manage their health, and success in making behavior change in relation to self-care recommendations.

Role of the Clinician

Across narratives, all participants discussed the influence of a clinician (physicians, nurses and dietitians), in relation to one or more of our identified themes. (Myers et al., 2020, pp. 819–820)

Discussion

Many of the components identified in our study are comparable to those seen in the Health Belief Model. ... There are also aspects of our study's findings that have clear parallels with the Situation-Specific Theory of HF Self-Care (Riegel et al., 2016)... [M]aking connections is an essential part of the interplay between knowledge and experience that underlies the naturalistic decision-making process. ... The qualitative design and sampling approach limit the generalizability of the findings. ... Another limitation is that recruitment relied on provider perceptions of behavior change, rather than objective measures. ... A follow up prospective longitudinal study with a larger sample size is warranted to examine the benefit of integrating these components into an educational intervention for HF. (Myers et al., 2020, p. 821–822).

Conclusions

The role of the clinician was a crosscutting theme, suggesting that the clinician may have importance in promoting a shift from non-adherence to adherence. Overall, our findings add new dimensions to our current understanding of HF self-care literature and theories, and provide important new directions for self-care interventions and research. (Myers et al., 2020, p. 822)

Critical Appraisal

The exploratory-descriptive qualitative study provided the expected outcome of useful information to modify patient care. The Introduction section contained the significance of the connections between self-care and HF

Continued

RESEARCH EXAMPLE 3.4—cont'd

outcomes. Myers et al. (2020) cited studies of self-care among patients with HF and concluded the findings were inconsistent. The researchers also identified two theoretical models that guided the interview questions and data analysis. Despite the research and theory related to HF self-care, a gap in knowledge existed about why persons with HF may transition from nonadherent to adherent with self-care behaviors. The purpose was clearly linked to the problem and stated at the end of the Introduction section.

The Methods section was divided with headings, such as Study Design and Sampling. The researchers detailed their procedures, including a paragraph on trustworthiness in which Myers et al. (2020) identified the steps they took to ensure the study's rigor.

The Results section began with a description of the sample's demographic characteristics, disease characteristics, and functional status. Each of five themes was supported with multiple quotations from the participants. Myers et al. (2020) also provided a figure displaying the components of each theme. Another figure was included showing the interconnectedness of the role of the clinician with the other themes.

In the Discussion section, Myers et al. (2020) linked the themes to the theoretical models and the findings of published studies. The limitations were also identified in this section. The researchers acknowledged that their sample did not included persons with HF who also had dementia, low health literacy, language barriers, and substance abuse. Despite the study being described as a pilot study, the researchers provided detailed clinical implications of the findings to their setting. They noted that their findings had been supported by other study findings as well. Myers et al. (2020) recommended a prospective longitudinal study with a larger sample as the next step to extend the findings.

Myers et al. (2020) delineated all the steps of the research process. Although the sample was small, even for a qualitative study, the researchers met their goal of learning how to motivate and support nonadherent patients with HF toward self-care behaviors.

SAMPLING

The methods used in conducting qualitative studies are different from the methods used in quantitative studies and are described in subsequent sections. The methods used to ensure rigor in qualitative research are explored also. Each aspect of the methods will include guidelines for critically appraising that aspect of the study.

Individuals in qualitative studies are referred to as participants because the researcher and participants carry out the study cooperatively. Sampling in qualitative research is purposeful. The researcher seeks participants for a study because of their knowledge, experience, or views related to the study (Moser & Korstjens, 2018). Additional sampling methods, such as network and theoretical, are used based on the focus of the study (see Chapter 9). For some studies, recruiting participants who are heterogeneous provides a wider range of experiences (Knechel, 2019). Heterogeneous samples, in which participants have different characteristics, are used frequently for grounded theory studies to support the development of a theory (Creswell & Poth, 2018). For other studies, participants may have similar characteristics (a homogeneous sample) because the central focus of the study is the phenomena (see Chapter 9 for more information on sampling).

RESEARCHER–PARTICIPANT RELATIONSHIPS

One of the important differences between quantitative and qualitative research lies in the degree of involvement of the researcher with the participants of the study. This involvement, considered to be a source of bias in quantitative research, is thought by qualitative researchers to be a critical element of the research process. The researcher–participant relationship has an impact on the collection, analysis, and interpretation of data, in fact, the entire qualitative research process (Denzin & Lincoln, 2018). The researcher creates a respectful relationship with each participant, which includes being honest and open about the purpose and methods of the study. The researcher's aims and means of achieving the aims need to be negotiated with the participants and honor their perspectives and values (Creswell & Poth, 2018; Gray & Grove, 2021). In various degrees, the researcher influences the people being studied and, in turn, is influenced by them. Without the support and confidence of participants, the researcher cannot complete the research. Skills in empathy and intuition may need to be cultivated, because the researcher must become closely involved in the participant's experience to interpret the data. Researchers must be aware of their own perceptions and be aware of the perceptions of the participants, rather than attach their own meaning to the experience.

📄 RESEARCH/EBP TIP

The researcher's relationship with participants in qualitative studies requires empathy and emotional awareness. The relationship is interactive and intertwined.

Researcher–participant relationships in qualitative studies may be brief when data collection occurs once in an interview or a focus group. Phenomenology and grounded theory studies may involve one or two interviews, although researcher–participant relationships may extend over time when the study design involves repeated interviews to study a lived experience or a process over time.

Ethnographic studies require special attention to the researcher–participant relationship. The ethnographic researcher observes behavior, communication, and patterns within groups in specific cultures. The researcher may form close bonds with participants who are key informants, persons with extensive knowledge and influence in a culture. The relationships between the researcher and participants can become complex, especially in ethnography studies in which the researcher lives for an extended time in the culture being studied.

❓ CRITICAL APPRAISAL GUIDELINES

Sampling and the Researcher–Participant Relationship

1. Did the researchers identify the specific type of sampling that was used, such as purposive, network, convenience, or theoretical sampling?
2. Were the participants' characteristics and life experiences appropriate to the qualitative approach?
3. Was the number of participants adequate to fulfill the purpose of the study?
4. Were the length and depth of the researcher–participant relationships in the study appropriate to the study approach and purpose?

In the grounded theory study conducted by Southby et al. (2019) with mothers of advanced maternal age (older than 35 years), the researchers conducted two phases of the study. This study was discussed previously in the chapter in greater detail (see Research Example 3.2). In Research Example 3.5, you will see that the researchers used different types of sampling in each phase. The maximum variation sampling meant the researcher recruited mothers with a wide range of characteristics and experiences. The theoretical sampling used in Phase Two meant the researcher sought mothers to expand on specific aspects of or add to the emerging theory.

RESEARCH EXAMPLE 3.5

Sampling and Researcher–Participant Relationship

Research/Study Excerpt

In Phase One, a purposive, maximum variation sample was sought in order to gain a broad spectrum of views and identify an emergent theory which could then be tested using a theoretical sample (Phase Two).... The author was not known to any of the participants prior to involvement in the study. (Southby et al., 2019, p. 2)

Nulliparous women aged 35 years or more, who were experiencing a straight-forward, singleton pregnancy were eligible to participate.... Recruitment ceased when no new categories emerged and it was considered that theoretical saturation had been reached.... Each participant engaged in one in-depth interview, lasting approximately one hour. (Southby et al., 2019, p. 2)

Critical Appraisal

Southby et al. (2019) identified that they used maximum variation sampling during Phase One of their study. When they realized that only two of the initial seven participants were older than 40 years, they specifically recruited more older mothers in the second phase. Phase Two mothers were asked questions based on the categories that emerged from the analysis of Phase One data. The researchers identified that they used theoretical sampling in Phase Two. Both types of sampling are purposeful or purposive.

Southby et al. (2019) recruited women with whom they could fulfill the study purpose without causing undue stress on potentially vulnerable mothers. They recruited women into the study until theoretical saturation was used. The PI conducted the interviews and specified that she was unknown to the participants before the study, indicating a short-term relationship with the mothers. The short relationship was not identified as a limitation and did not interfere with meeting the study objectives.

DATA COLLECTION

The data in most qualitative research studies are text and images collected through "observations, interviews, document, media, and artifacts" (Miles et al., 2020, p. 7). Creswell and Poth (2018) noted that the use of audiovisual data and media is growing. Media encompasses photographs, recordings, and artifacts. Artifacts are objects made by people that have meaning within a culture. We will discuss the data collection methods in the following order: (1) interviewing participants, (2) conducting focus groups, (3) observing participants and activities, and (4) examining documents and media materials. These methods, as they are used in qualitative studies, are described in the following sections in some detail; examples from the literature are provided. Guidelines for critically appraising each type of qualitative data collection are provided, along with a brief critical appraisal of that method.

Interviews

Differences exist between interviews conducted for a qualitative study and those conducted for a quantitative study. In quantitative studies, the researcher structures interviews to collect participants' responses to questionnaires or surveys (see Chapter 10). Interviews range from structured interviews on one end of a continuum to unstructured interviews on the other end (Fig. 3.3) (Brinkmann, 2018). Structured interviews have a prepared set of questions and answers. For example, the researcher may ask participants to rate their relationship with the provider on a scale of 1 to 10. The responses from structured interviews are often converted to numbers for statistical analysis (see Chapter 9 for more on structured interviews). Most qualitative interviews are less structured and are called semistructured interviews. Semistructured interviews are those for

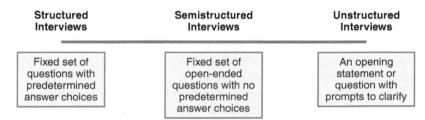

Structured Interviews	Semistructured Interviews	Unstructured Interviews
Fixed set of questions with predetermined answer choices	Fixed set of open-ended questions with no predetermined answer choices	An opening statement or question with prompts to clarify

FIG. 3.3 Continuum of Interview Structure.

which the researcher has prepared a set of questions. The interviews will have some similarities, but the responses will vary according to the participants' perspectives (Fig. 3.3). The interviewer can adjust the questions or ask clarifying questions. Unstructured interviews, also called open-ended interviews, are those for which the researcher may have only an initial question or statement to start the interview, such as "Tell me about a time that you received bad news about a diagnostic test," or "After your diagnosis, how did you learn about diabetes?" Although the researcher defines the focus of the interview, the participant's responses will lead to additional questions or probes. The questions or probes addressed in interviews tend to change as the researcher gains insights from previous interviews and observations. Probes are queries made by the researcher to obtain more information from the participant about a specific interview question. Data from semistructured and unstructured interviews are analyzed as text.

The researcher's goal is to obtain an authentic insight into the participant's experiences (Creswell & Poth, 2018). Although data may be collected in a single interview, dialogue between researcher and participant may continue at intervals across weeks or months and provide rich data for analysis. A researcher may design a study in which each participant is interviewed two times. During the second interview, the researcher may share a summary of the results of the initial analysis for the participant to either refute or validate, a process called member checking. Member checking is when the researcher provides the participant with the interview transcript or results of the data to review. Member checking increases the rigor of the study by ensuring that the researcher understood what the participant was saying.

📄 RESEARCH/EBP TIP

The implementation of interviews may vary depending on the qualitative study's design. Some researchers use a single interview to collect data, whereas others may choose to interview the same participant more than once. Most interviews are audio recorded. The recording is transcribed to provide a written record of the interview.

Other researchers plan multiple interviews to study a process that is evolving over time. For example, a researcher could interview participants 1 month, 3 months, 6 months, and 1 year after a significant loss. The researcher–participant relationship has time to develop as they discuss the grieving process. As the relationship develops and trust grows, the participant may reveal the emotional and value-laden aspects of the process more freely.

The purpose of the interview may vary, depending on the type of qualitative approach. Interviews in a phenomenology study may have one main question, with follow-up questions used as needed to elicit the participant's perspective on the phenomenon. Interviews in grounded theory studies are similar in that only one or two questions may be asked, but the follow-up questions will focus on the social processes of the phenomenon. Interviewing in ethnography studies may be used to obtain information and explanations about aspects of the culture that the researcher has witnessed. In an exploratory-descriptive qualitative study, the interviewer may ask more structured questions to achieve the purpose of the study.

Some strategies used to record information from interviews include writing notes during the interview, writing detailed notes immediately after the interview, and recording the interview. Video may be recorded, as well as audio. In their exploratory-descriptive qualitative study among persons with HF that was discussed previously in Research Example 3.4, Myers et al. (2020, p. 818) collected data using "60-minute audio-recorded interviews."

Ideally, the location for an interview is distraction-free (Creswell & Poth, 2018) and a place where both the researcher and the participant feel safe. Meeting in a clinic, for example, may not be appropriate if the interview involves describing the care being received. A person living with an infection caused by the human immunodeficiency virus may not want to be interviewed in a place where he or she may be seen by friends or family. You also want a place that is quiet enough to allow for effective audio recording. For the study conducted by Myers et al. (2020, p. 818), the interviews were conducted in "private exam rooms in the clinic or in patients' homes." Shaban et al. (2020, p. 1446) conducted the interviews with patients who had COVID-19 and were isolated "at the bedside" (see Research Example 3.1).

? CRITICAL APPRAISAL GUIDELINES

Interviews

1. Do the interview questions address concerns expressed in the research problem?
2. Are the interview questions relevant for the research purpose and objectives or questions?
3. Were the interviews adequate in length and number to address the research purpose or answer the research question?

Lundquist et al. (2019) conducted a phenomenological study among young women with advanced breast cancer that was previously cited to illustrate the steps of the research process. Excerpts from the study will be provided and then critically appraised (Research Example 3.6). Box 3.2 contains some of the interview questions used by the researchers.

BOX 3.2　INTERVIEW QUESTIONS POSED TO YOUNG WOMEN WITH ADVANCED BREAST CANCER

- What has living with the knowledge that you have advanced breast cancer been like for you?
- What is your daily life like?
- What has changed for you in relation to how you experience your ability to do things, your sense of time, your health, and your relationships?
- Can you tell me what the experience of living with breast cancer is like for you?
- How has this affected you from the perspective of your day-to-day life?
- What is a typical day like for you?
- Does how you feel physically restrict you from doing the things you want to do?
- Are you able to do everything you want to do? If not, why?

List of interview questions are from Lundquist, D., Berry, D., Boltz, M., DeSanto-Madeya, S., & Grace, P. (2019). Wearing the mask of wellness: The experience of young women living with advanced breast cancer. *Oncology Nursing Forum*, *46*(3), 329–337 (p. 331, Figure 1).

◢ RESEARCH EXAMPLE 3.6

Research/Study Excerpt

Although women may have common and shared experiences of living with advanced breast cancer, these experiences can be specific to their age, life stage, and familial responsibilities. According to the limited research available, younger women with advanced breast cancer face unique challenges in their daily lives...(Lundquist et al., 2019, p. 330)

The intent was to conduct two interviews two to six weeks apart; however, not all participants were able to complete the second interview for various reasons, including worsening symptoms. ...The first interview focused on exploring daily life experiences. The second interview drew on insights from the initial interview and focused primarily on additional elaborating on experiential or circumstantial changes related to living with advanced breast cancer. A third interview was conducted two to six months after the second encounter to validate findings with participants (member checking). ...Interviews were digitally audio recorded, and professionally transcribed. ...All interviews took place via telephone, Skype, or FaceTime based on participant preference. ...Participants were asked various questions regarding their experience of living with advanced breast cancer, and probes were used, as needed, to gain more detail, clarifications, or example. (Lundquist et al., 2019, p. 330–331)

Critical Appraisal

Lundquist et al. (2019) designed their longitudinal phenomenology study to describe the lived experience of advanced breast cancer from the perspective of young women. The statement of the research problem indicated the lack of knowledge about daily life of this unique sample. The interview questions elicited information about different aspects of daily life and how breast cancer had changed their lives. The questions addressed the research problem and study purpose. By conducting multiple interviews over a longer time, the researchers were able to gather adequate data to address the study purpose.

Focus Groups

Focus groups were designed to obtain the participants' perceptions of a specific topic in a permissive and nonthreatening setting. Focus groups were given the name because the interaction was around a narrow topic, a focused discussion (Guerrero & Xicola, 2018). One of the assumptions underlying the use of focus groups is that group dynamics can help people express and clarify their views in ways that are less likely to occur in a one-to-one interview (Morgan, 2019). The group may give a sense of safety in numbers to those wary of researchers or those who are anxious. Researchers may select this method to generate more information for a lower cost and in less time.

Focus groups are conducted by a moderator, who may or may not be the researcher. The moderator is the person who will identify the ground rules of the focus group, ask preselected questions, and guide the discussion. For focus groups to be effective, the moderator may have similar characteristics as the desired participants, such as race/ethnicity and socioeconomic class. An example would be the urban researcher who hires a health professional who grew up in a rural farming community to moderate a focus group on preventing agricultural injuries. Moderators or focus group leaders should be thoroughly trained in nonthreatening communication, understand the study's purpose, and be able to balance staying on the topic and responding to spontaneous comments related to the topic (Guerrero & Xicola, 2018).

The logistics of implementing a focus group include selecting a location or online meeting software, identifying a desired length of the interaction, and determining the composition and size of the group. Natural settings are ideal for focus groups if outside noise and interruptions can be prevented. Whenever possible, the researcher should visit the room or location in advance to ensure that the participants' confidentiality can be maintained. When an online group meeting software, such as Google Meet or Zoom, will be used, the researcher may want to have a person responsible for the technical aspects of the meeting. Convening a group meeting online has the advantage of increasing convenience for more participants and the researcher without the expense and time involved in travel (Oates & Alevizou, 2019).

Confidentiality and comfort may result in richer dialogue and data. Most researchers recommend that focus groups last 1 to 2 hours; however, convening the group and obtaining informed consent will take a portion of that time. Inclusion and exclusion criteria should be determined for group members, as you would do for any study (see Chapter 9). The recommended size of a focus group ranges from 4 to 12 participants (Morgan, 2019; Oates & Alevizou, 2019). Larger focus groups are sometimes used but may be more difficult to moderate. Because larger focus groups have more voices to hear, transcribing the recording can be challenging. All participants should have the opportunity to speak. The entire interaction is audio recorded and, in some cases, video recorded (Guerrero & Xicola, 2018). In addition to the recordings, members of the research team may serve as observers and take notes during the meeting.

Focus groups are used frequently to understand a clinical phenomenon, develop measurement methods, such as questionnaires or checklists, and evaluate the feasibility and acceptability of an intervention. Agitation is a common behavior seen in mental health settings. Tucker et al. (2020) conducted focus groups with nurses to identify how they recognized agitation in patients and strategies for responding. Correa et al. (2020) wanted to understand how and when screening for intimate partner violence was implemented. Seventeen female survivors participated in one of three focus groups to help health professionals improve intimate partner violence screening. The women reported not being screened or not being effectively screened when they encountered healthcare personnel, and they made suggestions of how screening could be implemented compassionately and effectively.

? CRITICAL APPRAISAL GUIDELINES

Focus Groups

1. Were the size, composition, and length of the focus group adequate to promote group interaction and to produce robust data?
2. Were the questions used during the focus group relevant to the study's research purpose and objectives or questions (Gray & Grove, 2021)?

Research Example 3.7 is a study conducted by Jiwani et al. (2021) to evaluate the acceptability of a behavioral health intervention developed for older adults with type 2 diabetes (T2D). The physical activity outcome of the intervention was tracked with a wearable device (Fitbit). After an excerpt from the research report, the use of focus groups will be appraised.

◢ RESEARCH EXAMPLE 3.7

Focus Groups

Research/Study Excerpt

Introduction

The Look AHEAD (Action for Health in Diabetes) study…tested a behavioral lifestyle intervention of weight loss and physical activity in overweight/obese adults with T2D….However, the effectiveness of behavioral lifestyle

---

RESEARCH EXAMPLE 3.7—cont'd

programs in community-dwelling overweight/obese older adults with T2D is inconclusive or uncertain. (Jiwani et al., 2021, p. 57–58)

Methods

This modified behavioral lifestyle intervention lasted 6 months. ...After completion, participants took part in focus group interviews about their experiences. ...These interviews lasted 30-60 min in length. The study's PI facilitated the focus group discussions using a semi-structured interview guide. Each of the focus group interviews was transcribed verbatim by a research assistant or by using NVivo version 1.1 transcription software...Focus groups were conducted via WebEx for groups 2, 3, and 4. Group 1 participated in an in-person focus group at their final study visit, before COVID-19 restrictions. (Jiwani et al., 2021, p. 58)

Results

Analysis of the focus group discussions...revealed six themes: 1) The Impact of COVID-19 on Behavioral Interventions and Program Acceptability; 2) Participant Logistics of Adherence with the Goal of Diabetes Management; 3) Impact of Technology (Fitbit) on Behavioral Intervention; 4) Perceptions of Program Participation on Quality of Life; 5) Impact of Intervention and Future Plans, and 6) Challenges and/or Resistance During the Program. ...These results demonstrate our participants' acceptability to the lifestyle changes encouraged by the program and how they responded to and integrated behavior changes into their lives. (Jiwani et al., 2021, p. 59)

Critical Appraisal

The 18 participants in the mixed methods study were interviewed in three focus groups, which kept the groups small enough for adequate interaction among the participants. The focus groups were long enough to collect the data needed to address the study's purpose. Focus groups were appropriately used by Jiwani et al. (2021) to collect data about the acceptability and feasibility of the behavior change intervention. Preferably all groups would have been conducted either face-to-face or using Web-based meeting software. However, the use of two modalities of interaction allowed the researchers to complete the study despite the intrusion of the COVID-19 pandemic.

Observation

Observation is a fundamental method of gathering data for qualitative studies, especially ethnography studies (Miles et al., 2020). The aim is to gather first-hand information in a naturally occurring situation. The researcher assumes the role of a learner to answer the question, "What is going on here?" The activities being observed may be automatic or routine for the participants, who may be unaware of some of their actions. The researcher seeks instances of the phenomenon being studied or the focus of the study, notices people and objects in the environment, and listens for what is said and unsaid. The researcher focuses on the details, including discrete events and the process of activities. Unexpected events occurring during routine activities may be significant and are carefully noted. As in any observation process, the qualitative researcher will attend to some aspects of the situation while disregarding others, depending on the focus of the study.

The researcher also needs to determine the observer role that will allow the research purpose and question to be addressed. The observer role is on a continuum from being a complete observer to being a complete participant (Fig. 3.4; Creswell & Poth, 2018). A good example of being a complete observer would be collecting data from a video recording of the events unfolding. The complete participant is when the researcher is fully engaged in the events, spending time after the observation reflecting on what happened. More often, the observer role is a mixture of participant and observer as shown in the middle of the continuum (see Fig. 3.4). The roles of observer and participant may switch back and forth during the time spent in observation.

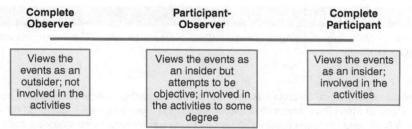

FIG. 3.4 Continuum of Researcher Involvement During Observation.

In studies that use observation, notes taken during or shortly after observations are called field notes. Waiting until the observation is over allows the researcher to focus entirely on the observational experience to avoid missing something meaningful, but that may result in not all pertinent data being recorded. You may want to create a checklist or an outline of key events you want to capture. Another useful strategy is to videotape the events, so that careful observations and detailed notes can be written later. From a human rights perspective, however, the actors must have given consent to be in a study and be aware that video recordings are being made.

The critical appraisal guidelines for observation are based on determining whether the data collected were adequate to address the study purpose. After the guidelines, an excerpt will be provided from a study of mothers' involvement in painful procedures of neonates. This study implemented by Hassankhani et al. (2020) in a NICU setting was described as an example of a focused ethnography (see Research Example 3.8).

CRITICAL APPRAISAL GUIDELINES

Observation

1. Did the researcher provide details about how much time was spent in observation, including at what times of the day, on which days of the week, and the cumulative amount of time spent?
2. Did the researcher describe how notes were made about the observations, such as were notes made during the observation or after the observation?
3. Were the observations of adequate length and implemented across days and times to provide rich data related to the study purpose?

RESEARCH EXAMPLE 3.8

Observation

Research/Study Excerpt

Fieldwork involved field notes, informal and formal individual interviews. …The principal investigator (PI), spent 200 h at different times, on different days and places on the ward, observing interactions between nurses and mothers over a period of 7 months (January to July 2017). During observations, 70 cases of painful procedures were observed. To clarify ambiguities during observations, informal discussion occurred, allowing questions to be asked about observed events and interactions as well as nurses and mothers engaging in spontaneous conversations with the PI. All participants gave written informed consent. (Hassankhani et al., 2020, p. 341)

Critical Appraisal

Hassankhani et al. (2020) supported the rigor of their methods by specifying that the observations occurred at different times of day on different days of the week. The cumulative length of 200 hours was achieved over 7 months. The specific events of interest, painful procedures, were observed 70 times. The PI noted that she made field notes and clarified what she observed through informal conversations. The observations were more than adequate to collect rich data and thoroughly describe mothers' involvement in painful procedures in the NICU.

Examination of Documents and Media

In qualitative studies, existing documents can be considered a rich source of textual data. The researcher may analyze the online comments made previously in a discussion group.

Other texts may be created for a study. For example, the researcher may ask participants to write an essay or journal entries about a topic related to the study's purpose. These written narratives may be solicited by mail or e-mail rather than in person. Text provided by participants may be a component of a larger study using a variety of sources of data.

Media may be photographs or recordings that researchers make during observations or online communication. Photovoice, a specific use of media in qualitative studies, involves participants taking photographs related to the research topic as a source of data. Researchers involved in studies to promote civic and environmental activism use photovoice more frequently than nurse researchers use this method of data collection.

CRITICAL APPRAISAL GUIDELINES

Examining Documents and Media as Data

1. Were the documents or media materials created specifically for the study?
2. For materials not created for the study, were their authenticity and authorship confirmed?
3. Were the human rights of any persons participating in the study or identified in the documents or media protected by informed consent? When possible, were identified persons assured that confidentiality was maintained?
4. Were the data from these sources used to address the study purpose or answer the research question in a meaningful way?

A therapeutic milieu is considered a desirable environment for mental health treatment. Theories and a few prior studies have documented that a therapeutic milieu protects the autonomy of patients. Grech et al. (2020) conducted a qualitative study that used annual evaluation documents of a mental health rehabilitation facility as the major source of data. The facility provided respite care in addition to residential and nonresidential care. Research Example 3.9 describes the document analysis in this study.

RESEARCH EXAMPLE 3.9

Examination of Documents and Media

Research/Study Excerpt

The...considerations have led to the formulation of the following research question: What are the perceptions of mental health service users on the therapeutic milieu in a rehabilitation unit?...Since previous research has prompted that quantitative measures might not fully capture a comprehensive understanding

Continued

> **RESEARCH EXAMPLE 3.9—cont'd**
>
> *of therapeutic milieu…its evaluations holds promise for the much needed delineations of what constitutes milieu therapy in international literature.* (Grech et al., 2020, p. 1020)
>
> *The documents included in this study consisted of annual evaluation reports issued by a mental health reha-bilitation unit within the community….The inclusion criterion for the data collection was that the documents must be service user evaluation reports compiled by the mental health organisation participating in the study within the past 10 years with regards to the rehabilitation unit under study….Permission for the study was sought from the organization which provided the documents for analysis. It was ensured that no respondent names appeared in the documents under study and any personal data which may have posed a threat to anonymity were not included in the study report….The documents were only available as a hard copy and so manual thematic analysis had to be used. This process was carried out independently by two researchers in order to enhance the coding accuracy and overall trustworthiness of the study.* (Grech et al., 2020, p. 1021)
>
> *The emergent conceptualisation of therapeutic milieu rested on four components: the facilitation of com-munity living, the relationships with professionals, the structure of the unit programme and the physical environment of the unit.* (Grech et al., 2020, p. 1026)
>
> **Critical Appraisal**
>
> Grech et al. (2020) used 10 years of existing evaluation reports that were provided by the facility, verifying that the documents were authentic. Before accepting the documents, the researchers confirmed that no patient names or identifiable data were included. The researchers analyzed the reports and found that community living included balancing the two human needs of attachment and autonomy (Grech et al., 2020). The docu-ments contained the information needed to answer the research question. Grech et al. (2020) noted a strength of the study to be that the evaluations of the unit had involved multiple types of data provided by service recipients. A limitation of the study was that the original data provided by the service recipients had been interpreted by the staff conducting the evaluation.

DATA MANAGEMENT

The limitations on the length of manuscripts for peer-reviewed journals may prevent the research-ers from reporting details of the processes of data management. However, having a general under-standing of this part of the process will allow you to critically appraise published studies and provide the background needed to evaluate study proposals being considered by your facility or institutional review board.

Transcribing Interviews and Field Notes

The most commonly used textual data in qualitative studies are transcripts of recorded interviews and focus groups. Transcripts are typed records of audio recordings, video recordings, and notes made during observation. The observations and interactions with participants may also be trans-formed into text for analysis, which may result in copious data for analysis. Typically, transcripts are prepared by typing the recording word for word, including audible noises, such as laughing, coughing, or hesitating. Computer transcription programs are now available that use voice recog-nition and can produce a written record of the recording. Even when computer software or a professional transcriptionist is used, the researcher will ensure accuracy by reading and correcting the transcript while listening to the recording.

Organization of Materials

Qualitative data analysis occurs concurrently with data collection and requires planning because qualitative studies generate a large amount of data. When qualitative researchers prepare to

---

BOX 3.3   ADVANTAGES AND DISADVANTAGES OF COMPUTER-ASSISTED QUALITATIVE DATA ANALYSIS SOFTWARE

Advantages
- Automatic creation of an audit trail
- Ease of retrieving text marked with the same code
- Maintenance of an organized storage file system
- Development of visual representations of the analyzed data
- Linkage of memos and journals to the text or code
- Ability to share analysis with fellow researchers

Disadvantages
- Time invested in selecting and learning the software
- Perceived distancing from the data
- Specific challenges with the selected software

Data are from Creswell, J., & Poth, C. (2018). *Qualitative inquiry and research design: Choosing among five approaches* (4th ed.). Sage.

conduct a study, their plan includes multiple locations in which data will be saved. Frequently, one of the locations is an online service or electronic network. The amount of data may be copious because a 1-hour interview may result in electronic (computer) files of a 25-page interview transcript, field notes, journaling related to codes or analysis, and a demographic form. Experienced researchers develop a standard way to name files before data collection begins. For example, the file name could include the name or pseudonym of the interviewee, the date the file was created, and what it is (i.e., transcript or field note). Other files may be generated from meetings of a research team or consultation with a qualitative expert. The researchers keep a record of how files are named and where they are stored, preventing wasted time looking for files during analysis, interpretation, and dissemination (Miles et al., 2020).

Nurse researchers are increasingly using computer-assisted qualitative data analysis software (CAQDAS) programs (Miles et al., 2020). The researcher reads the transcripts, identifies codes, and combines similar codes into themes. The computer software does not do the analysis but can record decisions that are made. The advantages and disadvantages of CAQDAS are listed in Box 3.3.

DATA ANALYSIS

Data analysis is a rigorous process. Because published qualitative studies may not contain the methodology in detail, many professionals believe that qualitative research is a free-wheeling process, with little structure. The data analysis process requires discipline, creativity, deep thought, and time. The researcher begins with a plan that is consistent with the qualitative design and adapts the plan as the study continues. In grounded theory studies, the researchers use constant comparison and begin data analysis with the first participant's interview. Constant comparison analysis means the ideas from the first interview are incorporated into the questions and probes in subsequent interviews. It also means that concepts identified through the analysis of each interview are compared with the concepts identified in data from previous and subsequent interviews. Qualitative researchers become immersed in the data, which means they spend considerable time reading, rereading, analyzing, and reflecting on the data, codes, and themes. In phenomenology, this immersion in the data is referred to as dwelling with the data.

Codes and Coding

Coding is the process of reading the data, breaking text down into subparts, and giving a label to that part of the text. These labels provide a way for the researcher to begin to identify patterns in the data because sections of text that were coded in the same way can be compared for similarities and differences (Miles et al., 2020). A code is a symbol or abbreviation used to classify words or phrases in the data. Codes may be handwritten on a printed transcript. In a word-processing program or CAQDAS, you code by highlighting a section of text and making a comment in the margin or sidebar. Codes may result in themes, processes, or exemplars of the phenomenon being studied. For example, during the interviews for a study of medication adherence, participants mentioned clocks, alarms, schedules, and the hours when doses were due. The researchers coded these sections of the transcript as "time." An exploratory-descriptive qualitative study about pain experiences of surgical patients may result in a taxonomy of types of pain, activities that resulted in pain, and types of pain relief strategies.

Themes and Interpretation

Themes emerge when codes are combined into more abstract phrases or terms. Sometimes there are several layers of themes, with each layer being another level of abstraction above the initial codes. Making links between these themes and the original data may become more difficult as the themes become more abstract. Displays such as tables, diagrams, and matrices may help organize the codes, themes, and their connections (Miles et al., 2020). The linkages between the data, codes, and themes are essential in maintaining the rigor of the study, and CAQDAS programs document these linkages automatically. However, CAQDAS cannot create the connections; it is the researcher who must create the links from the themes back to codes and from the codes to the original data. If you are critically appraising a qualitative study that includes themes, you will assess whether the researcher provided appropriate participant quotations to support the themes and determine whether the themes are consistent with the study purpose.

An audit trail is one way that a researcher can assure a reader that the methods of the study were implemented appropriately. An audit trail is the documentation of how data were collected, analyzed, and interpreted. Specifically, an audit trail allows you to check for the connections among the study components. CAQDAS contains detailed records that allow the researcher to easily produce an audit trail. When CAQDAS is not used, the researcher must record each aspect of the data collection and analysis in a diary or journal.

During interpretation, the researcher places the findings in a larger context and may link different themes or factors in the findings to each other. The researcher is explaining what the findings mean in the context of theories and previous research. The researcher compares the study's findings with the findings of published studies, identifying similarities and inconsistencies. The usefulness of the findings for clinical practice are also described.

? CRITICAL APPRAISAL GUIDELINES

Data Management, Analysis, and Interpretation

1. Were data analysis and interpretation consistent with the philosophical orientation, research problem, methodology, research question, and purpose of the study?
2. Did the researchers describe how they recorded decisions made during analysis and interpretation?
3. Did the researchers link the codes and themes used with participants' quotations?
4. Did the researchers provide adequate description of the data analysis and interpretation processes?

Weber et al. (2020, p. 52) conducted a grounded theory study, the purpose of which was to "describe the experiences of a sample of homeless male veterans" as they attempted to obtain care in an emergency department. Within a table in the report, the researchers identified the types of coding they used and other methodological terms common to grounded theory. They also provided a thorough description of data analysis and interpretation as cited in Research Example 3.10.

RESEARCH EXAMPLE 3.10

Data Management, Analysis, and Interpretation

Research/Study Excerpt

Semi-structured interviews with participants, lasting between 30 and 60 minutes, were audio-recorded, transcribed, and verified...Field notes allowed the researcher to follow up with any clarifying questions and record any general impressions of the environment and/or the participant. Memos were written congruently while data collection and analysis took place to enhance the development of emerging themes.... The transcripts from the 34 participants were analyzed for text units pertaining to self-reported ED visits while homeless.... The grounded theory technique of constant comparative analysis was used to analyze the resulting text units. Line-by-line coding, then substantive coding, and finally theoretical coding were used.... The research team met weekly to discuss the coded transcripts, analyze the data to reach group consensus and ensure rigor, and review the resulting categories to ensure theoretical saturation was achieved and theoretical sensitivity was maintained. The qualitative software MAXQDA (MAXQDA Analytics Pro, VERBI GmbH, Berlin, Germany) was used to assist with data analysis procedures. (Weber et al., 2020, p. 54)

The lack of health insurance did play a role in homeless veterans accessing the emergency department for care. One participant described using the emergency department for treatment of his chronic obstructive pulmonary disease: "I have lung disease, and it's not reversible. When I get sick, I normally do go to the emergency room because I don't have any health insurance, and so I can get my treatments by going to the emergency room." (Weber et al., 2020, p. 55)

The findings suggest that homeless veterans perceive the emergency department as their best option for care rather than primary or ambulatory care services because of convenience, accessibility, and time constraints. (Weber et al., 2020, p. 56)

Critical Appraisal

The data analysis and interpretation were consistent with grounded theory methodology and the purpose of the study. The researchers describe thoroughly how they coded the data from interviews and field notes, and how they recorded their decisions in a computer analysis software. Weber et al. (2020) provided multiple quotations from the veterans to support the components of each theme. The researchers described in detail their analysis and interpretation, which documented the quality and rigor of the study.

RIGOR AND VALUE OF QUALITATIVE RESEARCH

Scientific rigor is valued because the findings of rigorous studies are credible and of greater worth. Studies are critically appraised as a means of judging rigor. Rigor is defined differently for qualitative research because the desired outcome is different from the desired outcome for quantitative research (Gray & Grove, 2021). For qualitative research, rigor is defined as the trustworthiness of the findings. Do the study findings accurately portray the perspectives of the participants? Were standards of qualitative research applied during the study? Rigor is assessed by evaluating the detail built into the design, carefulness of data collection, and thoroughness of analysis.

The steps of the research process from research problem to conclusions must be consistent with each other. All steps must also be accurately and completely reported so that readers can assess the rigor of the study (Johnson et al., 2020). The fit between these key elements of a study (problem, purpose, questions, methods) is important for quantitative and qualitative research, but has special significance in qualitative research because of the evolving nature of studies.

The biases and preconceptions of a qualitative researcher influence every aspect of a study (Johnson et al., 2020). The researcher's self-awareness and intellectual honesty promote reflexivity. Reflexivity is a researcher's acknowledgment of personal experiences and expectations that influence the study. Along with the acknowledgment, the researcher attempts to set these preconceptions aside and be open during data collection and analysis.

When you critically appraise a study, you are evaluating the rigor of the study. The guidelines for critical appraisal of qualitative studies identified indicators of rigorous studies, such as checking the accuracy of a transcript by reading it while listening to the audio recording of the interview or focus group. Other strategies included maintaining an audit trail, ensuring interviews and focus groups were adequate in length, keeping field notes during observations, and returning interview descriptions to participants to check whether the essence of the experience was captured. Chapter 12 will include a comprehensive guideline for critical appraisal of qualitative research and an example of applying the guideline to a qualitative study.

With the current focus on EBP in health care, findings of qualitative research may be undervalued or even disregarded. It is true that qualitative studies produce a lower level of research evidence on the triangle of evidence (see Fig. 1.3). However, remember that EBP requires the integration of the best research evidence, the clinical expertise of the healthcare provider, and the values and circumstances of the patient. Qualitative study findings reflect the values and circumstances of the patient and provide insight into the acceptability and effectiveness of nursing actions from the perspective of the patient and family.

KEY POINTS

- Qualitative research is a systematic approach used to collect textual and visual data related to the phenomenon the study addresses.
- A phenomenological researcher examines an experience and interprets its meaning while staying true to the perspective of those who have lived the experience.
- Grounded theory researchers explore underlying social processes and describe the deeper meaning of an event as a theoretical framework.
- Ethnographic researchers observe and interview people within a culture to understand the environment, people, power relations, and communication patterns of a work setting, community, or ethnic group.
- Exploratory-descriptive qualitative studies are conducted to promote understanding of an experience or environment from the perspective of the people involved and possibly solve a problem.
- Data may be collected through interviews, focus groups, observation, and examination of documents and images.
- Qualitative data are analyzed to allow the participants' perspectives and the multiple realities of the persons experiencing a phenomenon to emerge.
- Data management, analysis, and interpretation require clear procedures to ensure methodological rigor and credibility of the findings.
- Rigor in qualitative research requires critically appraising the study for congruence with the philosophical perspective; appropriateness of the collection, analysis, and interpretation of data; and the reflexivity of the researcher.

REFERENCES

Brinkmann, S. (2018). The interview. In N. Denzin & Y. Lincoln (Eds.), *The Sage handbook of qualitative research* (5th ed., pp. 576–579). Sage.

Butcon, J., & Chan, E. (2017). Certainty in uncertainty: Our position on culture, focused ethnography, and researching older people. *International Journal of Qualitative Methods, 16*, 109. https://doi.org/10.1177/1609406917734471

Cooke, A., Mills, T., & Lavender, T. (2010). 'Informed and uninformed decision making'—women's reasoning, experiences and perceptions with regard to advanced maternal age and delayed childbearing: A meta-synthesis. *International Journal of Nursing Studies, 47*(10), 1317–1329. https://doi.org/10.1016/j.ijnurstu.2010.06.001

Correa, N., Cain, C., Bertenthal, M., & Lopez, K. (2020). Women's experiences of being screened for intimate partner violence in the health care setting. *Nursing for Women's Health, 24*(3), 185–196. https://www.doi.org/10.1016/j.nwh.2020.04.002

Creswell, J. W., & Creswell, J. D. (2018). *Research design: Qualitative, quantitative, and mixed methods approaches* (5th ed.). Sage.

Creswell, J., & Poth, C. (2018). *Qualitative inquiry and research design: Choosing among five approaches* (4th ed.). Sage.

Denzin, N., & Lincoln, Y. (2018). Introduction: The discipline and practice of qualitative research. In N. Denzin & Y. Lincoln (Eds.), *The Sage handbook of qualitative research* (5th ed., pp. 1–25). Sage.

Erickson, F. (2018). A history of qualitative inquiry in social and educational research. In N. Denzin & Y. Lincoln (Eds.), *The Sage handbook of qualitative research* (5th ed., pp. 36–65). Sage.

Fawcett, J., & McFarland, J. (2012). Madeleine Leininger (1925-2012): In memoriam. *Nursing Science Quarterly, 25*(4), 384–385. https://doi.org/10.1177/0894318412462316

Fernandez, A. (2020). Embodiment and objectification in illness and health care: Taking phenomenology from theory to practice. *Journal of Clinical Nursing, 29*(21/22), 4403–4412. http://doi.org/10.1111/jocn.15431

Glaser, B. G., & Strauss, A. (1967). *The discovery of grounded theory: Strategies for qualitative research.* Aldine.

Gray, J., & Grove, S. K. (2021). *The practice of nursing research: Appraisal, synthesis, and generation of evidence* (9th ed.). Elsevier.

Grech, P., Scerri, J., Vinceti, S., Sammut, A., Galea, M., Bitar, D., & Sant, S. (2020). Service users' perceptions of the therapeutic milieu in a mental health rehabilitation unit. *Issues in Mental Health Nursing, 41*(11), 1019–1026. https://doi.org/10.1080/01612840.2020.1757797

Guerrero, L., & Xicola, J. (2018). New approaches to focus groups. In G. Ares & P. Varela (Eds.), *Methods in consumer research: New methods to classic methods* (Vol. 1, pp. 49–77). Woodhead Publishing. http://dx.doi.org/10.1016/B978-0-08-102089-0.00003-0

Hassankhani, H., Negarandehb, R., Abbaszadehc, M., & Jabraeilid, M. (2020). The role of mothers during painful procedures on neonates: A focused ethnography. *Journal of Neonatal Nursing, 26*, 340–343. https://doi.org/10.1016/j.jnn.2020.03.002

Hennink, M., Kaiser, B., & Weber, M. (2019). What influences saturation? Estimating sample sizes in focus group research. *Qualitative Health Research, 29*(10), 1483–1496. https://doi.org/10.1177/1049732318821692

Jiwani, R., Dennis, B., Bess, C., Monk, S., Meyer, K., Wang, J., & Espinoza, S. (2021). Assessing acceptability and patient experience of a behavioral lifestyle intervention using Fitbit technology in older adults to manage type 2 diabetes amid COVID-19 pandemic: A focus group study. *Geriatric Nursing, 42*, 57–64. https://doi.org/10.1016/j.gerinurse.2020.11.007

Johnson, J., Adkins, D., & Chauvin, S. (2020). Qualitative research in pharmacy education: A review of quality indicators of rigor in qualitative research. *American Journal of Pharmaceutical Education, 84*(1), 7120. https://doi.org/10.5688/ajpe7120

Kelle, U. (2019). The status of theories and models in grounded theory. In A. Bryant & K. Charmaz (Eds.), *The Sage handbook of current developments in grounded theory* (pp. 68–88). Sage.

Knechel, N. (2019). What's in a sample? Why selecting the right research participants matters. *Journal of Emergency Nursing, 45*(3), 332–334. https://doi.org/10.1016/j.jen.2019.01.020

Laging, B., Kenny, A., Bauer, M., & Nay, R. (2018). Recognition and assessment of resident' deterioration in the nursing home setting: A critical ethnography. *Journal of Clinical Nursing, 27*, 1452–1463. https://doi.org/10.1111/jocn.14292

Leininger, M. M. (Ed.). (1985). *Qualitative research methods.* Grune and Stratton.

Leininger, M. M. (1988). Leininger's theory of nursing: Cultural care diversity and universality. *Nursing Science Quarterly, 1*(4), 152–160. https://doi.org/10.1177/089431848800100408

Leininger, M. M. (2002). Culture care theory: A major contribution to advance transcultural nursing knowledge and practices. *Journal of Transcultural Nursing, 13*(3), 189–192. https://doi.org/10.1177/10459602013003005

Lundquist, D., Berry, D., Boltz, M., DeSanto-Madeya, S., & Grace, P. (2019). Wearing the mask of wellness: The experience of young women living with advanced breast cancer. *Oncology Nursing Forum, 46*(3), 329–337. http://doi.org/10.1188/19.ONF.329-337

Marcil, L., Campbell, J., Silva, K., Hughes, D., Salim, S., Nguyen, H.,…Kistin, C. (2020). Women's experiences of the effect of financial strain on parenting and mental health. *Journal of Obstetric, Gynecologic, & Neonatal Nursing, 49*, 581–592. https://doi.org/10.1016/j.jogn.2020.07.002

Markham, A. (2018). Ethnographic in the digital internet era: From fields to flows, descriptions to interventions. In N. Denzin & Y. Lincoln (Eds.), *The Sage handbook of qualitative research* (5th ed., pp. 650–668). Sage.

Meadows-Oliver, M. (2019). Critically appraising qualitative evidence for clinical decision making. In B. Melnyck & E. Fineout-Overholt (Eds.), *Evidence-based practice in nursing and healthcare: A guide to best practice* (4th ed., pp. 189–218). Wolters Kluwer.

Miles, M., Huberman, A., & Saldaña, J. (2020). *Qualitative data analysis: A methods sourcebook* (4th ed.). Sage.

Miller, J. (2019). Reflecting on transcultural nursing. *Journal of Transcultural Nursing, 30*(4), 420. https://doi.org/10.1177/1043659619840410

Morgan, D. (2019). *Basic and advanced focus groups.* Sage Publications. https://dx.doi.org/10.4135/9781071814307

Moser, A., & Korstjens, I. (2018). Series: Practical guidance to qualitative research. Part 3: Sampling, data collection and analysis. *European Journal of General Practice, 24*(1), 9–18. https://doi.org/10.1080/13814788.2017.1375091

Myers, S., Siegel, E., Hyson, D., & Bidwell, J. (2020). A qualitative study exploring the perceptions and motivations of patients with heart failure who transitioned from non-adherence to adherence. *Heart & Lung, 49*, 817–823. http://doi.org/10.1016/j.hrtlng.2020.09.010

Newman, B., & Newman, P. (2020). Cultural theories. In B. Newman, & P. Newman (Eds.), *Theories of adolescent development* (pp. 363–393). Elsevier. https://doi.org/10.1016/B978-0-12-815450-2.00013-9

Nieto-Eugenio, I., Ventura-Puertos, P., & Rich-Ruiz, M. (2020). S.O.S! My child is at school: A hermeneutic of the experience of living a chronic disease in the school environment. *Journal of Pediatric Nursing, 53*, e171–e178. https://doi.org/10.1016/j.pedn.2020.03.016

Oates, C., & Alevizou, P. (2019). *Conducting focus groups for business and management students.* Sage. https://dx.doi.org/10.4135/9781529716610

Ranse, J., Arbon, P., Cusack, L., Shaban, R., & Nicholls, D. (2020). Obtaining individual narratives and moving to intersubjective lived-experience description: A way of doing phenomenology. *Qualitative Research, 20*(6), 945–959. https://doi.org/10.1177/1468794120905988

Riegel, B., Dickson, V., & Faulkner, K. (2016). The situation-specific theory of heart failure self-care: Revised and updated. *Journal of Cardiovascular Nursing, 31*(3), 226–235. https://doi.org/10.1097/JCN.0000000000000244

Roper, J., & Shapira, J. (2000). *Ethnography in nursing research.* Sage.

Rozario, P.A., & Derienzis, D. (2009). 'So forget how old I am!' Examining age identities in the face of chronic conditions. *Sociology of Health and Illness, 31*, 540–553. https://doi.org/10.1111/j.1467-9566.2008.01149.x

Sandelowski, M. (2000). Whatever happened to qualitative description? *Research in Nursing & Health, 23*(4), 334–340. https://doi.org/10.1002/1098-240x(200008)23:4<334::aid-nur9>3.0.co;2-g

Sandelowski, M. (2010). What's in a name? Qualitative description revisited. *Research in Nursing & Health, 33*(1), 77–84. https://doi.org/10.1002/nur.20362

Shaban, R., Nahidi, S., Sotomayor-Castillo, C., Li, C., Gilroy, N., O'Sullivan, M.,…Bag, S. (2020). SARS-CoV-2 infection and COVID-19: The lived experience and perceptions of patients in isolation and care in an Australian healthcare setting. *American Journal of Infection Control, 48*, 1445–1450. https://doi.org/10.1016/j.ajic.2020.08.032

Smith, A., McDonald, A., & Sasangohar, F. (2020). Night-shift nurses and drowsy driving: A qualitative study. *International Journal of Nursing Studies, 112*, 103600. https://doi.org/10.1016/j.ijnurstu.2020.103600

Southby, C., Cooke, A., & Lavender, T. (2019). 'It's now or never'—nulliparous women's experience of pregnancy at advanced maternal age: A grounded theory study. *Midwifery, 68*(1), 1–8. https://doi.org/10.1016/j.midw.2018.09.006

Tucker, J., Whitehead, L., Palmarara, P., Rosman, J., & Seaman, K. (2020). Recognition and management of agitation in acute mental health services: A qualitative evaluation of staff perceptions. *BMC Nursing, 19*, 106. https://doi.org/10.1186/s12912-020-00495-x

van Manen, M. (2017). But is it phenomenology? *Qualitative Health Research, 27*(6), 775–779. https://doi.org/10.1177/1049732317699570

Weber, J., Lee, R., & Martsolf, D. (2020). Experiences of care in the emergency department among a sample of homeless male veterans: A qualitative study. *Journal of Emergency Nursing, 46*(1), 51–58. https://doi.org/10.1016/j.jen.2019.06.009

Young, R., & Collin, A. (2004). Introduction: Constructivism and social constructivism in the career field. *Journal of Vocational Behavior, 64,* 373–388. https://doi.org/10.1016/j.jvb.2003.12.005

Examining Ethics in Nursing Research

Jennifer R. Gray

LEARNING OUTCOMES

After completing this chapter, you should be able to:

1. Describe the role of nurses in ensuring ethical research.
2. Identify the historical events that influence the development of ethical codes and regulations for nursing and biomedical research.
3. Describe the ethical principles and human rights that require protection in research.
4. Identify the essential elements of the informed consent process in research.
5. Describe the levels of review that an institutional review board (IRB) may use in reviewing a study.
6. Describe the challenges of protecting the rights of participants in genomic studies.
7. Explore the issues of research misconduct and its effect on evidence-based practice (EBP).
8. Critically appraise ethical sections in research reports, with emphasis on IRB and informed consent processes.

Ethical research is essential for generating credible and trustworthy knowledge for EBP, but what does ethical conduct of research involve? The necessity of conducting research ethically became apparent when the scientific community and the public were confronted with reports of unethical studies. Unethical studies that violate participants' rights have been implemented in the United States and other countries since biomedical research began. As these studies came to light, international and national codes were developed to promote the ethical conduct of research (Thakur & Lahiry, 2019). These codes and regulations dramatically reduced the number of unethical studies, but, unfortunately, ethical violations and research misconduct persist today.

In this chapter, elements of ethical research are described, including protecting human rights during research, understanding informed consent, and examining institutional review of research. Guidelines for critically appraising the ethical aspects of a study are provided. The chapter concludes with a discussion of current ethical issues surrounding genomics research and research misconduct.

THE NURSE'S ROLE IN ETHICAL RESEARCH

Nursing students and practicing nurses need the ability to critically appraise the ethical aspects of published studies and of research conducted in clinical agencies. The Methods section of most published studies includes information about the ethical selection of study participants and their treatment during the study. You will also find details about the study being approved by an IRB. Institutional review boards (IRBs) are organized in universities and clinical agencies to examine the ethical aspects of studies before they are conducted (Maloy & Bass, 2020). IRBs are responsible for initial and continuing approval of studies, as well as addressing any research violations that may occur during a study (Martien & Nelligan, 2018). When you are a practicing nurse, you may have the opportunity to be a member of an IRB and participate in the review of study proposals submitted for approval. You will need the ability to critically appraise the ethical aspects of research, which requires knowledge of ethical codes and regulations. Developed in response to unethical studies, these ethical codes and regulations guide the conduct of biomedical and behavioral research.

UNETHICAL RESEARCH: 1930s THROUGH THE 1980s

Four research projects have been highly publicized for their unethical treatment of human subjects and will be briefly described in this section. Nurses were involved in implementing these studies, although the primary researchers were physicians. These studies, as well as more recent unethical studies, demonstrate the importance of ethical conduct for nurses when they review or participate in research (Schroeter, 2020). These studies also influenced the formulation of ethical codes and regulations that continue to direct the conduct of research today.

Nazi Medical Experiments

From 1933 to 1945, the Third Reich in Europe was engaged in atrocious and unethical medical research. Medical experiments were conducted on Jews, prisoners of war, persons with disabilities, and other people in the concentration camps. The researchers tested how well people could tolerate extreme conditions, including torture, high altitudes, freezing temperatures, poisons, infections, untested drugs, and surgery without anesthesia (Artal & Rubenfeld, 2017). The Nazi experiments violated numerous rights of the research subjects. Subjects were selected based on their race/ethnicity, forced to participate, and exposed to pain and permanent harm. Because these studies were poorly conceived and conducted, this research was not only unethical but also generated little, if any, useful scientific knowledge (Berger, 1990; Steinfels & Levine, 1976).

Tuskegee Syphilis Study

In 1932 the US Public Health Service initiated a study of the natural history of syphilis in black men in and around the small rural town of Tuskegee in Macon County, Alabama (Alsan et al., 2020; Rothman, 1982). When the study began, there were few treatments for syphilis, and none that were curative. Men with and without syphilis were recruited to be in the study. Many of the subjects were not informed they were participating in a study. If they were told they were in a study, the study's purpose and procedures were not explained. By 1936, the researchers had shown that men with syphilis developed more complications than the men without syphilis. Ten years later, the death rate of the men with syphilis was twice as high as it was for the men without syphilis, and still the study continued. The subjects were examined periodically but were not treated for syphilis, even when penicillin was determined to be an effective treatment for the disease in the 1940s. Information about an effective treatment for syphilis was withheld from the subjects, and deliberate steps were taken to deprive them of treatment (Brandt, 1978).

Published reports of the Tuskegee Syphilis Study started appearing in medical journals in 1936, and additional papers were published every 4 to 6 years. No effort was made to stop the study. In 1969 the Centers for Disease Control and Prevention reviewed the 37-year study and decided that it should continue. The study was finally stopped in 1972 when a newspaper article about the study was widely disseminated by the Associated Press and sparked public outrage (Alsan et al., 2020). Because of the public outrage, the US Department of Health, Education, and Welfare stopped the study. The study was investigated and found to be ethically unjustified (Brandt, 1978). Researchers today have linked the racial ramifications of the study to the mistrust of research among black people and even lower life expectancies of black men in the United States (Alsan et al., 2020).

Willowbrook Study

Willowbrook, located on Staten Island in New York, was a facility for children who were mentally disabled. From the mid-1950s to the early 1970s, Dr. Saul Krugman conducted research on hepatitis at Willowbrook (Rothman, 1982). The facility was overcrowded, and the administrators had stopped admitting new residents. However, the research ward continued to admit new residents. Parents could admit their children only if they were willing to give permission for their child to be in the study and be injected with the hepatitis virus.

While the study was still in progress, Beecher (1966) cited the Willowbrook Study in the *New England Journal of Medicine* as an example of unethical research. The researchers defended injecting the children with the hepatitis virus because they believed that most of the children would acquire the infection naturally soon after admission to the institution. They also stressed the benefits the subjects received on the research ward, such as a cleaner environment, better supervision, and a higher nurse-to-patient ratio (Rothman, 1982). Despite the controversy, this unethical study continued until the early 1970s.

Jewish Chronic Disease Hospital Study

Researchers conducted a study at the Jewish Chronic Disease Hospital in New York in the 1960s. The hospital provided long-term care for older persons with chronic illnesses, including dementia. The purpose of this study was to determine whether older persons' bodies would reject cancer cells. A suspension containing live cancer cells was injected into 22 patients (Levine, 1988). The patients were neither informed they were participating in research nor that they were receiving live cancer cells. This lack of disclosure violated their rights to self-determination and protection from harm. In addition, the study was never presented for review to the research committee of the Jewish Chronic Disease Hospital, and the physicians caring for the patients were unaware that the study was being conducted (Hershey & Miller, 1976).

This unethical study was conducted without the informed consent of the subjects and institutional review and had the potential to injure, disable, or cause the death of the human subjects. When patients' families became aware of what was happening, the unethical study was stopped. Steps were immediately taken to provide appropriate care to the persons exposed to cancer. Precautions were put into place to ensure that all future proposed research conducted in the agency was properly reviewed and approved.

> ### 📄 RESEARCH/EBP TIP
>
> Unethical studies, such as the Tuskegee Syphilis Study, left a legacy of people who mistrust health-related research. Nursing researchers must intentionally develop and maintain relationships of respect and trust with research participants to overcome this legacy.

ETHICAL STANDARDS FOR RESEARCH

Because of these unethical studies, international standards, US standards, and laws were developed to delineate ethical research involving human participants. For the remainder of the chapter, we will refer to the people in a study as participants to emphasize their voluntary agreement to the conditions of the study. The first standard was developed in the aftermath of World War II.

International Standards

A list of ethical research principles was published after the Doctors' Trial at Nuremberg, Germany (Artal & Rubenfeld, 2017). Those perpetrators of the Nazi experiments were tried for murder and torture, which brought international attention to their unethical research. In 1949 after the trial ended, the Nuremberg Code was released (Eastwood, 2015). Box 4.1 presents the key components of the Nuremberg Code. The code emphasized voluntary consent and contains guidelines related to protecting subjects from harm and balancing the benefits and risks of a study.

The Declaration of Helsinki was written and adopted by the World Medical Association in 1964 (Shuster, 1997; World Medical Association, 2013). The declaration clarified the differences between therapeutic research and nontherapeutic research. Therapeutic research provides research participants with the opportunity for a potential benefit from an experimental treatment. Nontherapeutic research generates knowledge for science. The research participants are not

---

BOX 4.1 THE NUREMBERG CODE: CRITICAL COMPONENTS OF AN ETHICAL STUDY

The Person: Voluntary Participant
- Has comprehensive information about the study, the legal capacity to consent, and is not under duress to participate
- Can stop his or her participation at any time

The Study: Beneficial and Credible
- Based on prior studies, including those with animals
- Planned only if possible to yield results beneficial to society
- Designed so that potential benefit exceeds potential harm
- Implemented to avoid or minimize potential harm

The Researcher: Qualified and Ethical
- Possesses the knowledge and ability to safely implement study
- Able to maintain standards of scientifically sound study
- Willing to terminate study if it becomes harmful

Based on Shuster, E. (1997). Fifty years later: The significance of the Nuremberg Code. *New England Journal of Medicine, 337*, 1436–1440. https://doi.org/10.1056/NEJM199711133372006

expected to benefit, but the results may help future patients. Researchers are responsible for protecting the health, privacy, and dignity of human subjects, as well as designing studies that provide benefits greater than the risks and burdens for subjects.

📄 **RESEARCH/EBP TIP**

Ethical standards were developed to protect the rights of study participants. Nurses reviewing a research proposal, obtaining informed consent, or collecting data will want to ensure compliance with these standards as part of their professional responsibilities.

Standards in the United States

In the United States, the Belmont Report was written by the National Commission for the Protection of Human Subjects of Biomedical and Behavioral Research (1979). The commission was formed because of the public outcry when the Tuskegee Syphilis Study was exposed. The Belmont Report identified ethical principles to guide selecting subjects, informing them of the risks and benefits of a study, and documenting their consent. The Belmont Report provides a strong foundation for conducting ethical research. As science has advanced, additional international and national bioethics commissions have been formed to consider ethical issues related to using stem cells in research, protecting privacy during genetic research, and other topics (Presidential Commission, 2012; World Health Organization Expert Advisory Committee, 2021).

Federal Regulations for the Protection of Human Subjects

After the Belmont Report, the initial federal regulations to protect human research subjects were developed and continue to be updated as needed, most recently in 2017. The regulations are part of the *Code of Federal Regulations* (CFR). Each department in the US Government that is involved in human research has a chapter in the CFR with regulations for research funded by the department. Because of the similarities among the chapters, the CFR is called the Common Rule. The goals of the most recent revision were to enhance protection of human participants and reduce the administrative burden of regulating research in healthcare organizations and universities (Menikoff et al., 2017). The final version of the revised rule was published in the *Federal Register* in January 2017 and was fully implemented by January 2019 (US Department of Health and Human Services [USDHHS], 2018a).

The Common Rule includes requirements related to the content of an informed consent document, processes for obtaining informed consent, maintaining an IRB, and implementing special precautions for studies with vulnerable persons (Table 4.1). Vulnerable populations are defined as persons who are susceptible to undue influence or coercion, such as children, prisoners, and persons who are economically or educationally disadvantaged (USDHHS, 2018b). Persons who have impaired decision making were also identified as being vulnerable. This might include persons with Alzheimer disease, traumatic brain injury, and those born with intellectual limitations.

During your clinical practice, you may facilitate obtaining patient consent to participate in clinical trials related to new drugs and medical devices. The US Food and Drug Administration (2020) is responsible for managing the elements of the Common Rule that involve testing drugs, medical devices, biological products, dietary supplements, and electronic products for human use. To summarize, the Common Rule, including the US Food and Drug Administration regulations, provides guidelines for federally and privately funded research to protect subjects, ensure their privacy, and maintain the confidentiality of the information obtained through research. Table 4.1 contains descriptions of the regulations applicable to human research.

TABLE 4.1	CLARIFICATION OF FEDERAL REGULATIONS RELATED TO HUMAN PARTICIPANTS RESEARCH		
COMMON NAME OF THE REGULATION	**KEY PHRASE**	**PURPOSE**	
Common Rule[a]	Human participants research	Protect the rights and welfare of human participants involved in research conducted or supported by the USDHHS	
FDA Protection of Human Subjects Regulations[b]	Medications and medical devices	Protect the rights, safety, and welfare of subjects involved in clinical investigations regulated by the FDA	
HIPAA or the Privacy Rule[c]	Protected health information	Privacy protections for most individually identifiable protected health information	

[a]US Department of Health and Human Services (USDHHS). (2018b). *Subpart A of 45 CFR Part 46: Basic HHS policy for the protection of human subjects*. Retrieved from https://www.hhs.gov/ohrp/sites/default/files/revised-common-rule-reg-text-unofficial-2018-requirements.pdf
[b]US Food and Drug Administration (FDA). (2020). *21 CFR Part 50: Protection of human subjects*. Retrieved from https://www.accessdata.fda.gov/scripts/cdrh/cfdocs/cfcfr/CFRSearch.cfm?fr=50.1
[c]Health Insurance Portability and Accountability Act (HIPAA).

Another law that affects research conducted with people is the Health Insurance Portability and Accountability Act (HIPAA) (USDHHS, 2002). HIPAA has become known as the Privacy Rule and focuses on protecting electronic storage and transfer of patient information generated through clinical care (see Table 4.1). The Privacy Rule defined protected health information (PHI) as data generated and collected for research that can be linked to an individual person (Ennever et al., 2019). With the recent revision of the Common Rule, some PHI can be used without obtaining specific HIPAA permission if the risk to loss of privacy is deemed to be minimal (Williams & Colomb, 2020). Legal and medical experts have voiced concerns that the Common Rule has diminished the protection of the privacy of human participants. Others argue that the changes will allow robust use of the clinical databases to improve health. These databases already exist because of the use of electronic health records. Although different, the Common Rule and Privacy Rule have the same goal of protecting the rights of human participants.

📄 RESEARCH/EBP TIP

Unethical studies resulted in the development of ethical standards such as the Belmont Report and federal regulations such as the Common Rule. Nurses have an ethical obligation to protect the rights of persons who participate in research.

PROTECTING HUMAN PARTICIPANTS

Protecting the people who participate in research requires more than standards and laws. A responsible researcher must be guided also by ethical principles that support the rights of research participants.

Application of Ethical Principles

Within the standards and laws that protect human participants, three ethical principles guide appropriately implemented research: respect for persons, beneficence, and justice (Fig. 4.1). The principle of respect for persons indicates that people should be treated as autonomous agents, with the right to choose whether to participate in research or withdraw from a study. In Fig. 4.1, the principle is linked to autonomy. Because of your respect for persons, you will allow a person to act without your interference, or autonomously. Below the circle labeled "autonomy" are three ways that autonomy is applied in a study. Persons who are considered more vulnerable to coercion are entitled to additional protection to ensure that the principle of respect of persons is protected.

The principle of beneficence encourages the researcher to do good, instead of harm. This principle is the foundation for analyzing the benefits and risks of a specific study. In Fig. 4.1, the principle is linked to the circle labeled "promote good." Researchers guided by this principle will reduce a study's risks and ensure the participants receive the benefits. For example, a diabetic patient participates in a study of an enhanced education intervention and is randomized to the control group. The study's results show that the treatment group participants improved their glucose control. A researcher, guided by beneficence, will want the persons in the control group to receive the benefit of improved glucose control and will provide them the enhanced educational intervention. Beneficent researchers also follow the study's procedures carefully to ensure the accuracy of the study's results. Findings of poorly conducted studies provide no benefit to the participants or the wider population.

The principle of justice states that human participants have a right to fair treatment. Fair treatment includes access to the potential benefits of a study and not overexposure to its risks. Fig. 4.1 displays the principle of justice leading to fairness. The inclusion and exclusion criteria (see Chapter 9) for study participants must have scientific and/or logical explanations to be fair. For example, when recruiting participants, the researchers will approach potential participants even when they appear unfriendly or are dressed in dirty clothing, unless there is a scientific reason for including only friendly and clean participants.

In summary, Fig. 4.1 shows how each ethical principle can be linked to human rights. Although ethical principles can be abstract, each can be demonstrated as specific procedures during a study, as shown in this figure and described in the following sections. Whether critically appraising published studies, reviewing research for conduct in their agencies, or collecting data for a study, nurses have an obligation to follow the ethical principles and ensure the rights of the research

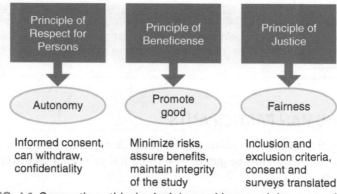

FIG. 4.1 Connecting ethical principles and human rights protection.

participants are being protected. The human rights that require protection in research are the rights to (1) self-determination, (2) privacy, (3) anonymity and confidentiality, (4) protection from pain and harm, and (5) fair selection and treatment.

> ### 📄 RESEARCH/EBP TIP
>
> Respect for persons is the basis for autonomy, beneficence results in promoting good through research, and justice supports fairness. The American Nurses Association (ANA, 2015) Code of Ethics for Nurses reiterates these rights and provides guidelines for ethical conduct of nurses in practice and research.

Right to Self-Determination

The right to self-determination is based on the ethical principle of respect for persons. Self-determination means that humans can make their own decisions. People should be given autonomy, which means having the freedom to conduct their lives as they choose, without external controls. Researchers protect the autonomy of potential participants by providing understandable information about a study and giving them a choice of whether to volunteer. In addition, a participant who consents to be in a study and begins a study can withdraw from the study at any time, without coercion or penalty (USDHHS, 2018b).

Participants' culture is a factor to consider related to autonomy. Autonomy has different interpretations and implications in different cultures (Roberts et al., 2017). Nurses are considered educationally prepared to advocate for potential research participants of different backgrounds because of nurses' knowledge of cultural values related to autonomy and decision making (Schroeter, 2020). Potential participants may be more open to discussing and consenting to a study when the researcher is a member of their culture (Jaiswal, 2019).

A participant's right to self-determination can be violated through coercion, covert data collection, and deception. Coercion occurs when one person presents an overt threat of harm or an excessive reward to another to obtain compliance. More often, research participants may respond to perceived coercion. They may participate because they fear harm or discomfort if they do not participate. Patients who are asked by their healthcare provider to participate in a study may fear that their care will be negatively affected if they do not agree to participate. Others feel coerced to participate in studies because they want the incentive that is being offered, such as access to experimental treatments. The Willowbrook study occurred because the only available admission to the hospital was to the research unit (Rothman, 1982). Parents who wanted to admit their children had no other option than to admit them to the research unit, even if they had concerns about the research being conducted.

With covert data collection, participants are unaware that research data are being collected (Reynolds, 1979). The Jewish Chronic Disease Hospital Study is an example. The participants were informed that they were receiving an injection of cells, but the word *cancer* was omitted (Beecher, 1966). The use of deception, the actual misinforming of participants for research purposes, can also violate a participant's right to self-determination. A classic example of deception is seen in the Milgram study (1963), in which the participants thought they were administering electric shocks to another person. However, the other person was an actor pretending to feel the shocks. To be acceptable, the use of deception must not potentially cause long-lasting harm. Also, the researchers should explain the deception to the participants as soon as possible. Based on the revision of the Common Rule, deception may be used ethically in a study only when the researcher informs potential participants that they will be unaware of or deliberately misguided about the true purpose of the study, and they agree to participate despite this condition (USDHHS, 2018b).

Persons With Diminished Autonomy as Participants

Persons have diminished autonomy when they cannot make decisions because of medications, mental illness, or mental capacity. Depending on the cause, diminished autonomy may be temporary or permanent. Persons with diminished autonomy require additional protection of their right to self-determination because of their decreased ability to give informed consent. In addition, they are vulnerable to coercion and deception.

Children are considered to have diminished autonomy because of their emotional immaturity and cognitive development. Children cannot consent to research as an adult until they reach legal age (USDHHS, 2019), which varies from state to state. Parents or guardians are the legal representative of the child and may, on a child's behalf, give their permission to participate in research. When children are developmentally able, they are provided an understandable explanation of the study and asked to assent to the research (Hodapp et al., 2020). Assent to participate in research means that the child has agreed to participate in the study (Brothers et al., 2020). Determining the appropriate age at which to include the child in decision making related to research is complex.

Because of the challenges of perceived risks with pediatric research, obtaining assent, and documenting consent, the research base for EBP with children and adolescents is limited. As a result, additional studies are needed with children and adolescents as participants (Brothers et al., 2020). Published studies need to indicate clearly that the child gave assent and the parents or guardians gave their permission before data were collected.

📄 RESEARCH/EBP TIP

When parents or guardians are reviewing a consent form for a pediatric study, they should be given adequate time to read and absorb the content of the document. They may need to ask questions and discuss the study with their child before deciding about the child's participation.

Right to Privacy

People have the freedom to determine who has access to their personal information. Privacy is being able to determine the time, extent, and general circumstances under which their private information is shared with others. Your private information includes your attitudes, beliefs, behaviors, opinions, and records. Your right to privacy is protected if you are informed about the study, consent to participate, and voluntarily share private information with a researcher. When private information is shared without a person's knowledge or against his or her will, this right has been violated. A research report often will indicate that the participant's privacy was protected but may not include the details of how this was accomplished.

The HIPAA Privacy Rule (USDHHS, 2002) expanded the protection of a person's privacy—specifically, his or her protected, individually identifiable health information. According to the Common Rule, identifiable private information is "private information for which the identity of the participant is or may be readily ascertained by the investigator or associated with the information" (USDHHS, 2018b, Section 102). Box 4.2 provides examples of the information considered to be identifiable and private. The revised Common Rule created a new type of consent called broad consent, through which a potential participant gives researchers permission to store, maintain, and use identifiable private information for other studies (USDHHS, 2018b). Broad consent does require that researchers protect confidentiality of the identity of the participants. In addition, broad consent applies to identifiable biospecimens collected for other studies or clinical care.

> ### BOX 4.2 TYPES OF IDENTIFIABLE PRIVATE INFORMATION AND SELECTED EXAMPLES
>
> | | |
> |---|---|
> | Demographic information | Physical and mental assessment findings |
> | Name | BP 174/102 |
> | Address | Arthritic changes in lumbar vertebrae |
> | Birthdate | Reduced airflow, left lower lobe |
> | Race/ethnicity | Pale first toe on right foot |
> | Previous and present medical diagnoses | Health care provided to the person |
> | Diabetes, type 2 | Uncomplicated delivery of male child |
> | Osteoarthritis | X-ray of the lower spine |
> | Hypertension | Removal of cyst from left breast |
> | Isolated psychotic event | Physical therapy services |

BP, Blood pressure.
From US Department of Health and Human Services (USDHHS). (2002). *45 CFR Parts 160 and 164. Standards for privacy of individually identifiable health information.* Retrieved from https://www.hhs.gov/hipaa/for-professionals/privacy/guidance/introduction/index.html

Broad consent and other regulations leave many questions unanswered. HIPAA (USDHHS, 2002) was enacted when mobile phones, social media platforms, and wearable devices were not widely used. Organizations heavily involved in research are working to integrate the multiple requirements of HIPAA and the Common Rule related to private health information (Ennever et al., 2019). Recognizing the limitations of HIPAA and data at risk for privacy breaches, additional or revised guidance is needed for researchers (Parasidis et al., 2019; Tovino, 2019).

Right to Anonymity and Confidentiality

Based on the right to privacy, the research participant has the right to anonymity and the right to assume that the data collected will be kept confidential. Complete anonymity exists when the researcher cannot link a participant's identity with her or his individual responses (Gray & Grove, 2021). In most studies, researchers know the identity of their participants, and they promise the participants that their identity will be kept anonymous from others and that the research data will be kept confidential. Confidentiality is the researcher's safe management of information or data shared by a participant to ensure that the data are kept private from others. The researcher agrees not to share the participants' information without their authorization. Confidentiality is grounded in two premises (ANA, 2015):

1. Because individuals own their personal information, they may share personal information to the extent that they wish and with whom they wish.
2. Accepting personal information comes with an obligation to maintain confidentiality, an obligation that is even greater for researchers and nurses.

A breach of confidentiality can occur when a researcher, by accident or by direct action, allows an unauthorized person to gain access to the raw data of a study. Confidentiality also can be breached in reporting or publishing a study if a participant's identity is accidentally revealed, violating his or her right to anonymity. In quantitative studies, results are presented for subgroups or groups, and a breach of confidentiality is less likely to occur. In qualitative studies, however, a breach of confidentiality is more likely because the researcher gathers data from fewer study participants and reports long quotes made by those participants. In ethnographic studies and collaborative research, researchers and participants often have relationships in which detailed stories of the participants' lives are shared, requiring careful management of study data to ensure confidentiality (Øye et al., 2019). Breaches of confidentiality are especially harmful to participants when factors such as their legal status, religious preferences, sexual practices, income, racial biases, drug use, or child abuse are shared (Rudolph et al., 2020). Participants' confidentiality should be maintained during data collection, analysis, and reporting (Gray & Grove, 2021). Research findings, whether quantitative, qualitative, or mixed methods, should be reported so that a participant or group of participants cannot be identified by their responses.

Right to Protection From Discomfort and Harm

The right to protection from discomfort and harm in a study is based on the ethical principle of beneficence, which states that one should do good and, above all, do no harm. According to this principle, members of society must take an active role in preventing discomfort and harm and promoting good in the world around them (ANA, 2015). In research, discomfort and harm is compared with what one might encounter in routine life activities. However, discomfort may vary from person to person because of personal characteristics, such as sexual orientation and prior life events (Alexander et al., 2018; Macapagal et al., 2019).

Studies range from no anticipated discomfort and harm to a high risk for discomfort and harm. Research designs that involve a review of medical records, student files, or secondary analysis of de-identified data collected for another study have no anticipated discomfort and harm. When there is no or minimal interaction between the researcher and participant, the study will usually be considered exempt when reviewed by an IRB (USDHHS, 2018b).

When temporary discomfort may occur, the study is described as a minimal risk study. The expected discomfort is like what the participant would encounter in his or her daily life and is temporary, ending when the study is complete (USDHHS, 2018b). Participants in a minimal risk study may complete questionnaires or participate in interviews. Physical discomfort in minimal risk studies may include fatigue, headache, or muscle tension. Anxiety or embarrassment might result from answering questions on sensitive topics. The only economic harm may be the costs of travel to the study site.

Most clinical nursing studies examining the effect of a treatment involve minimal risk. For example, you are recruiting participants for a study of exercise and serum glucose among persons with insulin-dependent diabetes. Physical discomfort or harm may be associated with obtaining blood specimens or participating in a prescribed exercise. To avoid economic harm, the researcher may reimburse the subject for the cost of any additional testing supplies. The participants encounter similar discomforts in their daily lives as they manage their disease. The discomfort of an extra finger stick will cease when the study ends.

Discomfort and harm during some studies may go beyond the minimal level and involve unusual levels of temporary discomfort. In studies with unusual levels of temporary discomfort, the participants may experience discomfort during and after the study. Unusual levels of discomfort or harm may occur when participants experience failure, extreme fear, or threats to their identity as part of a study. Qualitative researchers may ask questions that cause participants to relive a life crisis, such as being diagnosed with colon cancer or being in a car crash. Reliving these experiences or acting in an unnatural way involves unusual levels of temporary discomfort. In studies with unusual levels of discomfort or harm, the researcher will carefully describe the exclusion criteria for the sample in the IRB protocol. The exclusion criteria are developed to prevent recruitment of participants who are at higher risk for long-term discomfort or harm (see Chapter 9). A potential participant for a qualitative study related to recovery after a sexual assault might be excluded if the participant currently receives counseling from a licensed professional. The research team would also indicate in the IRB proposal and the subsequent research report the ways in which they assessed participants' discomfort and the resources they made available.

Studies in which there is the risk for permanent damage will undergo additional scrutiny by the IRB. The rationale for doing the study must establish reasons why the knowledge from the study cannot be gained in another way and what will be done to prevent or minimize damage. Biomedical studies involving new medications and devices are more likely to cause permanent damage than studies that nurses more typically initiate. Some topics investigated by nurses have the potential to cause permanent damage to participants, emotionally and socially. Studies examining sensitive information, such as sexual behavior, child abuse, HIV/AIDS status, or drug use, can be very risky for participants. These studies have the potential to cause permanent damage to a participant's personality or reputation. There also are potential economic risks, such as those resulting from a decrease in job performance or loss of employment.

The Nazi medical experiments and the Tuskegee Syphilis Study are examples of studies in which those in the study had a certainty of experiencing permanent damage. Conducting research that has a certainty of causing permanent damage to study subjects is highly questionable, regardless of the benefits that will be gained. Frequently, the benefits gained from such a study are experienced not by the research participants, but by others in society. Studies causing permanent damage to subjects violate the principles of the Nuremberg Code and should not be conducted (see Box 4.1).

📄 RESEARCH/EBP TIP

When assisting with studies that involve potential discomfort and harm, you must follow the study procedures exactly to minimize the risks to the participants. Ask the researcher about the participants' access to informational and support resources. These actions are part of your ethical responsibilities as a professional nurse.

Right to Fair Selection and Treatment

The right to fair selection and treatment is based on the ethical principle of justice. Justice demands that people be treated fairly and receive what they were promised. It also demands that people be treated in a way that is equitable to the treatment of other persons in the same situation. Inclusion criteria should reflect the research problem and study purpose and not the preferences or biases of the researcher. For example, you are studying the effects of a smart phone app on health behaviors of persons with hypertension but decide to collect data only at clinics in high-income neighborhoods. You live in one of these preferred neighborhoods. In this situation, you are unfairly excluding potential participants at clinics affiliated with a county-supported hospitals or participants unable to own a home. You are unfairly excluding persons who could potentially benefit from the app.

Another concern with participant selection is that some researchers select participants because they like them and want them to receive the benefits of a study. Other researchers have been swayed by incentives or money to ensure that certain patients become participants so that they can receive potentially beneficial treatments. Random selection of participants can eliminate some of the researchers' biases that may influence participant selection and strengthen the design of the study (see Chapter 9). When critically appraising a study, assess how the participants were selected and determine whether it was fair.

Fairness is not limited to participant recruitment. While conducting the study, the researcher must treat participants fairly and follow the procedures that were described in the study protocol and documented in the consent form. For example, the activities or procedures that participants are to perform should not be changed without the IRB's approval. The benefits promised to participants should be provided and distributed without regard for age, race, or socioeconomic level.

The report of a study needs to indicate that the selection and treatment of the participants were fair. For example, a team of researchers are testing the effects of meditation on work-related stresses of RNs in acute care who are in the first 5 years of their career. The inclusion criteria would be RNs employed in acute care for at least 1 year and less than 6 years. Exclusion criteria should be justified to protect potential participants who are at higher risk for harms or to avoid the unintentional influence of a participant's characteristics on the study results. An exclusion criterion for this study might be nurses who were working at more than one hospital or pursuing an advanced degree. Either of these conditions could influence the results of the study.

The responsible researcher designs the study to minimize discomfort and the risk of harm for potential participants, as well as protect their rights to self-determination, privacy, confidentiality, and fair selection and treatment. Details are usually not provided in the research report about how each of these was accomplished, but it should indicate the basic measures taken, such as keeping data confidential by assigning code numbers to participants' records. The guidelines that follow will assist you in critically appraising a study to ensure the protection of human rights, especially obtaining informed consent from persons vulnerable to undue influence or coercion. The informed consent aspects of protecting the human right of self-determination will be addressed in the next set of critical appraisal questions.

? CRITICAL APPRAISAL GUIDELINES

Protection of Human Rights

1. Were the participants' right to privacy protected and confidentiality of research data maintained during data collection, analysis, and reporting?
2. Was the participant's identifiable protected health information protected in compliance with the Common Rule and Privacy Rule (USDHHS, 2018b)?
3. Were the inclusion and exclusion criteria consistent with the study purpose?
4. Was participant selection conducted fairly? Were the participants treated equitably?
5. What aspects of the study could have been uncomfortable or harmful, if any? If so, what measures were in place to diminish discomfort and the potential for harm (USDHHS, 2018b)?

Mulholland et al. (2020) conducted a qualitative study of military families' experiences with deployment. The researchers were interested in how parents comforted their children and helped them adapt to the stressors of the experience. Because the study's open-ended questions were delivered to the participants online, the recruitment of potential participants was also conducted through Facebook, Instagram, and e-mail. The research excerpt in Research Example 4.1 includes the ethical aspects of the study related to protection from harm and maintenance of privacy and fairness.

RESEARCH EXAMPLE 4.1

Protection of Human Rights

Research Study Excerpt

This study was approved by the affiliated Institutional Review Board in November 2019. The researchers upheld the policies outlined in the Declaration of Helsinki, including the Federal Policy for the Protection of Human Subjects...Select demographic questions were used as a screening tool to determine the eligibility of the participant to be a part of the sample. Inclusion and exclusion criteria were established before obtaining data and were necessary to gather information that was current and relevant to the military community, but more specifically to military families with children that have experienced parental deployment...Data were recorded and initially stored on the web through a Google account, which was password protected and all information was obtained anonymously to ensure security. These data were transcribed into a Word document and Excel sheet, which was printed and distributed only to the researchers. (Mulholland et al., 2020, p. 36)

Critical Appraisal

One of the strengths of the study was that the inclusion criteria were congruent with the research problem and study purpose and were established before the study. Using internet-based recruitment strategies was appropriate because data were also going to be collected via the same media, and military families are more likely to have internet available. However, the researchers noted that their participants were primarily female and white. Potentially, the recruitment methods excluded some persons who were eligible for the study. The data were collected anonymously on a password-protected account. The ethical aspect of the study that received less attention was protection from discomfort and harm. There was no acknowledgment of the possibility that completing the questions may have been emotionally upsetting. More information about resources made available to participants if they become upset would have been helpful in determining whether the risks of the study were minimized.

RESEARCH/EBP TIP

In the same way that nurses maintain the confidentiality of patients' private information, nurses assisting with studies are expected to maintain the confidentiality of participants' data.

UNDERSTANDING INFORMED CONSENT

What is informed consent for research? It is very similar to informed consent for surgical procedures. Informed consent is providing information to a potential participant and giving the person the opportunity to participate in the study. The process does not end with the participant's signature on a document agreeing to be in a study (Farmer & Lundy, 2017). The researcher or the nurse obtaining consent is guided by the principle of beneficence and committed to the protection of the right to self-determination. The nurse describes the study and what participants will be asked to do. A potential participant's decision about whether to participate is the consenting part of the process. When obtaining consent, nurses need to be knowledgeable of the culture of potential participants. In some cultures a potential participant is expected to consult the family before consenting, or a woman is expected to ask her husband for permission. As a nurse, you may need to remember what you have learned about different cultures when you approach potential participants. If the risks and benefits of participating change during the study, the researcher and

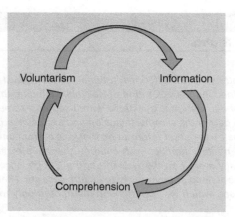

FIG. 4.2 Required elements of consent.

nurses assisting with the study maintain trust by sharing that information with participants. Participants provide ongoing consent by continuing to participate in the study, with the assurance that they can withdraw at any time.

Four Elements of Informed Consent

Informed consent is incomplete or unethical unless four required elements are incorporated (Fig. 4.2). The researcher must *disclose* essential information about the study to potential participants in a way that can be understood. The second element is the extent to which the potential participant *comprehends* the information. The final elements are the *competence* of the potential participant and the person's *voluntary agreement* to take part in the study (Scholton & Gather, 2021). The connections among these required elements are shown in Fig. 4.2.

Disclosure

The revision to the Common Rule changed the focus of the consent process from sharing every possible detail of a study to providing understandable and relevant information on which to decide about participation (USDHHS, 2018b). Box 4.3 contains the characteristics of a quality informed consent document. HIPAA authorization and broad consent for future use of research specimens, discussed earlier in the chapter, may be included in the consent for a study or may be separate.

You must document the information that was shared with participants, and their signatures denote they have volunteered to participate. A **consent form** is a written document that includes the elements of informed consent required by the Common Rule (USDHHS, 2018b). A consent form may also include other information required by the institution in which the study is to be conducted or by the agency funding the study. For federally funded clinical trials, a copy of the IRB-approved consent form must be posted on a publicly available website (USDHHS, 2018b).

Comprehension

Informed consent implies not only that the researcher has imparted information to the persons being recruited to be in the study but also that the prospective participants have comprehended that information. In their systematic review, Pietrzykowski and Smilowska (2021) included 14 studies of participants' understanding of different components of the informed consent. They found that about half of the participants did not understand one or more aspects of consent, such as the freedom to withdraw without penalty. Health literacy was correlated with the participant's

BOX 4.3 **CHARACTERISTICS OF INFORMED CONSENT**
General Requirements
Comprehendible
• Language that is understandable • Opportunity provided to discuss and make a deliberate decision without pressure
Complete but Concise
• Information that a reasonable person would want to decide whether to participate
Comprehensive
• Purpose and procedures of the research study • Length of participant's involvement • Benefits and risks or discomforts • Compensation, if any, for research-related injury • Disclosure of alternative treatments if available • Confidentiality of records • Contact persons • Right to refuse or withdraw without loss of benefits

From US Department of Health and Human Services (USDHHS). (2018b). *Subpart A of 45 CFR Part 46: Basic HHS policy for the protection of human subjects.* Retrieved from https://www.hhs.gov/ohrp/sites/default/files/revised-common-rule-reg-text-unofficial-2018-requirements.pdf

ability to comprehend the content of the informed consent document. The Common Rule, as well as other standards, requires that specific language be included in the informed consent document, which makes adjusting the reading level to the expected reading level of the sample challenging (Ennever et al., 2019).

The researcher must take the time to teach the participants about the study. The amount of information to be taught depends on the participant's prior knowledge of research and the specific research topic. Researchers need to discuss the benefits and risks of a study in detail, with examples that the potential participants can understand. Nurses often serve as patient advocates in clinical agencies and need to assess participants' understanding of the purpose and potential risks and benefits of the study (ANA, 2015; Axson et al., 2019; Barlow, 2020).

Competence

Autonomous persons, who can understand the benefits and risks of a proposed study, are competent to give consent. Persons with diminished autonomy because of legal or mental incompetence or confinement to an institution are not legally competent to consent to participate in research. In a study involving older persons who may have cognitive decline or other participants with possible decreased competence, the researchers must report how the competence of the participants was determined before the informed consent process (Scholton & Gather, 2021).

Voluntary Agreement

Voluntary agreement means that the prospective participant has decided to take part in a study of his or her own volition, without coercion or any undue influence (USDHHS, 2018b). Researchers ask potential participants who are competent to make the decision to volunteer to be in a study. However, a researcher cannot allow a person to volunteer without the person comprehending essential information about the study. All these elements of informed consent need to be documented in a consent form and discussed in the research report.

> **📄 RESEARCH/EBP TIP**
>
> The informed consent process includes providing a potential participant the essential information about the study, ensuring that the person comprehends the purpose and procedures of the study, and assessing the competence of the person to decide whether to participant. When these three components are present and the person agrees to participate, the consent document can be signed.

Documentation of Informed Consent

The documentation of informed consent may vary depending on a study's level of risk and the requirements of a specific IRB. Most studies require a written consent form that the participant signs. The participant also receives a copy of the consent form. There are three categories of situations in which the process of obtaining and documenting consent may be altered.

When recruiting participants with diminished autonomy, the informed consent may need to be signed by the legal authorized representative. When a participant has some comprehension of the study and volunteers to participate, the participant and the representative sign the informed consent document. The representative indicates his or her relationship with the participant under the signature. Sometimes nurses are asked to sign a consent form as a witness for a biomedical study. To ethically witness a signature on a consent form, the nurse must assess the participant's understanding of the study and its potential risks (Barlow, 2020).

When potential participants may not be able to read but can comprehend the risks and benefits of a study, the IRB may approve an oral presentation of the study. The researcher will prepare a summary of the study that is read aloud and explained as needed. A witness observes the consent process and ensures that the presentation includes the required content of the study summary approved by the IRB. The participant signs a short statement that he or she was provided the summary of the study information and volunteers to participate. The researcher and the witness also sign the statement and the written summary of the study that was orally presented. The participant is given a copy of the short form and the written summary.

In some minimal risk studies, the requirement for written consent is waived. Studies in which a signed consent can be waived usually involve procedures that do not normally require a signature outside of the research context. An example is anonymously answering questions about your family structure or the social support you receive from friends. An IRB may also approve a waiver when the signed document would be the only connection between the person and the study in situations in which confidentiality is especially a concern. For example, a waiver might be approved when the sample is women living with HIV infection and the topic is disclosing HIV status to friends and family members. The researcher provides information to the potential participants, answers their questions, and obtains their verbal agreement. Signed consent may also be waived if the potential participants are members of a culture or community in which signing documents is not the norm (USDHHS, 2018b). An ethical researcher will talk with the members of the group to identify an alternative mechanism to document the consent, such as using a thumbprint instead of a signature or stating aloud one's agreement to participate.

> **📄 RESEARCH/EBP TIP**
>
> Nurses practicing in community organizations can facilitate studies being conducted with their patients by introducing researchers to key community leaders. To effectively implement studies in potentially vulnerable communities, nurse researchers must involve community leaders and nurses familiar with the culture of the community in determining the best way to obtain informed consent.

Studies in which the researcher or data collector interacts with the participants require obtaining informed consent. The content of the consent document and the process of obtaining consent must meet the Common Rule requirements for ethical conduct of research. Research reports often discuss the consent process and identify some of the essential consent information that was provided to the potential participants. Reports should include some information about the consent process, but the depth of the discussion will vary according to the research purpose and types of participants included in the study. The consent process is usually presented in the "Methods" section under a discussion of study procedures or the data collection process. The following critical appraisal guidelines will assist you in examining the consent process of a published study or for a study to be conducted in your clinical agency. The purpose of the questions is to ensure that the participant's right to self-determination is protected.

? CRITICAL APPRAISAL GUIDELINES

Informed Consent Process

1. How was informed consent obtained from the participants?
2. Did the participants have diminished autonomy because of legal or mental incompetence, physical condition, or imprisonment? If the participants were not competent to give consent, did their legally authorized representatives give consent?
3. Were children included as participants in the study? If so, was assent obtained? Did the parents or guardians give permission for the child to participate?
4. Were the participants vulnerable to undue influence or coercion? If so, what precautions were taken to avoid potential participants feeling pressured to participate?
5. Was the essential information for consent provided and comprehended by the participants? Were measures taken to ensure that low-literacy participants and participants with diminished autonomy understood the study requirements?
6. Did it seem that the participants voluntarily consented to be in the study?

Mastel-Smith et al. (2019) conducted a pilot study to determine the effect of Tai Chi and electronic tablet interventions on older adults, specifically their health and cognition. The study is described in Research Example 4.2. The participants were recruited from assisted living centers. The initial study was a randomized trial with a planned sample of 60 older adults to be divided into three groups. One group was to participate in Tai Chi, another was to receive an electronic tablet with an explanation of how it could be used, and the third group was to be the control group. However, the researchers were able to recruit only 26 participants who were randomized into two intervention groups. A qualitative component was added to understand the quantitative results. This research report was like most reports in that there was minimal discussion about the informed consent process.

◢ RESEARCH EXAMPLE 4.2

Informed Consent

Research Study Excerpt

The research, including recruitment materials, was approved by the university's institutional review board where the authors are employed and the residence vice president of program development. To ensure understanding, participants reflected study purpose and procedures. All participants provided signed
Continued

◢ RESEARCH EXAMPLE 4.2—cont'd

informed consent....A second institutional review board application was approved for the qualitative strand and written consent obtained. (Mastel-Smith et al., 2019, p. 166)

Critical Appraisal

Minimal details of the informed consent process were described. The researchers used the Modified Mini-Mental Examination (Bland & Newman, 2001) to assess the residents' cognitive status before the informed consent process. They also requested consent from residents to refer them to the director of nursing if they scored less than the required score of 79 on the Modified Mini-Mental Examination and did not have any diagnosis of cognitive impairment. Referring participants for additional health-related evaluation and seeking their permission for the referral are consistent with nursing's ethical standards. However, the score on the examination was not used to exclude potential participants. The report included a flowchart of participants from recruitment to study completion. The flowchart indicated that the researchers excluded two of the recruited participants because they could not describe the study process and procedures after reading the consent form. The inability to comprehend the informed consent was an appropriate reason for not including these prospective participants.

The sample for the study did not include any children but rather adults residing in assisted living centers. The older adults did not seem to be coerced to participate because seven of them refused to participate for different reasons. The IRB reviewed the informed consent as part of the researchers' application for study approval, and they deemed the informed consent to meet the appropriate standards. In addition, the researchers obtained a second IRB approval for the qualitative part of the study. Participation was preceded by voluntary consent.

UNDERSTANDING INSTITUTIONAL REVIEW

An IRB is a committee that reviews research to ensure that the researcher who is proposing a study has a plan for ethical implementation. IRBs have the authority to approve, require modifications, and disapprove studies they review. If unforeseen problems occur during a study, the IRB is notified, the study is stopped until the issue is resolved, and the IRB approves the continuation of the study. Universities, hospitals, corporations, and other healthcare organizations have IRBs to promote the conduct of ethical research and protect the rights of prospective participants at their institutions. Federal regulations provide details about the composition and functions of IRBs (USDHHS, 2018b).

Institutional Review Board Composition and Function

Each IRB has at least five members of varying backgrounds—cultural, economic, educational, gender, and racial—to promote complete, scholarly, and fair review of research conducted in an institution (USDHHS, 2018b). At least one member has scientific expertise, and at least one member is a community member without scientific training. The same member or another member is not affiliated with the institution in any way. If an institution regularly reviews studies with participants who may be vulnerable to coercion or undue influence, one or more members of the IRB should have experience working with persons who are like the potential participants. All members are expected to be sensitive to the attitudes of the community it serves. Before serving on an IRB, the members are provided training on protecting the rights of human participants (USDHHS, 2018b).

Before a hospital or university can receive a federal grant to conduct research, its IRB must register with the Office of Human Research Protection (USDHHS, 2017) and obtain a federal-wide assurance (FWA). An FWA indicates that an institution's IRB has identified its ethical standard and agrees to comply with the Common Rule. To receive an FWA, an IRB must have written policies for membership and processes, and maintain records of all studies reviewed and the subsequent decisions (USDHHS, 2018b).

Levels of Reviews for Studies

The chairperson of the IRB determines the level of a review that a study must have to be approved. The level of research depends on the potential risks to the study participants. The revised Common Rule expanded the types of study that are exempt from review. Studies that are exempt from review include anonymous completion of surveys, interviews with participants in a government project, and analysis of de-identified data collected for another purpose. Box 4.4 contains a list of some of the types of studies that are exempt from review. Once evaluated to be an exempt study, the IRB does not require a continuing review of the study.

Studies that involve minimal risks to participants undergo expedited review. Instead of all the IRB's members reviewing the study, the IRB chairperson or one or more experienced IRB members conduct the expedited review (USDHHS, 2018b). The person conducting an expedited review can approve the study but cannot disapprove a study. If the reviewer does not approve a study, the study will be reviewed by all IRB members during a meeting. Examples of studies that may receive expedited review are provided in Box 4.5. Descriptive studies usually need only expedited review. Studies approved by expedited review do not require a continuing review every year.

Any study that involves more than minimal risk is reviewed by the IRB during a convened meeting. A full review of a study allows the researcher to describe their study, including how they can minimize the risks of the study and ensure fair selection of participants. Researchers proposing studies that require full IRB review may be asked questions about how they will obtain informed

---

BOX 4.4 SELECTED CHARACTERISTICS AND EXAMPLES OF STUDIES EXEMPT FROM REVIEW BY AN INSTITUTIONAL REVIEW BOARD

Will Be Conducted in Established Education Settings
- Correlational study of the relationship between the effectiveness of an innovative teaching strategy with class characteristics

Will Use Education Tests, Surveys, Interviews, or Observation of Public Behavior With Participant Not Identified and Minimal Risks With the Data Not Linked to the Participant
- Descriptive study with anonymous online data collection using a social support scale and demographic questionnaire

Will Use a Benign Behavioral Intervention[a] and Data That Were Not Linked to Participants
- Quasi-experimental study comparing knowledge of diabetes gained through playing an online game with knowledge gained through an oral presentation

Will Use Data That Were Publicly Available, De-Identified, or Collected to Evaluate Government Projects or Public Services
- Exploratory-descriptive qualitative study of program participants' written evaluation of the services of a federally supported clinic

[a]The Common Rule describes benign behavioral interventions as short noninvasive actions that are not expected to be offensive, embarrassing, or have a lasting adverse effect (USDHHS, 2018b).
Adapted from US Department of Health and Human Services (USDHHS). (2018b). *Subpart A of 45 CFR Part 46: Basic HHS policy for the protection of human subjects.* Retrieved from https://www.hhs.gov/ohrp/sites/default/files/revised-common-rule-reg-text-unofficial-2018-requirements.pdf

---

BOX 4.5 SELECTED CHARACTERISTICS AND EXAMPLES OF STUDIES ELIGIBLE FOR EXPEDITED REVIEW BY INSTITUTIONAL REVIEW BOARD

Data Collected by One of the Following Means
Small Amounts of Blood Collected by Venipuncture or Finger Stick
• Quasi-experimental study comparing fasting blood sugar readings of persons with diabetes receiving weekly phone calls about diet and exercise compared with those receiving usual care

Voice, Video, or Digital Recordings of Interviews and Focus Groups
• Grounded theory study of the experience of mothering adopted children with data collected by interview

Medical Records, When Participants Can Potentially Be Identified
• Descriptive comparative study of nutritional status of patients with community-acquired pressure ulcers to that of patients with hospital-acquired pressure ulcers

Questionnaires or Surveys of Cultural Beliefs, Communication, Perception, and Social Behavior
• Predictive correlational study of cultural beliefs and use of emergency department by underinsured and uninsured persons

---

consent and protect the confidentiality of the participants. Studies involving participants that may be more susceptible to coercion or undue influence will undergo full board review. Other studies that are likely to require full board review may involve safety risks or treatments that may potentially cause harm.

Researchers proposing studies with more than minimal risks for participants will have a plan to monitor the results related to safety concerns and to provide resources that may be needed. For example, a nurse researcher interviewing women who have experienced a sexual assault might have a counselor who can be called if a participant becomes distressed or provide a list of community support groups for all participants. If the ongoing monitoring of safety concerns raises a concern, participants must be notified and asked if they wished to continue in the study. Participants also must be notified if preliminary results might influence a participant's decision to continue participation (USDHHS, 2018b). For example, in a study comparing two medications, the researcher identifies that one medication is causing dramatic improvements in the health of the participants in the treatment group. Participants who are in the other group would need to be notified. They may choose to withdraw from the study, or the researcher may stop the study and collaborate with the participants' healthcare providers to offer the effective medications to all participants.

A major factor in determining whether an IRB can approve a study is whether the risks to participants are reasonable in relation to anticipated benefits (USDHHS, 2018b). To determine this balance, or benefit/risk ratio, the benefits and risks associated with the study's procedures and potential outcomes of the study are assessed. Whether the research is therapeutic or nontherapeutic affects the potential benefits for participants. In therapeutic research, participants benefit from the study procedures in areas such as skin care, range of motion, touch, and other nursing or medical interventions. The benefits might include improved confidence, physical well-being, and decreased anxiety. Nontherapeutic research does not benefit participants directly but is needed to generate knowledge that can be used to help other patients or communities. If the risks outweigh the benefits, the study may be unethical and will not be approved. If the benefits outweigh the risks, the study has passed one of the tests for being ethical research.

> ### 📄 RESEARCH/EBP TIP
>
> Before assisting with a study, nurses should ask the level of IRB review the study received. Exempt and expeditated levels of review indicate participants are expected to experience only minimal or temporary discomfort. Studies that receive full IRB review are those with greater risks for discomfort and harm.

Most published studies indicate that IRB approval was obtained but do not indicate whether the study was exempt from review, received an expedited review, or was reviewed by the full IRB. Researchers are required to identify in a published research report the IRBs that reviewed and approved the study. When studies are conducted in multiple locations, the revised Common Rule allows a single IRB to be designated to review the study for the other locations (USDHHS, 2018b). Another approach is that the multiple IRBs may conduct a joint review or accept the review of another institution. The revision to the Common Rule that allows one IRB to approve the study for multiple sites was implemented to increase efficiency by reducing duplication of effort (USDHHS, 2018b).

The following questions can be used to critically appraise the ethical aspects of a study. These critical appraisal questions build on the previous guidelines and are intended to help you summarize or draw conclusions about the ethical conduct of the study.

❓ CRITICAL APPRAISAL GUIDELINES

Overall Ethical Aspects of a Study

1. Was IRB approval documented in the research report?
2. Which level of review (exempt, expedited, or full) did the study warrant, in your opinion?
3. What were the benefits and risks of participating in the study?
4. What measures did the researchers take to minimize the risks and ensure the benefits?
5. Using the previous guidelines about consent, was informed consent ethically obtained from the participants?
6. Using the previous guidelines about protecting participants' rights, were the rights of the participants protected during the study?
7. Summarize your conclusions about the ethical aspects of the study.

Omran and Callis (2021) conducted a qualitative study of bereavement among 10 critical care nurses. After IRB approval, data were collected through a focus group. The researchers explored the death of critically ill patients and the nurses' perceptions of how they processed their grief. The person conducting the focus group knew all the participants before the study. An excerpt from the study is provided followed by the critical appraisal of the ethical aspects of the study in Research Example 4.3.

⚔ RESEARCH EXAMPLE 4.3

Overall Ethical Aspects of a Study

Utilizing purposeful sampling, the critical care bedside nurses were asked to talk about their experiences in a focus group on the topic of bereavement related to the death of patients under their care...All participants were employed at the same facility. (Omran & Callis, 2021, p. 85)

Because of the sensitive nature and emotional vulnerability of this topic, participants were informed there may be some discomfort. The likelihood of the participants recently experiencing a loss was high because of the nature of their job....The researcher gained approval from the university institutional review board

Continued

RESEARCH EXAMPLE 4.3—cont'd

prior to conducting the focus group. The researcher created a participation letter, which explained the research topic, purpose of the study, and that participation was optional and all data would be kept confidential....Each participant chose a pseudonym to go by during the session. No birth names or personal identifiers were associated with any data. (Omran & Callis, 2021, p. 86)

Critical Appraisal

IRB approval was noted in the report. A qualitative study on a more benign topic would have been deemed to be an exempt study. However, a study on the topic of bereavement would have warranted an expedited, or possibly a full, review. The benefits of participating included the opportunity to process grief in a supportive environment. The researchers noted the potential for discomfort in the participation letter so that participants would have that information before deciding to volunteer for the study. No specific mention was made of informed consent documents being signed. Risks were minimized by the researcher by using pseudonyms during the focus group, which prevented the loss of confidentiality when other people read the transcripts or the study report. A threat to confidentiality that was not addressed by Omran and Callis (2021) was that the participants knew each other and worked in the same facility. It is likely that, at the beginning of the focus group, the researcher asked participants to agree not to talk to anyone outside the focus group about what was shared during the group. Being vulnerable among people with whom you will continue to interact poses some emotional risk that was not mentioned in the report. Overall the rights of the participants were protected during and after the study, supporting the conclusion that the study was ethical.

CURRENT ISSUES IN RESEARCH ETHICS

The constant changes in health care and technology create new challenges in research ethics. In this section, two areas that continue to evolve are issues related to genomics research and research misconduct.

Genomics Research

Genomic research is an area of science with great potential to expand human knowledge and create new treatments for diseases. However, genomic research also has great potential for harm. Your genetic code is unique, which allows you to be identified. This ability to be identified makes it difficult to protect confidentiality and prevent future discrimination related to employment and approval for health insurance. Conducting research using the DNA contained in those specimens collected for clinical purposes can make protecting the participants' rights of self-determination and informed consent uniquely challenging. From the beginning of the Human Genome Project, the funding agencies have invested millions of dollars in the study of the legal, ethical, and social challenges related to genetic research. Despite these investments, many issues remain, and some segments of the public mistrust healthcare research involving DNA because of cases in which genetic materials were misused.

An example of unethical research occurred in the 1990s, when researchers began collecting blood from members of the Havasupai tribe for a study of genetics and diabetes (Caplan & Moreno, 2011). Unfortunately, the researchers used the blood specimens to study other topics, such as schizophrenia and tribal origin (Garrison, 2013). The tribe sued Arizona State University, the sponsor of the original study, and was awarded a settlement in 2010. Part of the settlement was the release of the remaining blood samples to the tribe to be disposed of in a culturally appropriate way.

In another example, Skloot (2010) published a book about Henrietta Lacks, a poor young black mother who was diagnosed with cervical cancer. Seen at a John Hopkins University clinic that accepted black patients (Sodeke & Powell, 2019), a portion of her cancerous tissue was given to a scientist, Dr. Gey. Dr. Gey was searching for human cells that would replicate themselves in a test tube. Much to his surprise, Henrietta's cells replicated themselves and kept replicating. Other researchers, building on Dr. Gey's work, developed a cell line from Mrs. Lacks's tissue that has become known as HeLa cells (Wolinetz & Collins, 2020). Major scientific discoveries and effective treatments, such as the polio vaccine and in vitro fertilization, have been developed using HeLa cells. Researchers and companies that used HeLa Cells to develop new treatments received literally billions of dollars from their innovations. In 2017 Mrs. Lacks's family sued John Hopkins University for compensation (Cassel & Bindman, 2019; McDaniels, 2017).

These two cases identify some of the unresolved issues in genetic research, such as de-identification of data. There is concern that by its very nature, genomic data cannot be completely de-identified (Terry, 2015). Genetic data, even when identifying information has been removed as required, can be combined with data from genetic genealogy databases and other publicly available demographic databases to identify a participant. Other unresolved issues include whether participants' DNA can be retrieved and removed should they choose to withdraw from the study and whether participants will be notified about other studies being conducted with their DNA. Potential participants may hesitate to consent to the use of the specimens because of concerns their genetic information would be available to future employers. The Genetic Information Nondiscrimination Act prohibits the use of genetic information in employment decisions, but knowing about the law may not alleviate participants' concerns (Wolf et al., 2019).

Broad consent was included in the revised Common Rule to address some of these concerns (USDHHS, 2018b). When individuals allow their biospecimens to be retained for future studies, the broad consent document will include information about possible studies that may be conducted using the specimens and whether the researchers will contact the individuals if the research reveals a preventable health problem (Wolf et al., 2020). Nurses involved in genetic studies need to be aware of the relevant state laws that may have stricter requirements, such as separate consent being required for each study using a person's genetic data. Some states have laws that allow a person access to his or her own genetic data (Wolf et al., 2020). Despite legal complexities, broad consent increases the capability of research institutes and universities to conduct genomic research. Critical appraisal of genomic research based on a research report includes understanding the decisions made by the researchers, the type of consent that was obtained, and discussion of the issues surrounding human protection from harm.

Research Misconduct

To generate sound scientific knowledge, research must involve rigorous methods and honest reporting and publication of the findings. The Office of Research Integrity (ORI) was created within the USDHHS in response to reports of altered data and study results. Research misconduct is defined as "the fabrication, falsification, or plagiarism in processing, performing, or reviewing research, or in reporting research results" (US Public Health Services [PHS], 2011). The prevalence of research misconduct is increasing in all disciplines, including nursing (Clark & Thompson, 2019). Research misconduct is an intentional act that involves a significant departure from the acceptable practice of the scientific community for maintaining the integrity of the research record.

Research misconduct does not include honest mistakes or differences of opinion but does include plagiarism, fabrication in research, and falsification of research (Gloviczki & Lawrence, 2021). Plagiarism is using the words or ideas of another person without citing the reference or otherwise giving that person credit. Plagiarism involves use of an idea or the word-for-word use of a sentence or paragraph without indicating the source. Fabrication occurs when researchers add data to the research record that were not collected from participants and create results that did not occur. For example, a researcher may create a figure for a research report from fabricated data. Falsification occurs when researchers manipulate equipment, alter statistical results, or omit results that do not support the study's hypotheses (PHS, 2011). Another type of falsification occurs when researchers add well-known experts or mentors to a grant proposal, even when that person has not contributed to the proposal, to increase the credibility and fundability of the proposal. This practice breaks several federal laws related to making false claims and statements to the federal government (Fong et al., 2020).

A review of case summaries from 2020 and 2021 indicated that most of the research misconduct involved cellular or animal research (ORI, 2021). However, one case included five grant applications submitted to the National Institute of Nursing Research that included falsified and fabricated data. Another case was proven to have begun with the respondent's dissertation, required the retraction of 14 published articles, and resulted in the university revoking his PhD (ORI, 2021). These instances are alarming because of the extent of the research misconduct.

One of the more common types of research misconduct is duplicate publications. Duplicate publication occurs when multiple papers report the same results from the same study. Researchers may recycle text from previous articles without referencing the source, a practice called self-plagiarism (Horbach & Halffman, 2019). The work of researchers in academic settings is evaluated by the number of articles they publish. Researchers may publish multiple articles from a single study to have the necessary publications to be promoted. During a literature review, you may find multiple articles by the same authors that report similar results. One article may describe the results of a subset of the sample, while another reports the results of a different group of participants. Duplicate publications magnify the effects of a single study and may skew the results when included in a systematic review or meta-analysis. Literature reviews should include the results of each study one time to avoid biasing the conclusions.

Even if you are never involved in seeking federal funding or publishing multiple research papers, there are steps you can take to avoid research misconduct in your scholarly work. Box 4.6 contains tips for maintaining the accuracy and veracity of the studies in which you are involved.

BOX 4.6 ACTIONS TO ENSURE THE ACCURACY AND TRUTHFULNESS OF STUDIES

1. Witness signatures on informed consent documents after you ensure the participants understand the benefits and risks of the study.
2. Be sure any data you collect are accurate and entered correctly into the database.
3. When providing a study's intervention, implement it exactly as prescribed in the protocol.
4. Participate in meetings of the research team.
5. Voice any concerns you have about the study to the primary investigator. If concerns are not addressed, communicate your concerns to the investigator's supervisor.
6. Become an author on a study's report only if you have contributed to the study and preparation of the report.

KEY POINTS

- Four experimental projects have been highly publicized for their unethical treatment of human subjects: the Nazi medical experiments, the Tuskegee Syphilis Study, the Willowbrook Study, and the Jewish Chronic Disease Hospital Study.
- Three documents were developed as the result of the unethical studies and have become the basis for ethical research: the Nuremberg Code, the Declaration of Helsinki, and the Belmont Report.
- The principles of respect for persons, beneficence, and justice are the foundation for the protection of human rights.
- Five human rights require protection during research: self-determination, privacy, anonymity and confidentiality, fair selection and treatment, and protection from discomfort and harm.
- The Common Rule, a set of federal regulations, guides the ethical conduct in research.
- Informed consent involves the disclosure of essential information about the study, comprehension of the information by a competent person, and voluntary agreement to participate.
- An IRB consists of a committee of peers who review research proposals to determine whether the researchers have designed their studies to protect the rights of human participants.
- The level of IRB review that a proposal requires—exempt, expedited, or full review—depends on the risk for harm and discomfort and the vulnerability of the proposed sample.
- Genomic research involves unique ethical challenges because of the potential that the participant can be identified by the data and the ability to store biospecimens for future studies.
- Research misconduct is defined as intentional acts that can be classified as plagiarism, falsification, or fabrication of data.

REFERENCES

Alexander, S., Pillay, R., & Smith, B. (2018). A systematic review of the experiences of vulnerable people participating in research on sensitive topics. *International Journal of Nursing Studies, 88*, 85–96. https://doi.org/10.1016/j.ijnurstu.2018.08.013

Alsan, M., Wanamaker, M., & Hardeman, R. (2020). The Tuskegee study of untreated syphilis: A case study in peripheral trauma with implications for health professionals. *Journal of General and Internal Medicine, 35*(1), 322–325. https://doi.org/10.1007/s11606-019-05309-8

American Nurses Association (ANA). (2015). *Code of ethics for nurses with interpretive statements.* Author.

Artal, R., & Rubenfeld, S. (2017). Ethical issues in research. *Best Practice & Research in Clinical Obstetrics & Gynaecology, 43*, 107–114. http://dx.doi.org/10.1016/j.bpobgyn.2016.12.006

Axson, S., Giordano, N., Hermann, R., & Ulrich, C. (2019). Evaluating nurse understanding and participation in the informed consent process. *Nursing Ethics, 26*(4), 1050–1061. https://doi.org/10.1177/0969733017740175

Barlow, C. (2020). Human subjects protection and federal regulations of clinical trials. *Seminars in Oncology Nursing, 36*, 151001. https://doi.org/10.1016/j.soncn.2020.151001

Beecher, H. K. (1966). Ethics and clinical research. *New England Journal of Medicine, 274*(24), 1354–1360. https://www.nejm.org/doi/full/10.1056/NEJM196606162742405

Berger, R. L. (1990). Nazi science: The Dachau hypothermia experiments. *New England Journal of Medicine, 322*(20), 1435–1440. https://doi.org/10.1056/NEJM199005173222006

Bland, R. C., & Newman, S. C. (2001). Mild dementia or cognitive impairment: The Modified Mini-Mental State Examination (3MS) as a screen for dementia. *Canadian Journal of Psychiatry, 46*, 506–510. https://doi.org/10.1177/070674370104600604

Brandt, A. M. (1978). Racism and research: The case of the Tuskegee syphilis study. *Hastings Center Report, 8*(6), 21–29. http://www.jstor.org/stable/3561468

Brothers, K., Clayton, E., & Goldenberg, A. (2020). Online pediatric research: Addressing consent, assent, and parental permission. *Journal of Law, Medicine, and Ethics, 48*(S1), 129–137. https://doi.org/10.1177/1073110520917038

Caplan, A., & Moreno, J. (2011). The Havasu 'Baaja tribe and informed consent. *Lancet, 377*(9766), 621–622. https://doi.org/10.1016/S0140-6736(10)60818-5

Cassel, C., & Bindman, A. (2019). Risks, benefits, and fairness in a big data world. *Journal of the American Medical Association, 322*(2), 105–106. https://doi.org/10.1001/jama.2019.9523

Clark, A., & Thompson, D. (2019). Editorial. How to minimize research misconduct? Priorities for academics in nursing. *Journal of Advanced Nursing, 76*, 751–753. https://doi.org/10.1111/jan.14273

Eastwood, G. (2015). Ethical issues in gastroenterology research. *Journal of Gasteroenterology and Hepatology, 30*(S1), 8–11. https://doi.org/10.1111/jgh.12755

Ennever, F., Nabi, S., Bass, P., Huang, L., & Fogler, E. (2019). Developing language to communicate privacy and confidentiality protections to potential clinical trial subjects: Meshing requirements under six applicable regulations, laws, guidelines and funding policies. *Journal of Research Administration, 50*(1), 20–44. Retrieved https://www.srainternational.org/blogs/martha-jack/2019/04/04/developing-language-to-communicate-privacy-and-con

Farmer, L., & Lundy, A. (2017). Informed consent: Legal and ethical considerations for advanced practice nurses. *Journal of Nurse Practitioners, 13*(2), 124–130. http://doi.org/10.1016/j.nurpra.2016.08.011

Fong. E., Wilhite, A., Hickman, C., & Lee, Y. (2020). The legal consequences of research misconduct: False investigators and grant proposals. *Journal of Law, Medicine, & Ethics, 48*, 331–339. https://doi.org/10.1177/1073110520935347

Garrison, N. (2013). Genomic justice for Native Americans: Impact of the Havasupai case on genetic research. *Science, Technology, & Human Values, 38*(2), 201–233. https://doi.org/10.1177/0162243912470009

Gloviczki, P., & Lawrence, P. (Eds.). (2021). Information for authors and editorial policy. *Journal of Vascular Surgery, 71*(1), e1–e12. https://doi.org/10.1016/S0741-5214(19)32743-0

Gray, J. R., & Grove, S. K. (2021). *The practice of nursing research: Appraisal, synthesis, and generation of evidence* (9th ed.). Elsevier.

Hershey, N., & Miller, R. D. (1976). *Human experimentation and the law.* Aspen.

Hodapp, J., Ali, S., & Drendel, A. (2020). Bringing it all together: A review of the challenges of measuring children's satisfaction as a key component of acute pain management. *Children, 7*, 243. https://doi.org/10.3390/children7110243

Horbach, S., & Halffman, W. (2019). The extent and causes of academic text recycling or 'self-plagiarism.' *Research Policy, 48*, 492–502. http://dx.doi.org/10.1016/j.respol.2017.09.004

Jaiswal, J. (2019). Whose responsibility is it to dismantle medical mistrust? Future directions for researchers and health care providers. *Behavioral Medicine, 45*(2), 188–196. https://doi.org/10.1080/08964289.2019.1630357

Levine, R. (1988). *Ethics and regulation of clinical research* (2nd ed.). Yale University Press.

Macapagal, K., Bettin, E., Matson, M., Kraus, A., Fisher, C., & Mustanski, B. (2019). Measuring discomfort in health research relative to everyday events and routine care: An application to sexual and gender minority youth. *Journal of Adolescent Health, 64*, 594–601. https://doi.org/10.1016/j.jadohealth.2018.10.293

Maloy, J., & Bass, P. (2020). Understanding broad consent. *Ochsner Journal, 20*, 81–86. http://doi.org/10.31486/toj.19.0088

Martien, N., & Nelligan, J. (2018). *The sourcebook for clinical research: A practical guide for study conduct.* Elsevier. https://doi.org/10.1016/B978-0-12-816242-2.00005-9

Mastel-Smith, B., Duke, G., & He, Z. (2019). A pilot randomized control trial examining the effects of Tai Chi and electronic tablet use on older adults' cognition and health. *Journal of Holistic Nursing, 37*(2), 163–174. https://doi.org/10.1177/0898010118792961

McDaniels, A. (2017, February). Henrietta Lacks's family wants compensation for her cells. *The Washington Post.* Retrieved from https://www.washingtonpost.com/local/henrietta-lackss-family-wants-compensation-for-her-cells/2017/02/14/816481ba-f302-11e6-b9c9-e83fce42fb61_story.html

Menikoff, J., Kaneshiro, J., & Pritchard, I. (2017). The Common Rule updated. *New England Journal of Medicine, 376*(7), 613–615. https://doi.org/10.1056/NEJMp1700736

Milgram, S. (1963). Behavioral study of obedience. *Journal of Abnormal and Social Psychology, 67*(4), 371–378. https://doi.org/10.1037/h0040525

Mulholland, E., Dahlberg, D., & McDowell, L. (2020). A two-front war: Exploring military families' battle with parental deployment. *Journal of Pediatric Nursing, 54*, 34–41. https://doi.org/10.1016/j.pedn.2020.05.019

National Commission for the Protection of Human Subjects of Biomedical and Behavioral Research. (1979).

Belmont Report: Ethical principles and guidelines for research involving human subjects [DHEW Publication No. (05) 78-0012]. U.S. Government Printing Office. Retrieved from https://www.hhs.gov/ohrp/regulations-and-policy/belmont-report/index.html

Office of Research Integrity (ORI). (2021). *Case summaries.* Retrieved from https://ori.hhs.gov/content/case_summary

Omran, T., & Callis, A. (2021). Bereavement needs of critical care nurses: A qualitative study. *Dimensions of Critical Care Nursing, 40*(2), 83–91. https://doi.org/1097/DCC.0000000000000460

Øye, C., Sørensen, N., Dahl, H., & Glasdam, S. (2019). Tight ties in collaborative health research puts research ethics on trial? A discussion on autonomy, confidentiality, and integrity in qualitative research. *Qualitative Health Research, 29*(8), 1227–1235. https://doi.org/10.1177/1049732318822294

Parasidis, E., Pike, E., & McGraw, D. (2019). A Belmont Report for health data. *New England Journal of Medicine, 380*(16), 1493–1495. https://doi.org/10.1056/NEJMp1816373

Pietrzykowski, T., & Smilowska, K. (2021). The reality of informed consent: Empirical studies on patient comprehension—systemic review. *Trials, 22*, 57. https://doi.org/10.1186/s13063-020-04969-w

Presidential Commission for the Study of Bioethical Issues. (2012). *Privacy and progress in whole genome sequencing.* http://www.bioethics.gov

Reynolds, P. D. (1979). *Ethical dilemmas and social science research.* Jossey-Bass.

Roberts, L., Jadalla, A., Jones-Oyefeso, V., Winslow, B., & Taylor, E. (2017). Researching in collectivist cultures: Reflections and recommendations. *Journal of Transcultural Nursing, 28*(2), 137–143. https://doi.org/10.1177/1043659615623331

Rothman, D. J. (1982). Were Tuskegee and Willowbrook "studies in nature"? *Hastings Center Report, 12*(2), 5–7. https://doi.org/10.2307/3561798

Rudolph, A., Young, A., & Havens, J. (2020). Privacy, confidentiality, and safety considerations for conducting geographic momentary assessment studies among persons who use drugs and men who have sex with men. *Journal of Urban Health, 97*, 306–316. https://doi.org/10.1007/s11524-018-0315-x

Scholton, M., & Gather, J. (2021). Equality in the informed consent process: Competence to consent, substitute decision-making, and discrimination of persons with mental disorders. *Journal of Medicine and Philosophy, 46*, 108–136. https://doi.org/10.1093/jmp/jhaa030

Schroeter, K. (2020). Research ethics: What nurses need to know. *American Nurse Today, 15*(11), 48. Retrieved from https://www.myamericannurse.com/research-ethics-what-nurses-need-to-know/

Shuster, E. (1997). Fifty years later: The significance of the Nuremberg Code. *New England Journal of Medicine, 337*, 1436–1440. https://doi.org/10.1056/NEJM199711133372006

Skloot, R. (2010). *The immortal life of Henrietta Lacks.* Crown Publishers.

Sodeke, S., & Powell, L. (2019). Paying tribute to Henrietta Lacks at Tuskegee University and at The Virginia Henrietta Lacks Commission, Richmond, Virginia. *Journal of Health Care for Poor and Underserved, 30*(Suppl. 4), 1–11. https://doi.org/10.1353/hpu.2019.0109

Steinfels, P., & Levine, C. (1976). Biomedical ethics and the shadow of Nazism. *Hastings Center Report, 6*(4), 1–20. https://doi.org/10.2307/3560386

Terry, N. (2015). Developments in genetic and epigenetic data protection in behavioral and mental health spaces. *Behavioral Sciences & Law, 33*(5), 653–661. https://doi.org/10.1002/bsl.2203

Thakur, S., & Lahiry, S. (2019). Research ethics in the modern era. *Indian Dermatological, Venereology, and Leprology, 85*(4), 351–354. https://doi.org/10.4103/ijdvl.IJDVL_499_18

Tovino, S. (2019). Privacy and security issues with mobile health research applications. *Journal of Law, Medicine, & Ethics, 47*(Suppl. 2), 154–158. https://doi.org/10.1177/1073110520917041

US Department of Health and Human Services. (2002). *45 CFR Parts 160 and 164. Standards for privacy of individually identifiable health information.* Retrieved from https://www.hhs.gov/hipaa/for-professionals/privacy/guidance/introduction/index.html

US Department of Health and Human Services. (2017). *Federalwide assurance (FWA) for the protection of human subjects.* Retrieved from https://www.hhs.gov/ohrp/register-irbs-and-obtain-fwas/fwas/fwa-protection-of-human-subjecct/index.html

US Department of Health and Human Services. (2018a). Federal policy for protection of human subjects: Six month delay of the general compliance date of revisions while allowing the use of three burden-reducing provisions during the delay period. *Federal Register, 83*(119), 28497–28520. Retrieved from https://www.govinfo.gov/content/pkg/FR-2018-06-19/pdf/2018-13187.pdf

US Department of Health and Human Services. (2018b). *Subpart A of 45 CFR Part 46: Basic HHS policy for the protection of human subjects.* Retrieved from https://www.hhs.gov/ohrp/sites/default/files/revised-common-rule-reg-text-unofficial-2018-requirements.pdf

US Department of Health and Human Services. (2019). *Research with children FAQs.* Retrieved from https://www.hhs.gov/ohrp/regulations-and-policy/guidance/faq/children-research/index.html

US Food and Drug Administration. (2020). *21 CFR Part 50: Protection of human subjects.* Retrieved from https://www.accessdata.fda.gov/scripts/cdrh/cfdocs/cfcfr/CFRSearch.cfm?fr=50.1

US Public Health Services. (2011). *42 CFR, § 93.103. Research misconduct.* Retrieved from https://www.govinfo.gov/content/pkg/CFR-2011-title42-vol1/pdf/CFR-2011-title42-vol1-sec93-103.pdf

Williams, K., & Colomb, P. (2020). Important considerations for institutional review board when granting Health Insurance Portability and Accountability Act authorizations waiver. *Ochsner Journal, 20,* 95–97. https://doi.org/10.31486/toj.19.0083

Wolf, L., Brown, E., Kerr, R., Razick, G., Tanner, G., Duvall, B., ... Posada, T. (2019). The web of legal protections for participants in genomic research. *Health Matrix, 29*(1), 3. https://scholarlycommons.law.case.edu/healthmatrix/vol29/iss1/3

Wolf, L., Hammack, C., Brown, E., Brelsford, K., & Beskow, L. (2020). Protection participants in genomic research: Understanding the "web of protections" afforded by federal and state law. *Journal of Law, Medicine, & Ethics, 48,* 126-144. https: doi, org/10.1177/1073110520917000

Wolinetz, C., & Collins, F. (2020). Recognition of research participants' need for autonomy. Remembering the legacy of Henrietta Lacks. *Journal of the American Medical Association, 324*(11), 1027–1028. https://doi.org/10.1001/jama.2020.15936

World Health Organization Expert Advisory Committee on Developing Global Standards for Governance and Oversight of Human Genome Editing (2021). Human genome editing: A framework for governance. World Health Organization. https://www.who.int/publications/i/item/9789240030060

World Medical Association. (2013). World Medical Association Declaration of Helsinki: Ethical principles for medical research involving human subjects. *Journal of the American Medical Association, 310*(20), 2191–2194. https://doi.org/10.1001/jama.2013.281053

Examining Research Problems, Purposes, and Hypotheses

Susan K. Grove

LEARNING OUTCOMES

After completing this chapter, you should be able to:

1. Identify research topics, problems, and purposes in published quantitative, qualitative, mixed methods, and outcomes studies.
2. Critically appraise the research problems and purposes in nursing studies.
3. Critically appraise the feasibility of research problems and purposes in studies.
4. Differentiate among the types of hypotheses (associative vs. causal, simple vs. complex, nondirectional vs. directional, and statistical vs. research).
5. Critically appraise the quality of objectives, questions, and hypotheses in published studies.
6. Differentiate the types of variables included in research reports.
7. Critically appraise the conceptual and operational definitions of variables in quantitative and outcomes studies.
8. Critically appraise the research concepts studied in qualitative and mixed methods research.

We are constantly asking questions to gain a better understanding of ourselves and the world around us. This human ability to wonder and ask creative questions is the first step in the research process. By asking questions, clinical nurses, researchers, and educators are able to identify significant research topics and problems to direct the generation of research evidence for practice. A research topic is a concept or broad issue that is important to nursing, such as chronic pain management, posttraumatic stress disorder assessment, prevention of coronavirus disease 2019 (COVID-19) spread, and health promotion strategies for children. Each topic contains numerous research problems that might be investigated through quantitative, qualitative, mixed methods, and outcomes studies. For example, chronic pain management is a research topic that includes

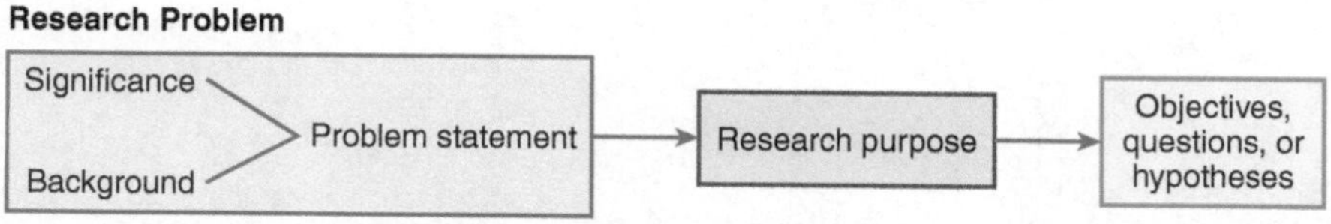

Research Problem

FIG. 5.1 Linking the Research Problem, Purpose, and Objectives, Questions, or Hypotheses.

research problems, such as "What is it like to live with chronic pain?" and "What strategies are useful in coping with chronic pain?" Different types of qualitative and mixed methods studies have been conducted to investigate these problems or areas of concern in nursing (Creswell & Clark, 2018; Creswell & Poth, 2018). Quantitative and outcomes studies have been conducted to address problems, such as "What is an accurate and concise way to assess and diagnose chronic pain?" and "What interventions are effective in managing chronic pain?" (Gray & Grove, 2021).

The problem provides the basis for developing the research purpose. The purpose is the goal or focus of a study that guides the development of the objectives, questions, or hypotheses that further focus the intent of the study (Fig. 5.1). Objectives, questions, or hypotheses can be developed to bridge the gap between the more abstractly stated problem and purpose and the detailed design for conducting the study. However, many studies do not include objectives, questions, or hypotheses and are guided by the study purpose. The study purpose, objectives, questions, and hypotheses include the variables, relationships among the variables, and often the population to be studied. In qualitative research, the purpose and, sometimes, broadly stated research questions or objectives guide the study of selected research concepts.

This chapter includes content that will assist you in identifying problems and purposes in a variety of quantitative, qualitative, mixed methods, and outcomes studies. Objectives, questions, and hypotheses are discussed, and the different types of study variables are introduced. Also presented are guidelines that will assist you in critically appraising the problems, purposes, objectives, questions, hypotheses, and variables or concepts in nursing studies.

WHAT ARE RESEARCH PROBLEMS AND PURPOSES?

A research problem is an area of concern in which there is a gap in the knowledge needed for nursing practice. Research is required to generate essential knowledge to address the practice concern, with the ultimate goal of providing evidence-based nursing care (Melnyk & Fineout-Overholt, 2019; Schuler et al., 2020). The research problem in a study (1) indicates the significance of the problem, (2) provides a background for the problem, and (3) includes a problem statement (Box 5.1). The significance of a research problem identifies the importance of the problem to

---

BOX 5.1   ELEMENTS OF THE RESEARCH PROBLEM

- Significance: Why the research problem is important to nursing and health care for the study population
- Background: What we know from previous research
- Problem statement: What we do not know (gap in nursing knowledge) that we need to know for practice; focus of the research purpose

nursing and to the health of individuals, families, and communities. Research problems are significant when many people are affected and their health conditions are complex and inadequately managed, resulting in high costs for individuals and society. The background for a problem briefly identifies what we know about the problem area, and the problem statement identifies the specific gap in the knowledge needed for practice (see Fig. 5.1). You can usually find the research problem on the first page of the research report. Typically, you will find the problem followed by the problem statement that is addressed by the study purpose.

The research purpose is a clear, concise statement of the specific goal or focus of a study. In quantitative studies, the goal of a study might be to identify and describe variables, examine relationships in a situation, or determine the effectiveness of an intervention (Creswell & Creswell, 2018). The purpose of an outcomes study is similar to that of a quantitative study, except it should include the word *outcomes*, such as research to determine the outcomes from a medication adherence program for community-dwelling elderly with heart failure (HF) (Moorhead et al., 2018). In qualitative studies, the purpose might be to describe perceptions of a phenomenon and give it meaning, develop a theory of a health situation or issue, describe aspects of a culture, or explore relevant concepts and concerns in nursing (Creswell & Poth, 2018). Mixed methods studies contain research problems and purposes that reflect the combined approach of quantitative and qualitative research (Creswell & Clark, 2018). A mixed methods study might include two purpose statements, one focused on quantitative research and the other on qualitative research, or might include a purpose and research questions that reflect both types of research.

📄 RESEARCH/EBP TIP

A clearly stated research purpose (1) captures the essence of a study in a single sentence; (2) is essential for directing the remaining steps of the research process; and (3) improves the credibility and quality of the study findings that might ultimately be used in practice.

Critically Appraising Research Problems and Purposes

When reading a research report, you need essential knowledge and skills for critically appraising the quality of a study problem and purpose. The guidelines for critically appraising the problems and purposes in studies are presented as follows.

❓ CRITICAL APPRAISAL GUIDELINES

Problems and Purposes in Studies

1. Is the problem clearly and concisely stated early in the study's report?
2. Does the problem include the significance, background, and problem statement?
3. Does the purpose clearly express the goal or focus of the study?
4. Is the purpose consistent with the knowledge gap identified in the problem statement?
5. Does the purpose include the study variables and population?

The research problem and purpose from the randomized controlled trial (RCT) conducted by Park and colleagues (2020) is presented as an example. Their study focused on the effects of a smartphone application (app)-based self-management program for people with chronic obstructive pulmonary disease (COPD). The problem and purpose from this study are identified and critically appraised in Research Example 5.1.

RESEARCH EXAMPLE 5.1

Problem and Purpose of a Quantitative Study

Research/Study Excerpt
Problem Significance

> [COPD] is characterized by limited airflow and persistent symptoms such as dyspnea, cough, and sputum production (Global Initiative for Chronic Obstructive Lung Disease, 2018). Despite advanced medical treatment, people with COPD become increasingly more dyspneic, which limits activity, and experience frequent exacerbations as their disease progresses, which severely affects them physically, psychologically, and socially. . . . Many attempts have been made to improve self-management skills and health-related outcomes in people with COPD. . . . Smartphone apps now enable healthcare providers to effectively manage the care of people with many chronic diseases (Lee et al., 2018). . . . However, research into the use of smartphone technology in a self-management program for people with COPD has been limited. (Park et al., 2020, Introduction section)

Research Purpose

> The purpose of this study was to examine the effect of a 6-month SASMP [smartphone app-based self-management program] on self-care behavior in people with COPD. (Park et al., 2020, Literature Review section)

Critical Appraisal

Park and colleagues (2020) presented a clear, concise research problem that included the significance, background, and problem statement. COPD is a significant, complex, chronic illness experienced by smokers that requires extensive knowledge to effectively manage. The background for the problem was presented in a systematic review by Lee et al. (2018) that addressed the effectiveness of smartphone technology in providing self-management programs to people with chronic diseases. The discussion of the problem concluded with a concise problem statement that identified a gap in the knowledge needed for practice and provided the basis for the study purpose.

The research purpose frequently is reflected in the title of the study, stated in the abstract, and restated after the literature review and before the methodology section. Park et al. (2020) included the purpose for their study in all three places. However, the statements of the purpose in the article were varied, which can be confusing to readers. The most clear, complete study purpose was stated before the methodology as: SASMP intervention (independent variable) was implemented over 6 months to determine its effect on self-care behavior (outcome or dependent variable) in people with COPD (population).

Park et al. (2020, Abstract section) found that a "self-management program, using a smartphone app, can effect behavioral change in people with COPD. This program could be a boon to patients with COPD who have limited access to a health care provider, no opportunities for pulmonary rehabilitation, and frequent exacerbations." However, the authors recognized the importance of additional studies with larger samples that include examining the effects of SASMP on other clinically relevant outcomes for individuals with COPD.

RESEARCH/EBP TIP

This RCT by Park et al. (2020) supports the Quality and Safety Education for Nurses (QSEN, 2020) prelicensure competencies of ensuring safe, quality, and cost-effective EBP for individuals with chronic disease. Research evidence supporting the effectiveness of technology, such as smartphone apps, can be used to assist individuals in managing their chronic illnesses.

IDENTIFYING THE PROBLEM AND PURPOSE IN QUANTITATIVE, QUALITATIVE, MIXED METHODS, AND OUTCOMES RESEARCH

Nursing knowledge is generated by conducting a variety of methodologies—quantitative, qualitative, mixed methods, and outcomes research—that are guided by problems and purposes formulated for these types of research. Quantitative and qualitative studies appear most often in the nursing literature. Two other important methodologies, mixed methods and outcomes research, have been appearing in the nursing literature more frequently from 2000 to the present. Examples of problems and purposes from these different types of studies are presented in Tables 5.1, 5.2, 5.3, and 5.4.

Research Problems and Purposes in Types of Quantitative Study

Example research problems and purposes for the different types of quantitative research—descriptive, correlational, quasi-experimental, and experimental—are presented in Table 5.1. When little is known about a topic, researchers usually conduct descriptive and correlational studies and progress to quasi-experimental and experimental studies as knowledge expands.

An examination of the problems and purposes in Table 5.1 will reveal the differences and similarities among the types of quantitative research (see Chapter 2). The research purpose usually

TABLE 5.1   QUANTITATIVE RESEARCH PROBLEMS AND PURPOSES

TYPE OF RESEARCH	RESEARCH PROBLEM AND PURPOSE
Descriptive research	*Title of study:* "Electronic cigarette use among heart failure patients: Findings from the Population Assessment of Tobacco and Health study (Wave 1: 2013-2014)" (Gathright et al., 2020)
	Problem: "Cigarette smoking is an important modifiable contributor to mortality among adults with heart failure (HF). Adults with HF are advised to discontinue and/or abstain from smoking due to the numerous deleterious effects of smoking on the cardiovascular system and disease process. Approximately 12% of adults with a HF hospitalization were recently documented to have tobacco use disorder. Given the increasing popularity of electronic cigarettes (e-cigarettes), HF patients may use e-cigarettes in an attempt to reduce or quit smoking. The prevalence, and reason for use, of e-cigarettes in HF patients is unknown." (Gathright et al., 2020, p. 229)
	Purpose: "Thus, the purpose of this study was to determine rates of and reasons for e-cigarette use among adults with HF." (Gathright et al., 2020, p. 229)
Correlational research	*Title of study:* "A complex population: Nurse's professional preparedness to care for medical-surgical patients with mental illness" (Avery et al., 2020)
	Problem: "In the United States one in six adults (45 million) has a diagnosable mental disorder (NIMH [National Institute of Mental Health], 2016). ... Sixty-eight percent of those diagnosed with mental illness have at least one medical condition and mental health disorders are the second most frequent co-occurring illness in Medicare recipients (Rice et al., 2019). ... An increasing number of patients are admitted to medical-surgical units with a secondary diagnosis of mental illness (MSMI). ... As implied from these studies many medical surgical nurses are not prepared to provide care for MSMI patients. Understanding the components of nurses' preparedness to care for this population is needed." (Avery et al., 2020, Introduction and Background sections)

Continued

TABLE 5.1	QUANTITATIVE RESEARCH PROBLEMS AND PURPOSES—cont'd
TYPE OF RESEARCH	**RESEARCH PROBLEM AND PURPOSE**
	Purpose: The purpose of this study was to examine "the components of nursing preparedness (nursing care self-efficacy and mental health care competency) to provide care for MSMI patients and explored characteristics of variables more frequently associated with and more predictive of nursing preparedness." (Avery et al., 2020, Background section)
Quasi-experimental research	*Title of study:* "Using the Engaging Parents in Education for Discharge (*e*PED) iPad application to improve parent discharge experience" (Lerret et al., 2020, p. 41)
	Problem: "High quality comprehensive preparation for discharge is essential for optimal recovery of children at home after hospitalization...(Lerret & Weiss, 2011). ...Nurses play a central role in discharge preparation, which involves the three interrelated processes of discharge planning, discharge coordination, and discharge teaching (Weiss et al., 2015). ...While disease-specific guidelines are used to prepare parents for the child's medical care and treatment needs at home after discharge, little research has been conducted to establish evidence-based practices for predischarge teaching methods. ...To address this gap, we developed the Engaging Parents in Education for Discharge (*e*PED) iPad application (app)." (Lerret et al., 2020, pp. 41–42)
	Purpose: "The purpose of this study was to evaluate the use of *e*PED in preparing for hospital discharge on parent experiences of hospital discharge teaching and care coordination." (Lerret et al., 2020, p. 42)
Experimental research	*Title of study:* "Effects of oral care with glutamine in preventing ventilator-associated pneumonia in neurosurgical intensive care unit patients" (Kaya et al., 2017, p. 10).
	Problem: "Ventilator-associated pneumonia (VAP) is one of the most frequent nosocomial infections in intensive care unit patients. ...One of the measures to prevent the development of VAP is applying good oral care. ...In recent studies, glutamine was reported to be an essential amino acid that is critical for the regulation of protein synthesis, respiratory fueling, and nitrogen shuttling. ...Different products and protocols in oral care have been the subject for research. However, the number of studies about glutamine is limited." (Kaya et al., 2017, pp 10–11)
	Purpose: The purpose of this study was "to determine the effects of oral care with glutamine in preventing ventilator-associated pneumonia in patients admitted to neurosurgical intensive care unit." (Kaya et al., 2017, p. 10)

reflects the type of study that was conducted (Gray & Grove, 2021). The purpose of descriptive research is to identify and describe concepts or variables, identify possible relationships among variables, and delineate differences between or among existing groups, such as males and females or ethnic/race groups (Kazdin, 2017).

Problem and Purpose for Descriptive Research

Gathright and colleagues (2020) conducted a descriptive study to determine the prevalence of and reasons for electronic cigarette (e-cigarette) use among adults with HF. Some patients with HF use e-cigarettes to assist them in reducing or abstaining from smoking. However, recent studies and clinical findings indicate e-cigarette use can result in increased lung and cardiovascular health problems (Ansari-Gilani et al., 2020). Gathright et al. (2020) identified a significant problem and clearly focused purpose to generate knowledge for practice. These researchers concluded that "e-cigarette use should be assessed and monitored to understand the safety and potential efficacy of e-cigarettes as a harm reduction approach for HF patients" (Gathright et al., 2020, p. 229).

Problem and Purpose for Correlational Research

The purpose of correlational research is to examine the type (positive or negative) and strength of relationships or associations among variables (Grove & Cipher, 2020; Leedy & Ormrod, 2019). Positive relationships (designated by a plus [+] sign) indicate that variables change in the same direction; they either increase or decrease together. For example, the more cigarettes an adult smokes each day, the greater his or her risk for lung cancer. Negative relationships (designated by a minus [−] sign) indicate that variables change in the opposite direction; as one variable increases, the other variable decreases. For example, the increased frequency of wearing a facial covering in public places and with groups decreases the potential of testing positive for COVID-19. The strength of a relationship may vary from −1 to 0 to +1, with −1 indicating a perfect negative relationship, 0 indicating no relationship, and +1 indicating a perfect positive relationship between variables (Grove & Cipher, 2020). Types of relationship are discussed in more detail in the later section Hypotheses.

Avery and colleagues (2020) conducted a correlational study to examine nurses' professional preparedness to care for medical-surgical patients with mental illness. This study included a significant problem, nurses' ability to care for mentally ill patients on medical-surgical units, and a clearly focused purpose (see Table 5.1). Avery et al. (2020, Abstract) found "three characteristics of professional experiences—mentoring, frequency of care, and continuing education—best prepare a registered nurse to care for this complex population."

Problem and Purpose for Quasi-Experimental Research

Quasi-experimental studies are conducted to determine the effect of a treatment or independent variable on designated dependent or outcome variables (Shadish et al., 2002). Research examining the effects of interventions has expanded in large healthcare systems, with a potential to generate knowledge for practice (Siedlecki & Albert, 2020). Lerret and colleagues (2020) conducted a quasi-experimental study to examine the effectiveness of an Education for Discharge (ePED) iPad app on parents' experiences with their children's hospital discharge. Quality discharge education is essential to promote continued healing of children at home. Lerret et al. (2020) cited four previous studies they had conducted in the area of discharge education and coordination, indicating their research expertise in this area and documenting how they built on previous research. The significant research problem and purpose for this study are presented in Table 5.1. The researchers found that nurses using the ePED iPad app were able to enhance the quality of the discharge experiences for parents. However, additional research was recommended to refine the ePED app to address different parents' educational needs and to examine different outcomes, such as quality of life (QoL) for parent and child.

Problem and Purpose for Experimental Research

Experimental studies are conducted in highly controlled settings using a structured design to determine the effect of one or more independent variables on one or more dependent variables (Gray & Grove, 2021; Kazdin, 2017). Kaya and colleagues (2017, p. 11) conducted a "randomized, controlled, experimental study to determine the effects of oral care with glutamine in preventing ventilator-associated pneumonia [VAP] in patients admitted to neurosurgical intensive care unit

[ICU] in New Jersey." They found that providing oral care with glutamine had no significant effect on the incidence of VAP in these ICU patients. Kaya et al. (2017) recommended additional research with a larger sample size over a longer time period.

Research Problems and Purposes in Types of Qualitative Study

The problems studied using qualitative research require investigation to gain new insights, expand understanding, and improve comprehension of the whole. The purpose of a qualitative study indicates the study's focus, which may be a concept such as dyspnea, an event such as loss of a child, or a facet of a culture such as the healing practices of a particular Native American tribe. In addition, the purpose often indicates the qualitative approach used to conduct the study (Creswell & Poth, 2018). Table 5.2 includes examples of research problems and purposes for the types of qualitative research—phenomenological, grounded theory, ethnographic, and exploratory-descriptive—commonly found in the nursing literature.

TABLE 5.2   QUALITATIVE RESEARCH PROBLEMS AND PURPOSES

TYPE OF RESEARCH	RESEARCH PROBLEM AND PURPOSE
Phenomenological research	*Title of study:* "A two-front war: Exploring military families' battle with parental deployment" (Mulholland et al., 2020)
	Problem: "Military families face unique challenges of prolonged separations, frequent relocations, and the uncertainty of a loved one's safety. In 2018, military families with children made up 38.8% of all military personnel, excluding families affiliated with the Coast Guard (US Department of Defense, 2018). . . . There is evidence of higher rates of marriage instability and family dysfunction in families with military deployment experience (Lester et al., 2016). . . . Further, there is limited research that directly asks the parents what they do to help their children cope during times of deployment and post-deployment." (Mulholland et al., 2020, p. 35)
	Purpose: "The purpose of this study was to identify ways parents comfort their children to help them cope and adapt to stresses during a parental military deployment, as well as the reintegration process of the parent returning home." (Mulholland et al., 2020, p. 34)
Grounded theory research	*Title of study:* "Parent-observed thematic data on quality of life in children with autism spectrum disorder" (Epstein et al., 2019)
	Problem: Population-based estimates of the prevalence of autism spectrum disorder (ASD) range from 5.1 to 15.5 per 1000 births (Bourke et al., 2016 . . .). The prevalence is increasing in part due to changing diagnostic criteria and assessment practices (Hansen et al., 2015) . . . Assessments of quality of life (QoL) are therefore important not only to paint an authentic picture of a child's life, but also to identify areas where support is needed and for evaluating treatment and intervention efficacy to promote successful outcomes . . . The QoL domains for children with ASD have not been explored and parent observations could provide a preliminary framework for understanding a child's QoL." (Epstein et al., 2019, pp. 71–72)
	Purpose: "This study therefore explored parental observations to identify QoL domains important to children with ASD with co-occurring intellectual disability. We also investigated whether different domains would be observed in childhood and adolescence." (Epstein et al., 2019, p. 72)

TABLE 5.2	QUALITATIVE RESEARCH PROBLEMS AND PURPOSES—cont'd
TYPE OF RESEARCH	**RESEARCH PROBLEM AND PURPOSE**
Ethnographic research	*Title of study:* "Using focused ethnography to explore and describe the process of nurses' shift reports in a psychiatric intensive care unit" (Salzmann-Erikson, 2018)
	Problem: "Shift reports and handoffs are an integral and routine activity among nurses in their everyday work. The tenet in this activity is to pass on and exchange between colleagues' vital information about the patients, health status. . . . Several studies stress the association between medical errors in hospital environments and the lack of communication between health-care staff. . . . To date, no studies have addressed nursing shift reports in psychiatric ICUs, hence this study." (Salzmann-Erikson, 2018, pp. 3104–3105)
	Purpose: "This study aimed to explore and describe the cultural routine of shift reports among nursing staff in a psychiatric ICU and further to develop a taxonomic, thematic and theoretical understanding of the process." (Salzmann-Erikson, 2018, p. 3105)
Exploratory-descriptive qualitative research	*Title of study:* "Identity and perceptions of quality of life in Alzheimer's disease" (Manson et al., 2020)
	Problem: "With life expectancy on the rise and the baby boomer generation growing older, it is predicted that by 2050, Alzheimer's disease (AD) will affect 13.8 million people in the United States, an increase of nearly 138% from present day (2019 Alzheimer's disease facts and figures, 2019) . . . It is important to understand adaptive strategies to maintain self-identity in early AD in order to facilitate continuity of the self as cognition continues to decline . . . It is possible that there is a gap in the literature regarding self-reported, subjective data on meaningful activities in AD because healthcare providers and caregivers hold implicit biases that person(s) with dementia (PwD) cannot accurately recall, assess, and discuss meaningful activities and subjective QoL." (Manson et al., 2020, Introduction section)
	Purpose: "This exploratory study aims to provide a preliminary and foundational understanding of the experiences and perceptions of people living with early- to mid-AD and their caregivers related to life satisfaction and QoL." (Manson et al., 2020, Abstract)

Problem and Purpose for Phenomenological Research

Phenomenological research is conducted to promote a deeper understanding of complex human experiences as they have been lived by the study participants (Creswell & Poth, 2018; see Chapter 3). Mulholland and colleagues (2020) conducted a phenomenological study to expand understanding of the lived experiences of families and the strategies they use to manage combat stressors during deployment and postdeployment. The problem and purpose for this study are presented in Table 5.2. Mulholland et al. (2020) detailed the challenges military families experience during deployment and reintegration and identified strategies they might use to manage them. These researchers recommended implementing their study findings in nursing practice so military families with children might receive education and guidance when planning for a parent's deployment.

Problem and Purpose for Grounded Theory Research

In grounded theory research, the problem identifies the area of concern, and the purpose indicates the focus of the model, framework, or theory developed to account for a pattern of behavior in study participants (Bryant & Charmaz, 2019). Epstein et al. (2019) conducted a grounded theory study to describe the QoL in children with autism spectrum disorder (ASD) (see Table 5.2). Data were collected by interviewing 22 parents who were primary caregivers and spoke on behalf of their child with ASD. Analysis of these data evolved into an initial framework for understanding QoL among these children. Epstein et al. (2019, p. 71) found the "Unique aspects of quality of life included varying levels of social desire, consistency of routines, and time spent in nature and the outdoors."

Problem and Purpose for Ethnographic Research

Ethnographic research involves examining individuals within cultures, identifying the member-ship requirements, expected behaviors, enacted behaviors, and rules of the shared culture. The problem and purpose statements identify the culture of interest. These cultures can be actual societal groups, loose associations of persons sharing common experiences, or unconnected individuals who share a common experience (Creswell & Poth, 2018). Salzmann-Erikson (2018) conducted a focused ethnography to describe the cultural routine of nursing shift reports in a psychiatric ICU (see Table 5.2). Data were obtained from 20 observational sessions conducted in a psychiatric ICU over a span of 5 months. Salzmann-Erikson (2018, p. 3104) found the process of shift reports included three phases: "(a) getting settled, (b) giving the report, and (c) engaging in the aftermath." These phases included different cultural activities, which take place in different areas of the ICU and at varied levels of formality.

Problem and Purpose for Exploratory-Descriptive Qualitative Research

Exploratory-descriptive qualitative research is being conducted by several nurse researchers to describe unique concepts, issues, health problems, or situations that lack clear description or definition. Exploratory-descriptive qualitative studies often provide the basis for future mixed methods and quantitative research (Kim et al., 2017). Manson and colleagues (2020) conducted an exploratory-descriptive qualitative study to detail the perceptions of patients with early- to mid-Alzheimer disease (AD) and their caregivers related to QoL and life satisfaction. The research problem and purpose for this study were clearly presented in the research report and indicated the type of qualitative study conducted (see Table 5.2). Manson et al. (2020, Abstract) concluded: "By accounting for individual levels of baseline engagement and taking each patient's perspective into account, nurses have the ability to identify individual changes overtime and positively impact the patient's QoL." The authors also recommended further study with a larger, more diverse sample to expand on these study findings.

Mixed Methods Research

Mixed methods research reports contain problems and purposes that reflect the combined approach of two methods, quantitative and qualitative research (Creswell & Clark, 2018). Table 5.3 presents an example of the problem and purpose for a mixed methods study of student performance during a low-stakes simulation. "Anxiety, self-efficacy, academic achieve-ment, and performance during simulations were measured quantitatively. Qualitative data were collected during post-simulation debriefing" and used to interpret the quantitative find-ings (Burbach et al., 2019, p. 44). The quantitative part of this study was correlational and identified significant relationships between knowledge of nursing care and simulation perfor-mance. The qualitative part of the study was exploratory-descriptive and detailed the students' lack of confidence, uncertainty, and heightened anxiety experienced during the simulation experience.

TABLE 5.3 MIXED METHODS STUDY PROBLEM AND PURPOSE

TYPE OF RESEARCH	RESEARCH PROBLEM AND PURPOSE
Mixed methods research	*Title of study:* "Correlates of student performance during low stakes simulation" (Burbach et al., 2019).
	Problem: "Low stakes simulation has been reported to effectively facilitate learning in an environment free from harm to live patients (Kolozsvari et al., 2011), and improve quality of learning, leading to safe and effective patient care (Alexander et al., 2015). …For simulation to be a valid and reliable evaluation tool, simulation performance needs to be correlated with what the student knows. …Students often report stress and anxiety during simulation as negatively affecting their performance (Burbach et al., 2016…). …Learning what modifiable factors influence simulation performance will make it possible to identify interventions to improve outcomes." (Burbach et al., 2019, pp. 44–45)
	Purpose: "To fill this gap in knowledge, the purpose of this study is to examine the relationship among anxiety, self-efficacy, and nursing knowledge and students' performance during low stakes simulation." (Burbach et al., 2019, p. 45)

TABLE 5.4 OUTCOMES RESEARCH PROBLEM AND PURPOSE

TYPE OF RESEARCH	RESEARCH PROBLEM AND PURPOSE
Outcomes research	*Title of study:* "Always InforMED: Nurse champion-led intervention to improve medication communication among nurses and patients" (Begum et al., 2020)
	Problem: "Providing effective communication regarding medications is an important responsibility of nurses that is related to both health outcomes and patient satisfaction. Studies have shown that while patients were more likely to understand the purpose of their new medications, only 14 to 25% of patients were able [to] recall any information about side effects. …To reduce the risk of adverse events, active patient involvement in treatment decisions is necessary, and is associated with increased satisfaction and better health outcomes. …While a unit-based nurse champion has been used with success to improve various health issues (…Hilken et al., 2017), evidence regarding the impact of this approach to improve communication related to medications is very limited." (Begum et al., 2020, Introduction section)
	Purpose: "The purpose of this project was to evaluate the effectiveness of a nurse champion-led, bundled intervention, 'Always InforMED,' to increase nurse utilization of hospital-based resources to improve nurse-to-patient communication regarding medications and increase patient satisfaction." (Begum et al., 2020, Introduction section)

Outcomes Research

Reports of outcomes studies contain problems and purposes that are similar to those found in quantitative research, except the word *outcomes* is usually included in the study purpose (Gray & Grove, 2021; Moorhead et al., 2018). An example of the problem and purpose for an outcomes study by Begum et al. (2020) is presented in Table 5.4. This study involved examining the effectiveness of a nurse champion intervention, *Always InforMED*, on the outcomes of nurse-to-patient communication regarding medications and patient satisfaction. The most common theoretical framework used for outcomes research is by Donabedian (1988), which focuses on three constructs of structure, process, and outcomes (see Chapter 14). Begum et al. (2020) conducted their study with hospital-based nurses (structure) to determine the effects of the *Always InforMED* intervention (process) on the outcomes of medication communications between nurse and patient and patient satisfaction. Begum et al. (2020) found that the medication communication score increased after the start of the intervention but decreased after 3 months. There was no significant difference between preintervention and postintervention medication communication scores. Additional research is needed in this area with larger samples and extended times for intervention implementation.

📄 RESEARCH/EBP TIP

Different types of problem and purpose are used to guide quantitative, qualitative, mixed methods, and outcomes research. Knowing the differences in the research problems and purposes examined in nursing studies will help you understand the knowledge generated and how it might ultimately be used in practice.

EXAMINING THE FEASIBILITY OF THE PROBLEM AND PURPOSE IN A PUBLISHED STUDY

Critical appraisal of research involves examining the feasibility of the study's problem and purpose. The feasibility of a study is determined by examining the researchers' expertise; money commitment; and availability of study participants, facilities, and equipment (Gray & Grove, 2021; Kazdin, 2017). The feasibility of the Gathright et al. (2020) study of e-cigarette use among patients with HF is presented as an example. You can review this study's problem and purpose in Table 5.1 and locate this article through your library. The critical appraisal involves addressing the following questions about the study's feasibility.

❓ CRITICAL APPRAISAL GUIDELINES

Examining the Feasibility of a Study's Problem and Purpose

1. Did the researchers have the research, clinical, and educational expertise to conduct the study?
2. Was the study funded? Did clinical agencies provide support for the study?
3. Did the researchers have access to adequate study participants, settings, and equipment to conduct their study?

Researcher Expertise

The research problem and purpose studied need to be within the area of expertise of the researchers. Research reports usually identify the education of the researchers and their current positions (academic or clinical), which indicate their expertise to conduct a study. Doctor of philosophy (PhD) and postdoctoral degrees indicate strong academic preparation for conducting research. Because universities provide strong support for research activities, many researchers are affiliated with academic institutions. Also, examine the reference list to determine whether the researchers have conducted additional studies in this area. Evaluate the researchers' clinical expertise because it is important for conducting studies relevant to practice. If you need more information, you can search the internet for the researchers' accomplishments and involvement in research (Gray & Grove, 2021).

Gathright has a PhD and works in the Department of Psychiatry and Human Behavior at Brown University in Rhode Island. Dr. Gathright has authored more than 25 publications, and several of them include patients with HF as participants. With Wu and Scott-Sheldon, she has published funded studies before that included patients with HF and other cardiovascular diseases. Dr. Wu is a cardiologist who is the director of a center for cardiac fitness and a professor of medicine at Brown University. One of the studies cited in the reference list is by Dr. Wu, and he has other funded studies with cardiac patients. Scott-Sheldon is PhD prepared and also a professor at Brown University. One of her primary areas of study includes novel tobacco products, such as e-cigarettes. All three authors have strong academic preparations and clinical expertise for conducting this study. They are affiliated with Brown University and are actively involved in nationally funded research that includes patients with HF using tobacco products.

Money Commitment

The problems and purposes studied are influenced by the funding available to the researchers. The cost of a research project can range from a few dollars for a student's small study to hundreds of thousands and even millions of dollars for complex projects. Critically appraising the feasibility of a study involves examining the financial resources used to conduct the study. A study's source of funding is usually identified on the front or back page of the article. Studies might be funded by grants from national institutions (e.g., National Institute of Nursing Research; Agency for Healthcare Research and Quality), professional organizations, or private foundations. Some researchers receive financial assistance from companies that provide necessary equipment, or they receive support from the agencies where the study is conducted. Receiving funding for a study indicates that it was reviewed by peers who chose to support the research financially. The study by Gathright et al. (2020) was funded by national organizations, including the Cardiovascular Behavioral Medicine Training Grant, and grants from the National Heart, Lung, and Blood Institute and the National Institute on Aging that were reported on the last page of their article.

Availability of Study Participants, Facilities, and Equipment

Researchers need to have an adequate number of participants and appropriate facilities, as well as equipment to implement their study (Aberson, 2019; Gray & Grove, 2021). Most studies indicate the sample size and setting in the Methods section of the research report. Often, nursing studies are conducted in natural or partially controlled settings, such as a home, school, hospital unit, or clinic. Many of these facilities are fairly easy to access, and the hospitals and clinics often provide access to adequate numbers of patients. Other studies involve conducting surveys through the internet or the secondary analysis of data from a primary study. Gathright et al. (2020) conducted a secondary analysis of data from the primary Population Assessment of Tobacco and Health (PATH) study. The PATH study included a nationally representative sample of 32,320 US noninstitutionalized adults older than 18 years. Gathright et al. (2020) analyzed the data from 484 individuals who completed the cigarette and e-cigarette data and had a diagnosis of HF. This descriptive study had a large, nationally representative sample that provided support for the findings (Kazdin, 2017).

A review of the Methods section of the research report will determine whether adequate and accurate equipment was available. Nursing and other health-related studies frequently require a limited amount of equipment, such as a video recorder for interviews; physiological measures, such as laboratory values, vital signs, or body mass index; and internet-based or hard copy scales (Bandalos, 2018; Waltz et al., 2017; see Chapter 10). This research was a secondary data analysis of the PATH study, which did not require data collection.

RESEARCH/EBP TIP

When critically appraising published studies, examine the feasibility of the problem and purpose directing the study. The authors need (1) relevant research and clinical expertise; (2) funding if possible; and (3) an appropriate sample, facility, and equipment.

CRITICALLY APPRAISING OBJECTIVES, QUESTIONS, AND HYPOTHESES IN STUDIES

Research objectives, questions, and hypotheses evolve from the problem, purpose, literature review, and often the study framework to direct the remaining steps of the research process (see Fig. 5.1). Many researchers only identify a problem and purpose to guide their quantitative or qualitative studies. However, some studies include specific objectives, questions, or hypotheses to guide the methodology, organize the results, and clarify the findings. Table 5.5 summarizes the use of objectives, questions, or hypotheses in different types of quantitative, qualitative, mixed methods, and outcomes studies. Objectives, questions, or hypotheses usually are presented after the literature review section and before the Methods section in a study. The following guidelines will assist you in identifying and critically appraising the objectives and questions in nursing studies.

? CRITICAL APPRAISAL GUIDELINES
Research Objectives and Questions

1. Are the objectives (aims) or questions clear and concise?
2. Are the study objectives or questions based on the study purpose?
3. Do the objectives or questions appear to direct the study methodology, organize the study results, and facilitate the interpretations of findings?

TABLE 5.5   **OBJECTIVES, QUESTIONS, OR HYPOTHESES USED IN DIFFERENT TYPES OF RESEARCH**

TYPE OF RESEARCH	OBJECTIVES, QUESTIONS, OR HYPOTHESES DEVELOPED TO GUIDE A STUDY
Qualitative research	Research purpose guides most qualitative studies; occasionally objectives or questions are stated
Quantitative research	
Descriptive studies	Research purpose guides many descriptive studies; occasionally objectives or questions are stated
Correlational studies	Objectives, questions, or hypotheses
Quasi-experimental studies	Hypotheses
Experimental studies	Hypotheses
Mixed methods research	Qualitative part of the study might be guided by purpose and an objective or question Quantitative part of the study might be guided by the purpose and objective, questions, or hypothesis based on the study design
Outcomes research	Objectives, questions, or hypotheses

Research Objectives

A research objective, also called an aim, is a clear, concise, declarative statement that identifies the goals of a study. Objectives are used more commonly in descriptive and correlational studies but also in other types of research (see Table 5.5). For clarity, an objective usually focuses on one or two variables and indicates whether they are to be identified or described. Sometimes the focus of objectives is to identify relationships among variables or determine differences between two or more existing groups, such as patients with and without HF (Kazdin, 2017).

Qualitative research is most appropriate when the focus of the study is to obtain a personal perspective of a situation, experience, or event (Creswell & Poth, 2018; Henson & Jeffrey, 2016). The research objectives formulated for quantitative, mixed methods, and outcomes studies have some similarities because they focus on exploration, description, and determination of relationships (see Table 5.5). However, the objectives directing qualitative studies are commonly broader in focus and include concepts that are more complex and abstract than those of quantitative studies. The aims in qualitative studies focus on theory development; understanding the cultures of groups and institutions; participants' experiences of certain events and health conditions; and description of challenges, reasons for behaviors, and perceptions of care in nursing practice (Kim et al., 2017). Mixed methods studies might include objectives to direct either the quantitative or qualitative aspect of a study (Creswell & Clark, 2018).

Lavoie and colleagues (2020) conducted a correlational study to examine nurses' judgments of patients' risk for deterioration at change-of-shift handoff in a university-affiliated hospital in Montreal, Canada. Aims were developed to direct this study regarding nurses' judgments of patients' conditions at handoff in relationship to early warning scores in surgical and medical units. Lavoie et al. (2020) included 62 nurses in their study of 444 handoffs of 158 patients. Research Example 5.2 demonstrated the logical flow from the research problem and purpose to the aims in this study.

🔌 RESEARCH EXAMPLE 5.2

Problem, Purpose, and Aims or Objectives

Research/Study Excerpt

Research Problem

> *In acute care settings, nurses are expected to determine whether patients are stable or are deteriorating—i.e., if patients are experiencing changes that could lead to a cardiac arrest or an unplanned transfer to an intensive care unit (ICU). ... In handoffs, nurses share crucial information regarding the condition of their patients and develop a shared picture of patient needs and priorities in care. Although there is much published research on nursing handoffs, little is known about how handoffs relate to nurses' clinical judgments.* (Lavoie et al., 2020, p. 420)

Research Purpose

> *The purpose of this study was to examine acute care nurses' judgments of patient risk of deterioration following a change-of-shift handoff.* (Lavoie et al., 2020, p. 421)

Research Aims

> *Specifically, we examined the degree of agreement between nurses in their judgments of stability/risk and compared these judgments to 'objective' numerical ratings of risk reflected in commonly used early warning scores. ... In addition, this study explored nurses' experiences of using a rating scale to express their judgments of patient risk of deterioration.* (Lavoie et al., 2020, p. 421)

Continued

RESEARCH EXAMPLE 5.2—cont'd

Critical Appraisal

Lavoie et al. (2020) identified a significant problem regarding patients' risk for deterioration during shift change. The problem statement identified what was not known and provided a basis for the purpose and aims of this study. The purpose clearly and concisely identified the study focus on nurses' clinical judgments about patients' status at change of shift. The study aims were linked to the study purpose and provided more clarity regarding the specific goals of the study. These aims were used to organize study results and interpret the findings. However, an aim was needed that focused on the relationships of the nurses' risk judgments with the early warning scores examined in this study. Lavoie et al. (2020, p. 420) concluded: "While the agreement between incoming and outgoing nurses was fair, correlations with the early warning scores were low. . . . Nurses shared information that influenced their clinical judgments at handoff; not all of these cues may necessarily be captured in early warning scores."

Research Questions

A research question is a clear, concise, interrogative statement that is worded in the present tense, includes one or more variables, and is expressed to guide the implementation of studies. The foci of research questions in quantitative and outcomes studies are description of variable(s), examination of relationships among variables, use of independent variables to predict a dependent variable (outcome), and determination of differences in a selected variable(s) between two or more groups. These research questions are usually narrowly focused and inclusive of the study variables and population. It is really a matter of choice whether researchers identify objectives or questions in their study, but, more often, questions are stated to guide quantitative and outcomes studies (see Table 5.5).

Akkayaoğlu and Çelik (2020) conducted a descriptive study to examine individuals' attitudes, body image perceptions, and QoL before and after bariatric surgery. The research purpose and questions to direct the implementation of this study are presented in Research Example 5.3. The critical appraisal guidelines for objective and questions, presented earlier, were applied in this example.

RESEARCH EXAMPLE 5.3

Purpose and Research Questions From a Quantitative Study

Research Excerpt

Research Purpose

This study examined eating attitudes, perceptions of body image, and quality of life of patients before and after bariatric surgery. (Akkayaoğlu & Çelik, 2020; Objective section)

Research Questions

This study investigated the following questions:

- *Are there differences between the eating attitudes of patients undergoing bariatric surgery during the preoperative period and the postoperative 1st, 3rd and 6th months?*
- *Are there differences between the body image perceptions of patients undergoing bariatric surgery during the preoperative period and the postoperative 1st, 3rd, and 6th months?*
- *Are there differences between the quality of life of patients undergoing bariatric surgery during the preoperative period and the postoperative 1st, 3rd and 6th months? (Akkayaoğlu & Çelik, 2020; Objective section)*

RESEARCH EXAMPLE 5.3—cont'd

Critical Appraisal

Akkayaoğlu and Çelik (2020) focused on the significant health problem of obese patients' and their responses before and after bariatric surgery. The purpose addressed the gap in nursing knowledge identified in the problem statement, identified the study variables (eating attitudes, body image perceptions, and patients' QoL), and reported the population was patients who were undergoing bariatric surgery. The research questions evolved from the purpose and clarified the goals of this study. The first question focused on a description of eating attitudes and a comparison of these attitudes before and after bariatric surgery. The second question focused on body image perceptions before and after bariatric surgery, and the third question focused on QoL before and after surgery. These questions were addressed by the study methodology and were used to organize the study results and findings.

Akkayaoğlu and Çelik (2020) found that eating attitudes, body image perceptions, and QoL were significantly improved from before to after bariatric surgery. "Based on these results, it is recommended that nurses should improve the quality of care for obese patients during the preoperative and postoperative periods. They also need to monitor physiological and psychological changes occurring in patients for the long run. This may facilitate patient follow up" (Akkayaoğlu & Çelik, 2020, Conclusions and Implications for Nursing section).

The research questions directing qualitative studies are often limited in number, broadly focused, and inclusive of concepts that are more complex and abstract than those of quantitative studies. Marshall and Rossman (2016) indicated that the questions developed to direct qualitative research might be theoretical, which can be studied with different populations or in a variety of sites, or the questions could be focused on a particular population or setting. The study questions formulated are important to the type of qualitative research used to conduct the study (Creswell & Poth, 2018). Ricks et al. (2020) conducted a phenomenological study to explore the health and disability among young black men. These researchers developed two questions to guide their study. The purpose and questions from this study are presented in Research Example 5.4.

RESEARCH EXAMPLE 5.4

Purpose and Research Questions From a Qualitative Study

Research/Study Excerpt

Research Purpose

The purpose of this study was to explore how young Black men experienced the onset of chronic disabling conditions while negotiating health-promoting activities in the context of gender, race, social class, disability positionalities, and culture. (Ricks et al., 2020, p. 13)

Research Questions

1. *What is the essence of losing abilities among young Black men in Western societies?*
2. *What is the context of learning health promotion reported by Black men living with disabilities?* (Ricks et al., 2020, p. 14)

Critical Appraisal

Ricks et al. (2020) identified a significant research purpose in a population of understudied young black men with disabilities from chronic conditions. The research questions flowed from the purpose and clarified the foci

Continued

> **🔎 RESEARCH EXAMPLE 5.4—cont'd**
>
> of the study. Research question 1 focused on the exploration of losing abilities in black men, and question 2 focused on describing the experience of young black men in learning health promotion activities. These questions were the focus of data collection and analysis and provided organization to the discussion of findings (Miles et al., 2020). Ricks and colleagues' (2020) study contributed to the understanding of the experiences of young black men living with disabilities. These men's personal challenges, health needs, and use of health promotion strategies were described.

Hypotheses

A hypothesis is a formal statement of the expected relationship(s) between two or more variables in a specified population. The hypothesis translates the research problem and purpose into a clear explanation or prediction of the expected results or outcomes of selected quantitative and outcomes studies. A clearly stated hypothesis identifies (1) the independent variables to be manipulated or measured, (2) the proposed outcomes or dependent variables to be measured, and (3) the population to be studied. (Types of variables are discussed in more detail later in this chapter.) Hypotheses also influence the study design, sampling method, data collection and analysis processes, and interpretation of findings. Quasi-experimental and experimental quantitative studies are conducted to test the effectiveness of an intervention and *should include hypotheses* to predict the study outcomes (Kazdin, 2017; Shadish et al., 2002).

Predictive correlational studies that focus on measuring independent variables to predict a dependent variable often include hypotheses. Some outcomes and mixed methods studies might include hypotheses to predict study results (see Table 5.5; Creswell & Clark, 2018; Gray & Grove, 2021). In this section, types of hypothesis are described, and the elements of a testable hypothesis are discussed so that you can critically appraise hypotheses in nursing studies.

Types of Hypothesis

Different types of relationships and numbers of variables are identified in hypotheses. A study might have one, four, or more hypotheses, depending on its complexity. The type of hypothesis developed is based on the problem and purpose of the study. Hypotheses can be described using four categories that are presented in Table 5.6 and discussed in this section.

Associative versus causal hypotheses. The relationships identified in hypotheses are associative or causal. An associative hypothesis proposes relationships among variables that occur or exist together in the real world so that when one variable changes, the other changes.

TABLE 5.6   TYPES OF HYPOTHESIS

TYPES OF HYPOTHESIS	FOCUS OF HYPOTHESES
Associative versus causal hypotheses	Type of relationship presented in the hypothesis
Simple versus complex hypotheses	Number of variables in each hypothesis
Nondirectional versus directional hypotheses	Direction or nondirectional relationship expressed in the hypothesis
Research versus null hypotheses	Relationship expressed in research hypothesis No relationship expressed in a null hypothesis

Fig. 5.2 includes a diagram for both an associative and a causal hypothesis. Associative hypotheses identify relationships among variables in a study but do not indicate that one variable *causes* an *effect* on another variable (Gray & Grove, 2021).

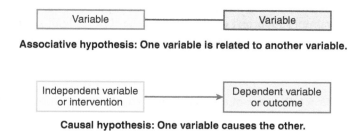

Associative hypothesis: One variable is related to another variable.

Causal hypothesis: One variable causes the other.

FIG. 5.2 **Associative Versus Causal Hypothesis.** The *straight line* indicates a relationship or association between two variables. The *causal arrow* points from the independent variable toward the dependent variable.

Castner et al. (2020) conducted a predictive correlation study to examine the effect of sleep disruption on women's asthma control. They "hypothesized that increased sleep disruption will predict increased lung obstruction" in women with asthma (Castner et al., 2020, p. 548). This associative hypothesis predicts a positive relationship between sleep disruption and lung obstruction that is diagrammed in Fig. 5.3. The line that connects the two variables is straight, without an arrow, which indicates a linear relationship or association. Castner et al. (2020) found that the sleep disruption data were predictive of women's daily asthma outcomes. However, some of the relationships were weak, and additional research with a larger sample is needed.

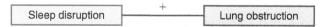

FIG. 5.3 **Diagram of an Associative Hypothesis from the Castner et al. (2020) Study.**

A causal hypothesis proposes a cause-and-effect interaction between two or more variables, referred to as independent and dependent variables (see Fig. 5.2). The independent variable (intervention) is manipulated by the researcher to cause an effect on the dependent variable. The dependent variable is then measured to determine the effect created by the independent variable. A format for stating a causal hypothesis is presented in Box 5.2.

BOX 5.2   FORMAT FOR STATING A CAUSAL HYPOTHESIS

Study participants in the experimental group, who are exposed to the independent variable (intervention), demonstrate greater change, as measured by the dependent variable, than those in the comparison group, who received standard care.

The quasi-experimental study by Lerret and colleagues (2020), presented earlier in Table 5.1, was conducted to examine the effects of the *e*PED iPad app (independent variable) on the quality of discharge teaching and care coordination (dependent variables). This study stated the following causal hypothesis: "Parents exposed to discharge teaching using *e*PED will report better coordination of care than parents exposed to usual discharge teaching" (Lerret et al., 2020, p. 42). This hypothesis included two variables: one independent variable (*e*PED) that was implemented to create an effect on the dependent variable (coordination of care). This causal hypothesis might be diagrammed as in Fig. 5.4, with an arrow (→) to indicate a cause-and-effect relationship.

Hypotheses are tested through research; when the study results are significant, the hypothesis is supported. If study results are nonsignificant, the hypothesis is not supported (Kazdin, 2017). Lerret et al.'s (2020) study result for this causal hypothesis was not significant. Therefore the hypothesis was not supported, which indicated the *e*PED did not significantly improve coordination of care in the intervention group versus the standard care group.

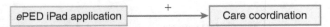

FIG. 5.4 Diagram of a Causal Hypothesis from the Lerret et al. (2020) Study.

Simple versus complex hypotheses. Hypotheses are either simple or complex (see Table 5.6). A simple hypothesis states the relationship (associative or causal) between two variables. Lerret et al. (2020) stated a simple causal hypothesis in their study of the effects of the *e*PED on the quality of discharge teaching scores. They hypothesized: "Parents exposed to discharge teaching using *e*PED will have higher quality [of] discharge teaching scores than parents exposed to usual discharge teaching" (Lerret et al., 2020, p. 42). This hypothesis might be diagrammed as in Fig. 5.5. These researchers found the parents receiving *e*PED intervention reported higher discharge teaching scores than the parents exposed to standard discharge teaching. The results were significant, supporting the hypothesis that *e*PED was effective in improving the quality of discharge teaching.

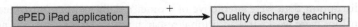

FIG. 5.5 Diagram of a Simple Causal Hypothesis from the Lerret et al. (2020) Study.

A complex hypothesis states the relationships (associative or causal) among three or more variables. Lerret et al. (2020, p. 42) included the following complex associative hypothesis in their study: "Quality of discharge teaching and care coordination will be inversely associated with readmission within 30 days for parents who receive teaching with the app." This hypothesis might be diagrammed as in Fig. 5.6 showing inverse or negative relationships. The variables quality discharge teaching and care coordination were only weakly associated with readmissions after 30 days. Thus the study results were nonsignificant, and the hypothesis was not supported. Lerret et al. (2020) had mixed results in their study with one hypothesis supported and three others not supported (Gray & Grove, 2021). Additional research was recommended with larger samples and other studies to examine the effects of the *e*PED app on additional healthcare outcomes for hospitalized children and their parents.

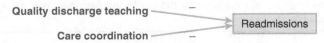

FIG. 5.6 Diagram of a Complex Associative Hypothesis from the Lerret et al. (2020) Study.

Nondirectional versus directional hypotheses. A nondirectional hypothesis states that a relationship exists, but it does not predict the nature (positive or negative) of the relationship. If the direction of the relationship being studied is not clear in clinical practice or in the theoretical or empirical literature, the researcher has no clear indication of the nature of the relationship (Chinn &

TABLE 5.7 EXAMPLE HYPOTHESES FROM PUBLISHED STUDIES

AUTHORS, YEAR	HYPOTHESIS	CAUSAL OR ASSOCIATIVE	SIMPLE OR COMPLEX	DIRECTIONAL OR NONDI-RECTIONAL	NULL OR RESEARCH
Lerret et al. (2020)	"Parents exposed to discharge teaching using *e*PED will have higher quality of discharge teaching scores than parents exposed to usual discharge teaching" (p. 42).	Causal	Simple	Directional	Research
Lerret et al. (2020)	"Parents of children with a chronic condition will report higher quality discharge teaching and care coordination than parents of children without a chronic condition" (p. 42).	Associative	Complex	Directional	Research
Theeke et al. (2019)	"Mean loneliness scores would differ based on diagnosis of depression" (p. 56).	Associative	Simple	Nondirectional	Research
Karasu & Aylaz (2020)	"Nursing care given to patients with COPD according to a health promotion model does not affect the meaning of life" (Introduction section).	Causal	Simple	Nondirectional	Null

Kramer, 2018; Gray & Grove, 2021). Under these circumstances, nondirectional hypotheses are developed. Theeke et al. (2019, p. 56) developed the following nondirectional hypothesis: "Mean loneliness scores would differ based on diagnosis of depression." This is an example of a simple (two variables), associative, nondirectional hypothesis (see Table 5.7). This hypothesis was supported because loneliness was significantly related to depression.

A directional hypothesis states the nature (positive or negative) of the interaction between two or more variables. The use of terms such as *positive, negative, less, more, increase, decrease, greater, higher,* or *lower* in a hypothesis indicates the direction of the relationship. Directional hypotheses are developed from theoretical statements (propositions), findings from previous studies, and clinical experience. As the knowledge on which a study is based increases, researchers are able to make a prediction about the direction of a relationship between the variables being studied. For example, Lerret et al. (2020, p. 42) stated a directional hypothesis: "Quality of discharge teaching and care coordination will be *inversely* [negatively] associated with readmission within 30 days for parents who receive teaching with the app." The italicized word indicates the nature of the relationship in this complex, associative, directional hypothesis. This inverse hypothesis predicts that as the quality of discharge teaching and care coordination increases, the number of readmissions within 30 days will decrease (see Fig. 5.6).

A causal hypothesis predicts the effect of an independent variable on a dependent variable; the independent variable increases or decreases each dependent variable. Therefore all causal hypotheses are directional (Kazdin, 2017). Chen and Hu (2019) conducted an RCT to determine the effects of a modified stretching exercise program (MSEP) on menstrual low back pain. One of the hypotheses examined in this study was: "The experimental group treated with the MSEP will score higher on the exercise self-efficacy scale (EXSE) than the control group" (Chen & Hu, 2019, p. 243). At 12 months, the young women in the MSEP group had significantly higher exercise self-efficacy scores than the control group, which supported the study hypothesis.

Statistical versus research hypotheses. Hypotheses are either research or statistical (see Table 5.6). The statistical hypothesis, also referred to as a null hypothesis (H_0), is used for statistical testing and interpretation of statistical results. Even if the null hypothesis is not stated, it is implied because it is the converse of the research hypothesis (Grove & Cipher, 2020). Some researchers state the null hypothesis because it is easier to interpret using the statistical results. The null hypothesis is also used when researchers believe that there is no relationship between two variables and when theoretical or empirical information is inadequate to state a research hypothesis. Null hypotheses can be simple or complex but are always nondirectional because the null hypothesis states there is no relationship between variables or differences between groups. Karasu and Aylaz (2020) examined the meaning of life and self-care in nursing care given to patients with COPD using a health promotion model. These researchers stated the following null hypothesis to direct their study: "Nursing care given to patients with COPD according to a health promotion model does not affect the meaning of life" (Karasu & Aylaz, 2020, Introduction section). This null hypothesis was not supported because the results were significant, indicating that nursing care applied to patients with COPD according to a health promotion model had increased self-care and meaning of life (Karasu & Aylaz, 2020, Abstract section).

A research hypothesis is the alternative hypothesis (H_1 or H_A) to the null or statistical hypothesis and states that a relationship exists between two or more variables. All the hypotheses stated earlier in this chapter were research hypotheses. Table 5.7 provides four hypotheses from nursing studies for you to review. Test yourself on the types of hypotheses that are presented—casual or associative, simple or complex, nondirectional or directional, and research or statistical.

📄 RESEARCH/EBP TIP

Hypotheses are tested in quasi-experimental and experimental studies to determine the effect of an intervention on a selected outcome. Determining the effectiveness of nursing interventions is essential for EBP.

❓ CRITICAL APPRAISAL GUIDELINES

Hypotheses in Studies

1. Are the hypotheses formally stated in the study? If the study is quasi-experimental or experimental, hypotheses are needed to direct the study.
2. Do the hypotheses clearly identify the relationships among the variables of the study?
3. Are the hypotheses associative or causal, simple or complex, directional or nondirectional, and research or null (see Table 5.6)?
4. If hypotheses are included in a study, are they used to organize research results and interpret study findings?

The Chen and Hu (2019) study, introduced earlier, identified three causal hypotheses to direct their study. The research purpose and two of the study hypotheses are presented and critically appraised in Research Example 5.5.

RESEARCH EXAMPLE 5.5

Hypothesis

Research/Study Excerpt

Purpose

The purpose of this study was to evaluate the effectiveness of a modified stretching exercise program (MSEP) on young women with low back pain during menstrual period. (Chen & Hu, 2019, p. 243)

Hypotheses

Hypothesis 2: The experimental group treated with a MSEP will score lower on the back pain disability questionnaire (Oswestry Low Back Pain Disability Questionnaire [ODI]) than the control group.

Hypothesis 3: The experimental group treated with a MSEP will score higher on the exercise self-efficacy scale (EXSE) than the control group. (Chen & Hu, 2019, p. 243)

Critical Appraisal

The research purpose clearly identified the intervention (MSEP) and the population studied (young women with menstrual low back pain). However, the study dependent variables were not identified, which reduced the logical flow from the purpose to the research hypotheses. Chen and Hu (2019) stated simple, directional, causal research hypotheses, which are appropriate for an RCT. An RCT is an experimental study that determines the effectiveness of an intervention on selected dependent variables (Gray & Grove, 2021). The hypotheses clearly identified the intervention and population, but not the dependent variables. The researchers identified measurement methods, Oswestry Low Back Pain Disability Questionnaire and EXSE, instead of the dependent variables, back pain disability and exercise self-efficacy, in their hypotheses. The Results section was not organized by the study hypotheses, but the findings did indicate that both hypotheses were supported, which strengthened the empirical evidence for the MSEP intervention in this population. With additional research, this intervention has the potential to be used in practice.

Testable Hypothesis

The value of a hypothesis ultimately is derived from whether it is testable in the real world. A testable hypothesis is one that clearly predicts the relationships among variables and contains variables that are measurable or able to be manipulated in a study. The independent variable must be clearly defined, often by a protocol. A protocol is a detailed plan for implementing an intervention and measuring its effects precisely and consistently (see Chapter 8). The dependent variable must be clearly defined to indicate how it will be precisely and accurately measured (see the next section on defining study variables).

A testable hypothesis also needs to predict a relationship that can be "supported" or "not supported," as indicated by the data collected and analyzed. If the hypothesis states an associative relationship, correlational analyses are conducted on the data to determine the existence, type, and strength of the relationship between the variables studied. A causal hypothesis is tested by conducting statistics, such as the *t*-test or analysis of variance, to determine differences between the means of the dependent variables for the experimental and comparison or control groups (Grove & Cipher, 2020; see Chapter 11). It is the statistical or null hypothesis (stated or implied) that is tested to determine whether the independent variable produced a significant effect on the dependent variable.

Hypotheses are clearer without specifying the presence or absence of a *significant difference* because determination of significance is only a statistical technique applied to sample data. In addition, hypotheses should not identify methodological points, such as techniques of sampling, measurement, and data analysis (Grove & Cipher, 2020). Therefore phrases such as *measured by*, *in a random sample of*, and *using analysis of variance* are inappropriate because they limit the hypothesis to the measurement methods, sample, or analysis techniques identified for one study.

📄 **RESEARCH/EBP TIP**

Objectives, questions, and hypotheses direct the methodology of a study, organize the study results, and provide direction for implementing findings in practice. A well-designed study increases the credibility of the findings and provides a basis for further research to generate sound knowledge for practice.

UNDERSTANDING VARIABLES AND CONCEPTS IN RESEARCH

The research purpose and objectives, questions, and hypotheses include the variables or concepts to be examined in a study. Variables are qualities, properties, or characteristics of persons, things, or situations that change or vary. Variables should be concisely defined to promote their measurement or manipulation in quantitative and outcomes studies (Bandalos, 2018; Kazdin, 2017). Research concepts are usually studied in qualitative research, are at higher levels of abstraction than variables, and are described, not manipulated, or measured (Creswell & Poth, 2018). The different types of variable are described, and the conceptual and operational definitions of variables in quantitative and outcomes studies are discussed.

Types of Variable in Quantitative Research

Variables are classified into a variety of types to explain their use in research. Some variables are manipulated; others are controlled. Some variables are identified, but not measured; others are measured with refined measurement devices. The types of variable presented in this section include research, independent, dependent, and extraneous variables.

Research Variables

Descriptive and correlational quantitative studies and mixed methods studies usually involve the investigation of research variables. Research variables are the qualities, properties, or characteristics identified in the research purpose and objectives or questions that are measured in a study. Research variables are included in a study when the intent is to observe or measure variables as they exist in a natural setting, without the implementation of a treatment. Gathright et al. (2020) conducted a descriptive study to identify the rates of and reasons for e-cigarette use among adults with HF (see Table 5.1 for the study problem and purpose). The research variables for this study are identified in Table 5.8 and linked to the concept of tobacco product use from the study framework.

Independent and Dependent Variables

The relationship between independent and dependent variables is the basis for formulating hypotheses for correlational, quasi-experimental, and experimental studies and sometimes outcomes studies. In predictive correlational studies, the independent variables are measured to predict a single dependent variable (Grove & Cipher, 2020). For example, Lerret et al. (2020) predicted quality of discharge teaching scores and care coordination would be negatively associated

TABLE 5.8	LINKING CONCEPTS TO VARIABLES AND IDENTIFYING TYPES OF VARIABLE		
RESEARCH ARTICLE	**CONCEPT**	**VARIABLE**	**TYPE OF VARIABLE**
Gathright et al. (2020)	Tobacco product use	Rate of e-cigarette use	Research
	Tobacco product use	Reasons for e-cigarette use	Research
Lerret et al. (2020)	Discharge education	Engaging Parents in Education for Discharge (ePED) iPad application	Independent
	Discharge experience	Quality of discharge teaching	Dependent
		Care coordination	Dependent

Data are from Gathright, E. C., Wu, W., & Scott-Sheldon, L. (2020). Electronic cigarette use among heart failure patients: Findings from the Population Assessment of Tobacco and Health Study (Wave 1: 2013-2014). *Heart & Lung*, *49*(3), 229–232. https://doi.org/10.1016/j.hrtlng.2019.11.006; and Lerret, S. M., Johnson, N. L., Polfuss, M., Weiss, M., Gralton, K., Gibson, C.,...Sawin, K. (2020). Using the engaging Parents in Education for Discharge (ePED) iPad Application to improve parent discharge experience. *Journal of Pediatric Nursing*, *52*, 41–48. https://doi.org/10.1016/j.pedn.2020.02.041

with readmission within 30 days of discharge. The independent variables discharge teaching and care coordination were used to predict the outcome or dependent variable readmissions (see Fig. 5.6 for a diagram of this hypothesis). This hypothesis was presented earlier and was not supported by the study results.

The term independent variable is more frequently used to identify an intervention that is manipulated or varied by the researcher to create an effect on the dependent variable. The independent variable is also called an intervention, treatment, or experimental variable. A dependent variable is the outcome that the researcher wants to predict or explain. Changes in the dependent variable are presumed to be caused by the independent variable. The Lerret et al. (2020) study hypothesis, presented in Fig. 5.5, focused on examining the effect of the ePED iPad app on parents' quality of discharge teaching scores. The independent variable was the ePED iPad app that was implemented to improve the quality of discharge teaching scores and care coordination (dependent variables) for parents with hospitalized children. The variables for this study are presented in Table 5.8 and linked to the concepts in the study framework. The concept discharge education was linked to the independent variable ePED iPad app. The concept discharge experience was linked to the dependent variables of quality of discharge teaching and care coordination. The study results were significant, and the hypothesis was supported. The researchers recommended "the use of the ePED by the discharging nurse to enhance parent-reported quality of discharge teaching" (Lerret et al., 2020, p. 41).

Extraneous Variables

Extraneous variables exist in all studies and can affect the measurement of study variables and the relationships among these variables. Extraneous variables are of primary concern in studies examining the effects of interventions because they can interfere with obtaining a clear understanding of the relational or causal dynamics in these studies (Kazdin, 2017). Extraneous variables are classified as recognized or unrecognized and controlled or uncontrolled. Some extraneous variables are not recognized until the study is in progress or has been completed, but their presence influences the study outcome.

Researchers attempt to recognize and control as many extraneous variables as possible in quasi-experimental and experimental studies. For example, specific designs, intervention protocols, and sample criteria have been developed to control the influence of extraneous variables. Lerret et al. (2020) conducted a pretest–posttest two-group design to examine the effect of the *e*PED on parent experiences of hospital discharge (see Table 5.1). This is a strong experimental design that includes random assignment of study participants to the experimental and comparison groups, reducing the potential effects of extraneous variables (see Chapter 8; Kazdin, 2017). The study sample of parents of hospitalized children was large ($N = 395$) with fairly equal numbers of participants in the experiment group ($n = 211$) and the comparison group ($n = 184$). The participants were obtained from two different units in a pediatric academic medical center, to reduce any communication about the intervention to the comparison group. The nurses implementing the intervention and collecting data were trained to reduce the potential for errors. However, the authors might have provided more detail about the *e*PED intervention or included the protocol for the intervention in the article. The scales used to measure quality of discharge teaching and care coordination were reliable and valid (Bandalos, 2018).

The extraneous variables that are not recognized until the study is in process or are recognized before the study is initiated but cannot be controlled are referred to as confounding variables. Sometimes, extraneous variables can be measured during the study and controlled statistically during analysis. However, extraneous variables that cannot be controlled or measured are a design weakness and can hinder the interpretation of findings. As control in correlational, quasi-experimental, and experimental studies decreases, the potential influence of confounding variables increases.

Environmental variables are a type of extraneous variable that compose the setting in which the study is conducted. Examples of these variables include climate, family, and healthcare system. If a researcher is studying people in an uncontrolled or natural setting, it is impossible and undesirable to control the extraneous variables. In qualitative and some quantitative (descriptive and correlational) and mixed methods studies, little or no attempt is made to control extraneous variables. The intent is to study participants in their natural environment, without controlling or altering that setting or situation.

The environmental variables in quasi-experimental and experimental research can be controlled by using a laboratory setting or a specially constructed research unit in a hospital (see Chapter 9). For example, Kaya and colleagues (2017) conducted an experimental study in a neurosurgical ICU, a highly controlled clinical setting (see Table 5.1). The controlled setting, structured intervention of oral care with glutamine, and detailed measurement of VAP reduced the potential for extraneous and environment variables to adversely affect the study outcomes.

Conceptual and Operational Definitions of Variables in Quantitative Research

A variable is operationalized in a study by the development of conceptual and operational definitions. A conceptual definition provides the theoretical meaning of a variable (Chinn & Kramer, 2018) and is often derived from a theorist's definition of a related concept. The framework in a study includes concepts and their definitions, and the variables are selected to represent these concepts (see Chapter 7). The variables are conceptually defined, indicating the link with the concepts in the framework.

An operational definition is derived from a set of procedures or progressive acts that a researcher performs to receive sensory impressions (e.g., sound, visual, tactile impressions) that indicate the existence or degree of existence of a variable (Kazdin, 2017; Waltz et al., 2017). An operational definition is developed so that a variable can be measured or manipulated in a concrete situation; the knowledge gained from studying the variable will increase the understanding of the theoretical concepts that this variable represents. Operational definitions need to be independent of time and setting so that variables can be investigated at different times and in different settings using the same operational definitions. Table 5.8 includes the concepts and variables from the Gathright et al. (2020) and Lerret et al. (2020) studies. Reading across the table, you can see the link of each concept to the appropriate variable(s), and the type of variable is identified. The conceptual and operational definitions for the independent variable *ePED* and one of the dependent variables, care coordination, from the Lerret et al. (2020) study are presented in Research Example 5.6. The guidelines identified in the following Critical Appraisal Guidelines box were used to critically appraise these variables and their definitions.

? CRITICAL APPRAISAL GUIDELINES

Study Variables

1. Are the variables clearly identified in the study purpose and/or research objectives, questions, or hypotheses?
2. What types of variables are examined in the study? Are independent and dependent variables or research variables examined in the study?
3. If a quasi-experimental or experimental study is conducted, are the extraneous variables identified and controlled?
4. Are the variables in quantitative and outcomes studies conceptually defined?
5. Are the variables operationally defined?

⑸ RESEARCH EXAMPLE 5.6

Conceptual and Operational Definitions of Variables

Independent Variable: Engaging Parents in *e*PED iPad App
Conceptual Definition
The ePED was based on the Tanner's Reflective Practitioner Theory and the Individual and Family Self-Management Theory (IFSMT). "The integration of these frameworks informed the content, as well as the process for this innovative ePED teaching tool…to guide an interactive conversation between the parent and discharging nurse" (Lerret et al., 2020, p. 42).

Operational Definition
The ePED app guides the nurse through the five domains by providing specific open-ended questions to assess, confirm, and encourage parents before going home, eliciting specific plans and potential concerns, gaps in knowledge and opportunities for additional teaching. (Lerret et al., 2020, p. 43)

Dependent Variable: Care Coordination
Conceptual Definition
Care coordination is an outcome of the IFSMT that focuses on the nurse's ability to promote a quality discharge experience, which includes the parent's and child's ability to manage their condition at home (Lerret et al., 2020).

Operational Definition
Care coordination was measured with the Care Transition Measure (CTM) that includes 15 items that measure four key domains (information, preparation of patient/caregiver, self-management support, and empowerment) of this variable. (Lerret et al., 2020)

Continued

⚡ RESEARCH EXAMPLE 5.6—cont'd

Critical Appraisal

These independent and dependent variables were identified in the research purpose and hypotheses stated earlier (see Table 5.1). The conceptual definitions for the *e*PED and care coordination were based on the theories and concepts presented in the study framework. The operational definitions for the variables were clear and relevant; they were found in the Methods section of the research report. The conceptual and operational definitions for *e*PED and care coordination were strong in this study.

📄 RESEARCH/EBP TIP

The conceptual definitions in research link the concepts in the framework to the study variables, expanding the knowledge generated for nursing. Operational definitions identify intervention protocols and measurement methods that might be used in practice. A protocol details the process for implementing an intervention. The measurement methods used in research provide a way to examine outcomes in practice.

Research Concepts Investigated in Qualitative Research

The variables in quasi-experimental and experimental research are narrow and specific in focus and can be quantified (converted to numbers) or manipulated using specified steps in a protocol. In addition, the variables are objectively defined to decrease researcher bias. Qualitative research is more abstract, subjective, and holistic than quantitative research and involves the investigation of research concepts. Research concepts include the ideas, experiences, situations, events, or cultures that are investigated in qualitative and mixed methods studies. For example, Manson et al. (2020) conducted an exploratory-descriptive qualitative study to increase understanding of the experiences and perceptions of people living with AD and their caregivers related to life satisfaction and QoL (see Table 5.2). The research concepts explored were experiences and perceptions of living with AD, including life satisfaction and QoL. In many qualitative studies, the focus of the study is to explore, identify, define, or describe the concept(s) being studied (Creswell & Poth, 2018). In this study, the concept of living with mild to moderate AD involves extensive hardships and challenges for the individual with AD and their caregivers and the need for many resources (Manson et al., 2020).

Demographic Variables

Demographic variables are attributes of study participants. Some common demographic variables include age, education, gender, marital status, income, and medical diagnosis. Once data are collected from participants on these demographic variables and analyzed, the results are called demographic or sample characteristics (see Chapter 9). The demographic characteristics are included in a research report to describe the sample and can be presented in table and/or narrative format. The demographic characteristics can be used to compare this sample with the samples from similar studies. When many samples have similar characteristics and findings, the credibility of the findings is expanded, as is their potential usefulness in practice. Mulholland et al. (2020) conducted a phenomenological study to explore military families' battles with parental deployment (see Table 5.2). They presented their demographic characteristics in a table (Table 5.9) and summarized key ideas about their sample in the study's narrative. Research Example 5.7 provides a critical appraisal of the demographic characteristics in this study.

TABLE 5.9 DEMOGRAPHICS OF STUDY SAMPLE

		NUMBER (N = 15)	PERCENTAGE (%)	AVERAGE
Gender	Female	14	93.3%	
	Male	1	6.7%	
Role	Spouse/significant other	13	86.7%	
	Military parent	2	13.3%	
Age (years)	20–29	5	33.3%	35.8 ≈ 36
	30–39	5	33.3%	
	40–49	4	26.7%	
	50–59	1	6.7%	
Race/ethnicity	White/Caucasian	10	66.7%	
	Hispanic/Latino	2	13.3%	
	Mixed race	2	13.3%	
	Native American	1	6.7%	
Military branch	Army	10	66.7%	
	Air force	5	33.3%	
Rank/paygrade[a]	Enlisted (E4–E6)	6	40%	
	Enlisted (E7–E9)	5	33.3%	
	Officer (O3–O5)	2	13.3%	
	Officer (W3)	1	6.7%	
	Not identified	1	6.7%	
# of deployments completed	1–2	3	20%	5
	3–4	6	40%	
	5–6	1	6.7%	
	7–8	1	6.7%	
	9–10	4	26.7%	
Duration of recent deployment (months)	5–9	9	60%	8.04 ≈ 8
	10–14	4	26.7%	
	Not disclosed	2	13.3%	
First deployment	Yes	2	13.3%	
	No	13	86.7%	
Number of children	1	3	20%	2.3 ≈ 2
	2	8	53.3%	
	3	2	13.3%	
	4+	2	13.3%	

Continued

TABLE 5.9	DEMOGRAPHICS OF STUDY SAMPLE—cont'd			
		NUMBER (N = 15)	PERCENTAGE (%)	AVERAGE
Single parent	No	15	100%	
Age of oldest/only child (years)	0–1	2	13.3%	9.01 ≈ 9
	2–3	2	13.3%	
	4–6	3	20%	
	7–12	1	6.7%	
	13–18	7	46.7%	

[a]US Department of Defense. (n.d.). U.S. military rank insignia. Retrieved from https://www.defense.gov/Resources/Insignias/

From Mulholland, E., Dahlberg, D., & McDowell, L. (2020). A two-front war: Exploring military families' battle with parental deployment. *Journal of Pediatric Nursing, 54*, 34–41. https://doi.org/10.1016/j.pedn.2020.05.019

RESEARCH EXAMPLE 5.7

Demographic Characteristics

Research/Study Excerpt

A total of 27 participants completed the survey, and 15 of those were selected for the study sample. Of the 12 participants that were not selected due to the exclusion criteria, nine participants had not completed a deployment within the past 5 years, two participants did not have children. ... The demographic characteristics of the study sample are presented in Table 5.9. The majority of the sample represented were female (93.3%), the spouse/significant other of someone in military service (86.7%), and of white/Caucasian race (66.7%). The Army and Air Force were the only branches of the military represented in the sample, in which the Army represented the majority (66.7%). (Mulholland et al., 2020, p. 36)

Critical Appraisal

The demographic variables included in this study were gender, role, age (years), race/ethnicity, military branch, rank/paygrade, number of deployments completed, duration of recent deployment (months), first deployment, number of children, single parent, and age of oldest/only child (years). Data for many of these demographic variables are commonly collected and analyzed to describe study samples. Other demographic variables, such as military branch, rank, and deployments, were specific to this study to describe important characteristics of this sample. Mulholland et al. (2020) clearly identified the sample size of 15 and the reasons for not including 12 individuals who had been initially recruited for the study. These researchers provided a quality description of their sample in table and narrative formats.

RESEARCH/EBP TIP

Studies require a clear, concise statement of a problem and purpose to ensure a quality study is conducted. The foci of some studies are clarified with objectives, questions, or hypotheses that include study variables. You need to critically appraise these elements in studies to determine the quality and credibility of the findings and potential use in practice.

KEY POINTS

- The research problem is an area of concern in which there is a gap in the knowledge base needed for nursing practice. The problem includes significance, background, and problem statement.
- The research purpose is a concise, clear statement of the specific study goal or focus.
- Research objectives, questions, or hypotheses are formulated to bridge the gap between the more abstractly stated research problem and purpose and the detailed quantitative design, results, and interpretation of findings.
- Qualitative and mixed methods studies often include the problem, purpose, and research questions or aims to direct a study.
- A hypothesis is the formal statement of the expected relationship(s) between two or more variables in a specified population in quantitative and outcomes studies.
- Quasi-experimental and experimental studies should include hypotheses that predicted the effect of an intervention on study outcomes.
- Variables are qualities, properties, or characteristics of persons, things, or situations that change or vary.
- An independent variable is an intervention or treatment that is manipulated or varied by the researcher to create an effect on the dependent variable. A dependent variable is the outcome that the researcher wants to predict or explain.
- A variable is operationalized in quantitative and outcomes studies by developing conceptual and operational definitions.
- A conceptual definition provides the theoretical meaning of a variable and is derived from a theorist's definition of a related concept.
- Operational definitions indicate how an independent variable will be implemented and how the dependent or outcome variable will be measured.
- Research concepts include the ideas, experiences, situations, events, or behaviors that are investigated in qualitative and mixed methods research.
- Demographic variables are collected and analyzed to determine sample characteristics for describing the study participants in all types of nursing research.

REFERENCES

2019 Alzheimer's Disease Facts and Figures (2019). *Alzheimer's & Dementia, 15*(3), 321–387. https://doi.org/10.1016/j.jalz.2019.01.010

Aberson, C. L. (2019). *Applied analysis for the behavioral sciences* (2nd ed.). Routledge Taylor & Francis Group.

Agency for Healthcare Research and Quality. (2021). *About AHRQ: Mission and budget.* Retrieved from https://www.ahrq.gov/cpi/about/mission/index.html

Akkayaoğlu, H., & Çelik, S. (2020). Eating attitudes, perception of body image and patient quality of life before and after bariatric surgery. *Applied Nursing Research, 53*, 151270. https://doi.org/10.1016/j.apnr.2020.151270

Alexander, M., Durham, C. F., Hooper, J. I., Jeffries, P. R., Goldman, N., Kardong-Edgren, S.,...Radtke, B. (2015).

NCSBN simulation guidelines for prelicensure nursing programs. *Journal of Nursing Regulation, 6*(3), 39–42. https://doi.org/10.1016/S2155-8256(15)30783-3

Ansari-Gilani, K., Petraszko, A. M., Teba, C. V., Reeves, A. R., Gupta, A., Gupta, A.,...Gilkeson, R. C. (2020). E-cigarette use related lung disease, review of clinical imaging. *Heart & Lung, 49*(2), 139–143. https://doi.org/10.1016/j.hrtlng.2020.01.005

Avery, J., Schreier, A., & Swanson, M. (2020). A complex population: Nurse's professional preparedness to care for medical-surgical patients with mental illness. *Applied Nursing Research, 52*, 151232. https://doi.org/10.1016/j.apnr.2020.151232

Bandalos, D. L. (2018). *Measurement theory and applications for the social sciences.* The Guilford Press.

Begum, R., Liu, J., & Sun, C. (2020). Always InforMED: Nurse champion-led intervention to improve medication communication among nurses and patients. *Applied Nursing Research, 53*, 51264. https://doi.org/10.1016/j.apnr.2020.151264

Bourke, J., de Klerk, N., Smith, T., & Leonard, H. (2016). Population-based prevalence of intellectual disability and autism spectrum disorders in Western Australia: A comparison with previous estimates. *Medicine 95*(21), e3737. https://doi.org/10.1097/MD.0000000000003737

Burbach, B. E., Struwe, L. A., Young, L., & Cohen, M. Z. (2019). Correlates of student performance during low stakes simulation. *Journal of Professional Nursing, 35*(1), 44–45. https://doi.org/10.1016/j.profnurs.2018.06.002

Burbach, B. E., Thompson, S. A., Barnason, S., Wilhelm, S., Kotcherlakota, S., Miller, C. L., & Paulman, P. M. (2016). Lived experiences during simulation: Student-perceived influences on performance. *Journal of Nursing Education, 55*(7), 396–398. https://doi.org/10.3928/01484834-20160615-07

Bryant, A., & Charmaz, K. (2019). *The Sage handbook of current developments of grounded theory.* Sage.

Castner, J., Jungquist, C. R., Mammen, M. J., Pender, J. J., Licata, O., & Sethi, S. (2020). Prediction model development of women's daily asthma control using fitness tracker sleep disruption. *Heart & Lung, 49*(5), 548–555. https://doi.org/10.1016/j.hrtlng.2020.01.013

Chen, H., & Hu, H. (2019). Randomized trial of modified stretching exercise program for menstrual low back pain. *Western Journal of Nursing Research, 41*(2), 238–257. https://doi.org/10.1177/0193945918763817

Chinn, P. L., & Kramer, M. K. (2018). *Knowledge development in nursing: Theory and process* (10th ed.). Mosby.

Creswell, J. W., & Clark, V. L. P. (2018). *Designing and conducting mixed methods research* (3rd ed.). Sage.

Creswell, J. W., & Creswell, J. D. (2018). *Research design: Qualitative, quantitative, and mixed methods approaches* (5th ed.). Sage.

Creswell, J. W., & Poth, C. N. (2018). *Qualitative inquiry & research design: Choosing among five approaches* (4th ed.). Sage.

Donabedian, A. (1988). The quality of care: How can it be assessed? *Journal of the American Medical Association, 260*(12), 1743–1748.

Epstein, A., Whitehouse, A., Williams, K., Murphy, N., Leonard, H., Davis, E.,…Downs, J. (2019). Parent-observed thematic data on quality of life in children with autism spectrum disorder. *Autism, 23*(1), 71–80. https://doi.org/10.1177/1362361317722764

Gathright, E. C., Wu, W., & Scott-Sheldon, L. (2020). Electronic cigarette use among heart failure patients: Findings from the Population Assessment of Tobacco and Health Study (Wave 1: 2013–2014). *Heart & Lung, 49*(3), 229–232. https://doi.org/10.1016/j.hrtlng.2019.11.006

Global Initiative for Chronic Obstructive Lung Disease. (2018). *Global strategy for the diagnosis, management, and prevention of chronic obstructive pulmonary disease.* Retrieved from https://goldcopd.org/wp-content/uploads/2017/11/GOLD-2018-v6.0-FINAL-revised-20-Nov_WMS.pdf

Gray, J. R., & Grove, S. K. (2021). *The practice of nursing research: Appraisal, synthesis, and generation of evidence* (9th ed.). Elsevier.

Grove, S. K., & Cipher, D. J. (2020). *Statistics for nursing research: A workbook for evidence-based practice* (3rd ed.). Elsevier.

Hansen, S. N., Schendel, D. E., & Partner, E. T. (2015). Explaining the increase in the prevalence of autism spectrum disorders: The proportion attributable to changes in reporting practices. *JAMA Pediatrics, 169*(1), 56–62. https://doi.org/10.1001/jamapediatrics.2014.1893

Henson, A., & Jeffrey, C. (2016). Turning a clinical question into nursing research: The benefits of a pilot study. *Renal Society of Australasia Journal, 12*(3), 99–105.

Hilken, L., Dickson, A., & Sidley, C. (2017). Nurse infection prevention champions: A model for success. *American Journal of Infection Control, 45*(6) S107. https://doi.org/10.1016/j.ajic.2017.04.176

Karasu, F., & Aylaz, R. (2020). Evaluation of meaning of life and self-care agency in nursing care given to chronic obstructive pulmonary patients according to health promotion model. *Applied Nursing Research, 51*, 151208. https://doi.org/10.1016/j.apnr.2019.151208

Kaya, H., Turan, Y., Tunali, Y., Aydin, G., Yüce, N., Gürbüz, S., & Tosun, K. (2017). Effects of oral care with glutamine in preventing ventilator-associated pneumonia in neurosurgical intensive care unit patients. *Applied Nursing Research, 33*, 10–14. http://dx.doi.org/10.1016/j.apnr.2016.10.006

Kazdin, A. E. (2017). *Research design in clinical psychology* (5th ed.). Pearson.

Kim, H., Sefcik, J. S., & Bradway, C. (2017). Characteristics of qualitative descriptive studies: A systematic review. *Research in Nursing & Health, 40*(1), 23–42. https://doi.org/10.1002/nur.21768

Kolozsvari, N. O., Feldman, L. S., Vassiliou, M. C., Demyttenaere, S., & Hoover, M. L. (2011). Sim one, do one, teach one: Considerations in designing training curricula for surgical simulation. *Journal of Surgical Education, 68*(5), 421–427. https://doi.org/10.1016/j.jsurg.2011.03.010

Lavoie, P., Clarke, S. P., Clausen, C., Purden, M., Emed, J., Mailhot, T.,…Frunchak, V. (2020). Nurses' judgements of patient risk of deterioration at change-of-shift handoff: Agreement between nurses and comparison with early warning scores. *Heart & Lung, 49*(4), 420–425. https://doi.org/10.1016/j.hrtlng.2020.02.037

Lee, J. A., Choi, M., Lee, S. A., & Jiang, N. (2018). Effective behavioral intervention strategies using mobile health applications for chronic disease management: A systematic review. *BMC Medical Informatics and Decision Making, 18*(1), 12. https://doi.org/10.1186/s12911-018-0591-0

Leedy, P. D., & Ormrod, J. E. (2019). *Practical research: Planning and design* (12th ed.) Pearson.

Lerret, S. M., Johnson, N. L., Polfuss, M., Weiss, M., Gralton, K., Gibson, C.,…Sawin, K. (2020). Using the Engaging Parents in Education for Discharge (*e*PED) iPad Application to improve parent discharge experience. *Journal of Pediatric Nursing, 52*, 41–48. https://doi.org/10.1016/j.pedn.2020.02.041

Lerret, S. M., & Weiss, M. E. (2011). How ready are they? Parents of pediatric solid organ transplant recipients and the transition from hospital to home following transplant. *Pediatric Transplantation, 15*(6), 606–616. https://doi.org/10.1111/j.1399-3046.2011.01536.x

Lester, P., Aralis, H., Sinclair, M., Kiff, C., Lee, K. H., Mustillo, S., & Wadsworth, S. (2016). The impact of deployment on parental, family, and child adjustment in military families. *Child Psychiatry & Human Development, 47*(6), 938–949. https://doi.org/10.1007/s10578-016-0624-9

Manson, A., Ciro, C., Williams, K. N., & Maliski, S. L. (2020). Identity and perceptions of quality of life in Alzheimer's disease. *Applied Nursing Research, 52*, 151225. https://doi.org/10.1016/j.apnr.2019.151225

Marshall, C., & Rossman, G. B. (2016). *Designing qualitative research* (6th ed.). Sage.

Melnyk, B. M., & Fineout-Overholt, E. (2019). *Evidence-based practice in nursing & healthcare: A guide to best practice* (4th ed.). Wolters Kluwer.

Miles, M. B., Huberman, A. M., & Saldaña, J. (2020). *Qualitative data analysis: A methods sourcebook* (4th ed.). Sage.

Moorhead, S., Swanson, E., Johnson, M., & Maas, M. L. (2018). *Nursing outcomes classification (NOC): Measurement of health outcomes* (6th ed.). Elsevier.

Mulholland, E., Dahlberg, D., & McDowell, L. (2020). A two-front war: Exploring military families' battle with parental deployment. *Journal of Pediatric Nursing, 54*, 34–41. https://doi.org/10.1016/j.pedn.2020.05.019

National Institute of Mental Health. (2016). *Mental illness.* Retrieved from https://www.nimh.nih.gov/health/statistics/mental-illness.shtml

National Institute of Nursing Research. (2021). *About NINR.* Retrieved from https://www.ninr.nih.gov/aboutninr/budgetandlegislation

Park, S. K., Bang, C. H., & Lee, S. H. (2020). Evaluating the effect of a smartphone app-based self-management program for people with COPD: A randomized controlled trial. *Applied Nursing Research, 52*, 51231. https://doi.org/10.1016/j.apnr.2020.151231

Quality and Safety Education for Nurses. (2020). *QSEN competencies: Pre-licensure knowledge, skills, and attitudes (KSAs).* Retrieved from http://qsen.org/competencies/pre-licensure-ksas/

Rice, M. J., Stalling, J., & Monasterio, A. (2019). Psychiatric-mental health nursing: Data-driven policy platform for a psychiatric mental health care workforce. *Journal of the American Psychiatric Nurses Association, 25*(1), 27–37. https://doi.org/10.1177/1078390318808368

Ricks, T. N., Frederick, A., & Harrison, T. (2020). Health and disability among young Black men. *Nursing Research, 69*(1), 13–21. https://doi.org/10.1097/NNR.0000000000000396

Salzmann-Erikson, M. (2018). Using focused ethnography to explore and describe the process of nurses' shift reports in a psychiatric intensive care unit. *Journal of Clinical Nursing, 27*(15–16), 3104–3114. https://doi.org/10.1111/jocn.14502

Schuler, E., Paul, F., Connor, L., Doherty, D., & DeGrazia, M. (2020) Cultivating evidence-based practice through mentorship. *Applied Nursing Research, 55*, 151295. https://doi.org/10.1016/j.apnr.2020.151295

Shadish, W. R., Cook, T. D., & Campbell, D. T. (2002). *Experimental and quasi-experimental designs for generalized causal inference.* Rand McNally.

Siedlecki, S. L., & Albert, N. M. (2020). The growth of nursing research within a large healthcare system. *Applied Nursing Research, 55*, 151291. https://doi.org/10.1016/j.apnr.2020.151291

Theeke, L., Carpenter, R. D., Mallow, J., & Theeke, E. (2019). Gender differences in loneliness, anger, depression, self-management ability, and biomarkers of chronic illness in chronically ill mid-life adults in Appalachia. *Applied Nursing Research, 45*, 55–62. https://doi.org/10.1016/j.apnr.2018.12.001

US Department of Defense. (2018). *2018 demographics report: Profile of the military community.* Retrieved from https://download.militaryonesource.mil/12038/MOS/Reports/2018-demographics-report.pdf

Waltz, C. F., Strickland, O. L., & Lenz, E. R. (2017). *Measurement in nursing and health research* (5th ed.). Springer.

Weiss, M. E., Bobay, K. L., Bahr, S. J., Costa, L., Hughes, R. G., & Holland, D. E. (2015). A model for hospital discharge preparation: From case management to care transition. *Journal of Nursing Administration, 45*(12), 606–614. https://doi.org/10.1097/NNA.0000000000000273

Understanding and Critically Appraising the Literature Review

Polly A. Hulme

LEARNING OUTCOMES

After completing this chapter, you should be able to:

1. Discuss the purposes of the literature review in quantitative, qualitative, mixed methods, and outcomes research.
2. Critically appraise the literature review section of a published study for current quality sources, relevant content, and synthesis of relevant content.

3. Conduct a computerized search of the literature.
4. Write a literature review from a synthesis of critically appraised sources to promote the use of evidence-based knowledge in nursing practice.

A high-quality review of literature contains the current theoretical and scientific knowledge about a specific topic. The review identifies what is known and unknown about that topic. Nurses in clinical practice review the literature to synthesize the available evidence to find a solution to a problem in practice or to remain current in their practice. As students and nurses read studies, they must critically appraise the literature review, as well as the other components of the study. Critically appraising a review of literature begins with understanding the purpose of the literature review in quantitative, qualitative, mixed methods, and outcomes studies and the relative quality of the different types of reference that are cited. The critical appraisal guidelines for literature reviews listed in this chapter can be applied to a variety of studies conducted in nursing. In addition, example critical appraisals of the literature reviews from research reports are provided.

A review of literature is the process of finding relevant research sources and theoretical sources, critically appraising these sources, synthesizing the results, and developing an accurate and complete reference list. As a foundation for this process, this chapter includes information on how to find references, select those that are relevant, organize what you find, and write a logical summary of the findings.

You may be required to review the literature as part of a course assignment or project in the clinical setting, especially projects in Magnet hospitals. Nurses in Magnet hospitals must implement evidence-based practice (EBP), identify practice problems, and assist with data collection for studies (American Nurses Credentialing Center, 2021; Brown, 2020). Reviewing the literature is a first step in implementing EBP and identifying practice problems.

PURPOSE OF THE LITERATURE REVIEW

Literature reviews in published research reports provide the background and significance for the problem studied. Such reviews include (1) describing the current knowledge of a practice problem, (2) identifying the gaps in this knowledge base, and (3) explaining how the study being reported has contributed to building knowledge in this area. The scope of a literature review must be broad enough to allow the reader to become familiar with the research problem and narrow enough to include only the most relevant sources (Gray & Grove, 2021).

Purpose of the Literature Review in Quantitative and Outcomes Research

The review of literature in quantitative and outcomes research is conducted to direct the planning and execution of a study. A major literature review is performed at the beginning of the research process (before the study is conducted). A limited review is conducted after the study is completed to identify studies published since the original literature review, especially if it has been 1 year or longer since the study began. Additional articles may be retrieved to find information relevant to interpreting the findings. The results of both reviews are included in the research report. The purpose of the literature review is similar for the different types of quantitative studies—descriptive, correlational, quasi-experimental, and experimental; outcomes studies; and the quantitative part of mixed methods studies.

Quantitative and outcomes research reports may include citations to relevant sources in all sections of the report. The researchers include sources in the Introduction section to summarize the background and significance of the research problem. The review includes theoretical and research references that document current knowledge about the problem studied. Citations about the number of patients affected; cost of treatment; and consequences in terms of human suffering, physical health, disability, and mortality may be included. The review of literature section may not be labeled but may be integrated into the introduction or background of a research report.

A quantitative researcher develops the framework section of a proposal or article from the theoretical literature and sometimes from research reports, depending on the focus of the study. Similar to the review of literature, the research framework may not be labeled but may be integrated into the introduction, literature review, or background of a study. A chosen theoretical framework is an organizational tool that places a study within a larger body of knowledge. A study is like a puzzle piece that has a place and context within the larger puzzle (the framework). Theoretical frameworks are described in detail in Chapter 7.

The Methods section of the research report describes the design, the sample and the process for obtaining the sample, measurement methods, treatment, the data collection process, and a list of the statistical analyses conducted. References may be cited in various parts of the Methods section as support for the appropriateness of the methods used in the study. The Results section includes the results of the statistical analyses but also includes sources to validate the analytical techniques that were used to address the research questions or hypotheses (Grove & Cipher, 2020). Sources might also be included to compare the analysis of the data in the present study with the results of previous studies. The Discussion section of the research report provides a comparison of the findings with other studies' findings, if not already included in the Results section. The Discussion section also incorporates conclusions that are a synthesis of the findings from previous research and those from the present study.

Purpose of the Literature Review in Qualitative and Mixed Methods Research

In qualitative and mixed methods research reports, the Introduction will be similar to the same section in the quantitative study report because the researchers document the background and significance of the research problem. Researchers often include citations to support the need to study the selected topic (Creswell & Clark, 2018; Creswell & Poth, 2018). Sometimes they include a theory or selected concepts for initial guidance of the study. However, additional review of the literature may not be cited for two reasons. One reason is that qualitative studies are often conducted on topics about which we know very little, so little literature is available to review. The other reason is that some qualitative researchers deliberately do not review the literature deeply before conducting the study because of not wanting their expectations about the topic to bias their data collection, data analysis, and findings (Creswell & Poth, 2018). This is consistent with the expectation that qualitative researchers remain open to the perspectives of the participants. In the Methods, Results, and Discussion sections, qualitative researchers will incorporate literature to support the use of specific methods and place the findings in the context of what is already known.

SOURCES INCLUDED IN A LITERATURE REVIEW

The literature is all sources relevant to the topic that you have selected, including articles published in periodicals or journals, internet publications, monographs, encyclopedias, conference papers, theses, dissertations, textbooks, and other books. Websites and reports developed by relevant and reliable government agencies, intergovernmental organizations, and professional organizations may also be included. Each source reviewed by the author and used to write the review is cited. A citation is the act of quoting a source, paraphrasing content from a source, using it as an example, or presenting it as support for a position taken. Each citation should have a corresponding reference in the reference list. The reference is documentation of the origin of the cited quote or paraphrased idea and provides enough information for the reader to locate the original material. This information typically consists of (1) author names, (2) date of publication, (3) title of publication, and (4) the publication's source (where it can be retrieved). The citation and reference style developed by the American Psychological Association (APA, 2020) is commonly used in nursing education programs and nursing journals. More information about APA style is provided later in this chapter.

Types of Publication

An article is a paper about a specific topic and may be published together with other articles on similar themes in journals (periodicals), encyclopedias, or edited books. As part of an edited book, articles may be called chapters. A periodical is a journal that is published over time and is numbered sequentially for the years published. This sequential numbering is seen in the year, volume, issue, and page numbering in periodicals that publish a print version only or both print and electronic versions. In periodicals that publish only electronic versions, an article number or article eLocator is used that takes the place of the page numbering and sometimes the issue number as well. A monograph, such as a book on a specific subject, a record of conference proceedings, or a pamphlet, is usually a one-time publication. Periodicals and monographs are available in a variety of media, including online and in print. An encyclopedia is an authoritative compilation of information on alphabetized topics that may provide background information and lead to other sources but is rarely cited in academic papers and publications. Some online encyclopedias are electronic publications that have undergone the same level of review as published encyclopedias. Other online encyclopedias, such as Wikipedia, are in an open, editable format; as a result, the credibility of the information is variable. When you are writing a review of the literature, Wikipedia may provide ideas for other sources that you may want to find, but check with your faculty about whether Wikipedia or any other encyclopedia may be cited for course assignments.

Major professional organizations may publish papers selected by a review process that were presented at their conference, called conference proceedings. These publications may be in print or online. Conference proceedings may include the findings of pilot studies and preliminary findings of ongoing studies. A thesis is a report of a research project completed by a graduate student as part of the requirements for a master's degree. A dissertation is a report of an extensive, mentored research project that is completed as the final requirement for a doctoral degree. Theses and dissertations can be cited in a literature review.

📄 RESEARCH/EBP TIP

Always search for a follow-up article of a conference proceeding, thesis, or dissertation that you are planning to cite. If an article is available by the same authors with the same content, it is preferable to cite the published article instead.

Academic journals are periodicals that include research reports and nonresearch articles related to a specific academic discipline and/or research methodology. Clinical journals are periodicals that include research reports and nonresearch articles about practice problems and professional issues in a specific discipline. Table 6.1 includes examples of academic and clinical nursing journals that publish a substantial amount of nursing research.

TABLE 6.1   NURSING JOURNALS THAT PUBLISH A SUBSTANTIAL AMOUNT OF RESEARCH

NUMBERS OF RESEARCH ARTICLES	ACADEMIC JOURNALS	CLINICAL JOURNALS
20–40 articles annually	*Clinical Nursing Research* *Journal of Research in Nursing* *Research in Nursing & Health*	*American Journal of Maternal Child Nursing*
40–60 articles annually	*Nursing Research* *Western Journal of Nursing Research* *Journal of Nursing Scholarship*	*Heart & Lung* *The Journal of Acute and Critical Care* *Journal of Psychiatric and Mental Health Nursing* *Archives of Psychiatric Nursing*
More than 60 articles annually	*International Journal of Nursing Studies* *Applied Nursing Research*	*Journal of Pediatric Nursing*

You are familiar with textbooks as a source of information for academic courses. Other books on theories, methods, and events may also be cited in a literature review. To evaluate the quality of a book, consider the qualifications of the author related to the topic, and review the evidence that the author provides to support the book's premises and conclusions. With textbooks and other books, chapters in an edited book might have been written by different people, which are cited differently than the book as a whole (addressed later in this chapter). This is important to note when checking citations and writing your own literature reviews.

Electronic access to articles and books makes many types of published and unpublished literature more widely available. In addition, websites are an easily accessible source of information. However, not all websites are valid and appropriate for citation in a literature review. Websites may contain information that is not scientifically sound or is biased by commercial interest. For example, the website of a pharmaceutical company that sells diuretic medications may not be an appropriate source for hypertension treatment statistics. In contrast, websites prepared and sponsored by government agencies, such as the Centers for Disease Control and Prevention (CDC), intergovernmental organizations, such as the World Health Organization, and professional organizations, such as the American Nurses Association, are considered appropriate references to cite.

📄 RESEARCH/EBP TIP

Be critical in appraising sources for knowledge to use in practice. The saying "you can't believe everything you read" is an old one, but it pertains as much today as ever before. You likely were not surprised to read here that some websites are not valid. But did you know that some journals pretend to be academic journals when they are not? You will find out more about these journals later in the Quality of Sources section.

Content of Publications

References cited in literature reviews contain two main types of content, theoretical and empirical. Theoretical literature includes concept analyses, models, theories, and conceptual frameworks that support a selected research problem and purpose. Theoretical sources can be found in books, periodicals, and monographs. Nursing theorists have written books to describe the development and content of their theories. Other books contain summaries of several theories (Smith & Liehr, 2018). In a published study, theoretical and conceptual sources are described and summarized to reflect the current understanding of the research problem and provide a basis for the study framework.

Empirical literature is composed of knowledge derived from research. In other words, the knowledge is data based. Research reports of quantitative, qualitative, mixed methods, and outcomes research are all considered empirical literature, as are articles in which the results of research reports are synthesized. Empirical sources can be located in periodicals, books, monographs, and unpublished works, such as master's theses and doctoral dissertations. In addition, government agencies, intergovernmental organizations, and professional organizations post original data at their websites, such as the US Census Bureau and the American Cancer Society. In a published study, current and relevant empirical sources are summarized and synthesized to describe what is known and unknown about a research problem, thus providing a basis for the study purpose.

Quality of Sources

Most references cited in quality literature reviews are primary sources that are peer reviewed and come from reputable journals. A primary source is written by the person or persons who originated or are responsible for generating the ideas published. A research report written by the researchers who conducted the study is a primary source. A theorist's development of a theory or other conceptual content is a primary source. A secondary source summarizes or quotes content from primary sources. Authors of secondary sources paraphrase the works of researchers and theorists and present their interpretation of what was written by the primary author. As a result, information in secondary sources may be misinterpretations of the primary authors' thoughts. Secondary sources are used only if primary sources cannot be located, or the secondary source provides creative ideas or a unique organization of information not found in a primary source.

Peer-reviewed means that the authors submitted a manuscript to a publication editor, who identified scholars familiar with the topic to review the manuscript. These scholars provide input to the editor about whether the manuscript in its current form is accurate, meets standards for quality, and is appropriate for the journal. A peer-reviewed paper in a reputable journal has undergone significant scrutiny, and its content is considered trustworthy. A reputable journal is an academic journal that uses peer-review and other quality-control measures that are transparently described on their website. In contrast, nonreputable journals—often called predatory journals—bypass or minimize quality-control measures, including peer review. As a result, predatory journals publish articles that are of poor to average quality and are sometimes not trustworthy (Oermann et al., 2018). Unfortunately, predatory journals often mimic reputable journals by using similar journal names and official-looking websites. Articles from predatory journals are not appropriate to include in literature reviews conducted for research, EBP, or student papers.

Quality literature reviews include relevant and current sources. Relevant studies are those with a direct bearing on the problem of concern. Current sources are those published within 5 years before publication of the manuscript. However, some studies 6 to 10 years old in a literature review might be considered current based on the focus of the study and delays in publication. Sources cited should be comprehensive and predominantly current. Some problems have been studied for decades, and the literature review often includes seminal and landmark studies that were conducted years ago. Seminal studies are the first studies on a particular topic that signaled the beginning of a new way of thinking on the topic and sometimes are referred to as classic studies. Landmark studies are significant research projects that have generated knowledge that influences a discipline and sometimes society as a whole. Such studies frequently are replicated or serve as the basis for the generation of additional studies. Some authors may describe a landmark study as being a groundbreaking study. Thus citing a few older studies significant to the development of knowledge on the topic being reviewed is appropriate. Most publications cited, however, should be current. Replication studies are reproductions or repetitions of a study that researchers conducted to determine whether the findings of the original study could be found consistently in different settings and with different study participants. Replication studies are important to build the evidence for practice. A replication study that supports the findings of the original study increases the credibility of the findings and strengthens the evidence for practice. A replication that does not support the original study findings raises questions about the credibility of the findings.

Syntheses of research studies, another type of data-based literature, may be cited in literature reviews. A research synthesis can be a systematic review of the literature, meta-analysis of quantitative studies, metasynthesis of qualitative studies, or a mixed methods research synthesis. These publications are valued for their rigor and contributions to EBP (see Chapters 1 and 13).

CRITICALLY APPRAISING LITERATURE REVIEWS

Appraising the literature review of a published study involves examining the quality of the content and sources presented. A correctly prepared literature review includes what is known and not known about the study problem and identifies the focus of the present study. As a result, the review provides a basis for the study purpose and may be organized according to the variables (quantitative or outcomes studies) or concepts (qualitative and mixed methods studies) in the purpose statement. The sources cited must be relevant and current for the problem and purpose of the study. The reviewer must locate and review the sources or respective abstracts to determine whether these sources are relevant. This is very time-consuming and usually is not done for appraising an article. However, you can review the reference list and determine the focus of the sources, the number of theoretical and research sources cited, and where and when the sources were published (Gray & Grove, 2021). Sources should be current, up to the date when the paper was accepted for publication. Most articles indicate when they were accepted for publication on the first page of the study.

Although the purpose of the literature review for a quantitative or outcome study is different from the purpose of the literature review for a qualitative or mixed methods study, the guidelines for critically appraising their literature reviews are the same. However, because the purposes of literature reviews are different, the types of sources and the extent of the literature cited may vary.

CRITICAL APPRAISAL GUIDELINES

Literature Reviews

1. Quality sources
   * Are most references from reputable peer-reviewed sources (Aveyard, 2019)?
   * Are most references primary sources?
   * Do the authors justify citing references that are not peer-reviewed, primary sources?
2. Current sources
   * Are the references current (number and percentage of sources published in the last 10 years and in the last 5 years)?
   * Are references older than 10 years landmark, seminal, or replication studies?
   * Are references older than 10 years cited to support measurement methods or theoretical content?
3. Relevant content
   * Is the content directly related to the study concepts or variables?
   * Are the types of sources and disciplines of the source authors appropriate for the study concepts or variables?
4. Synthesis of relevant content
   * Are the studies critically appraised and synthesized (Aveyard, 2019; Gray & Grove, 2021; Hart, 2018; Machi & McEvoy, 2016)?
   * Is a clear, concise summary presented of the current theoretical and empirical knowledge in the area of the study, including identifying what is known and not known (Fineout-Overholt & Stevens, 2019; Garrard, 2022; Machi & McEvoy, 2016)?
   * Does the study address a gap in the literature or knowledge base identified in the literature review?

Critical Appraisal of a Literature Review in a Quantitative Study

McDonald and colleagues (2021) conducted an experimental study (randomized controlled trial [RCT]) to test the effectiveness of a behavioral intervention designed to reduce inattention to the roadway by adolescent drivers. The intervention targeted adolescents 16 to 17 years old who had obtained a driver's license within the past 90 days. The interactive web-based intervention was completed individually by participants, who were randomly assigned to intervention and control groups. Control participants received an interactive web-based activity but on a different health topic. Outcome variables included (1) cell phone use, (2) use of a peer passenger to help manage distractions, and (3) eyes off the forward roadway for 2 or more seconds. Outcomes were measured by a simulated driving assessment and by self-report. Because it was relatively short, the literature review in the Introduction section is excerpted in its entirety in Research Example 6.1.

RESEARCH EXAMPLE 6.1

Literature Review: Quantitative Study

Research/Study Excerpt

Motor vehicle crashes (MVCs) are the leading cause of adolescent death and disability (Centers for Disease Control and Prevention, [n.d.]). Adolescent drivers are at highest MVC risk in the first 6 months of licensure, making it a vitally important period for interventions (Curry et al., 2015; Williams & Tefft, 2014). Inattention to the roadway is a major contributor to adolescent driver MVCs (Curry et al., 2011; Regan et al., 2011) and includes not looking at the roadway, hands not on the wheel, and mind off the task of driving (US Department of Transportation, 2013). Adolescents are particularly susceptible to driver inattention, notably owing to cell phone use and presence of peer passengers in the vehicle. Adolescent drivers disproportionately account for distraction-related crashes, with cell phones involved in 23% of distracted-related fatal crashes with adolescent drivers (US Department of Transportation, 2019). A higher number of peer passengers also increases fatal MVC risk among adolescent drivers (Ouimet et al., 2015; Tefft et al., 2013). Both cell phones and peer passengers can take attention away from the roadway, including eyes off the roadway. Eye glances > 2 seconds off the roadway by teenagers is associated with an odds ratio of 5.5 increased risk of a crash (Simons-Morton et al., 2014).

Few theoretically grounded, behavioral interventions exist to reduce teenage driver inattention. (McDonald et al., 2021, p. 89)

Critical Appraisal

Quality Sources

Quality sources were chosen by McDonald et al. (2021) for their literature review. They cited a total of 31 references in their research report, the majority of which were original research and primary sources. Twenty-four references (77%) were from reputable academic or clinical journals, all of which were peer reviewed. References not from journals were obtained from credible sources, such as the CDC and the US Department of Transportation. In the review of literature located in the Introduction section, 10 references were cited. The remaining references were cited in the Methods and Discussion sections to support methodological choices and recommendations for future research and nursing practice.

Current Sources

The appraisal of currency revealed that the literature cited was not sufficiently current. Only 8 references (26%) were published in the past 5 years (in or since 2016). All the remaining references were published within the past 10 years (in or since 2011) except for one. The older reference was a 192-page research report published in 2006 by the National Highway Safety Administration. Thus the bulk of sources were published between 2011 and 2015, which made them outdated. A literature review for a current problem as significant as MVCs in adolescents needs to be based on literature that is primarily published in the prior 5 years (Gray & Grove, 2021).

Relevant Content

The appraisal of relevant content for this quantitative study focused on the references from the Introduction section. The cited literature directly addressed the research problem, as demonstrated by its focus on contributors to MVCs in adolescents. In addition, the journals cited were from disciplines with expertise on the topic: public health and adolescent health. However, one area of relevant content was missing. This area was the methods and findings of other behavioral interventions that have been tested to reduce MCVs in adolescents. The existence of such interventions was acknowledged in the last sentence of the excerpt, but the researchers chose not to include them in their literature review, a noteworthy omission.

Synthesis of Relevant Content

The review of literature in the Introduction section was well synthesized in its delivery of relevant content as demonstrated by a logical flow that was organized by the main variables. First, the significance of the research problem was succinctly stated using CDC evidence. The time of greatest vulnerability of adolescents to MVCs

RESEARCH EXAMPLE 6.1—cont'd

was pinpointed in the second sentence. The literature review continued with what is known about this phenomenon, beginning with inattention to the roadway as a major contributor. Three behaviors were identified that signify inattention: not looking at the roadway, hands not on the wheel, and mind off the task of driving. Documented reasons for inattention were also presented and included cell phone use and multiple peer passengers. Finally, a measurable behavior that signifies driver inattention—eye glances off the roadway for more than 2 seconds—was shown to highly increase risk for MVCs in adolescents.

This synthesis of relevant content contained key (but dated) evidence required for the researchers' choice of the (1) targeted population (adolescents licensed to drive for 90 or fewer days), (2) behavioral intervention with its focus on reducing cell phone use and distraction from peer passengers, and (3) outcome variables (cell phone use, help from a peer passenger to maintain attention, and eyes off the roadway). The last sentence in the literature review is the statement on what is not known: "Few theoretically grounded, behavioral interventions exist to reduce teenage driver inattention" (McDonald et al., p. 47). The accuracy of this statement is difficult to assess due to no other intervention studies being included in the literature review, as noted previously. An additional drawback of this literature review is that the researchers did not include an overall appraisal of the quality of the studies that were cited.

Critical Appraisal of a Literature Review in a Qualitative Study

The phenomenological study conducted by Kelsick et al. (2021) is presented as an example critical appraisal of a qualitative literature review. The purpose of the study was to explore the lived experience of a person with dementia viewing themselves in the mirror. Informal and formal caregivers were interviewed for the study. Such knowledge is important because there is little professional guidance for the use of mirrors for individuals with dementia living in their own homes or in long-term care facilities. As background, the researchers pointed out that mirrors are important for dressing and personal grooming. Further, viewing the reflection of oneself in a mirror plays a role in self-awareness, which in turn can contribute to overall well-being. In contrast, individuals in the later stages of dementia may become upset when viewing their reflection in a mirror, and later not respond at all. Because of this, many informal and formal caregivers cover up or eliminate mirrors. Key literature review content for the Kelsick et al. (2021) study is presented in Research Example 6.2. The excerpts were drawn from both the Introduction and Discussion sections.

RESEARCH EXAMPLE 6.2

Literature Review: Qualitative Study

Research/Study Excerpts

Mirrors are reflective surfaces that have been around since the beginning of time and serve multiple purposes such as: viewing one's image, decorative purposes, scientific instruments such as telescopes, and even entertainment (Enoch, 2006). Duval and Wicklund's (1972) Theory of Objective Self-Awareness suggests that reflection of one's self in the mirror contributes to an increased sense of self-awareness. In general, this awareness contributes to our overall well-being.... In 2010, Freysteinson conducted a preliminary survey on the availability and access of mirrors in 10 long-term care facilities and found access and availability of mirrors in long-term care facilities were challenging. Mirrors were either lacking, or the placement of mirrors were not accessible for patients in [a] wheelchair or those who were bed-bound. (Kelsick et al., 2021, Introduction section)

[Di] et al. (2014) found mirror visual fixation (staring) in 29 of 81 patients in a minimally conscious state. The authors theorized that visual self-recognition in a mirror is a higher-level self-referential stimulus, like responding to one's own name. In our study, caregivers said the persons with dementia in the latent stage

Continued

RESEARCH EXAMPLE 6.2—cont'd

stared into the mirrors, providing us with a reason to pause and wonder if there may be a degree of mirror self-recognition in the last stages of dementia. (Kelsick et al., 2021, Discussion section)

Critical Appraisal
Quality Sources

Kelsick et al. (2021) chose quality sources for their literature review. They cited a total of 28 references in their research report, of which 12 (43%) were from reputable peer-reviewed academic or clinical journals. These journal articles were primary sources of (1) original research, (2) clinical scholarship, or (3) theory. Ten references (36%) were from reputable web sources, such as the National Alliance for Caregiving and the Alzheimer's Association. These Web references laid the groundwork for the background and significance of the research problem. The remaining references included a theory book, four books on phenomenology, and one lay website for caregivers.

Current Sources

The researchers noted that the literature on the topic is not current. Of the 12 references from academic or clinical journals, none was published in the prior 5 years (in or since 2016). Only 3 of 12 journal references (25%) were published in the prior 10 years (in or since 2011). Picking up threads of evidence from sparse and dated studies can help breathe new life into a still timely topic like this one. Thus the incorporation of older research references was appropriate in this case. The theory and phenomenology books referenced were published in the 1960s, 1970s, and 1980s. The age of these nonresearch references is not unusual because referencing original sources is preferred over referencing secondary sources. Finally, the 10 web sources cited to support the significance of the topic were suitably current, with 8 (80%) published within the prior 5 years.

Relevant Content

The appraisal of relevant content for this qualitative study focused on references from the entire article. The sources cited in the Introduction section were all relevant for providing a background on the (1) significance of mirrors to those with dementia and their caregivers, (2) the history and uses of mirrors, and (3) a theoretical perspective on mirror use and its connection to self-awareness. Research reports on the topic were not reviewed in the Introduction section but rather in the Discussion section. Kelsick et al. (2021) read these reports only after they completed their phenomenological study to not be influenced by prior findings (Creswell & Poth, 2018). All research reports in the Discussion section focused on studies of mirror use and response in persons with dementia, which was relevant content for the study purpose. Besides nursing, the disciplines of the cited journal articles were appropriate, such as gerontology and neurology.

Synthesis of Relevant Content

Kelsick et al. (2021) demonstrated synthesis of relevant content from prior research reports in a somewhat different manner than synthesis is used in quantitative reviews of literature. In the Discussion section, they briefly described each study one by one and then compared their own findings with those of that particular study. Because the literature was scant on the topic (as is often the case in qualitative research), briefly describing each study before comparing its findings with their own study was appropriate in this case. This technique satisfactorily placed their study findings in the context of what is already known. However, the synthesis of relevant background content in the Introduction section was incomplete, because the authors did not identify the gap in the literature the study was designed to address.

REVIEWING THE LITERATURE

Reviewing the literature is a frequent expectation in nursing education programs. Students may be intimidated by this expectation, a feeling that can be overcome with information and a checklist of steps to follow in the process. The steps of the literature review are discussed one by one as presented in Box 6.1; these steps provide an outline for the rest of the chapter. In addition, this section will include common student questions with answers.

BOX 6.1 STEPS OF THE LITERATURE REVIEW

1. Preparing to review the literature
   - Clarify the purpose of the literature review.
   - Select electronic databases and search terms.
2. Conducting the search
   - Search the selected databases.
   - Use a table to document the results of your search.
   - Refine your search.
   - Review the abstracts to identify relevant studies.
   - Obtain full-text copies of relevant articles.
   - Ensure that information needed to cite the source is recorded.
3. Processing the literature
   - Read the articles.
   - Appraise, analyze, and synthesize the literature.
4. Writing the review of the literature
   - Develop an outline to organize information from the review.
   - Write each section of the review.
   - Create the reference list.
   - Check the review and the reference list.

Preparing to Review the Literature

Preparation before a complex task can give structure to the process and increase the efficiency and effectiveness of these efforts. This section provides information about the purpose of a literature review and selecting the databases to be searched (see Box 6.1).

Clarify the Purpose of the Literature Review

Your approach to reviewing the literature will vary according to the purpose of the review. Reviewing the literature for a course assignment requires a clear understanding of the assignment. These reviews will vary depending on the level of educational program, purpose of the assignment, and expectations of the instructor. Note the acceptable length of the written review of the literature to be submitted. Usually the focus of course assignment literature reviews will be a summary of information on the selected topic and the implications of the information for clinical practice (Fineout-Overholt & Stevens, 2019).

Students repeatedly ask, "How many articles should I include in the review? How far back in years should I go to find relevant information?" The answer to both those questions is an emphatic "It depends." Faculty for undergraduate courses may provide you with guidelines about the number and types of article you are required to include in an assignment or project. Graduate students are expected to conduct a more extensive review for course papers and research proposals for theses or dissertations. How far back in the literature you need to search depends on the topic. You need to locate the seminal and landmark studies and other relevant sources in the field of interest. A librarian or course faculty member may be able to assist you in determining the range of years to search for a specific topic.

Another reason you may be conducting a review of the literature is to examine the strength of the evidence and synthesize the evidence related to a practice problem. EBP guidelines are developed through the synthesis of the literature on the practice problem. The purpose of this type of literature review is to identify all studies that included a particular intervention, critically appraise the quality of each study, synthesize the studies, and draw conclusions about the effectiveness of a particular intervention (Gray & Grove, 2021; Fineout-Overholt & Stevens, 2019). When available, replication studies, systematic reviews, meta-analyses, meta-syntheses, and mixed methods research syntheses are important publications to include. Other types of literature syntheses related to promoting evidence-based nursing practice are described in Chapter 13.

📄 RESEARCH/EBP TIP

When reviewing relevant studies, identify authors who are experts in developing the evidence for a particular intervention to promote EBP and note their conclusions.

Select Databases and Search Terms

Because electronic access to the literature is so readily available, reviewing the literature can be overwhelming. General internet search engines such as Google, Google Scholar, or Microsoft Bing will identify scholarly publications but also include sources that are not trustworthy. In addition, the sources you identify from a general search engine may not be the most current. To find trust-worthy and current literature, learn to use professional bibliographical databases, such as the Cumulative Index to Nursing and Allied Health Literature and Science Direct. These databases are valuable tools to easily search for relevant empirical or theoretical literature, but different databases contain citations for articles from different disciplines. Table 6.2 includes professional bibliographical databases valuable for nursing literature reviews. Depending on the focus of your review, you will be able to select relevant professional bibliographical databases to search.

Searching professional bibliographical databases has many advantages, but one challenge is that you will have to select relevant sources from a large number of articles. You can narrow the number of articles and retrieve fewer by using keywords or subject terms to search. When a keyword is typed into the search box of a professional bibliographical database, each reference on the resultant list contains that keyword. Subject terms are standardized phrases and more formal than keywords. For example, a quasi-experimental study focused on providing text message reminders to patients living with heart failure who are taking five or more medications might be found by searching with keyword phrases, such as "electronic communication," "instant messaging," "medication adherence," "patient teaching," "quasi-experimental designs," and "heart failure." The quote marks will keep the search to that combination of words only. When you find one article on your topic, look below its abstract to determine whether the subject terms are listed. Using keywords or subject terms to search is a skill you can teach yourself, but also remember that a librarian is an information special-ist. Consulting a librarian may save you time and make searching more effective.

📄 RESEARCH/EBP TIP

Scrutinize all sources obtained from general search engines, including Google Scholar, to determine whether they are from a reputable journal. Only sources from reputable journals should be used for EBP. If a source is not found in any of the professional databases listed in Table 6.2, it is likely not from a reputable journal (Oermann et al., 2021).

Conducting the Search

Preparation leads to actual conduct of the search. This section spans from the initial step of search-ing the selected database to the last step of obtaining full-text copies of articles with adequate

TABLE 6.2   PROFESSIONAL BIBLIOGRAPHICAL DATABASES FREQUENTLY USED FOR NURSING LITERATURE REVIEWS

NAME OF DATABASE	DATABASE CONTENT
Cumulative Index to Nursing and Allied Health Literature (CINAHL)	Nursing and allied health journals that publish clinical, theoretical, and research articles, including many full-text articles
MEDLINE	Biomedical journals relevant to healthcare professionals deemed reputable by the National Library of Medicine; includes abstracts with links to some full-text sources
PubMed	Free access to MEDLINE available to patients and other consumers
PsycArticles	Journals published by the American Psychological Association (APA) and affiliated organizations
Academic Search Complete	Multidisciplinary databases, including articles from many disciplines
Health Source: Nursing/Academic Edition	Journals published for physicians, nurses, and other healthcare professionals; includes many full-text articles and medication education materials for patients
Psychological and Behavioral Sciences Collection	Psychiatry, psychology, and behavioral health journals

information for referencing them. Keeping organized throughout the steps of the search is key to identifying and retrieving articles that are relevant for the literature review's purpose.

Search the Selected Databases

The actual search of the databases may be the easiest step of the process (see Box 6.1). One method of decreasing search time is to search multiple databases simultaneously, an approach that is possible when several databases are available within a search engine, such as the Elton B. Stephens Company host (EBSCOhost). Setting the format of the results to "date newest" will order the results from most recent to oldest, and thus will ensure that you are viewing the most current articles first. To avoid duplicating your work, keep a list of searches that you have completed. This is especially important if you have limited time and will be searching in several short sessions, instead of a single long one.

Use a Table or Other Method to Document the Results of Your Search

A very simple way to document your search is to use a table. On the table, you will record the search terms, time frame you used, and the results. With most professional bibliographical databases, you can sign up for an account and keep your search history online. Reference management software, such as RefWorks (http://www.refworks.com) and EndNote (http://www.endnote.com), can make tracking the references you have obtained through your searches considerably easier. You can use reference management software to conduct searches and store the information on all search terms for each reference obtained in a search. Within the software, you can store articles in folders with other similar articles. For example, you may have a folder for theory sources, another for methodological sources, and a third for relevant research sources. You likely will also want to create a folder for sources on the significance of the topic, such as morbidity and mortality and associated societal costs. As you read the articles, you can also insert comments into the reference file about each one. By exporting search results from the bibliographical database to your reference management software, all the needed citation information and abstract are readily available to you electronically when you write the literature review.

Refine Your Search

A search may identify thousands of references, many more than you can read and include in any literature review. Open a few articles that were identified, and see what key terms were used. Reconsider the topic and determine how you can narrow your search. One strategy is to decrease the range of years you are searching. Some professional bibliographical databases allow you to limit the search to certain types of articles, such as scholarly, peer-reviewed articles. Combining search terms or searching for the terms only in the abstracts will decrease the number of articles identified. For undergraduate course assignments, it may be appropriate to limit the search to only full-text articles. The recommendation would be, however, that graduate students avoid limiting searches to full-text articles because doing so might result in missing sources that are needed. Narrowing a search tightly, you can end up with too few results. When that occurs, you can retry the search with one or more search terms and limitations removed.

Review the Abstracts to Identify Relevant Studies

The abstract provides pertinent information about the article. You can easily determine whether the article is a research report, description of a practice problem, or theoretical article, such as a concept analysis. You will identify the articles that seem to be the most relevant to your topic and the purpose of the review. If looking for evidence on which to base clinical practice, you can identify the research reports and select those conducted in settings similar to yours. If writing a literature review for a course assignment, you will review the abstracts to identify different types of information. For example, you may need information on mortality and morbidity, as well as descriptions of available treatments or interventions. Mark the abstracts of the relevant studies or save them in an electronic folder.

Obtain Full-Text Copies of Relevant Articles

Using the abstracts of relevant articles, you will retrieve and save the electronic files of full-text articles to review more thoroughly. You may want to rename the electronic file using a file name that includes the first author's last name and the year or a file name with a descriptive phrase. For articles not available as full-text online, you may be able to obtain the article through interlibrary loan. Check with your library's website or a librarian to learn the process for using the interlibrary loan system. If you prefer reading print materials to electronic materials, print the articles and create a paper folder system to organize them. It is important to obtain the full text of the article because the abstract does not include the details needed for your literature review.

Ensure That Information Needed to Cite the Source Is Recorded

As you retrieve and save the articles, note whether the article includes all the information needed for the citation. The bibliographical information on a source should be recorded in a systematic manner, according to the format that you will use in the reference list. The purpose for carefully citing sources is that readers can retrieve the reference for themselves, confirm your interpretation of the findings, and gather additional information on the topic. For each reference, you will need author names, year of publication, article title, journal name, journal volume, journal issue number (if present), page numbers or article number or eLocator, and digital object identifier (DOI). If a book chapter has been photocopied or retrieved electronically, ensure that the year of publication and the publisher's name are recorded. Notice specifically whether the chapter is in an edited book and if the chapter has an author other than the editor. If you are using reference management software such as RefWorks, the software records the citation information for you.

Processing the Literature

Processing the literature is among the more difficult phases of the literature review. This section includes reading the articles and appraising, analyzing, and synthesizing the literature (see Box 6.1).

Read the Articles

As you look at the stack of printed articles or scan the electronic copies of several articles, you may be asking yourself, "Am I expected to read every word of the available sources?" The answer is no. Reading every word of every source would result in you being well read and knowledgeable, but with no time left to prepare the course assignment or paper. Becoming a skilled reviewer of the literature involves finding a balance and learning to identify the most pertinent and relevant sources. However, you cannot critically appraise and synthesize what you have not read. Skim over information provided by the author that is not relevant to your task. Learn what is normally included in different sections of an article so you can read the sections pertinent to your task more carefully. Chapter 2 provides ideas on how to read the literature.

Comprehending and critically appraising sources leads to an understanding of the current state of knowledge related to a research problem. Although you may skim or read only selected sections of some references that you find, you will want to read the articles that are most relevant to your topic word for word and probably more than once. Comprehending a source begins by reading and focusing on understanding the main points of the article or other sources. Highlight the content that you consider important or make notes in the margins of your electronic files or photocopies. The type of information you highlight or note in the margins of a source depends on the type of study or source. With theory articles, you might make note of concepts, definitions, and relationships among the concepts. For a research article, the research problem, purpose, framework, major variables, study design, sample size, intervention (if appropriate), measurement methods, data collection, analysis techniques, results, and findings are usually highlighted. You may wish to record quotes (including page numbers) that might be used when you write your review of the literature assignment or paper. The decision to paraphrase these quotes can be made later. Also, make notes about what you think about the article, such as how this content fits with other information that you have read.

Appraise, Analyze, and Synthesize the Literature

Analysis is required to determine the value of a reference as you make the decision about what information to include in the review. First, you need to appraise the individual studies critically (see Chapter 12). To critically appraise a study, you need to identify relevant content in the articles and make value judgments about the validity or credibility of the findings. However, the critical appraisal of individual studies is only the first step in developing an adequate review of the literature. The studies that have been found to be valid and credible next must be further analyzed in a systematic manner, a process that leads seamlessly into synthesis. Synthesis entails clustering and interrelating ideas from several studies to promote a new understanding or provide a description of what is known and not known in an area (Gray & Grove, 2021).

Analysis and synthesis require manipulation of what you are finding, literally making it your own (Garrard, 2022). Pinch (1995, 2001) was the first nurse to publish a strategy to analyze and synthesize research findings using a literature summary table. An example of a literature summary table is provided in Table 6.3. This table contains key information from the McDonald et al. (2021) quantitative study, plus key information from two studies that McDonald et al. (2021) included in their own review of literature. As you examine the literature summary table, note that each article has its own row in the table. Also note the table's column headings, which are topics useful for summarizing key information for each study. Column topics may vary depending on the purpose of the literature review. For example, the column topic of Design/Approach could be added to the table or substituted for another column topic. If using reference management software, it may allow you to generate summary tables from information you record about each study.

Another way to manipulate the information you have retrieved and transform it into knowledge is known as *mapping* (Hart, 2018; Machi & McEvoy, 2016). Your nursing faculty may have taught you how to map what you are studying conceptually to make connections between facts and principles (Eisenmann, 2021). The same strategy can be applied to a literature review to classify the sources by key concepts and arrange them into a graphic or diagrammatic format (Hart, 2018; Machi & McEvoy, 2016). The map may connect studies with similar methodologies or key ideas.

As you continue to analyze the literature you have found, you will make comparisons among the studies. Look for connections, similarities, and themes in the literature. This analysis allows you to appraise the existing body of knowledge critically in relation to the research problem. You may want to record the theories and methods that have been used to study the problem and any flaws with these theories and methods. You will begin to work toward summarizing what you have found by describing what is known and not known about the problem. The information gathered by using the table format shown in Table 6.3 or displayed in a conceptual map can be useful in making these comparisons. Pay special attention to conflicting findings and recommendations for future research because they may provide clues for gaps in knowledge that represent researchable problems.

The synthesis of sources involves thinking deeply about what you have found and identifying the main themes of information that you want to present. Through synthesis, you will cluster and describe connections among what you have found (Hart, 2018). From the clusters of connections, you can begin to draw some conclusions about what is known, and you can make additional connections to the topic being examined. Any written literature review that simply appraises individual studies paragraph by paragraph is inadequate. A literature review that is a series of paragraphs, in which each paragraph is a description of a single study, with no link to other studies being reviewed, does not provide evidence of adequate analysis or synthesis of the literature (Aveyard, 2019).

Note the review of literature paragraph in McDonald et al. (2021), the quantitative study used for Research Example 6.1. Synthesis of what is known is illustrated by the following two sentences:
- "Inattention to the roadway is a major contributor to adolescent driver MVCs (Curry et al., 2011; Regan et al., 2011) and includes not looking at the roadway, hands not on the wheel, and mind off the task of driving (US Department of Transportation, 2013)" (McDonald et al., 2021, p. 89).
- "A higher number of peer passengers also increases fatal MVC risk among adolescent drivers (Ouimet et al., 2015; Tefft et al., 2013)" (McDonald et al., 2021, p. 89).

In these two excerpted sentences, you can observe that five sources were synthesized to support the researchers' statements about the consequences and contributors to roadway inattention in adolescents.

TABLE 6.3   LITERATURE SUMMARY TABLE

ARTICLE	QT/QL?	PURPOSE	FRAMEWORK	SAMPLE	MEASURES	INTERVENTION	RESULTS
McDonald et al. (2021)	QT	To pilot test a theoretically grounded intervention to reduce teenage driver inattention to the road as a result of cell phone engagement	Theory of Planned Behavior	61 adolescents 16–17 years old who were licensed for ≤90 days in Pennsylvania, USA	• **Cell phone engagement:** video of visual or manual interaction with a cell phone during a simulated driving assessment • **Driver inattention to the road:** eye-tracking videos during a simulated driving assessment	*Let's Choose Ourselves:* an interactive Web-based intervention	When the intervention and control groups were compared, there were no significant differences in outcome measures.
Simons-Morton et al. (2014)	QT	To examine the relationship between crash (or near-crash) risk and duration of driver's eyes off the road among newly licensed teenage drivers	None	42 adolescents 16.4 years old on average who were licensed for ≤3 weeks in Virginia, USA	• **Crash (or near crash):** car video footage showing crash (or near crash) • **Driver's eyes off road:** car video footage of driver's eyes ≤6 seconds before crash or near crash	None	Crash (or near crash) risk increased with duration of the single longest glance off the road during the 18-month observation period.
Curry et al. (2015)	QT	To examine monthly crash rates by (1) age at full licensure and (2) time since full licensure in 17- to 20-year-olds	None	All adolescents 17–20 years old who were granted an intermediate level license from 1/1/2006 through 12/31/2009 in New Jersey, USA	• **Monthly crash rates:** New Jersey Department of Transportation's crash database • **Age at full licensure and time since full licensure:** New Jersey Motor Vehicle Commission's licensing database	None	Initial crash risk was higher for the youngest drivers than for older adolescent novice drivers. Adolescent drivers with more driving experience had lower crash rates.

QL, Qualitative; *QT,* qualitative.

One strategy for synthesizing is to review the summary tables or conceptual maps that you have developed and make a list of findings that are similar and those that are different. For example, you have read five intervention studies of end-of-life care in children with leukemia. As you review your notes, you notice that four studies were conducted in home settings with samples of children from ages 7 to 10 years and had similar statistically significant results when using a parent-administered intervention. The remaining study, with nonsignificant results, also used a parent-administered intervention but was set in an inpatient hospice unit and had a sample of younger children. The main ideas that you identify may be that the effectiveness of parent-administered interventions can vary, depending on the setting and age of the child. Another strategy for synthesis is to talk about the articles you have reviewed with another student, nurse, or friend. Verbalizing the characteristics of the studies and explaining them to another person can cause you to think differently about the studies than when you are just reading your notes. Your enhanced thinking may result in the identification of main ideas or conclusions of the review.

RESEARCH/EBP TIP

You may wonder why articles that come from reputable journals need to be critically appraised for the validity or credibility of their findings. Simply put, blindly accepting researchers' statements about findings and suggestions for their use in practice can lead to costly mistakes—both in enacting EBP changes and in formulating research hypotheses.

Writing the Review of the Literature

Talking about the main ideas of the review can prepare you for the final steps of writing the literature review (see Box 6.1). The final steps begin with organizing your information by developing an outline before writing the major sections of the review. After writing each section of the review and creating the reference list, the last steps are to complete a final check of your review and the reference list.

Develop an Outline to Organize the Review

Before beginning to write your review, develop an outline based on your synthesis of what you have read, using the sections of the review as major headings in the outline. Depending on the purpose of the written literature review, you will determine what the major sections of the paper will be. Frequently, a comprehensive literature review has four major sections: (1) Introduction, (2) Discussion of theoretical literature, (3) Discussion of empirical literature, and (4) Summary (Box 6.2). The Introduction and Summary are standard sections, but the Discussion sections should be organized by the main themes that you have identified or the concepts of the theoretical framework that you want to include in the review. Under the major headings of the outline, make notes about which sources you want to mention in the different sections of the paper. The Introduction section will include the focus or purpose of the review and the significance of the topic and will present the organizational structure of the review. In this section, you should make clear what you will be covering.

The Discussion section may be divided into theoretical and empirical literature as described in the prior paragraph, or divided by the themes of the review findings. A theoretical literature section might include concept analyses, models, theories, or conceptual frameworks relevant to the topic. The empirical section, if it is a separate section, will include the research findings from the

---

BOX 6.2   MAJOR SECTIONS OF A LITERATURE REVIEW WITH TYPICAL CONTENT

1. Introduction
   - Focus or purpose of the review
   - Significance of the topic
   - Organizational structure of the review
2. Discussion of theoretical literature
   - Introductory paragraph: the concept analyses, models, theories, and/or conceptual frameworks that best promote understanding of the topic
   - Body of the theoretical section: concept definitions and relationships among concepts, theory assumptions
   - Summary paragraph: current theoretical understanding of the topic
3. Discussion of empirical literature
   - Introductory paragraph: search terms, databases searched, and number of research reports reviewed
   - Body of the empirical literature section: synthesis of the research reports organized by the concepts from the theoretical literature or by the main themes identified from analysis of the research reports
   - Strengths and weaknesses of overall body of knowledge on the topic
   - Summary paragraph: what is known and unknown about the topic
4. Summary
   - Conclusion: state of knowledge in relation to the topic

---

studies reviewed. In addition to the synthesis, you want to incorporate the strengths and weaknesses of the overall body of knowledge, rather than a detailed presentation and critical appraisal of each study. In the Summary section of the outline, make notes of your conclusions. A conclusion is a statement about the state of knowledge in relation to the topic area, which includes what is known and not known about the area.

Write Each Section of the Review

Start each paragraph with a theme sentence that describes the main idea of the paragraph. Present the relevant studies in each paragraph that support the main idea stated in the theme sentence. End each paragraph with a concluding sentence that transitions to the next paragraph. Each paragraph can be compared with a train with an engine (theme sentence), freight cars connected to each other (sentences with evidence), and caboose (summary sentence linking to the next paragraph). Avoid using direct quotes from an author. Your analysis and synthesis of the sources will allow you to paraphrase the authors' ideas. Paraphrasing involves expressing the ideas clearly and in your own words. The meanings of these sources are then connected to the purpose of the literature review. If the written review is not clear or cohesive, you may need to look at your notes and sources again to ensure that you have synthesized the literature adequately. The defects of a study or body of knowledge need to be described but maintain a respectful tone and avoid being highly critical of theorists' or researchers' work.

As you near the end of the review, write the Summary section as a concise presentation of the current knowledge base for the research problem. The findings from the studies will have been logically presented in the previous sections so that the reader can see how the body of knowledge in the research area evolved. You will also make conclusions about the gaps in the knowledge base. The Summary section should end with the potential contribution of your literature review to the body of nursing knowledge (Aveyard, 2019).

Create the Reference List

Many journals and academic institutions use the format developed by the APA (2020). The seventh edition of the *APA Publication Manual* (2020) provides the latest guidelines for citing print and electronic sources (including websites), directly quoting from these sources, and creating a reference list. The sources included in the list of the references are only those sources that were cited in the paper. Within each of the elements of a reference (see APA, 2020, p. 283), there are standardized formatting rules. The manual walks you through just about any variation in these elements you may come upon in writing a reference for your reference list. You may have noticed that the reference lists in this text are presented in APA format.

The source element in a reference must include all the proper information for retrieving that reference. As noted previously, journal articles usually include a DOI. Each journal article has a unique DOI that contains a persistent link to its internet location. An older journal article may require the use of Crossref (http://www.crossref.org) to find its assigned DOI. Most references other than journal articles and books will end with a URL (uniform resource locator) to readily link the reader to the source's location on the internet. You can review the reference list at the end of this chapter to find examples of journal, book, and website references in APA format.

Each citation on an APA-style reference list is formatted as a paragraph with a hanging indent, meaning that the first line is at the left margin and subsequent lines are indented. If you do not know how to format a paragraph this way, search the Help tool in your word processing program to find the correct command to use. EBSCO provides an APA style reference citation for each article located in its databases. Alternatively, reference management software will automatically create a reference list in APA style of all in-text citations in a paper. However, you will need to check each reference citation from EBSCO or your reference management software for APA style accuracy. For example, only the first word of a journal title starts with a capitalized letter in APA style. If you find all words of a journal title start with capital letters in an automated APA style reference, you will need to manually change all but the first word to lower case to conform with APA style. Table 6.4 presents the components of common references with the correct formatting.

Check the Review and the Reference List

You may complete the first draft of your review of the literature and feel a sense of accomplishment. Before you leave the review behind, a few tasks remain that will ensure the quality of your written review (see Box 6.1). Begin by rereading the review. It is best to delay this step for a day or at least for a few hours to allow you to take a fresh look at the final written product. One way to identify incorrect grammar, awkward sentences, or disjointed paragraphs is to read the review aloud. Ask a fellow student or trusted colleague to read the review and provide constructive feedback.

A critical final step is to compare the sources cited in the paper with the reference list. Be sure that the author names and year of publication match. If you are missing sources on the reference list, add them. If you have sources on the reference list that you did not cite, you must remove them. Downloading citations from a bibliographical database directly into a reference management system and using the system's manuscript formatting functions will reduce some errors but will not eliminate all of them, as noted previously. You want your references to be accurate as a reflection of your attention to detail and quality of your work.

TABLE 6.4   **AMERICAN PSYCHOLOGICAL ASSOCIATION FORMATTING OF CITATIONS**

REFERENCE COMPONENT	TYPE OF FONT	CAPITALIZATION	EXAMPLE
Article title	Regular font	• First word of title and subtitle • Proper nouns	Grounded theory methods: Similarities and differences Nursing students' fears of failing the National Council Licensure Examination (NCLEX)
Journal title	Italicized font	• All key words	*Journal of Clinical Information Systems* *Health Promotion Journal*
Book title	Italicized font	• First word of title and subtitle • Proper nouns	*Qualitative methods: Grounded theory expanded* *Human resources for health in Uganda*

RESEARCH/EBP TIP

Quality literature reviews are essential for determining the current research evidence that might be implemented in practice. Thus literature reviews are an important step in promoting EBP for nursing.

KEY POINTS

- The review of literature in a research report is a summary of current knowledge about a particular practice or research problem and includes what is known and not known about this problem.
- Reviews of the literature in published studies can be critically appraised for current quality sources, relevant content, and synthesis of relevant content (see the critical appraisal guidelines).
- A review of literature may be necessary to complete an assignment for a course or summarize knowledge for use in practice.
- A checklist for reviewing the literature includes preparing, conducting the search, processing the literature, and writing the review.
- Professional bibliographical databases allow for the identification of a large number of sources quickly, and the use of keywords and subject headings can refine the search to the most relevant sources.
- Reference management software is recommended for tracking the references obtained through the searches.
- A literature summary table or conceptual map can be used to help you process the information in numerous studies and identify the main ideas.
- A written review of literature should be grammatically correct, with a logical flow, and contain a reference list that is accurate and complete.

REFERENCES

American Nurses Credentialing Center. (2021). *Magnet Model: Creating a magnet culture.* Retrieved from https://www.nursingworld.org/organizational-programs/magnet/magnet-model/

American Psychological Association. (2020). *Publication manual of the American Psychological Association* (7th ed.). American Psychological Association.

Aveyard, H. (2019). *Doing a literature review in health and social care: A practical guide* (4th ed.). Open University Publishing.

Brown, R. E. (2020). Empowering nurses with an online roadmap for evidence-based practice. *Journal of Hospital Librarianship, 20*(4), 309–322. https://doi.org/10.1080/15323269.2020.1819748

Centers for Disease Control and Prevention. (n.d.). *Leading causes of death and injury.* Retrieved from http://www.cdc.gov/injury/wisqars/leadingcauses.html

Creswell, J. W., & Clark, V. L. P. (2018). *Designing and conducting mixed methods research* (3rd ed.). Sage.

Creswell, J., & Poth, C. N. (2018). *Qualitative inquiry & research design: Choosing among five approaches* (4th ed.). Sage.

Curry, A. E., Hafetz, J., Kallan, M. J., Winston, F. K., & Durbin, D. R. (2011). Prevalence of teen driver errors leading to serious motor vehicle crashes. *Accident Analysis and Prevention, 43*(4), 1285–1290. https://doi.org/10.1016/j.aap.2010.10.019

Curry, A. E., Pfeiffer, M. R., Durbin, D. R., & Elliott, M. R. (2015). Young driver crash rates by licensing age, driving experience, and license phase. *Accident Analysis and Prevention, 80*, 243–250. https://doi.org/10.1016/j.aap.2015.04.019

Di, H., Nie, Y., Hu, X., Tong, Y., Heine, L., Wannez, S.,... Laureys, S. (2014). Assessment of visual fixation in vegetative and minimally conscious states. *BMC Neurology, 14*(1), 147. https://doi.org/10.1186/1471-2377-14-147

Duval, S., & Wicklund, R. A. (1972). *The theory of objective self-awareness.* Academic Press.

Eisenmann, N. (2021). An innovative clinical concept map to promote clinical judgment in nursing students. *Journal of Nursing Education, 60*(3), 143–149. https://doi.org/10.3928/01484834-20210222-04

Enoch, J. M. (2006). History of mirrors dating back 8000 years. *Optometry and Vision Science: Official Publication of the American Academy of Optometry, 83*(10), 775–781. https://doi.org/10.1097/01.opx.0000237925.65901.c0

Fineout-Overholt, E., & Stevens, K. R. (2019). Critically appraising knowledge for clinical decision making. In B. M. Melnyk & E. Fineout-Overholt (Eds.), *Evidence-based practice in nursing and healthcare: A guide to best practice* (4th ed., pp. 109–188). Wolters Kluwer.

Freysteinson, W. M. (2010). Assessing the mirrors in long-term care homes: A preliminary survey. *Journal of Gerontological Nursing, 36*(1), 34–40. https://doi.org/10.3928/00989134-20091204-05

Garrard, J. (2022). *Health sciences literature review made easy: The matrix method* (6th ed.). Jones & Bartlett Learning.

Gray, J. R., & Grove, S. K. (2021). *The practice of nursing research: Appraisal, synthesis, and generation of evidence* (9th ed.). Elsevier.

Grove, S. K., & Cipher, D. J. (2020). *Statistics for nursing research: A workbook for evidence-based practice* (3rd ed.). Elsevier.

Hart, C. (2018). *Doing a literature review: Releasing the social science imagination* (2nd ed.). Sage.

Kelsick, J. R., Freysteinson, W. M., Young, A., & Nurse, R. (2021). Experiences of viewing self in the mirror for men and women with dementia as perceived by their caregivers: A phenomenological study. *Applied Nursing Research, 58*, 151398. https://doi.org/10.1016/j.apnr.2021.151398

Machi, L., & McEvoy, B. (2016). *The literature review: Six steps to success* (3rd ed.). Corwin.

McDonald, C. C., Fargo, J. D., Swope, J., Metzger, K. B., & Sommers, M. S. (2021). Initial testing of a web-based intervention to reduce adolescent driver inattention: A randomized controlled trial. *JEN: Journal of Emergency Nursing, 47*(1), 88–100.e3. https://doi.org/10.1016/j.jen.2020.07.012

Oermann, M. H., Nicoll, L. H., Chinn, P. L., Ashton, K. S., Conklin, J. L., Edie, A. H., Amarasekara, S., & Williams, B. L. (2018). Quality of articles published in predatory nursing journals. *Nursing Outlook, 66*(1), 4–10. https://doi.org/10.1016/j.outlook.2017.05.005

Oermann, M., Wrigley, J., Nicoll, L., Ledbetter, L. S., Carter-Templeton, H., & Edie, A. H. (2021). Integrity of databases for literature searches in nursing: Avoiding predatory journals. *Advances in Nursing Science, 44*, 102–110. https://doi.org/10.1097/ANS.0000000000000349

Ouimet, M. C., Pradhan, A. K., Brooks-Russell, A., Ehsani, J. P., Berbiche, D., & Simons-Morton, B. G. (2015). Young drivers and their passengers: A systematic review of epidemiological studies on crash risk.

Journal of Adolescent Health, 57(1), S24–S35.e6. https://doi.org/10.1016/j.jadohealth.2015.03.010

Pinch, W. J. (1995). Synthesis: Implementing a complex process. *Nurse Educator, 20*(1), 34–40. https://doi.org/10.1097/00006223-199501000-00013

Pinch, W. J. (2001). Improving patient care through the use of research. *Orthopaedic Nursing, 20*(4), 75–81. https://doi.org/10.1097/00006416-200107000-00012

Regan, M. A., Hallett, C., & Gordon, C. P. (2011). Driver distraction and driver inattention: Definition, relationship and taxonomy. *Accident Analysis and Prevention, 43*(5), 1771–1781. https://doi.org/10.1016/j.aap.2011.04.008

Simons-Morton, B. G., Guo, F., Klauer, S. G., Ehsani, J. P., & Pradhan, A. K. (2014). Keep your eyes on the road: Young driver crash risk increases according to duration of distraction. *Journal of Adolescent Health, 54*(Suppl. 5), S61–S67. https://doi.org/10.1016/j.jadohealth.2013.11.021

Smith, M. J., & Liehr, P. R. (2018). *Middle range theory for nursing* (4th ed.). Springer Publishing Company.

Tefft, B. C., Williams, A. F., & Grabowski, J. G. (2013). Teen driver risk in relation to age and number of passengers, United States, 2007-2010. *Traffic Injury Prevention, 14*(3), 283–292. https://doi.org/10.1080/15389588.2012.708887

US Department of Transportation. (2013, April). *Distracted driving 2011* (Traffic Safety Facts Research Note, DOT HS 811 737). National Highway Traffic Safety Administration. Retrieved from https://crashstats.nhtsa.dot.gov/#!/PublicationList/41

US Department of Transportation. (2019, April). *Distracted driving in fatal crashes, 2017* (Traffic Safety Facts Research Note, DOT HS 812 700). National Highway Traffic Safety Administration. Retrieved from https://crashstats.nhtsa.dot.gov/#!/Publication-List/41

Williams, A. F., & Tefft, B. C. (2014). Characteristics of teens-with-teens fatal crashes in the United States, 2005–2010. *Journal of Safety Research, 48*, 37–42. https://doi.org/10.1016/j.jsr.2013.11.001

Understanding Theory and Research Frameworks

Jennifer R. Gray

LEARNING OUTCOMES

After completing this chapter, you should be able to:

1. Define theory and the elements of theory (concepts, relational statements, and propositions).
2. Distinguish among the levels of theoretical thinking.
3. Describe the use of middle range theories as frameworks for studies.
4. Describe the purpose of a research framework.
5. Identify research frameworks developed from nursing, physiological, and other theories.
6. Critically appraise the frameworks in published studies.

Theories are essential to the sciences, including the science of nursing. In a developmental psychology course, you may have learned about Erikson's theory of psychosocial development (Dunkel & Harbke, 2017) or Piaget's theory of cognitive development (Barrouillet, 2015). If you assess a child guided by Erikson's theory, you will focus on stages of psychosocial development. If you are guided by Piaget's theory, your assessment conclusion might be the degree to which the child can make decisions or think abstractly. The theory that you use in a specific situation will shape your understanding, responses, and goals in the situation.

In nursing, we also have theories that shape our understanding and guide our practice. Our theories explain human responses to illness and other phenomena that you encounter in clinical practice. Some of our theories are more abstract, such as Roy's Adaptation Model (RAM; Roy & Andrews, 2009), which is one of several grand nursing theories. Other theories are specific to a situation or one phenomenon. For example, the middle range theory of transition provides guidance to nurses as they support patients during life transitions, such as moving from acute care to palliative care (Meleis, 2010).

In addition to guiding the care of patients in clinical settings, nursing theories are also used to provide frameworks for studies. To assist you in learning about theories and their use in research, the elements of theory are described, types of theories are identified, and how theories provide frameworks for studies are discussed. You are also provided with guidelines for critically appraising research frameworks, and these guidelines are applied to a variety of frameworks from published studies.

UNDERSTANDING THE ELEMENTS OF THEORY

The core ideas that guide practice and research within a scientific discipline are called theory (Im & Meleis, 2021). A theory is defined as a set of concepts and statements that present a view of a phenomenon. Fig. 7.1 is a diagram of a theory's structure. Note that within the definition of theory are the words concepts, statements, and phenomena. Concepts are terms that abstractly describe and name an object, idea, experience, or phenomenon, providing it with a separate identity or meaning. Concepts are defined to present the ideas relevant to a theory (see Fig. 7.1). The statements in a theory describe how the concepts are connected to each other. For example, Thomas et al. (2020) analyzed the concept of self-advocacy of women with cancer and conducted five related studies to develop a middle range theory for this specific group of patients. The researchers determined that the woman's precursors (personality and previous life experiences) affected her perspective of the challenge or problem, in this case a diagnosis of cancer. From the perspective of the woman, Thomas et al. (2020) identified the components of self-advocacy to be informed decision making, effective communication with health professionals, and connected strength. Self-advocacy influenced the outcomes of person-centered care, symptom burden, quality of life, and healthcare utilization/care management. Box 7.1 displays the concepts of self-advocacy. The statements connecting the concepts are listed in the second column.

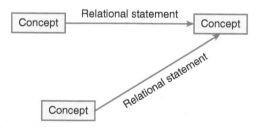

FIG. 7.1 Concepts, Statements, and Theory Diagram.

BOX 7.1 **CONCEPTS AND STATEMENTS OF SELF-ADVOCACY**	
Concepts	**Statements**
Individual precursors	Individual precursors are associated with challenge.
Challenge	
Informed decision making	Challenge is related to self-advocacy.
Effective communication	An informed decision is related to effective communication and connected strength.
Connected strength	
Outcomes	Self-advocacy is related to outcomes.

A concept, a statement, or a theory may be used to describe a phenomenon, the conscious awareness of an experience that comprises the lives of humans (van Manen, 2017). The plural form is phenomena. You may understand the phenomenon of anxiety because of giving your first injections or the phenomenon of joy when you were accepted into nursing school. Our patients experience many phenomena during a hospitalization, such as pain, uncertainty, fear, and relief, and many other emotions. Our nursing actions are designed to relieve the stress and anxiety of patient experiences and move the patients toward improved health.

Theory

Theories are abstract, rather than concrete. When you hear the term *social support*, you have an idea about what the concept means and how you have observed or experienced social support in different situations. The concept of social support is abstract, which means it is the expression of an idea, apart from any specific instance. An abstract idea focuses on a general view of a phenomenon. Family social support has been defined by one group of researchers as "an interpersonal process that is centered on the exchange of information...one has the perception or belief of being connected to and feeling loved and esteemed by others" (Gomes et al., 2017, p. 69). Concrete refers to realities or actual instances—it focuses on a specific instance rather than a general idea. In the study conducted by Gomes et al. (2017), the abstract concept of family social support is provided by a person, a family caregiver. The concept of family caregiver is concrete, referring to a person living with and assisting a person who was diagnosed with diabetes mellitus. Like concepts, some theories are abstract and others are concrete. Later in this chapter, we will provide examples of abstract and concrete theories.

📄 RESEARCH/EBP TIP

What theories do you use in practice? Nurses in practice may use a theory of adaptation when they attempt to decrease the stress of the intensive care environment. They may use a theory of caring when they spend additional time with patients and listen to their concerns.

Philosophy

At the abstract level, you may also encounter a philosophy. Philosophies are rational intellectual explorations of truths or principles of being, knowledge, or conduct. Philosophies describe viewpoints on what reality is, how knowledge is developed, and which ethical values and principles should guide our practice. Other abstract components of philosophies and theories are assumptions, which are statements that are taken for granted or considered true, even though they have not been scientifically tested. For example, a common assumption made by nurses is that "people want to provide the necessary self-care related to their health problems." When confronted with patients in denial about their health problems, this assumption may seem untrue. Regardless of whether you agree, it is true that theories are based on assumptions. Some theorists will clearly identify their assumptions, but others will not.

Concepts

Nursing's theories describe what is known about person, environment, health, and nursing because these four concepts are the essence of nursing. Person, environment, health, and nursing are known as the metaparadigm concepts of our discipline (Meleis, 2018). The phenomenon labeled earlier as *social support* is a concept. A concept is the basic element of a theory or the building blocks of theories (Peterson, 2020). Each concept in a theory needs to be defined by the theorist. The definition of a concept might be detailed and complete, or it might be vague and incomplete and require further development (Chinn & Kramer, 2018). Theories with clearly identified and defined concepts provide a stronger basis for a research framework.

Two terms closely related to concept are *construct* and *variable*. In more abstract theories, concepts have very general meanings that may be a label for a complex idea and are sometimes referred to as constructs. A construct is a broader category or idea that may encompass several concepts. For example, a construct for the concept of social support might be resources. Another concept that is a resource might be household income. At a more concrete level, terms are referred to as variables and are narrow in their definitions. Variables are defined so that they are measurable and suggest that numerical values of variables can differ (vary) from one instance to another. The levels of abstraction of constructs, concepts, and variables are illustrated in Fig. 7.2. The left column is a vertical sequence of construct, concept, and variable, with construct being the most abstract and variable being the most concrete. The other two vertical sequences are examples of a construct, concept, and variable.

One aspect of social support might be emotional social support, which could be a variable. Researchers might define emotional social support as a person's perceived emotional encouragement or affirmation that he or she receives during a stressful time. The measurement of the variable is a specific method for assigning numerical values to varying amounts of emotional social support. To measure the variable, the researcher asks participants to respond to questions on a survey. For example, the Enhancing Recovery in Coronary Heart Disease (ENRICHD) Social Support Instrument (ESSI) was used to measure social support among persons with heart failure (ENRICHD Investigators, 2001; Park et al., 2021). The ESSI has seven questions that measure instrumental, emotional, and informational aspects of the concept. The total score of these questions is the measurement of the variable emotional social support. Chapter 10 provides a detailed discussion of measurement methods.

Defining concepts allows consistency in the way the term is used. Concepts from theories have conceptual definitions that are developed by the theorist and differ from the primary or dictionary definition of a word. A conceptual definition is more comprehensive than a typical dictionary definition and includes associated meanings that the word may have. A conceptual definition is referred to as connotative because the term recalls memories, moods, or images, subtly or indirectly. For example, a conceptual definition of school might include feelings of confidence and

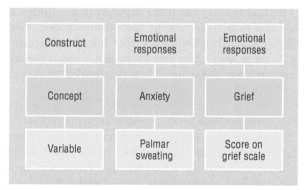

Construct	Emotional responses	Emotional responses
Concept	Anxiety	Grief
Variable	Palmar sweating	Score on grief scale

FIG. 7.2 Abstract to Concrete: Constructs, Concepts, and Variables.

excitement associated with education, the desire to learn new information, or the lack of confidence because of unsuccessful educational experiences. The dictionary definition is narrower and more specific—a school is a building or group of buildings in which adults teach courses to children and adolescents to increase their knowledge. Some of the words or terms that are used frequently in nursing language, such as coping and presence, have not been clearly defined. Terms used in theory or research need connotative meanings based on professional literature.

Conceptual definitions are clear statements of the concepts' meaning in a specific theory or study. The conceptual definition that a researcher identifies or develops for a concept comes from a theory and provides a basis for the operational definition. Remember that in quantitative studies, each variable is ideally associated with a concept, conceptual definition, and operational definition. The operational definition is how the concept can be *manipulated*, such as an intervention or independent variable, or *measured*, such as a dependent or outcome variable (see Chapter 5). The researchers do not always explicitly define the study's concepts but may imply what the concepts mean. When you critically appraise a study, you will need to identify the researcher's conceptual definitions of the study variables.

Martínez-Santos et al. (2021) used Virginia Henderson's human needs theory to describe the needs met by 423 family caregivers of persons with dementia. The instrument used to collect data, the ICUB97-R, measured the types and intensity of care needed and the repercussions on the caregivers. Table 7.1 contains the conceptual and operational definitions for these variables. The conceptual definitions were based on the theory and the operational definitions were the related questions on the ICUB97-R.

RESEARCH/EBP TIP

For a measurement to be valid, the operational definition must be consistent with the conceptual definition. You will be looking for the consistency of the two definitions when you are critically appraising a study.

Statements

A statement clarifies the type of relationship that exists between or among concepts. For example, in the study just mentioned, Martínez-Santos et al. (2021) identified several statements among the concepts. One statement was "caring has negative effects on the caregiver's physical and mental health" (Martínez-Santos et al., 2021, Background).

The statements of relationships are what are tested through research. The researcher obtains data for the variables that represent the concepts in the study's framework. Then the researcher analyzes the data for possible significant relationships among the variables using specific statistical tests (Grove & Cipher, 2021). Testing a theory involves determining the truth of each statement in the theory. As more researchers provide evidence about the relationships among concepts, the accuracy or inaccuracy of the statements is determined. Many studies are required to validate all the statements in a theory.

In theories, propositions are statements explaining the concepts that are related to each other. General propositions are broad and abstract and can be applied across many types of nursing care and settings. Stating a relationship in an even narrower way moves the abstract to a concrete level and makes the statement testable. A statement indicating a relationship between concepts that can be tested is called a specific proposition. Specific propositions in less abstract frameworks (middle range theories) may lead to hypotheses. Hypotheses, written at a lower level of abstraction, are developed to be tested in a study (see Chapter 5). Statements at varying levels of abstraction that express relationships between or among the same conceptual ideas can be arranged in hierarchical

TABLE 7.1	CONCEPTUAL AND OPERATIONAL DEFINITIONS OF SELECTED* NEEDS OF PERSONS LIVING WITH DEMENTIA IN SPAIN AND THE REPERCUSSIONS FOR CAREGIVERS	
CONCEPT/VARIABLE	**CONCEPTUAL DEFINITION**	**OPERATIONAL DEFINITION**
Physical care provided	Meeting the physical needs of a person who cannot meet them independently, which includes dressing/undressing, keeping the body clean, protecting the skin, moving and maintaining body postures, and eliminating body wastes.	Total of Yes answers to the 17 items on the ICUB97-R related to meeting the patient's physical needs, such as accompanying patient to the bathroom, giving medications or enemas to regulate bowel movements, and preventing skin injuries.
Environmental care provided	Meeting the environmental needs of a persons who cannot meet them independently, which includes ensuring fluid and food intake, promoting breathing, avoiding dangers, and maintain body temperature.	Total of Yes answers to the 11 items on the ICUB97-R related to the environmental needs, such as buying and preparing food, giving medication to regulate temperature, and helping with respiratory rehabilitation.
Psychophysical repercussions	Effects of family caregiving on the caregiver in the areas of sleep, breathing, and avoidance of danger.	Total of Yes answers to 15 items on the ICUB97-R that include smoking more, sleeping less, feeling depressed, taking medications, and feeling short of breath.
Socioeconomic repercussions	Effect of family caregiving on the caregiver in the areas of recreation, personal hygiene and dress, and sense of accomplishment.	Total of Yes answers to 11 items on the ICUB97-R that include having less free time, working outside the home less or not at all, and modifying leisure activities.

*ICUB97-R has 65 items with 3 types of needs for care (physical, environmental, and psychosocial and 3 types of repercussions for the caregiver (psychophysical, socioeconomic, and emotional). The table includes definitions for 2 types of needs and 2 types of repercussions.
From Martínez-Santos, A-E, de la Fuente, N., Facal, D. Vilanova-Trillo, L., Gandoy-Crego, M., & Rodríguez-González, R. (2021). Care tasks and impact of caring in primary family caregivers: A cross-sectional study from a nursing perspective. *Applied Nursing Research, 62,* 151505. https://doi.org/10.1016/j.apnr.2021.151505

form, from general to specific. Table 7.2 provides examples of relationships between two concepts that are written as general propositions, specific propositions, and hypotheses.

LEVELS OF THEORETICAL THINKING

Theories can be abstract and broad, or they can be more concrete and specific. Between abstract and concrete, there are several levels of theoretical thinking. Understanding the degree of abstraction or level of theoretical thinking will help you to critically appraise whether a theory is applicable to the research problem in a study.

Grand Nursing Theories

Early nurse scholars labeled the most abstract theories as conceptual models or conceptual frameworks. Today, we refer to the more abstract nursing theories as grand nursing theories because they encompass nursing actions, patient responses, and healthcare outcomes in multiple settings (Meleis, 2018). For example, Roy and Andrews (2009) developed a theory in which adaptation was

TABLE 7.2	EXAMPLES OF A GENERAL PROPOSITION, SPECIFIC PROPOSITION, AND HYPOTHESIS
General proposition	Health-related quality of life is related to depression.
Specific proposition	Among persons with osteoarthritis, physical functioning, a component of health-related quality of life, is related to depressive symptoms.
Hypothesis	Among Hispanic patients older than 85 years with osteoarthritis, those who need assistance with activities of daily living report higher frequency and intensity of depressive symptoms than persons who do not need assistance with activities of daily living.

TABLE 7.3	SELECTED GRAND NURSING THEORIES	
NAME	AUTHOR (YEAR)	BRIEF DESCRIPTION
Adaptation Model	Roy and Andrews (2009)	In response to focal, contextual, and residual stimuli, people adapt by using a variety of processes and systems, some of which are automatic and some of which are learned. The overall goal is to return to homeostasis and promote growth.
Self-Care Deficit Theory of Nursing	Orem (2001) Orem & Taylor (2011)	Individuals' ability to care for themselves is affected by developmental stage, presence of disease, and available resources and may result in a self-care deficit. The goal of nursing is to provide care in proportion to the person's self-care capacity.
Science of Unitary Human Beings	Rogers (1970)	Persons, who are unitary human beings, and the environment around them are energy fields that interact as open systems. The energy fields may produce patterns that can be used for assessment.
Theory of Goal Attainment	King (1992)	Within systems, persons are goal oriented. The nurse and the patient set mutually agreed-on goals. Through interaction, the nurse educates, supports, and guides the patient toward the goals.

the primary phenomenon of interest to nursing. This theory identifies the elements considered essential to adaptation and describes how the elements interact to produce adaptation and thus health. Another view of nursing is presented by Orem and Taylor (2011), who describes health phenomena in terms of self-care, self-care deficits, and nursing systems. Table 7.3 lists four well-known grand nursing theories, with a brief explanation of their content.

Building a body of knowledge related to a particular grand nursing theory requires an organized program of research and a group of scholars. The Roy Adaptation Association is a group of researchers who "analyze, critique, and synthesize all published studies in English based on the RAM [Roy's Adaptation Model]" (Roy, 2011, p. 312). An example of RAM's continued use in nursing research is a randomized controlled trial (RCT) with a sample of persons diagnosed with Alzheimer disease (AD) (Lok et al., 2020). The study's intervention, Cognitive Stimulation Therapy (CST), was based on RAM. At the end of the study, the persons in the experimental group had higher cognitive functioning than those in the control group.

The Society of Rogerian Scholars continues to conduct studies and develop knowledge related to Martha Rogers' Science of Unitary Human Beings. The society publishes an online journal called *Visions: The Journal of Rogerian Nursing Science* (https://www.societyofrogerianscholars.org/). The International Orem Society publishes an issue each year of their online journal, *Self-Care, Dependent-Care & Nursing*, to disseminate research and clinical applications of Dorothea Orem's theory of self-care. These are examples of researchers who maintain a network to communicate with each other and other nurses about their work with a specific theoretical approach.

Middle Range Theories

Middle range theories are less abstract and narrower in scope than grand nursing theories but are more abstract than theories that apply to only a specific situation (Meleis, 2018). These types of theories describe experiences such as comfort (Kolcaba, 1994), uncertainty in acute or chronic illness (Mishel, 1988, 1990), and self-transcendence as a person ages (Reed, 1991). Because middle range theories are more closely linked to clinical practice and research than grand nursing theories, nurses providing patient care and nurse researchers find them to be helpful. They may emerge from a grounded theory study, be deduced from a grand nursing theory, or be created through a synthesis of the literature on a topic (Liehr & Smith, 2017). Table 7.4 lists middle range theories that continue to be used to guide studies. Middle range theories are sometimes called substantive theories because they are closer to the substance of clinical practice. Substantive theories have clearly identified concepts, definitions of concepts, and relational statements. Thus they are more commonly applied as frameworks in nursing studies.

Situation-specific theories are more concrete than middle range theories and limited to a population and phenomenon or a nursing specialty (Fawcett, 2021). They are designed to propose approaches to specific nursing practice situations. Despite significant research and theory development related to self-care for heart failure, nurses have found it difficult to effectively promote self-care in persons living with heart failure. Herber et al. (2019) synthesized previous theoretical publications and the research findings of 31 qualitative studies (Herber et al., 2017). From this work, they developed a situation-specific theory of barriers and facilitators of self-care for self-care in patients with heart failure. In the theory, the concept of self-efficacy is related to the persons' view of their disease, and their view of the disease affects their self-efficacy, forming a two-way

TABLE 7.4	SELECTED MIDDLE RANGE THEORIES FOR NURSING USED TO GUIDE STUDIES
THEORY	**RELEVANT THEORETICAL SOURCES**
Caring	Swanson (1991)
Comfort	Kolcaba (1994)
Heat stress	Byrne and Ludington-Hoe (2021)
Nursing intellectual capital	Covell (2008)
Self-care in chronic illness	Riegel et al. (2012, 2019)
Self-transcendence	Reed (1991)
Transitions	Meleis (2010)
Uncertainty in illness	Mishel (1988, 1990)
Unpleasant symptoms	Lenz et al. (1997)

relationship. The person's view of the disease leads to naturalistic decision making, which leads to effective self-care. Herber et al. (2019) identified barriers and facilitators that exert influence on the person's view of the disease and the decision-making process.

RESEARCH/EBP TIP

Patients discharged from the hospital may need to implement new self-care behaviors because of a surgery or illness exacerbation. Do you agree with the conclusion of Herber et al. (2019) that patients' views of their surgery or illness affect their decisions and ability to provide self-care?

Research Frameworks

Research and theory have a cyclic relationship (Meleis, 2018). A research framework is an abstract and logical structure of meaning, such as a portion of a theory, which guides the development of the study and enables the researcher to link the findings to nursing's body of knowledge (Lor et al., 2017). For clarity, we are using the term *research framework* to refer to the concepts and relationships being addressed in a study. Lor et al. (2017) provided guidance on how theories can be used to guide descriptive and experimental studies. For descriptive studies, researchers can use "concepts from the theory to inform data collection"; researchers conducting experimental studies will find that "concepts from the theory guide overall design" (Lor et al., 2017, p. 583). Perhaps the researcher expects one variable to cause a change in another variable, such as the independent variable of an aerobic exercise program affecting the dependent variable of weight. In a well-developed quantitative study, the researcher explains abstractly in the framework why one variable is expected to influence the other. The idea is expressed concretely as a hypothesis to be tested during the study.

Every quantitative study, no matter its focus, has an implicit or explicit framework. A clearly expressed framework is one indication of a well-developed quantitative study. The researcher develops or applies the framework to explain the concepts contributing to or partially causing an outcome. The researcher cites articles and books, preferably primary sources, in support of the explanation.

One strategy for expressing a theory or research framework is a diagram with the concepts and relationships graphically displayed. These diagrams are sometimes called maps or models (Gray & Grove, 2021). A model includes all the major concepts in a research framework. Arrows between the concepts indicate the proposed linkages between them. Each linkage shown by an arrow is a graphic illustration of a relational statement (proposition) of the theory. Lor et al. (2017) described how they choose a theory to guide their research and presented a model for the Theory of Care-Seeking Behavior (Fig. 7.3). In Fig. 7.3, clinical and sociodemographic factors are seen to influence affect, beliefs, norms, and habits. Care-seeking behaviors are affected by clinical and sociodemographic factors and by affect, beliefs, norms, and habit. The relationships between affect, belief, norms, and habits and care-seeking behavior are moderated by external conditions.

Unfortunately, in some quantitative studies the ideas that compose the framework remain nebulous and are vaguely expressed. Although the researcher believes that the variables being studied are somehow related, this notion is expressed only in concrete terms, such as hypotheses. The researcher may make little attempt to explain why the variables are thought to be related. However, a research framework assumes that one or more variables are linked to other variables. The researcher may describe the relationships among variables found in previous studies, but then the researcher stops, without fully developing the ideas as a framework. These ideas are referred to as implicit frameworks. In most cases a careful reader can extract an implicit framework from the text of the research report. When researchers do not clearly describe the framework, you may want

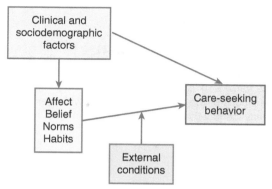

FIG. 7.3 Theory of Care-Seeking Behavior. (Redrawn from Lor, M., Backonja, U., & Lauver, D. [2017]. How could nurse researchers apply theory to generate knowledge more efficiently? *Journal of Nursing Scholarship, 49*(5), 580–589.)

to draw a model based on the information provided. Having a model helps you visualize the framework and how the variables in the study are linked. Implicit frameworks provide limited guidance for developing and implementing a study and limit the contribution of the study findings to nursing knowledge.

Research frameworks may be based on relationships found in grand nursing theories, middle range theories, and theories from other disciplines, or a combination of these (Meleis, 2018). In some quantitative studies the framework that is newly proposed can be called a tentative theory. Frameworks for physiological studies are usually derived from physiology, genetics, pathophysiology, and physics. This type of theory is called scientific theory. Scientific theory has extensive research evidence to support its claims. Many of these theories are physiological theories. Framework concepts are clearly linked to study variables, and valid and reliable methods exist for measuring each concept, related variable, and relational statement in scientific theories. Because the knowledge in these areas has been well tested through research, the theoretical relationships are often referred to as physiological laws and principles. In addition, propositions can be developed and tested using these laws and principles and then applied to nursing problems.

Scientific theories must remain open, however, to possible contrary evidence that would require their revision. For example, before this century, scientists believed that they knew the functions and interactions of various genes. The knowledge gained through the Human Genome Project (National Human Genome Research Institute, 2020) has required that scientists revise some of their theories.

📄 RESEARCH/EBP TIP

Think about the scientific theories related to respiration, cardiac muscle contractility, and metabolism of medications that influence your practice. You may also unconsciously or consciously use concepts and propositions from grand nursing theories, such as Orem's Self-Care Theory, to promote understanding of a patient's rehabilitation after a myocardial infarction.

CRITICAL APPRAISAL GUIDELINES FOR RESEARCH FRAMEWORKS

The research framework in a quantitative study needs to be critically appraised to determine its usefulness for directing the study and interpreting the study findings. The following questions provide guidelines for evaluating the quality of a study's framework.

? CRITICAL APPRAISAL GUIDELINES

Framework of a Study

1. Is a research framework explicitly identified and described in the study? If so, what is the name of the theory and theorist used for the framework?
2. Are the concepts in the framework conceptually defined?
3. Are the operational definitions of the variables consistent with their associated conceptual definitions?
4. Do the researchers clearly identify the relationship statement(s) or proposition(s) from the framework being examined by the study design?
5. Are the study findings linked back to the framework?

Critically appraising a framework of a quantitative study requires that you go beyond the framework itself to examine how it is reflected in other components of the study, such as the design, measurement of the variables, and implementation of an intervention, if applicable. Begin by identifying the concepts and conceptual definitions from the written text in the introduction, literature review, or discussion of the framework. Then you must judge the adequacy of the linkages of concepts to variables, measurement of research or dependent variables, and implementation of independent variables. In the discussion section, determine whether the researchers linked the results back to the research framework. In the remaining sections of the chapter the critical appraisal guidelines are applied to frameworks that have been derived from a grand nursing theory, middle range theory, tentative theory, and a scientific (physiological) theory.

FRAMEWORK FROM A GRAND NURSING THEORY

The primary challenge with using a grand nursing theory as a research framework is its abstractness and the difficulty measuring its concepts. To overcome this challenge, some researchers have deduced middle range theories from grand nursing theories and used middle range theories to guide their studies. Other researchers have used a grand nursing theory as an overall framework but have not directly linked the variables to the theory constructs.

Some researchers have made their use of the grand theory explicit, as in Research Example 7.1. The study conducted by Lok et al. (2020) was described earlier in the chapter as an example of a study explicitly using a grand nursing theory. Among persons with AD, RAM was used as the basis for the intervention, which was called CST. The researchers also used an instrument developed to be consistent with RAM, the Coping and Adaptation Processing Scale (Roy et al., 2016). The study excerpt includes the study aim and examples of the study components being linked to RAM.

⚡ RESEARCH EXAMPLE 7.1

Grand Nursing Theory as a Framework

Research/Study Excerpt

This study aims to specify the effects of RAM-based CST, which is to be applied as a nursing procedure to enhance AD patients' deteriorated cognitive functions, coping and adaptation skills, and QOL [quality of life] on AD patients' cognitive functions, coping and adaptation skills, and QOL. (Lok et al., 2020, p. 583) The experimental group was treated using RAM-based CST, and routine treatment (monthly polyclinic monitoring) was provided to the control group. (Lok et al., 2020, p. 585)

RESEARCH EXAMPLE 7.1—cont'd

Coping and Adaptation Processing Scale (CAPS), which was developed by SC [Sister Callista] Roy... helps define the coping and adaptation strategies of the people under the critical and challenging conditions. (Lok et al., 2020, p. 586)

RAM-based CST enhanced the cognitive functions of the patients in the experimental group. Cognitive functions of the control group patients who did not receive RAM-based CST regressed. Following the application of RAM-based CST, the coping and adaptation functions of the patients in the experimental group were found to be better than those of the patients in the control group in all subdimensions. Similarly, following the application of RAM-based CST, QOL of the patients in the experimental group was found to be better than the cognitive functions of the control group. (Lok et al., 2020, p. 590)

Critical Appraisal

RAM was explicitly identified as the study's framework. The intervention was a revision of CST to reflect Roy's theoretical principles. Lok et al. (2020) conceptually defined AD to be the focal stimulus in RAM, and the degree of adaptation and coping as the person's response. Coping and adaptation were operationally defined as the participants' scores on the subdimensions of the Coping and Adaptation Processing Scale. The congruence of the conceptual and operational definitions to each other was demonstrated by RAM being the foundation for both. The relationships among the concepts were shown in a diagram as the research framework. The findings of the study were clearly linked to RAM framework. Lok et al. (2020) provided an example of the explicit use of a grand nursing theory in a quality RCT.

FRAMEWORK BASED ON MIDDLE RANGE THEORY

Research frameworks for nursing are frequently based on middle range theories. These studies test the validity of the middle range theory and examine the parameters within which the middle range theory can be applied (Peterson, 2020). Some nursing researchers have used middle range theories developed by non-nurses. Other researchers have used middle range theories that have been developed through grounded theory studies. In either case, middle range theories should be tested before being applied to nursing practice.

Persons living with chronic renal disease require hemodialysis and restrictions on diet and fluid intake. Vicdan (2020) conducted an RCT with an intervention developed using the principles of Kolcaba's Theory of Comfort (Kolcaba, 1994; Kolcaba, 2003). The 68 participants were randomly assigned to a control group and a treatment group. Vicdan (2020) collected pretest and posttest data using the General Comfort Questionnaire developed by Kolcaba (1992). The middle range theory provided a strong foundation for the study, as indicated in Research Example 7.2.

RESEARCH EXAMPLE 7.2

Middle Range Theory as a Framework

Research/Study Excerpt

There is a limited number of studies in which the comfort theory of Kolcaba is used in hemodialysis patient training (Tabiee et al., 2017). This study is considered to guide the nurses in the evaluation of individuals' comfort that is applied in hemodialysis treatment. This study was conducted to determine the effect of training that is given in accordance with the Comfort Theory to hemodialysis patients. (Vicdan, 2020, p. 31)

Continued

> ### RESEARCH EXAMPLE 7.2—cont'd
>
> *The data of the research were collected with the Patient Evaluation Form and the General Comfort Questionnaire (GCQ).... The GCQ was developed by Kolcaba (1992) to determine the comfort needs and to evaluate the nursing initiatives that provide comfort and the increase in comfort (Dowd, 2006; Kolcaba, 2003). (Vicdan, 2020, p. 31)*
>
> *In this study, the training given to the hemodialysis patients in accordance with the Comfort Theory of Kolcaba was evaluated. It was determined that there was an increase in all of the mean scores on the General Comfort Questionnaire subdimensions, the mean score on the overall questionnaire, and the mean scores of the comfort level of hemodialysis patients in the experimental group at the end of the training. Based on these findings, it is considered that providing training to hemodialysis patients in accordance with the Comfort Theory would positively affect the comfort of the patients. (Vicdan, 2020, p. 36)*
>
> **Critical Appraisal**
>
> Vicdan (2020) explicitly identified and described Kolcaba's Comfort Theory (Kolcaba, 1994) as the research framework. The study variables were clearly linked to the theory and carefully defined and operationally defined (measured) by using the General Comfort Questionnaire. The intervention was developed based on the theory. Vicdan (2020) did not identify a specific proposition that was tested. The lack of a proposition or hypothesis prevented directly testing the theory. However, the findings were linked back to the Comfort Theory (Kolcaba, 1994).

> ### RESEARCH/EBP TIP
>
> Kolcaba's Comfort Theory (Kolcaba, 1994) is considered a middle range theory but can be widely applied in research and in practice. Being comfortable allows a person to implement health-seeking behaviors, such as adhering to medications and following dietary recommendations.

FRAMEWORK FROM A TENTATIVE THEORY

Findings from completed studies reported in the literature can be a rich source of frameworks when synthesized into a coherent, logical set of relationships. The findings from studies, especially when combined with concepts and relationships from middle range theories or non-nursing theories, can be synthesized into a tentative theory. Another approach to developing a tentative theory is to combine two or more middle range theories into a new framework and test the propositions of the framework. Boamah et al. (2018) developed their framework by applying the theory of transformation leadership (Bass, 1985) and the theory of structural empowerment (Kanter, 1993) to nurses in their clinical settings (Research Example 7.3).

> ### RESEARCH EXAMPLE 7.3
>
> #### Tentative Theory as a Framework
>
> **Research/Study Excerpt**
>
> *The present study draws from theory and research to propose a theoretical model linking transformational leadership to workplace empowerment and, subsequently, to nurse job satisfaction and nurse-assessed adverse patient outcomes. The hypothesized model illustrating the proposed relationships is depicted in Fig. 7.4 [Figure 1]. Overall, it is hypothesized that higher staff ratings of their manager's transformational leadership would be related to greater structural empowerment (hypothesis 1), which in turn, would contribute to increased job satisfaction (hypothesis 2), and lower adverse events (hypothesis 3). Higher job satisfaction would lead to lower adverse patient outcomes (hypothesis 4). (Boamah et al., 2018, p. 182–183)*

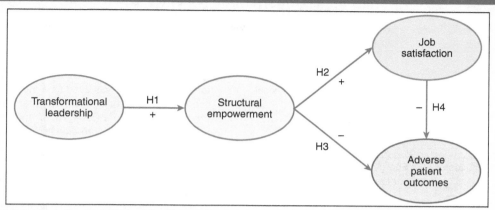

RESEARCH EXAMPLE 7.3—cont'd

FIG. 7.4 Hypothesized Theoretical Model. (Reproduced from Boamah, S., Laschinger, H., Wong, C., & Clarke, S. [2018]. Effect of transformational leadership on job satisfaction and patient safety outcomes. *Nursing Outlook,* 66, 180–189. https://doi.org/10.1016/j.outlook.2017.10.004)

A cross-sectional predictive survey design was used to test the hypothesized model....A total of 378 nurses responded to the questionnaire for a response rate of 38%. (Boamah et al., 2018, p. 183)
   The findings of this study are consistent with transformational leadership theory....By developing strong relationships, transformational leaders understand and anticipate the needs of their staff and make great efforts to influence the acquisition of resources needed to increase nurses' feelings of empowerment. Empowered nurses seek innovative approaches to perform their job, and thereby improving patient care outcomes and generating a greater sense of job satisfaction. (Boamah et al., 2018, p. 187)

Critical Appraisal
Boamah et al. (2018) explicitly described their research framework and cited the primary sources for the two theories from which the tentative theory's propositions were developed. The conceptual and operational definitions of the variables were consistent with each other, indicating the theory's concepts are linked to the study variables. The researchers proposed hypotheses that linked the four concepts. Because the relationship in the tentative theory were tested, the results indicated the strength and direction of the relationships among the concepts. The researchers explicitly linked the findings to the research framework.

RESEARCH/EBP TIP

Developing a tentative theory from the findings of prior studies is one strategy for linking research back to the knowledge base of theories that guide nursing practice. Synthesizing research findings related to a clinical problem can generate a tentative theory that becomes the research framework for a study.

FRAMEWORK FROM A PHYSIOLOGICAL STUDY

As nurses, we assess symptoms and responses to treatment that result from physiological and pathological processes. Studies that examine these processes must be guided by physiological frameworks that express the logic on which the study is based. Among persons living with T2D, fatigue was frequently reported, especially among women. Clinicians typically attributed fatigue to

TABLE 7.5 **CONCEPTUAL AND OPERATIONAL DEFINITIONS OF SELECTED VARIABLES FROM A STUDY OF FATIGUE AND REAL-TIME GLUCOSE LEVELS AMONG PERSONS WITH TYPE 2 DIABETES**

VARIABLE	CONCEPTUAL DEFINITION	OPERATIONAL DEFINITION
Fatigue	The person's "a subjective perception of a decreased capacity to perform physical and/or mental tasks" (Fritschi et al., 2020, p. 197)	Actiwatch-Score® (Philips Respironics, Bend, OR) from the accelerometer placed on the nondominant wrist was used as a measure of sleep and activity. Also, accelerometer randomly reminded participants to self-report their fatigue, one a scale of 0–10, six to eight times a day (Fritschi et al., 2020).
Serum glucose	Energy source available in the blood	Measurement of real-time glucose using Medtronic CGMS iPro®2 continuous glucose monitoring system with the sensor in the abdomen collecting interstitial fluid (Fritschi et al., 2020).

From Fritschi, C., Park, C., Quinn, L., & Collins, E. (2020). Real-time associations between glucose levels and fatigue in Type 2 diabetes: Sex and time affects. *Biological Research for Nursing, 22*(2), 197–204. https://doi.org/10.1177/1099800419898002

abnormal glucose levels, but research findings were inconclusive. Fritschi et al. (2020) conducted a study among persons with T2D to learn more about fatigue and its relationship to changes in serum glucose levels. Participants wore glucometers and accelerometers to collect data over 6 days. The researchers did not explicitly define the variables measured during the study. However, we have inferred the conceptual and operational definitions of the key variables from the article (Table 7.5). You may notice that the conceptual definitions of physiological variables are less abstract than those of the psychosocial variables. In Research Example 7.4, the technology used by Fritschi et al. (2020), their results, and their conclusions are described.

RESEARCH EXAMPLE 7.4

Physiological Theory as a Framework

Research/Study Excerpt

Advancing our knowledge of physiological factors that cause fatigue is the first step in designing interventions to treat fatigue.... Wearable technology, including continuous glucose monitoring systems (CGMS) and real-time symptom monitoring using actigraphy, have made it possible to gather real-time and objective data under free-living conditions, thus overcoming the problems associated with traditional research methods. Thus, the aim of the present study was to use this technology to examine real-time momentary relationships between glucose and fatigue levels by week, day, and time of day in adults with type 2 diabetes. Additionally, we explored how these relationships differed by sex.... We measured real-time glucose using the Medtronic CGMS iPro®2 continuous glucose monitoring system (CGMS; Medtronic, Northridge, CA).... We collected real-time, self-reported fatigue data using a wrist accelerometer (Actiwatch-Score®; Philips Respironics, Bend, OR) placed on the nondominant wrist. (Fritschi et al., 2020, p. 198)

This study is the first to use ecological momentary assessment to study the real-time relationships between glucose levels and fatigue symptoms in adults with type 2 diabetes. The findings provide evidence that real-time glucose levels and fatigue symptoms are associated. In ecological momentary analyses,

RESEARCH EXAMPLE 7.4—cont'd

using CGM and real-time fatigue ratings, glucose and fatigue were related when the data were averaged by day and by time of day but not by week. When we ran separate analyses by sex, these relationships remained significant only in women. (Fritschi et al., 2020, p. 201)

This finding is relevant for nursing practice as it suggests both the need to assess fatigue in the clinic setting and the possibility that effective interventions may differ by sex. Improving glucose levels across hours and days may improve fatigue levels in women, while in men the presence of fatigue symptoms may indicate the presence of underlying depression. Future studies should address momentary fatigue levels in relationship to the ability to carry out self-care activities in aging adults with type 2 diabetes. (Fritschi et al., 2020, p. 202)

Critical Appraisal

Fritschi et al. (2020) did not identify a specific theory when they described the conflicting findings about fatigue and serum glucose of persons living with diabetes. The researchers conceptually defined fatigue, but not serum glucose, and operationally defined both as the primary variables of the study. The conceptual definition of fatigue included a subjective component, which the researchers measured by asking participants to rate their fatigue when prompted by the accelerometer. Fritschi et al. (2020) linked their findings to the growing body of evidence linking serum glucose and fatigue among persons living with T2D. However, the implicit framework and lack of stated propositions were serious study weaknesses.

KEY POINTS

- A theory is an integrated set of concepts, definitions, and statements that presents a view of a phenomenon.
- The elements of theories are concepts and relational statements.
- Grand nursing theories are very abstract and broadly explain nursing, making them applicable to a wide range of clinical phenomena.
- Middle range and tentative theories are less abstract and narrower in scope than grand nursing theories. As a result, they apply to a specific phenomenon or a narrow range of phenomena.
- Theory is essential to research because it provides the framework for developing a study and links the study findings back to the knowledge of the discipline.
- A research framework is an abstract, logical structure of meaning, such as a portion of a theory, which guides the development of the study and enables the researcher to link the findings to nursing's body of knowledge.
- Every study has a framework, although some research frameworks are poorly expressed or are implicit.
- To be used effectively, the research framework must include the concepts that are linked to the study variables. The study variables also must have clear conceptual and operational definitions.
- The relational statements or propositions being examined need to be clear and represented by a model or map. These propositions are tested through the development of hypotheses in the study.
- Frameworks for studies may come from grand nursing theories, middle range theories, research findings, non-nursing theories, tentative theories, and scientific theories.
- Scientific theories are derived from physiology, genetics, pathophysiology, and physics and are supported by extensive evidence.
- Critically appraising a framework requires the identification and evaluation of the concepts, their definitions, and the statements linking the concepts. The study findings should be linked back to the research framework to determine its usefulness in describing reality.

REFERENCES

Barrouillet, P. (2015). Theories of cognitive development: From Piaget to today. *Developmental Review, 38*, 1–12. http://dx.doi.org/10.1016/j.dr.2015.07.004

Bass, B. M. (1985). *Leadership and performance beyond expectations.* Collier Macmillan.

Boamah, S., Laschinger, H., Wong, C., & Clarke, S. (2018). Effect of transformational leadership on job satisfaction and patient safety outcomes. *Nursing Outlook, 66*, 180–189. https://doi.org/10.1016/j.outlook.2017.10.004

Byrne, J., & Ludington-Hoe, S. (2021). Theory of heat stress management: Development and application in the operating room. *Journal of Advanced Nursing, 77*, 1218–1227. https://doi.org/10.1111/jan.14668

Centers for Disease Control and Prevention. (2017). *Behavioral risk factor surveillance system: Annual survey data.* Retrieved from https://www.cdc.gov/brfss/annual_data/annual_data.htm

Chinn, P., & Kramer, M. (2018). *Knowledge development in nursing: Theory and process* (10th ed.). Elsevier.

Covell, C. (2008). The middle-range theory of nursing intellectual capital. *Journal of Advanced Nursing, 63*(1), 94–103. https://doi.org/10.1111/j.1365-2648.2008.04626.x

Dowd, T. (2006). Theory of comfort. In A. Tomey & M. Alligood (Eds.), *Nursing theorists and their work* (6th ed., pp. 726–742). Elsevier.

Dunkel, C., & Harbke, C. (2017). A review of measures of Erikson's stages of psychosocial development: Evidence of a general factor. *Journal of Adult Development, 24*, 58–76. https://doi.org/10.1007/s10804-016-9247-4

ENRICHD Investigators. (2001). Enhancing Recovery in Coronary Heart Disease (ENRICHD) study intervention: Rationale and design. *Psychosomatic Medicine, 63*(5), 747–755.

Fawcett, J. (2021). Middle range and situation specific theories: Similarities and differences. In E. O. Im & A. Meleis (Eds.), *Situation specific theories: Development, utilization, and evaluation in nursing* (pp. 39–47). Springer.

Fritschi, C., Park, C., Quinn, L., & Collins, E. (2020). Real-time associations between glucose levels and fatigue in Type 2 diabetes: Sex and time affects. *Biological Research for Nursing, 22*(2), 197–204. https://doi.org/10.1177/1099800419898002

Gomes, L., Coelho, A., dos Santos Gomides, D., Foss-Freitas, M., Foss, M., & Pace, A. (2017). Contribution of family social support to the metabolic control of people with diabetes mellitus: A randomized controlled clinical trial. *Applied Nursing Research, 36*(1), 68–76. https://doi.org/10.1016/j.apnr.2017.05.009

Gray, J. R., & Grove, S. K., (2021). *The practice of nursing research: Appraisal, synthesis, and generation of evidence* (9th ed.). Elsevier.

Grove, S. K., & Cipher, D. J. (2021). *Statistics for nursing research: A workbook for evidence-based practice* (3rd ed.). Elsevier.

Herber, O., Bücker, B., Metzendorf, M. I., & Barroso, J. (2017). A qualitative meta-summary using Sandelowski and Barroso's method for synthesizing qualitative research to explore barriers and facilitators to self-care in heart failure patients. *European Journal of Cardiovascular Nursing, 16*, 662–677. https://doi.org/10.1177/1474515117711007

Herber, O., Kastaun, S., Wilm, S., & Barroso, J. (2019). From qualitative meta-summary to qualitative meta-synthesis: Introducing a new situation-specific theory of barriers and facilitators for self-care in patients with heart failure. *Qualitative Health Research, 29*(1), 96–106. https://doi.org/10.1177/1049732318800290

Im, E., & Meleis, A. (Eds.). (2021). *Situation-specific theories: Development, utilization, and evaluation in nursing.* Springer.

Kanter, R. M. (1993). *Men and women of the corporation* (2nd ed.). Basic Books.

King, I. (1992). Interpersonal relations: A theoretical framework for application in nursing practice. *Nursing Science Quarterly, 5*(1), 13–18. https://doi.org/10.1177/089431849200500106

Kolcaba, K. (1992). Holistic comfort: Operationalizing the construct as a nurse sensitive outcome. *Advances in Nursing Science, 15*(1), 1–10. https://doi.org/10.1097/00012272-199209000-00003

Kolcaba, K. (1994). A theory of holistic comfort for nursing. *Journal of Advanced Nursing, 19*(6), 1178–1184. https://doi.org/10.1111/j.1365-2648.1994.tb01202.x

Kolcaba, K. (2003). *Comfort theory and practice: A vision for holistic health care and research.* Springer.

Lenz, E. R., Pugh, L. C., Milligan, R., Gift, A., & Suppe, F. (1997). The middle range theory of unpleasant symptoms: An update. *Advances in Nursing Science, 19*(3), 14–27. https://doi.org/10.1097/00012272-199703000-00003

Liehr, P., & Smith, M. (2017). Middle range theory: A perspective on development and use. *Advances in Nursing Science, 40*(1), 51–63. https://doi.org/10.1097/ANS.0000000000000162

Lok, N., Buldukoglu, K., & Barcin, E. (2020). Effects of the cognitive stimulation therapy based on Roy's adaptation model on Alzheimer's patients' cognitive functions, coping, adaptation skills, and quality of life: A randomized controlled trial. *Perspectives in Psychiatric Care, 56*, 581–592. https://doi.org/10.1111/ppc.12472

Lor, M., Backonja, U., & Lauver, D. (2017). How could nurse researchers apply theory to generate knowledge more efficiently? *Journal of Nursing Scholarship, 49*(5), 580–589.

Martínez-Santos, A-E, de la Fuente, N., Facal, D. Vilanova-Trillo, L., Gandoy-Crego, M., & Rodríguez-González, R. (2021). Care tasks and impact of caring in primary family caregivers: A cross-sectional study from a nursing perspective. *Applied Nursing Research, 62*, 151505. https://doi.org/10.1016/j.apnr.2021.151505.

Meleis, A. I. (2010). *Transitions theory: Middle range and situation specific theories in nursing research and practice.* Springer Publishing.

Meleis, A. I. (2018). *Theoretical nursing: Development and progress* (6th ed.). Wolters Kluwer.

Mishel, M. H. (1988). Uncertainty in illness. *Journal of Nursing Scholarship, 20*(4), 225–232. https://doi.org/10.1111/j.1547-5069.1988.tb00082.x

Mishel, M. H. (1990). Reconceptualization of the uncertainty in illness theory. *Journal of Nursing Scholarship, 22*(3), 256–262. https://doi.org/10.1111/j.1547-5069.1990.tb00225.x

National Human Genome Research Institute. (2020). *The human genome project.* Retrieved from https://www.genome.gov/human-genome-project

Orem, D. E. (2001). *Nursing: Concepts of practice* (6th ed.). Mosby.

Orem, D. E., & Taylor, S. G. (2011). Reflections on nursing practice science: The nature, the structure, and the foundation of nursing science. *Nursing Science Quarterly, 24*(1), 35–41. https://doi.org/10.1177/0894318410389061

Park, C., Won, M., & Son, Y. J. (2021). Mediating effects of social support between Type D personality and self-care behaviours among heart failure patients. *Journal of Advanced Nursing, 77*(3), 1315–1324. https://doi.org/10.1111/jan.14682

Peterson, S. (2020). Introduction to the nature of nursing knowledge. In S. Peterson & T. Bredow (Eds.), *Middle range theories: Application to nursing research and practice* (5th ed., pp. 1–36). Wolters Kluwer.

Reed, P. (1991). Toward a nursing theory of self-transcendence: Deductive reformulation using developmental theories. *Advances in Nursing Science, 13*(4), 64–77. https://doi.org/10.1097/00012272-199106000-00008

Riegel, B., Jaarsma, T., Lee, C., & Strömberg, A. (2012). A middle-range theory of self-care of chronic illness. *Advances in Nursing Science, 35*(3), 194–204. https://doi.org/10.1097/ANS.0b013e318261b1ba

Riegel, B., Jaarsma, T., Lee, C., & Strömberg, A. (2019). Integrating symptoms into the middle-range theory of self-care of chronic illness. *Advances in Nursing Science, 42*(3), 206–215. https://doi.org/10.1097/ANS.0000000000000237

Rogers, M. E. (1970). *An introduction to the theoretical basis of nursing.* F. A. Davis.

Roy, C. (2011). Research based on the Roy Adaptation Model: Last 25 years. *Nursing Science Quarterly, 24*(4), 312–320. https://doi.org/10.1177/0894318411419218

Roy, C., & Andrews, H. A. (2009). *Roy Adaptation Model* (3rd ed.). Prentice Hall Health.

Roy, C., Bakan, G., Li, Z., & Nguyen, T. (2016). Coping measurement: Creating short form of Coping and Adaptation Processing Scale using item response theory and patients dealing with chronic and acute health conditions. *Applied Nursing Research, 32*, 73–79. https://doi.org/10.1016/j.apnr.2016.06.002

Swanson, K. M. (1991). Empirical development of a middle range theory of caring. *Nursing Research, 40*(3), 161–166.

Tabiee, S., Momeni, A., & Alireza Saadatjoo, S. (2017). The effects of comfort-based interventions (back massage and patient and family education) on the level of comfort among hemodialysis patients. *Modern Care Journal, 14*(3), e64687. https://doi.org/10.5812/modernc.64687

Thomas, T., Donovan, H., Rosenzweig, M., Bender, C., & Schenker, Y. (2020). A conceptual framework of self-advocacy in women with cancer. *Advances in Nursing Science, 44*(1), E1–E13. https://doi.org/10.1097/ANS.0000000000000342

van Manen, M. (2017). Phenomenology in its original sense. *Qualitative Health Research, 27*(6), 810–825. https://doi.org/10.1177/1049732317699381

Vicdan, A. (2020). The effect of training given to hemodialysis patients according to the Comfort Theory. *Clinical Specialist, 34*(1), 30–37. https://doi.org/10.1097/NUR.0000000000000495

8

Clarifying Quantitative Research Designs

Jennifer R. Gray

LEARNING OUTCOMES

After completing this chapter, you should be able to:

1. Describe the concepts relevant to quantitative research designs, including causality and control.
2. Examine study designs for threats to design validity.
3. Identify the noninterventional designs (descriptive and correlational) and interventional designs (quasi-experimental and experimental) commonly used in quantitative nursing studies.
4. Critically appraise descriptive, correlational, quasi-experimental, and experimental designs in studies.
5. Examine the quality of randomized controlled trials conducted in nursing.

A building begins with a blueprint. How many stories will it have? Where will the entrance be? How many rooms will there be? A building blueprint is developed by an architect who understands the purpose of the proposed building, knows construction rules and design principles, and ensures the plan meets relevant laws and requirements. The builder cannot obtain a building permit unless the plan meets these standards. Much like architects, researchers develop a plan for their study before they begin. The plan for a study is called a research design.

When you read an article about a study, notice the decisions the researchers have made. What is the purpose of the study? How many groups are in the study? Is there an intervention? Descriptive and correlational research designs are focused on describing variables and examining relationships among the variables in natural settings. The researcher does not intervene to change the variables or relationships, making these designs noninterventional studies. Quasi-experimental and experimental research designs have been developed to examine causality, or the cause-and-effect relationship between an intervention and an outcome. These study designs are interventional designs.

This chapter provides information about the principles that researchers follow when designing a study and different types of research design. Identifying the design is an essential step in critically appraising the study. We have provided algorithms or decision trees to help you in identifying a study's design. In addition to the algorithms, we provide figures that display the structure of common research designs. Analyzing a study also involves identifying weaknesses of different study designs, which are called threats to design validity. To critically appraise a study, you will examine its characteristics and determine whether there are threats to the validity, or credibility, of its findings.

CONCEPTS RELEVANT TO QUANTITATIVE RESEARCH DESIGNS

To understand specific research designs, you need to be familiar with several key concepts, including causality, multicausality, probability, prospective, retrospective, bias, control, and manipulation. These concepts are used when describing studies and provide a foundation for understanding the strengths of specific designs and the threats to design validity.

Causality

Causality basically means that things have causes, and causes lead to effects (York, 2021). Studies that describe variables (descriptive designs) and examine relationships among variables (correlational designs) do not examine causality. Studies that test the effect of interventions on specific outcomes do examine causality. You may be able to determine whether the researchers were examining causality by reading the purpose of the study and examining its hypotheses. The hypotheses (see Chapter 5) may have been developed from propositions of the study's theoretical framework (see Chapter 7). For example, the purpose of a causal study may be to examine the effect of an early postsurgical ambulation program on the length of hospital stay. The framework proposition may state that early physical activity after surgery decreases recovery time. However, the early ambulation program is not the only factor affecting the length of hospital stay. Other important factors or extraneous variables that affect the length of hospital stay include the diagnosis, type of surgery, patient's age, physical condition of the patient before surgery, and complications that occurred after surgery. Researchers usually design quasi-experimental and experimental studies to examine causality or the effect of an intervention (independent variable) on a selected outcome (dependent variable), using a design that controls for relevant extraneous variables (Gray & Grove, 2021).

Multicausality

Think about the grade you received on your last examination. Was there only one cause of your exam grade (effect)? Likely, you can identify several factors that caused your grade, such as study time and understanding the content. Few phenomena in nursing can be linked to a single cause and a single effect. Most often, interrelating variables produce an effect. When researchers recognize the multiple causes, they develop studies that include more variables than those using a strict causal orientation. The presence of multiple causes for an effect is referred to as multicausality. As in the previous example, patient diagnosis, age, presurgical condition, and complications after surgery are interrelated causes of the length of a patient's hospital stay. Because of the complexity of causal relationships, a theory is unlikely to identify every element involved in causing the specified outcome. However, the greater the proportion of causal factors that can be identified and examined or controlled in a single study, the clearer the understanding will be of the overall phenomenon (Kazdin, 2017). This greater understanding is expected to increase the ability to predict and control the effects of study interventions.

Probability

Probability addresses relative rather than absolute causality. A cause may not produce a specific effect each time that it occurs. As a result, researchers recognize that the cause *probably* will result in a specific effect. Using a probability orientation, researchers design studies to examine the probability that a given effect will occur under a defined set of circumstances. The circumstances may be variations in multiple variables that have been identified as possible causes. Researchers who are examining the probability of a hospital stay of 48 hours after surgery may select specific sets of circumstances that are causes. They might select circumstances such as patients who have undergone a partial knee replacement, have no chronic illnesses, and experienced no complications after surgery. The inclusion and exclusion criteria for the sample would specify the patients to be recruited to control most of the extraneous variables (see Chapter 9). The probability of a given length of hospital stay could be expected to vary as the set of circumstances are varied or controlled in the design of the study.

📄 **RESEARCH/EBP TIP**

Researchers recognize that multicausality and probability apply to most life events, especially those related to nursing care of patients and families. To conduct studies that are applicable to clinical practice, they frequently design studies to examine the probability that selected causes have a specified effect.

Prospective Versus Retrospective

Prospective is a term that means looking forward, whereas the term retrospective means looking backward, usually in relation to time. In research, these terms are used most frequently to refer to the timing of data collection. Are the data collected in real time by the research team, or are the study's data obtained from information collected at a previous time? Data collection in noninterventional research can be either prospective or retrospective because, by definition, it lacks researcher intervention. Many noninterventional studies in health care use retrospective data obtained from national electronic databases and clinical and administrative databases of healthcare agencies. Secondary analysis of data from a previous study to address a newly developed study purpose is also considered retrospective. When using retrospective data, the researchers have no control over the accuracy of the data. However, prospective data collection is usually more accurate than retrospective data collection (Kazdin, 2017). The researchers are passionate about the topic of study and are rigorous in the implementation of the data collection process.

Data collection in interventional studies must be prospective because the researcher enacts an intervention in real time. However, the researchers may not collect all the data themselves in a real-time study. An example is a study that includes the variables of arterial blood pressure and position in critically ill adults. The researchers may establish a baseline by collecting data for 24 hours before the intervention with the patient in supine position. Each day, the researchers will collect the hourly readings of arterial blood pressure recorded by the nurses in the electronic chart. Although information retrieval of the electronic chart data does look back in time over the preceding 24-hour period, this study would be considered prospective because data are generated and recorded during the time the adults are hospitalized (Pole & Bondy, 2012). After the baseline period, the intervention of prone position would be implemented twice a day by the nurses followed by additional data collection.

Bias

The term *bias* means a slant or deviation from the true or expected. Bias in a study distorts the findings from what the results would have been without the bias. Because studies are conducted to determine what is real and true, quantitative researchers highly value identifying, removing, and controlling the effects of sources of bias in their study. Any component of a study that deviates or causes a deviation from a true measurement of the study variables contributes to distorted findings (Kazdin, 2017).

Many factors related to research can be biased, such as the attitudes or motivations of the researcher (conscious or unconscious) and components of the environment in which the study is conducted. Many other study conditions can be biases, including the selection of the participants, assignment of the participants to groups, measurement methods, data collection process, and statistical analyses (Gray & Grove, 2021; Grove & Cipher, 2020). For example, a research assistant recruiting potential study participants at a health center may approach only patients who seemed friendly. Researchers might use a scale with limited reliability and validity to measure a study variable (Waltz et al., 2017). Each of these situations introduces bias to nonintervention and intervention studies.

An important focus in critically appraising a study is to identify possible sources of bias. This requires careful examination of the Methods section in the research report, including the strategies for obtaining study participants, methods of measurement, implementation of a study intervention, and data collection process. However, not all biases can be identified from the published study report. The article may not provide enough detail about the methods of the study to detect possible biases.

Control

One method of reducing bias is to increase the amount of control in the design of a study. Control means having the power to direct or manipulate factors to achieve a desired outcome. For example, Reaves and Angosta (2021) conducted a single-group intervention study with persons who had chronic obstructive pulmonary disease (COPD). The intervention was teaching the participants the relaxation response mediation technique (RRMT) with the goal that participants would implement the RRMT on their own and manage their anxiety and respiratory symptoms. The researchers increased the control in the study by recruiting patients with COPD from one pulmonary rehabilitation clinic and by excluding patients who also had lung cancer, pneumonia, or asthma. They also scheduled intervention visits to be completed when participants returned to the clinic for their next appointments. The standardization of the study procedures also increased the control of the study and minimized potential biases. Because of the controls implemented during the study, the researchers could be confident in the study's results, which were decreases in anxiety, perceived dyspnea, and respiratory rate after the intervention (Reaves & Angosta, 2021).

Control also can be enhanced when patients serve as their own controls. Low-molecular-weight heparin (LMWH) requires two subcutaneous injections at the same clinic visit. Unal et al. (2021) tested the effect of a vapocoolant spray on pain during the LMWH injection and the degree of ecchymosis at the site 2 days later. The participants were randomly selected from patients who were eligible for the study. Vapocoolant spray was applied before the LMWH injection in one arm and plain water was sprayed on the skin before the injection in the other arm, to mimic the actual intervention. This use of an action that was similar to the intervention was called the *placebo* method. The placebo method controlled for patient differences related to injections and pain. Unal et al. (2021) found the vapocoolant spray reduced injection pain but not ecchymosis.

Manipulation

Manipulation is a form of control used in quasi-experimental and experimental studies during the implementation of the intervention and its characteristics as they exist in a natural environment or setting. The researchers must manipulate the intervention under study. Researchers need to develop quality interventions that are implemented in consistent ways (Kazdin, 2017). For example, Reaves and Angosta (2021) did not rely on the nurse consistently teaching participants how to use the RRMT. Instead, the researchers recorded the instructions and delivered the recording to each participant using a headset and an MP4 player. This controlled implementation of the study's intervention (manipulation) decreased the potential for bias and increased the validity of the study findings.

DESIGN VALIDITY OF QUANTITATIVE STUDIES

You read the report of a study and wonder, "Are these findings accurate?" or "Can I trust these findings?" These are questions about the design validity of the study. A study has design validity when it is conducted with rigorous methods. As a result, the findings are considered accurate and credible. Design validity encompasses the strengths and threats to the quality of a study design. Critical appraisal of studies requires that you identify the design strengths and think through the threats to validity or the possible weaknesses in a study's design. When researchers recognize threats to design validity in their study, these threats are often identified as limitations in the Discussion section of the study report. The four types of design validity relevant to nursing research are construct validity, internal validity, external validity, and statistical conclusion validity (Gray & Grove, 2021; Shadish et al., 2002). We have provided tables, one for each of the four types of design validity, that summarize the threats common to each. You need to understand the types of validity and their possible threats so that you can critically appraise quantitative studies (Grainger, 2021).

Construct Validity

When reading a study, the first thing you want to know is whether the methods and process used to collect the data were valid. Did the researchers measure what they thought they were measuring? Construct validity begins with the fit between the conceptual and operational definitions of variables (Gravetter & Forzano, 2018). Theoretical constructs or concepts are defined within the study framework when a framework is identified. When the researchers do not identify a specific study framework, the variables may be defined according to definitions used in other studies or in clinical practice. The conceptual definitions are abstract statements about the variables, which provide the basis for the operational definitions of the variables (see Chapter 5). Operational definitions (methods of measurement) must be congruent with the conceptual definitions of the theoretical constructs or concepts. The process of developing construct validity for an instrument often requires years of scientific work. Researchers need to discuss the construct validity of the instruments that they use in their studies (see Chapter 10). The process of measuring the variables must be carefully planned and implemented to avoid threats to construct validity. Threats to construct validity are described here and summarized in Table 8.1.

Inadequate Definitions of Constructs

Ideally, the conceptual definition should emerge from a concept analysis, which is an in-depth study of the meanings of a construct or concept as used by theorists, clinicians, and researchers.

TABLE 8.1   CONSTRUCT VALIDITY: THREATS AND EXAMPLES

Questions to answer: Did the researchers measure what they thought they were measuring? Were the operational definitions of the variables congruent with the conceptual definitions?

THREAT TO VALIDITY AND DESCRIPTION	EXAMPLES OF THE THREAT
Inadequate definitions of variables: The lack of clear conceptual and operational definitions may result in noncongruent or inappropriate measurements.	The study report lacks explicit conceptual definitions of the variables. If there is a clear definition or you can infer what the definition is, examine whether the measurement of the variable fits its conceptual definition.
Mono-operation bias: Each variable is measured using one instrument or scale.	Measuring the dependent (outcome) variable one way may be a threat, especially when that measurement is a researcher-developed instrument. Complex constructs, such as pain or adherence, are measured using one scale.
Mono-method bias: Only one measurement method is used to measure the study variable.	All the measurements in the study require the participants to complete scales delivered by a computer. Measuring all variables by self-report can increase risk that social desirability influenced responses.
Experimenter expectancies: Researchers' expectations or bias may influence data collection.	The primary author of the study report collects the data in the study. The researchers do not mention using a protocol or script to ensure the instructions to participants are consistent. In intervention studies, the data collectors know the group assignment of the participants, which means they were not blinded.
Social desirability: Participants select answers based on wanting the researcher to like them or based on behaviors that are perceived as positive.	The study report does not acknowledge the limitation of self-report as a method of data collection. Data are collected in a way that the data are linked to the participant's identity. The researchers do not mention that the data are kept confidential (or anonymous).

Researchers should include an explicit definition of the concept in the study's report. The method of measurement (operational definition) should be carefully selected to be consistent with the conceptual definition. A deficiency in the conceptual or operational definition leads to low construct validity.

Mono-Operation Bias

Mono-operation bias is the potential for incomplete measurement when only one tool, questionnaire, or assessment is used to measure a construct. When only one method of measurement is used, fewer dimensions of the construct are measured. Construct validity greatly improves if the researcher uses more than one instrument, such as two scales to measure depression (Waltz et al., 2017). For example, for a study in which pain is a dependent variable, more than one measure of pain could be used, such as a pain rating scale, verbal reports of pain, and observations of behaviors that may reflect pain, such as crying or reacting when a painful area is touched. The measurement of pain is enhanced using multiple operations. It is sometimes possible to apply more than one measurement of the dependent variable with little increase in time, effort, or cost (Gray & Grove, 2021).

Mono-Method Bias

Mono-method bias is the potential for inaccurate measurement when only one type of measurement is used to assess a construct (Gray & Grove, 2021). For example, when all the variables in a study are self-report measures, the participants' concerns about confidentiality and social desirability may interfere with accurate measurements. Another example is when an instrument measuring depression is delivered on an iPad. The participant may report a low score, not because the participant is depressed, but because the participant is unsure in how to use the iPad. One solution would be to include a set of sample questions, and the research assistant could demonstrate the use of the iPad in answering the sample questions. A quality of life instrument and other scales delivered on paper that require extensive reading may be measuring the participant's ability to read and comprehend rather than quality of life. Having a research assistant read the scales aloud to all participants and record their answers would be one solution.

Experimenter Expectancies

The expectancies of the researcher can bias the data. For example, experimenter expectancy occurs when a researcher knows which participants received the intervention and collects the data. The data that he or she collects may be biased to reflect the expectation of improvement. The opposite can be true when a data collector knows which participants received the intervention and does not believe that the intervention is effective. The extent to which expectancies influence studies is not known. Because of their concern about experimenter expectancy, some researchers choose not to be involved in the data collection process. In other studies, data collectors are blinded to group assignment, which means they do not know who has received the intervention and who is in the control or placebo group. Using nonbiased data collectors or those who are blinded to group assignment increases the construct design validity of a study.

Social Desirability

People are social beings and we want others to think highly of us. Nurses participating in a study on health behaviors might underestimate the number of cigarettes they smoke, the frequency of eating high-calorie foods, or the hours spent playing video or computer games. They might also overestimate the steps walked and the time spent in sleep and exercise. Other participants in studies might do the same thing. They will tend to answer in ways that are perceived as being desirable or healthy. When the topic of a study is sensitive or stigmatized, social desirability may be a greater concern. Collecting data confidentially so that the researcher cannot link the participant to his or her data may decrease social desirability, but not completely. Researchers attempt to minimize this threat by telling participants that there are no wrong or right answers and to answer as honestly as possible (see Table 8.1).

📄 RESEARCH/EBP TIP

When critically appraising a study's quality, read the Methods section very carefully. Identify the validity of the instruments, the methods used for data collection, and whether data collectors knew the participants' group assignments. Did the researchers measure what they thought they were measuring?

Internal Validity

Internal validity is the extent to which the study findings are a true reflection of reality, rather than the result of extraneous variables. Any study can contain threats to internal design validity, and these validity threats can lead to inaccurate conclusions (York, 2021). Internal validity is a greater concern in interventional studies. The researcher must determine whether the dependent variables were changed by the independent variable (the intervention) or by a third variable (an extraneous variable). A researcher committed to quality considers whether there is an alternative explanation for the findings. Some of the common threats to internal validity, such as study participant selection and assignment to groups, participant attrition, history, and maturation, are discussed in this section, and examples are summarized in Table 8.2.

TABLE 8.2   INTERNAL VALIDITY: THREATS AND EXAMPLES

Question to answer: Are the study findings accurate or the result of extraneous variables?

THREAT TO VALIDITY AND DESCRIPTION	EXAMPLES OF THE THREAT
Participant selection: Participants are selected by nonrandom sampling methods. The participants have unique characteristics that may influence the study findings.	Convenience or other nonrandom sampling methods are used. The participants have one or more demographic characteristics in common, such as predominantly one race or highly educated.
Participant assignment to groups: Participants are placed in groups using nonrandom methods in an interventional study. Characteristics of the groups may influence the findings.	In an interventional study, participants are assigned to receive the treatment or the control condition based on their location, such as the clinic where they receive care. In an interventional study, participants are assigned to groups based on which day of the week they are recruited.
Participant attrition: The percentage of participants withdrawing from a longitudinal study is high (>20%). The participants who withdrew may be different in some way from those who complete the study.	This threat occurs in studies where data are collected at multiple points in time. The number of participants who complete the study is 20% less than the number who begin the study.
History: An unrelated event occurs during the study that may have an effect on the findings.	The study limitations include a note about a significant event that occurred in the communities where the study was conducted. The researchers acknowledge changes in the study setting that may influence the results, such as a provider leaving whom patients liked.
Maturation: Participants become more experienced, wiser, or tired over the course of a study, which may influence the data collected.	The data collection procedure includes the multiple instruments the participants complete. The data collection required more than an hour for each participant. In longitudinal studies, data collection is extensive at each research visit. In pediatric longitudinal studies, the researchers fail to acknowledge that changes over time may be a result of normal developmental, rather than the intervention.

Participant Selection

Selection addresses the process whereby participants are chosen to take part in a study. A selection threat is more likely to occur in studies in which randomization is not possible (see Chapter 9; Gray & Grove, 2021; Shadish et al., 2002). When selected nonrandomly, study participants may differ in some important way from people not selected for the study. One example would be a descriptive study of nurses' commitment to the profession with a convenience sample recruited from the membership list of the American Nurses Association. The nurses paying for membership in a professional organization may have a higher commitment to the profession than nurses who do not pay for membership. One might question the internal validity of the findings because of how the participants were selected (York, 2021).

Patient Assignment

Internal validity also can be threatened when patients are not randomly assigned to groups during intervention studies. For example, you decide that the participants recruited from one location will comprise the treatment group; the participants recruited from a second location will comprise the control group. The participants in the control group may be different in some important way from the participants assigned to the intervention group. This difference in selection could cause the two groups to react differently to the intervention. The groups' outcomes may not be caused by the intervention, but by the differences in the individuals selected for the two groups. Random selection of participants for nursing studies is often not possible, and the number of participants available for studies may be limited. However, randomly assigning participants to the treatment and control groups decreases the possibility of this threat to internal validity (Kazdin, 2017).

Participant Attrition

Attrition involves participants dropping out of a study before it is completed. Ideally, all the participants who begin a study will complete the study. Participant attrition becomes a threat to internal validity when those who drop out of a study are different in some way from those who remain in the study. Participant attrition also may be a problem when there are differences in the number and characteristics of the people who drop out of the intervention group and the people who drop out of the control or comparison group (see Chapter 9). If the attrition in a study is high (>20%), the accuracy of the study results may be affected (Gray & Grove, 2021).

History

Despite everything that researchers do to control the conditions of a study, an unexpected event may occur. This threat to internal validity is called history (see Table 8.2). History is an event that occurs during a study and may influence a participant's response to the intervention or alter how a participant answers the questions on a scale or survey. The event can occur in the immediate environment or in the political/social environment. For example, a study is being conducted at a cardiac rehabilitation center to test the effect of a nurse-implemented intervention on the participants' physiological outcomes and completion of their rehabilitation. During the study, a well-respected medical director is replaced by another director with an authoritarian leadership style. The work environment becomes stressful, and several nurses resign. This historical event threatens the study's internal design validity. Participants who had worked closely with the nurses who left may stop participating, or working with different nurses may change the study outcomes.

Another example is a longitudinal study of the effects of an educational intervention on participants being screened for breast and prostate cancer. The study is being conducted in a low-income clinic where most of the participants do not have health insurance. Due to a change in state laws, some of the participants in the study become eligible for health insurance and enroll in a health plan. This change in insurance status may make determining the effect of the intervention difficult.

Maturation

In research, maturation is defined as growing older, wiser, stronger, hungrier, more tired, or more experienced during the study. These unplanned and unrecognized changes are a threat to the study's internal validity and can influence the findings of the study. Maturation is more likely to occur in longitudinal studies with repeated measures of study variables. Maturation may also be an issue when normal development affects the findings of studies conducted with children or adolescents (see Table 8.2).

📄 **RESEARCH/EBP TIP**

The internal validity of a study may be threatened by how the participants are selected and assigned to groups, whether they complete the study, how they change during the study, and how unrelated events may have influenced the participants.

Statistical Conclusion Validity

In noninterventional studies, after the data have been collected and the statistical analyses completed, the researchers may use the results of the analyses to answer research questions about the presence of relationships among the variables or differences in the variables between naturally occurring groups. In interventional studies, the researchers' goal is to determine whether the group who received the intervention had different outcomes than the group who did not receive the intervention. Statistical conclusion validity is concerned with whether the conclusions about relationships or differences drawn from statistical analyses are an accurate reflection of the real world (Grove & Cipher, 2020).

Researchers want to reduce the potential for inaccurately concluding that relationships between variables and differences between groups have been found. There are some common reasons why inaccurate conclusions may be drawn. These reasons are threats to statistical conclusion validity that are presented in Table 8.3. In this chapter, we have included the threats of low statistical power, unreliable measurement methods, limited intervention fidelity, and extraneous variances in the study setting. Shadish et al. (2002) have provided a more detailed discussion of statistical conclusion validity.

Low Statistical Power

Low statistical power increases the probability of concluding that there is no significant relationship between variables or significant difference between groups when there is a relationship or difference. When nonsignificant statistical results are inaccurate, a Type II error occurs. A Type II error is most likely to occur when the sample size is small or when the power of the statistical test to determine differences is low (Grove & Cipher, 2020). You need to ensure that the study has adequate sample size and power to detect relationships and differences. The concepts of sample size, statistical power, and Type II error are discussed in detail in Chapters 9 and 11.

Reliability or Precision of Measurement Methods

The technique of measuring variables must be reliable to reveal true differences. A measure is reliable if it gives the same result each time that the same situation or variable is measured. If a scale

TABLE 8.3   STATISTICAL CONCLUSION VALIDITY: THREATS AND EXAMPLES

Question to answer: Are the conclusions drawn based on the statistical analyses an accurate reflection of the real world?

THREAT TO VALIDITY AND DESCRIPTION	EXAMPLES OF THE THREAT
Low statistical power: A conclusion is drawn that there are no significant differences or relationships when one exists (Type II error).	The researchers acknowledge the limitation of a small sample or power <80% (see Chapter 9). The sample size is <30 participants per group. The researchers recommend that in future studies the intervention be delivered more than once or strengthened.
Unreliable measurement methods: Scales or physiological measures used in a study are not consistently measuring study variables.	Cronbach's alpha of the scales or subscales are calculated as <0.70. The researchers do not mention the calibration of physiological equipment according to the manufacturer's instructions. For laboratory tests, the study report does not include information about the accreditation of the laboratory or the methods used to collect specimens.
Intervention fidelity concerns: The intervention in a study is not consistently implemented, which may make detecting differences in the outcome difficult.	The researchers do not report an intervention protocol or training of the individuals implementing the intervention. The report does not mention any spot checks or ongoing monitoring of whether the intervention was being delivered correctly.
Extraneous variables in study setting: Extraneous variables in the setting are not controlled in an interventional study, which may affect participants' responses to the intervention.	The researchers do not mention efforts to control the setting. Limitations related to the setting are identified.

used to measure depression is reliable, it should give similar scores when depression is repeatedly measured over a short time period (Kazdin, 2017; Waltz et al., 2017). Another measure of reliability is an instrument's internal consistency, often reported as Cronbach's alpha. Physiological measures that consistently measure physiological variables are considered precise. For example, a thermometer is precise if it shows the same reading when being used repeatedly on the same patient within a limited time period (see Chapter 10). You need to examine the measurement methods in a study and determine whether they are reliable.

Intervention Fidelity

Intervention fidelity ensures that the research intervention is standardized by a protocol and is applied consistently each time it is implemented in a study (Bova et al., 2017). If the method of administering a research intervention varies from one person to another, detecting a true difference becomes difficult (see Table 8.3; Bonar et al., 2020). For example, one nurse might implement the study intervention to the first 20 participants and spend more time with them than was designated by intervention protocol; another nurse might implement the intervention protocol exactly as was planned to the next 20 participants. The persons delivering the intervention must be trained to ensure consistent or reliable implementation of a study intervention to prevent threats to the statistical conclusion validity.

Extraneous Variances in the Study Setting

Extraneous variables in complex settings such as hospital units and busy clinics can influence scores on the dependent variable. These variables increase the difficulty of detecting differences between the experimental and control groups. Consider the activities that occur on a nursing unit. The numbers and variety of staff, patients, health crises, and work patterns merge into a complex arena for the implementation of a study. Any of the dynamics of the unit can influence manipulation of the independent variable or measurement of the dependent variable. You might review the Methods section of the study and determine how extraneous variables were controlled in the study setting.

📄 RESEARCH/EBP TIP

Experimental studies are designed to minimize threats to statistical conclusion validity by selecting reliable instruments, recruiting a large sample, ensuring intervention fidelity, and minimizing extraneous variances.

External Validity

External validity is concerned with the extent to which study findings can be generalized beyond the sample used in the study (Gray & Grove, 2021; Kazdin, 2017). When a serious threat to external validity is present, the findings are meaningful only for the group studied. Sometimes, the factors influencing external validity are subtle and may not be reported in the study; however, the researchers implementing the study are responsible for these factors. Generalization is usually narrower for a single study than for multiple replications of a study using different samples, perhaps from different populations in different settings. For external validity, we have included two threats for noninterventional studies and three threats for interventional studies in Table 8.4.

Homogenous Sample

When designing noninterventional studies (descriptive and correlational studies), researchers who want to be able to generalize their findings recognize the need to have a large, diverse sample. A larger, more diverse sample is more likely to provide data with a wide range of values on the key variables. Consider a study of the relationships among spirituality and different aspects of health. If a researcher recruits only 30 participants, aged 50 to 70 years, from one religion, the range of values on a spirituality variable would be narrower than if 200 participants were recruited, aged 20 to 70 years, from multiple religious and nonreligious groups. Relationships among variables are more likely to be found when the variables have a wide range of values. The researcher can generalize significant findings to other groups when the sample is larger and more diverse. Consequently, a homogenous sample is considered a threat to external validity for noninterventional studies (Grove & Cipher, 2020).

Interaction of Selection and Setting

Another threat to external validity for noninterventional studies is an interaction of the sample selection and setting. For example, a group of researchers selected a large healthcare system as the setting for a descriptive study because the setting provided care to a community of people from multiple racial and ethnic groups, those educated at different educational levels, and those who

TABLE 8.4 EXTERNAL VALIDITY: THREATS AND EXAMPLES

Question: Are the findings generalized beyond the sample used in the study?

THREAT TO VALIDITY AND DESCRIPTION	EXAMPLES OF THE THREAT
Homogeneity of the sample in a noninterventional study: The sample recruited was unique and does not reflect the larger population.	The participants who are recruited are different from the persons to whom you want to generalize the findings.
Interaction of sample and setting in a noninterventional study: The sample and the setting combined in a way that resulted in a unique sample that does not reflect the larger population.	The participants available in the setting have unexpected unique characteristics, different from those to whom you want to generalize the findings.
Interaction of selection and intervention (interventional designs): Participants decline to participate because of the commitment or effort the intervention requires. The sample recruited does not reflect the larger population.	The refusal rate is high (>20%) and/or the intervention requires excessive time and effort. The intervention involves painful or psychologically uncomfortable procedures.
Interaction of setting and intervention (interventional designs): The setting influences the implementation of the intervention and data collection process.	The study limitations include characteristics of the setting (culture, physical environment) that affected how the intervention and data collection were implemented.
Interaction of history and intervention (interventional designs): An event that occurs in the setting affects the implementation of the intervention and data collection.	The study limitations include an event in the setting that may have affected the intervention or data collection. Examples include a change in ownership, closure of a hospital unit, change in leadership, or high nursing staff attrition.

were native and internationally born. One of the inclusion criteria was being able to read and write English. Efforts were made to recruit a diverse sample. However, when the researchers analyzed the demographic data, they found the sample was composed of predominantly native-born participants who had finished high school. The selection of the sample interacted with the setting and produced a sample that was unrepresentative of the persons receiving care in the health system and in the larger population.

Interaction of Selection and Intervention

Finding individuals who are willing to participate in an interventional study can be difficult, particularly if the study requires extensive amounts of time and energy (see Table 8.4). Researchers must report the number of persons who were approached and refused to participate in the study (refusal rate) so that those examining the findings can identify any threat to external validity. If the refusal rate for a study is high, there is a greater potential for threats to external design validity. For example, if greater than 25% of the persons asked to participate decline, the sample may be limited in ways that might not be evident to the researchers without deeper review. The participants may be persons who are unemployed, retired, or otherwise have more discretionary time to complete the study. In this case, generalizing the findings to all members of a population is unjustified.

When you read the report of a study in which there was a high refusal rate or high attrition rate, assess the amount of time required to participate in the study. Did the researchers ask participants to report glucose levels every 4 hours? Did the intervention involve 10 visits to the health facility? Ideally, studies are developed that limit the demands on people and increase their interest in participation, while collecting all needed data and implementing an effective intervention. For example, researchers should consider the reliability, validity, and participant burden when selecting the instruments or data collection methods. A researcher may find a 100-item instrument that takes 60 minutes to complete and a second 25-item instrument that takes 20 minutes to complete but has a slightly lower reliability. The shorter instrument may be a better choice because it decreases the time and energy the participants will expend. The study intervention must be skillfully developed and clearly communicated to individuals to increase their participation in the study. Enough data need to be collected on the participants to allow researchers to be familiar with their characteristics and, to the greatest extent possible, the characteristics of those who decline to participate (see Chapter 9).

Interaction of Setting and Intervention

Bias can exist in the types of setting and organization that agree to participate in studies (Gray & Grove, 2021). For example, a hospital seeking Magnet designation may have a stronger commitment to serving as the setting for nurse-led studies. Other hospitals may be resistant to the conduct of nursing research. These two types of hospital may be different in ways that affect the intervention. In this case, there may be an interaction of setting and intervention that limits the generalizability of the findings. Different settings may also serve different types of patient or potential study participants. For example, a clinic in a low-resource community may have patients with lower health literacy, whereas a clinic that accepts only patients with insurance might have a larger portion of college-educated patients. The intervention and measurement methods to be implemented may interact with the ability to read and comprehend written materials by the patients in different settings. The interactions of settings and interventions can influence study outcomes. Researchers should cautiously consider the characteristics of the study's setting and the patients served in the setting when making statements about the population to which their findings can be generalized.

Interaction of History and Intervention

The extent to which a study's findings are generalizable is affected by the events that occur during the study. A researcher implementing a suicide-prevention intervention in two high schools must consider the interaction of history and intervention should a suicide occur in one of the high schools during the study. Another example would be a study of a medication adherence intervention being conducted when a large manufacturing plant lays off most of its workforce and stops their health insurance coverage immediately. The interaction of the event (history) and the intervention in these examples may affect the generalization of the findings. Replicating studies during various time periods and in different communities strengthens the usefulness of findings over time. In critically appraising studies, you need to consider the effects of nursing practice and societal events that occurred during the time the study was conducted.

Understanding construct validity, internal validity, statistical conclusion validity, and external validity provides a foundation for evaluating the quality of a study's findings. This discussion of design validity was presented to assist you in critically appraising the designs in the quantitative studies presented as examples in the following sections (Grainger, 2021).

IDENTIFICATION OF QUANTITATIVE RESEARCH DESIGNS IN NURSING STUDIES

A variety of quantitative research designs are implemented in nursing studies; the four most common types are descriptive, correlational, quasi-experimental, and experimental. These designs are categorized in different ways in textbooks (Kazdin, 2017; Kerlinger & Lee, 2000; Shadish et al., 2002). Because descriptive and correlational designs do not involve a treatment or intervention, they are referred to as noninterventional designs. Some authors call them nonexperimental designs. The focus of descriptive and correlational designs is examining variables as they occur in natural environments.

Some of the noninterventional designs include a time element, such as the cross-sectional designs, which involve collecting data at one point in time. The participants in cross-sectional designs may be in various stages of development, levels of education, severity of illness, or stages of recovery to describe changes in a phenomenon across stages. For example, in a cross-sectional study about people who are living with kidney disease, some of the participants would be older, diagnosed 15 or more years ago, and experienced with managing the symptoms of the disease. Other participants may be younger, recently diagnosed with kidney disease, and learning about the symptoms. Some participants would be between the two. The assumption is that the phenomenon being studied is part of a process that will progress over time. Selecting participants at various points in the process provides important information about the totality of the process, even though the same subjects are not monitored throughout the entire process (Gray & Grove, 2021).

Another design with a time element is the longitudinal design. Longitudinal designs involve collecting data from the same study participants at multiple points in time. The participants are recruited and initial data collected. Then, at prescheduled points in time, data are collected again, which is why the design is also called repeated measures. Repeated measures might be included in descriptive, correlational, quasi-experimental, or experimental study designs. Han et al. (2020) collected sleep disturbance data every 6 months from novice nurses ($N = 435$) who worked rotating shifts during the first 2 years of their careers. With four data points for each nurse, the researchers compared the sleep trajectories of nurses who remained employed at the hospital to the trajectories of those who left. The study conducted by Han et al. (2020) was a comparative descriptive longitudinal study.

Quasi-experimental and experimental studies are designed to examine causality or the cause-and-effect relationship between a researcher-implemented intervention and selected study outcomes. The designs for these studies are sometimes referred to as interventional or experimental designs because the focus is on examining the differences in dependent variables thought to be caused by independent variables or interventions. For example, the quasi-experimental study conducted by Reaves and Angosta (2021) with persons living with COPD examined differences in the dependent variables of anxiety, dyspnea, and respiratory rate after the implementation of the RRMT intervention, the independent variable. Reaves and Angosta (2021) implemented a quasi-experimental design in their study. This chapter introduces you to quasi-experimental and experimental designs and provides examples of these designs from published nursing studies. Details on other study designs can be found in a variety of methodology sources (Creswell & Creswell, 2018; Gray & Grove, 2021; Kazdin, 2017; Kerlinger & Lee, 2000; Shadish et al., 2002).

Algorithm for Identifying Designs in Nursing Studies

The algorithm shown in Fig. 8.1 may be used to determine the type of design (e.g., descriptive, correlational, quasi-experimental, experimental) used in a study. This algorithm includes a series of yes or no responses to specific questions about designs to enable you to identify the design in a study. The algorithm starts with the question, "Is there an intervention controlled by the researcher?" The answer leads to the next question, with the four types of design being identified in the algorithm. For example, if researchers conducted a study to identify the characteristics of nurses who either passed or failed their registered nurse licensure on the first try, Fig. 8.1 indicates that a descriptive design would be used. If the researchers examined the relationships among the student nurses' characteristics and their GPAs at the end of their degree, a correlational design would be implemented. If researchers tested the effectiveness of a relaxation intervention on whether graduates pass the registered nurse licensure examination, either a quasi-experimental or experimental design would be implemented. Experimental designs have the greatest control because (1) a highly controlled intervention is implemented and (2) study participants are randomly assigned to either the intervention or the control group (Stone et al., 2019; see Fig. 8.1).

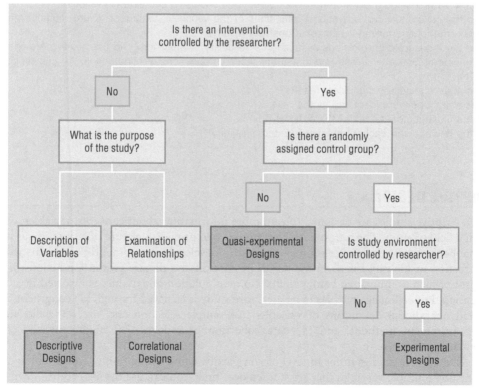

FIG. 8.1 Algorithm for Determining the Type of Quantitative Study Design.

Descriptive Designs	**Correlational Designs**
Simple descriptive design	Descriptive correlational design
Comparative descriptive design	Predictive correlational design

Noninterventional Study Designs

The next section of this chapter will explore common noninterventional study designs that are presented in Box 8.1. For each design, we will provide an example study to help you understand the unique characteristics that distinguish the designs. We will also provide a critical appraisal of the example study. For noninterventional designs (descriptive and correlational), the critical appraisal will be guided by the questions that follow.

? CRITICAL APPRAISAL GUIDELINES

Noninterventional Designs

1. What is the specific design of the study? Use the algorithms in Figs. 8.1, 8.2, and 8.5 to identify the specific type of design (descriptive or correlational) implemented in the study.
2. Does the study design address the study purpose and/or objectives or questions?
3. Was the sample appropriate for the study? How were the participants selected? (Internal validity)
4. Was the sample large and heterogenous? (Statistical conclusion and external validity)
5. Were the conceptual and operational definitions of the variables congruent? Were multiple methods of measurement used for the variables? (Construct validity)
6. Were the measurement methods assessed for reliability or precision? Did the researchers conduct the appropriate statistical analyses to address the research questions or hypotheses? (Statistical conclusion validity)
7. Were there statistically significant results?
8. What limitations were identified by the researchers?
9. Are the findings generalizable? (External validity)
10. Are the findings applicable to practice? (External validity)

DESCRIPTIVE DESIGNS

Descriptive studies are designed to gain more information about concepts, variables, or elements in a field of study. The purpose of these studies is to provide a picture of a situation as it naturally happens. A descriptive design may be used to develop theories, identify problems with current practice, or identify trends in the health promotion and disease prevention actions of a specific group, such as uninsured young adults. No manipulation of variables is involved in a descriptive design. Protection against bias in a descriptive study is achieved through (1) congruent conceptual and operational definitions of variables, (2) sample selection and size, (3) valid and reliable measurement methods, and (4) data collection procedures that might partially control the environment or setting.

Descriptive studies differ in level of complexity. Some contain only two variables; others may include multiple variables that are studied over time. You can use the algorithm shown in Fig. 8.2 to determine which descriptive design was used in a published study. Simple descriptive and

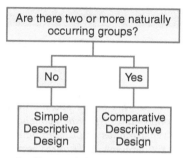

FIG. 8.2 **Algorithm for Determining the Type of Descriptive Design.**

comparative descriptive designs are discussed in this chapter. More complex descriptive designs are described in Gray and Grove (2021).

Simple Descriptive Design

A simple descriptive design is used to examine variables in a single sample (Fig. 8.3). This descriptive design includes identifying the variables within a phenomenon of interest, measuring these variables, and describing them. The description of the variables leads to an interpretation of the theoretical meaning of the findings and the development of possible relationships or hypotheses that might guide future correlational or quasi-experimental studies. Papermaster and Champion (2021) conducted a descriptive study of the beliefs and values of 402 nurse practitioners (NPs) related to curbside consultations (CCs). They described CCs as the "informal discussions with colleagues about the care of a patient" that "occur commonly and are favored by clinicians as an information-seeking resource" (Papermaster & Champion, 2021, Introduction section). The researchers developed a Web-based survey that they shared with potential participants through social media. They consulted research reference books and determined a sample of 400 NPs was needed (5 participants per each of 80 items). Key aspects of this study's design are presented in Research Example 8.1.

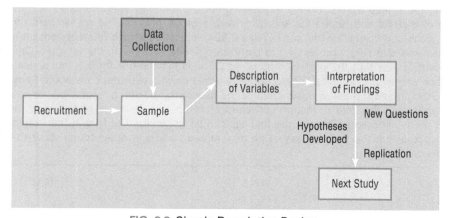

FIG. 8.3 **Simple Descriptive Design.**

RESEARCH EXAMPLE 8.1

Simple Descriptive Design

Research/Study Excerpt

Aims

> The aim of this study was to describe the process for CC among a nationally representative sample of NPs. Research questions included: (1) How do NPs define specific CC processes discerning from FC [formal consultation]? (2) Is the CC process different for NPs when collaborating with physicians as experts versus a nonphysician colleague? And (3) What modes of CC communication are useful and do these vary by clinical circumstance? (Papermaster & Champion, 2021, Aims section)

Design

> This exploratory, descriptive, cross-sectional study required creation of a survey for assessment of CC.... The final survey included 80 questions concerning CC familiarity, use, overall experience, and definition. In addition, there were questions regarding the work environment, personal and interpersonal qualities, mode of communication, and patient engagement. (Papermaster & Champion, 2021, Design section)

Data Collection

> In this cross-sectional online survey, 617 surveys were viewed and initiated with 402 (65%) eligible and completing the survey. (Papermaster & Champion, 2021, Data Collection section)

Conclusions

> These survey findings advance an understanding of the CC process including overall beliefs and values of the experience, advantages and disadvantages, decision-making and approach. Dimensions of CC including personal and interpersonal, environmental, and patient-centered were explored. (Papermaster & Champion, 2021, Conclusions section)

Critical Appraisal

Papermaster and Champion (2021) conducted a simple descriptive study. The methods, including the design, were appropriate for the study purpose and the findings directly related to the research questions. The sample was recruited through online social media and e-mail lists of professional organizations. The heterogenous sample was appropriate for a descriptive study design and reflected the NP population in the United States. During its development, the survey was evaluated for content validity by a group of experts and tested for feasibility with a group of NPs. The researchers noted that the Cronbach's alpha coefficient for the survey was 0.804, indicating strong internal consistency. The only potential bias was that NPs who wanted to participate needed access to the internet. One statistically significant finding was that the preferred mode of CC was in-person if the NP had a relationship with the consultant and by phone if the NP did not have a relationship with the consultant. Papermaster and Champion (2021) noted the following limitations: the descriptive design did not allow for causal interpretation of trends, and the data collection consisted of self-report. Because of the large, heterogenous sample and the well-designed survey, the findings can be generalized to NPs in the United States. The researchers noted that the findings cannot be generalized to NPs in other countries or to other health professionals.

Comparative Descriptive Design

A comparative descriptive design is used to describe variables and examine differences in variables in two or more groups that occur naturally in a setting. Fig. 8.4 presents a comparative descriptive design's structure. The researcher collects data from participants who were not randomly assigned to groups but can be placed in groups based on an existing characteristic, such as age or gender. The groups might be formed also using ethnicity and race, educational level, medical diagnosis, location of care, or presence of health insurance (Gray & Grove, 2021). Shajrawi et al. (2019) conducted a comparative descriptive study in Jordan among persons who survived their first acute myocardial infarction (AMI). The researchers compared the physical activity for three treatment groups in the early recovery period. The three groups were (1) ST-elevation myocardial infarction (STEMI) patients treated with percutaneous coronary intervention (PCI), (2) STEMI patients treated with thrombolytic therapy, and (3) non-ST elevation myocardial infarction (NSTEMI) patients treated with medications. There was no study intervention to increase physical activity. Physical activity was measured by an accelerometer-based device worn on the thigh for 24 hours for 7 days at weeks 1 and 6 after the AMI. Although Shajrawi et al. (2019, p. 286) called their study a "descriptive repeated measures research design," it meets our definition of a comparative descriptive design. Research Example 8.2 includes excerpts from the Results and Discussion sections of the study report.

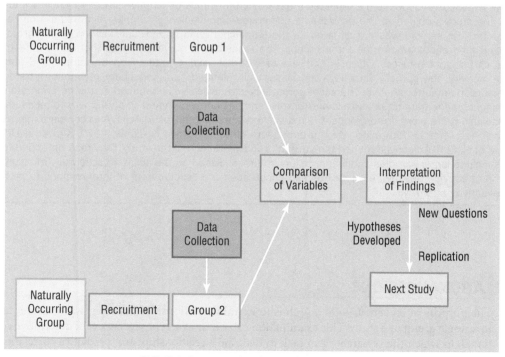

FIG. 8.4 Comparative Descriptive Design.

RESEARCH EXAMPLE 8.2

Comparative Descriptive Design

Research/Study Excerpt

Results

The data analysis showed there were statistically significant differences between the 3 types of AMI treatment modalities at time 1, as determined by 1-way ANOVA test in mean steps count per day.…and also mean stepping time per day. … Repeated-measures ANOVA test was used to examine the impact of different types of AMI treatment modalities on changes in physical activity outcomes between time 1 and time 2. (Shajrawi et al., 2019, p. 288–289)

Discussion

Physical activity outcomes…showed that AMI patients treated with primary PCI have better physical activity outcomes than AMI patients treated with thrombolytic therapy, and with PCI and NSTEMI. … This study was conducted in Jordan, where there was no cardiac rehabilitation and limited secondary prevention strategy. (Shajrawi et al., 2019, p. 290)

This present study has a number of strengths, which include the comparison of objectively measured physical activity outcomes across 3 groups of AMI patients following treatment…this study also has many limitations, notably its small sample size. … The study did not examine the influence of other risk factors in physical activity…more than 50% of screened AMI patients were ineligible. Also, about 30% of eligible AMI patients refused to participate. (Shajrawi et al., 2019, p. 291)

Critical Appraisal

Shajrawi et al. (2019) conducted a repeated measures comparative descriptive study, which was appropriate for the study's objective. The participants comprised a convenience sample, recruited at one cardiac care center. The sample was not as large as the researchers had hoped, but was large enough to find significant differences among the three groups. The researchers, however, noted that about 30% of the eligible participants refused, which is a threat to external validity (interaction of sample and setting). Physical activity, the primary variable, was conceptually defined as a secondary prevention strategy to decrease mortality after an AMI. The accelerometer-based device was identified as the criterion standard for measuring sedentary time, had a low error rate, and has been identified as a valid way to measure motion. Because there were three groups, the researchers appropriately used ANOVA to compare the groups with post hoc tests to determine which groups were different (Grove & Cipher, 2020; Kim et al., 2022). Shajrawi et al. (2019) clearly identified the strengths and limitations of the study. They recommended future studies include larger samples and longer follow-up times. Based on the ability to accurately measure the outcome of activity, Shajrawi et al. (2019) also encouraged the development of interventions to promote physical activity after AMI.

CORRELATIONAL DESIGNS

The purpose of a correlational design is to examine relationships between two or more variables in a single group in a study. This examination can occur at any of several levels: descriptive correlational, in which the researcher can seek to describe a relationship; and predictive correlational, in which the researcher can predict relationships among variables. Model testing is also a correlational design, in which the relationships proposed by a theory are tested simultaneously (see Gray & Grove, 2021, pp. 255–257, for a discussion of this design).

In correlational designs, a large range in the variable scores is necessary to determine the existence of a relationship. Therefore the sample should be large to reflect the full range of scores possible on the variables being measured (Grove & Cipher, 2020). Some study participants should have very high scores and others very low scores, and the scores of the rest should be distributed throughout the possible range.

> ### 📄 RESEARCH/EBP TIP
>
> The distinction between descriptive and correlational designs is whether the researchers are describing characteristics of the sample (descriptive design) or identifying the presence and strength of relationships among the variables (correlational design).

The diagram in Fig. 8.5 can be used to identify the specific correlational design included in a study. Sometimes, researchers combine elements of different designs to accomplish their study purpose. For example, researchers might conduct a cross-sectional, descriptive, correlational study design to examine the relationship of body mass index to blood lipid levels in early adolescence (age, 13–16 years) and late adolescence (age, 17–19 years). It is important that researchers clearly identify the specific design that they are using in their research report. More details on correlational designs are available from other research sources (Gray & Grove, 2021; Kazdin, 2017).

Descriptive Correlational Design

The purpose of a descriptive correlational design is to describe variables and examine relationships among these variables. Using this design facilitates the identification of many interrelationships in a situation. The study may examine variables in a situation that has already occurred or is currently occurring. Researchers make no attempt to control or manipulate the situation. As with descriptive studies, variables must be clearly identified and defined conceptually and operationally (see Chapter 5).

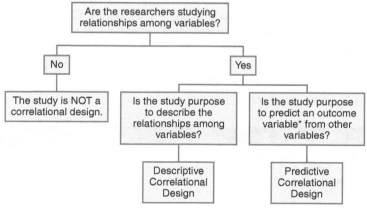

FIG. 8.5 Algorithm for Determining the Type of Correlational Design.
*Outcome variable may be called the dependent variable. The predictor variables may be called independent variables.

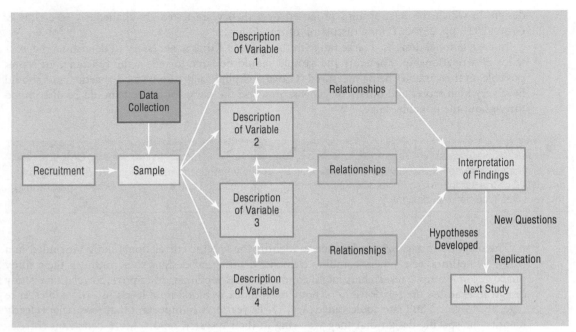

FIG. 8.6 Descriptive Correlational Design.

As shown in Fig. 8.6, the variables are measured, described, and examined for relationships. The findings from descriptive correlational studies are interpreted and provide the basis for further research.

Telemedicine allows healthcare providers to have access to the knowledge and experience of off-site experts. Kaplow and Zellinger (2021) conducted a descriptive correlational study at Emory University Hospital, which had recently opened additional intensive care units (ICUs). The ICUs were needed to provide care for patients with complex health needs who needed more care than could be provided in medical-surgical settings. The providers and nurses at the hospital had access to experts through Emory e-ICU Center. Kaplow and Zellinger (2021) were interested in the relationships among nurse characteristics and their perceptions of the e-ICU Center. The study was conducted in an ICU with experienced critical care nurses (cardiovascular surgery ICU [CVICU]) and a second unit with nurses newer to critical care (acute respiratory ICU [ARICU]). Research Example 8.3 includes key aspects of this study.

RESEARCH EXAMPLE 8.3

Descriptive Correlational Design

Research/Study Excerpt
Methods

We collected data for 2 months…Each participant provided written informed consent, and completed a demographic form…and a questionnaire regarding their perceptions of the Emory e-ICU Center. (Kaplow & Zellinger, 2021, p. 124)

RESEARCH EXAMPLE 8.3—cont'd

Results

Sixty participants completed the study (30 nurses from each of the 2 units). ... Most nurses were female, had 5 or fewer years of experience in an ICU, and worked the night shift. ... half of respondents had only 1 year of experience or less. (Kaplow & Zellinger, 2021, p. 125)

We computed an average perception score across all 8 items, with a final average score ranging from 1 (strongly disagree) to 5 (strongly agree); a higher score indicates a more positive or favorable perception. The average perception scores were significantly higher for the nurses in the ARICU than for those in the CVICU. ... The correlation between respondents' years of experience in the ICU and their average perception scores was not statistically significant ($p = -0.137$, $p = 0.30$). This correlation was also not significant within each unit (ARICU: $p = 0.103$, $p = 0.59$; CVICU: $p = -0.300$, $p = 0.11$). Years of e-ICU experience did not correlate significantly with average perception scores either ($p = -0.192$, $p = 0.14$). (Kaplow & Zellinger, 2021, p. 126)

Critical Appraisal

The study's purpose focused on differences between the nurses' perceptions on the two units, despite the researchers specifying the design as being descriptive correlational. The convenience sampling method was appropriate for this study but resulted in a homogenous and relatively small sample ($N = 60$). The conceptual definition of the primary variable was not explicit. The content validity of the questionnaire measuring perceptions of the e-ICU was supported by the five ICU experts. Internal consistency reliability was supported by a Cronbach's alpha of 0.80. The appropriate statistical analyses were conducted; however, no statistically significant relationships were identified. Kaplow and Zellinger (2021) noted that they did not examine how the e-ICU Center was implemented on each unit. The single application to practice was the recommendation to share examples of how telemedicine improved patient outcomes with the ICU nurses. The findings from the convenience sample recruited from two ICUs in one hospital are not generalizable.

RESEARCH/EBP TIP

As you learn about different designs, you will sometime detect discrepancies between the design the researchers have indicated they used and what they did in the study. Include this information in your critical appraisal as a possible threat to design validity.

Predictive Correlational Design

The purpose of a predictive correlational design is to predict the value of one variable based on the values obtained for another variable or variables. Prediction is one approach for examining causal relationships between the independent and dependent variables. The variable to be predicted is classified as the dependent or outcome variable, and all other variables are independent or predictor variables. A predictive correlational design attempts to predict the level of a dependent variable from the measured values of the independent variables. For example, the dependent variable of medication adherence among patients with hypertension could be predicted using the independent variables of age, number of medications, and medication knowledge. The independent variables that are most effective in prediction are significantly correlated with the dependent variable but are not highly correlated with other independent variables used in the study (Grove & Cipher, 2020; Kim et al., 2022). The predictive correlational design structure is presented in Fig. 8.7.

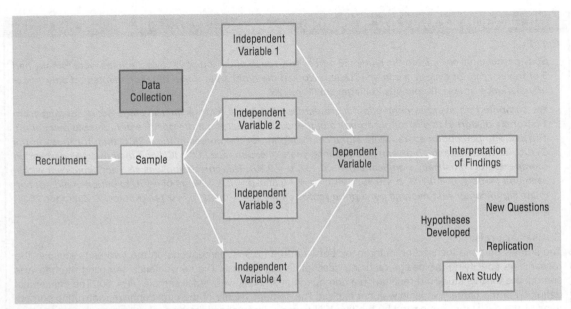

FIG. 8.7 Predictive Correlational Design.
The relationship between each independent variable and the dependent variable are combined with the relationships between the other independent variables and the dependent variable to predict the dependent variable.

Predictive correlational designs require the development of a theory-based hypothesis proposing variables expected to effectively predict the dependent variable. Researchers then use regression analysis to test the hypothesis (see Chapter 11). The Joint Commission has raised concerns about alarm fatigue in critical care settings, with alarm fatigue being defined as desensitization to responding to monitor alarms. Storm and Chen (2021) noted that false alarms can deplete compassion and contribute to burnout. The researchers conducted a predictive correlational study to determine factors predicting alarm fatigue of critical care nurses in three Philadelphia hospitals. Research Example 8.4 includes major elements of this predictive correlational design based on Watson's caring theory (Watson, 2011).

🔍 RESEARCH EXAMPLE 8.4

Predictive Correlational Design

Research/Study Excerpt

The current study purpose was to...identify to what extent compassion fatigue, burnout, compassion satisfaction and personal characteristics can predict alarm fatigue in critical care nurses. (Storm & Chen, 2021, p. 445)

The operational definition of alarm fatigue used for observation in this study was an elapsed time greater than 10 min between the time a monitor alarm sounds and the time a critical care nurse responds (Bridi et al., 2014). Data of compassion fatigue, burnout and compassion satisfaction were gathered using the Professional Quality of Life (ProQOL) measure. ...In total, 52 critical care nurses voluntarily participated in this study. (Storm & Chen, 2021, p. 446)

> ### ◢ RESEARCH EXAMPLE 8.4—cont'd
>
> *Forty per cent of the participants were observed to have alarm fatigue (n = 21). … Binary logistic regression statistical test was used to examine which of the independent variables predict the dependent variable of alarm fatigue. …The results indicated that the variables of gender…, nursing unit…and age…remained in the regression equation but were not significant predictors ($r^2 = 0.046$) to the variable of alarm fatigue.* (Storm & Chen, 2021, p. 447–449)
>
> **Critical Appraisal**
> The predictive correlational design was appropriate to address the study's purpose and research questions. The sample of critical care nurses ($n = 52$) from three different hospitals volunteered to participate. Participating involved completing a demographic questionnaire and the ProQOL and being observed for the length of time that elapsed between monitor alarms going off and the nurse responding. Participants had been in nursing for 1 to 50 years, had a wide range of ages, and 21.1% were nonwhite, indicating a heterogeneous sample. The conceptual and operational definitions of the variables were explicit and congruent. Each variable was measured using a single method. The researchers reported that prior studies had found the ProQOL measure reliable and valid. They also reported interrater reliability for the observations and the reliability coefficients for the instrument used in this study. The researchers provided detail about measures taken to ensure the data were correctly entered into the database. They found significant relationships among alarm fatigue and some demographic variables, but did not find significant relationships among alarm fatigue, burnout, compassion fatigue, and compassion satisfaction. Storm and Chen (2021) noted that the small sample size may have caused a Type II error (see Chapter 9), resulting in the nonsignificant results of the regression analysis. Their sample represented only 16% of the critical care nurses in the three hospitals, which negatively affected the study's internal validity. The researchers were appropriately cautious about generalizing the findings. Nurses at the bedside may want to reflect on their personal characteristics and the potential for alarm fatigue. Another possible application to practice would be that nurse leaders develop strategies to prevent alarm fatigue.

EXAMINING CAUSALITY AND STUDY INTERVENTIONS

Quasi-experimental and experimental designed studies are implemented to obtain an accurate representation of cause and effect by the most efficient means. The design should provide the greatest amount of control with the least error possible. The effects of some extraneous variables are controlled in a study by using specific sampling criteria, a highly controlled setting, and a structured independent variable or intervention (see Box 8.2). For a study to have an experiment design, the researcher must (1) have maximum control over the intervention and setting, (2) include both intervention and control groups, and (3) randomly assign participants to receive or not receive the intervention (Kazdin, 2017). A randomized controlled trial (RCT) is one type of true experimental design; RCTs are discussed later in this chapter. To critically appraise experimental and quasi-experimental studies, you need to understand some key components of these studies: interventions, intervention fidelity, and types of group. These components are described in the following sections.

Examining Interventions in Nursing Studies

In studies examining causality, investigators develop an intervention that is expected to result in differences in posttest measures between the treatment and control groups. Interventions may be physiological, psychosocial, educational, or a combination of these. The therapeutic intervention

BOX 8.2   REQUIRED ELEMENTS OF RESEARCH TO EXAMINE CAUSALITY

Sampling and Setting
Sampling criteria (inclusion and exclusion) are clearly identified and appropriate for the study (see Chapter 9).
Researchers control the experimental situation and setting.

Groups
Study has a control, comparison, or placebo group.
Participants are randomly assigned to groups.

Treatment or Intervention
Independent variable or intervention is clearly defined.
Researchers control or manipulate the intervention.
Researchers ensure the intervention was implemented consistently.

Measurement
Dependent or outcome variable is carefully measured (see Chapter 10).

implemented in a nursing study needs to be carefully designed, clearly described, and appropriately linked to the outcomes (dependent variables) in the study. The intervention needs to be provided consistently to all study participants in the treatment group. The research report should describe the strategies used by the researchers to maintain intervention fidelity. Intervention fidelity is ensuring the intervention is implemented completely and consistently with every participant assigned to receive it (Bonar et al., 2020; Holtrop et al., 2021). A research report should include a detailed description of the essential elements of the intervention, including who is implementing it and how they were trained (Hasson et al., 2021). Sometimes, researchers provide a table of the intervention content and/or the protocol used to implement the intervention to each participant consistently.

Increasing physical activity among primary care patients at risk for cardiovascular disease is an ongoing challenge for nurses. One approach has been to change the nurses' behavior from teaching patients about the importance of physical activity to coaching patients to increase their physical activity. Westland et al. (2020) implemented the Activate intervention in general care clinics in the Netherlands that included nurse consultations with patients related to physical activity. The intervention is described in Research Example 8.5.

RESEARCH EXAMPLE 8.5

Nursing Intervention

Research/Study Excerpt

The Activate intervention consisted of four prestructured, standardised nurse-led consultations to enhance patients' level of physical activity. Consultations were offered at weeks 1, 3, 7 and 12 in patients' own general practice, with a duration of 20–30 minutes. ... At the first consultation, patients received activity logs, forms for action planning, information about the trial, useful websites, apps and tips and tricks for physical activity.... In the second consultation, nurses briefly repeated the information provided at the first consultation. In the second, third and fourth consultations, nurses reviewed and gave feedback on patients' level of goal attainment and, when needed, adjusted the goals and action plans.

RESEARCH EXAMPLE 8.5—cont'd

The standardised comprehensive training programme for nurses consisted of a one-day skills training supplemented with two individual coaching sessions from a health psychologist, instructional videos showing how to apply the BCTs [behavior change techniques] in the consultations, a handbook which provided a structure of the consultations and included example sentences and checklists (what to do when). (Westland et al., 2020, p. 723)

Critical Appraisal of the Intervention

Westland et al. (2020) briefly described the training and support the nurses received before the beginning of the study. No evidence was provided that the nurses were observed during the implementation the intervention or provided additional training if needed. Six months after the intervention, the treatment group patients did not have a significant increase in their physical activity compared with the usual care patients. Several patient characteristics were identified that moderated the effect of the intervention. The desired sample size was not achieved, so a Type II error may have occurred. The researchers also concluded that intervention fidelity (Bonar et al., 2020) needed to be explored in more depth in future studies.

RESEARCH/EBP TIP

Critically appraising quasi-experimental and experimental studies includes careful examination of the intervention. Were adequate details provided so that researchers can replicate the intervention in other studies? Interventions must be based on strong research evidence before they are used in practice.

Experimental and Control or Comparison Groups

The group of participants who received the study intervention is referred to as the intervention, treatment, or experimental group. The group that is not exposed to the study intervention is referred to as the control, comparison, or placebo group. Some researchers distinguish between the types of group by how the groups are formed. For these researchers, a group to which participants are randomly assigned would be called a control group. Groups that are formed naturally or involve nonrandom assignment are called comparison groups. However, the terms *control group* and *comparison group* are frequently used interchangeably in nursing studies.

In some disciplines, the control groups receive no care or action. However, to implement ethical nursing studies, patients must receive care. For examples, nurses must provide preoperative education to all patients, not just those in the intervention group. When the comparison or control group is to receive standard nursing care, the researchers should describe in detail what that care entails. For example, a hospital's standard care for unconscious patients is that the patient is repositioned every 2 hours. Because the quality of this standard care is likely to vary considerably among study participants, variance in the control or comparison group is likely to be high and needs to be considered in the discussion of findings. Researchers studying loss of muscle tone among unconscious patients might include a group placed on a specialized air mattress (intervention group) and a comparison group being repositioned every 2 hours (standard care). To distinguish the effect of the specialized mattress from standard care, the intervention group would have the mattress and be repositioned on the 2-hour schedule.

Another type of a group is called a placebo group. A placebo group receives an intervention that is like the intervention being tested. Because study interventions frequently involve the nurse spending additional time with the participant, separating the effects of an intervention from the effects of time and attention can be difficult. The personal interaction itself may cause a change in the dependent variable. To overcome this challenge, nursing studies often include a placebo group receiving a nursing action so that both groups (intervention and placebo) receive time and attention. For example, the treatment group in an osteoporosis study may receive an intervention to increase physical activity with the dependent variable being bone density in women older than 70 years. The comparison or placebo group in the study may receive an instructional session about the normal aging process. This design structure allows the researchers to differentiate between the effect of time and attention and the effect of the intervention (Gray & Grove, 2021; Kazdin, 2017).

The following critical appraisal guidelines provide questions to guide your appraisal of intervention studies. When you appraise a study, read the Methods and Discussion sections closely, especially the limitations. Researchers will often acknowledge threats to the validity of the findings in the limitations in the Discussion section. They may also identify strengths of the study in the Discussion section.

? CRITICAL APPRAISAL GUIDELINES

Quasi-Experimental and Experimental Designs

1. Is the study design quasi-experimental or experimental? Review the algorithm in Fig. 8.8 to determine the type of study design.
2. Review designs represented by Figs. 8.9 to 8.12 to determine the specific type of intervention design.
3. Construct validity (see Table 8.1)
   a. Were the dependent variables measured with valid measurement methods?
   b. What were the study's strengths related to construct validity?
   c. What were the threats to construct validity?
4. Internal validity (see Table 8.2)
   a. What were the strengths related to internal validity, such as were the participants randomly assigned to groups?
   b. What were the threats to internal validity, such as attrition or history?
5. Statistical conclusion validity (see Table 8.3)
   a. Were the research variables measured with reliable scales or precise physiological methods?
   b. What were the study's strengths related to statistical conclusion validity, such as intervention fidelity?
   c. What were the threats to statistical conclusion validity, such as potential for Type II error?
6. External validity (see Table 8.4)
   a. What were the strengths related to external validity?
   b. What were the threats to external validity, such as interaction of selection and intervention?
7. Summarize the validity of the study findings.

QUASI-EXPERIMENTAL DESIGNS

Experiments require that the researchers have maximum control over the intervention and setting and randomly assigned participants to the treatment and comparison groups. Ideally, the participants also are randomly selected. Quasi-experimental designs facilitate the search for knowledge and examination of causality in situations in which complete control is not possible. Box 8.3 includes the quasi-experimental and experimental designs that we will cover in this chapter. Quasi-experimental studies are developed to control as many threats to validity as possible when the conditions of a true experiment are not possible (Kazdin, 2017; Shadish et al., 2002). Most quasi-experimental studies include a sample of convenience, meaning the participants are recruited to

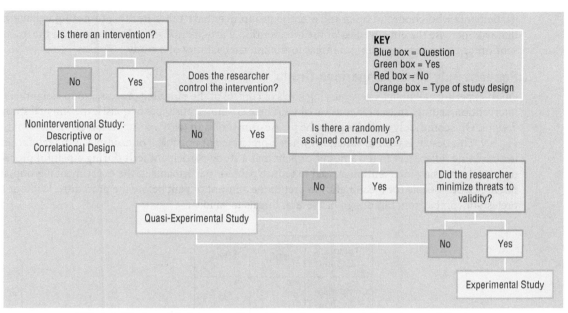

FIG. 8.8 Distinguish Between Quasi-Experimental and Experimental Designs.

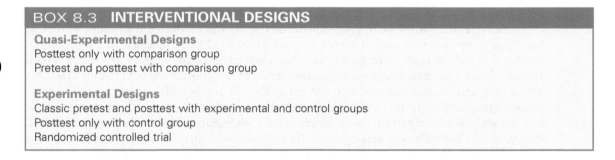

BOX 8.3   INTERVENTIONAL DESIGNS

Quasi-Experimental Designs
Posttest only with comparison group
Pretest and posttest with comparison group

Experimental Designs
Classic pretest and posttest with experimental and control groups
Posttest only with control group
Randomized controlled trial

be in a study because they are in the right place at the right time (see Chapter 9). The participants selected are usually randomly assigned to receive the experimental intervention or standard care.

Random assignment of participants from the original sample to either the intervention or comparison group promotes internal validity. Occasionally, comparison and intervention groups may occur naturally. For example, four primary care practices are selected for an intervention study because they have similar patients. The researchers randomly select two practices to be the settings for recruitment of participants to the treatment group. Participants will be recruited from the remaining two practices to be in the comparison group.

In other quasi-experimental studies, groups may include study participants who choose to be in the intervention group and those who choose not to receive the intervention as the comparison group. These groups cannot be considered equivalent because the participants who choose to be in the intervention group may differ in important ways from those who prefer the comparison group. These differences are likely to affect the dependent variables. For example, if researchers were implementing an intervention of a structured exercise program to promote weight loss, the participants who choose to be in the exercise group may have other health-promoting behaviors that will increase the effectiveness of the intervention. Participants' self-selecting to be in the intervention or comparison group is a threat to the internal validity of a study.

Posttest Only With Comparison Group

Quasi-experimental designs have varying levels of control of the sampling process, group assignment, intervention, setting, and extraneous variables. There are numerous types of quasi-experimental study designs. One commonly used design is the posttest-only design with a comparison group, shown in Fig. 8.9. This design is used in situations when a pretest is not possible. For example, if the researcher is examining differences in the amount of pain that a study participant feels during a painful procedure, and a nursing intervention is used to reduce pain for participants in the experimental group, it might not be possible (or meaningful) to pretest the amount of pain before the procedure. Without a pretest for comparison, this design has several threats to validity.

Treatment Group	TX	M
Comparison Group		M

FIG. 8.9 Quasi-Experimental Posttest-Only Design With a Comparison Group. *M*, Measurement; *TX*, treatment.

An example of a posttest-only quasi-experimental study was conducted with adults who cared for a family member who died of cancer. Petursdottir et al. (2020) implemented a psychosocial intervention with 26 family caregivers before their close relative died of cancer and then 1 month after the death. The researchers recruited a comparison group from among other family caregivers whose close relative had died and who did not receive the psychosocial intervention. The comparison group caregivers did receive usual care, which included a home visit 1 month after their loss. Because the 25 comparison group members were not recruited until the bereavement period, the researchers had no pretest measurements for comparison. Both groups completed instruments measuring anxiety, depression, stress, and grief reactions at 3, 5, and 6 months after the death. Although the intervention group had lower anxiety scores than the comparison group did, the difference must be considered with caution because of threats to design validity.

Pretest and Posttest Designs With Comparison Group

The most frequently used design in social science research is the untreated comparison group design, with a pretest and posttest (Fig. 8.10). With this design, the study has a group of participants who received the experimental intervention and a comparison group of participants who received standard care. The following research example is a study with this design. For information about other quasi-experimental designs, consult other sources (Gray & Grove, 2021; Kazdin, 2017; Shadish et al., 2002).

Fard et al. (2021) conducted a study among women with breast cancer in Iran. Although medical and surgical interventions for women with breast cancer are routinely implemented in Iran, the mental health of the women has received less attention. Specifically, the researchers noted that women with breast cancer frequently experienced depression, anxiety, and hopelessness that decreased their quality of life. Hope therapy was selected as the intervention for this pretest/posttest

Treatment Group	M	TX	M
Comparison Group	M		M

FIG. 8.10 Quasi-Experimental Pretest and Posttest Design With a Comparison Group. *M*, Measurement; *TX*, treatment.

quasi-experimental study with a comparison group. The dependent variable was happiness as measured by the Oxford Happiness Questionnaire, which had been evaluated for validity and reliability in Iran by other researchers. The internal consistency coefficient for this study was Cronbach's alpha 0.85, indicating strong reliability for this scale in the study (see Chapter 10; Grove & Cipher, 2020). Excerpts from the study are presented in Research Example 8.6.

RESEARCH EXAMPLE 8.6

Quasi-Experimental Pretest/Posttest Design With a Comparison Group

Research/Study Excerpt

Participants were selected using convenience sampling techniques and randomly assigned to two groups of intervention (n = 50) and control (n = 50). ... Hope therapy training is a treatment program...to enhance positive thinking and strengthening goal-directed activities. Participants in the program first get familiar with the principles of hope theory, and they are then instructed on how to apply these principles in their lives. ... The hope therapy training program was held...in eight sessions (two sessions per week)...[and] led by a psychiatric nurse. (Fard et al., 2021., Methods section)

The mean score of happiness for patients in the intervention group increased from 70.68 ± 13.98 to 76.46 ± 11.86 after providing the intervention. Besides, the mean score of happiness for patients in the control group was 68.62 ± 13.98 before the study and decreased to 66.04 ± 12.76 after the study. The results of the independent samples t-test revealed no significant difference concerning the mean scores of happiness between the two groups before providing the intervention (p = 0.55). However, there were significant differences in the mean scores of happiness between the two groups after providing the intervention (p = 0.001). (Fard et al., 2021, Results section)

The findings pointed to the effectiveness of hope therapy-based training on happiness in women with breast cancer. This finding was consistent with the results of previous studies...it can be argued that this intervention increases individuals' positive self-concept and encourages them to actualize their positive potentials. This can increase hope for cancer patients who see themselves at the end of life and offer them a form of palliative care. ... One of the limitations of the present study was that the research sample did not include patients with disease metastasis....caution should be exercised in generalizing the results to patients with metastasis. (Fard et al., 2021, Discussion section)

Critical Appraisal

One strength of this pretest/posttest quasi-experimental study with a comparison group was that the researchers measured the dependent variable using a validated instrument, supporting the study's construct validity. The conceptual and theoretical definitions of happiness were congruent. However, it was unclear whether the data collectors were blinded to group assignment, which may have increased the risk for experimenter expectancy. Fard et al. (2021) did not acknowledge the risk for social desirability with using a self-report measurement for the dependent variable.

Continued

RESEARCH EXAMPLE 8.6—cont'd

Related to internal validity, a strength was that the women were randomly assigned to the groups. Fard et al. (2021) acknowledged the threat of history, noting that the coronavirus disease 2019 (COVID-19) outbreak occurred during the time when the intervention was being delivered. Also, all the women were receiving chemotherapy during the study. There was no mention of attrition.

Supporting the statistical conclusion validity, the intervention was implemented by the same nurse for all sessions. Women were excluded if they missed even one of the hope therapy sessions. In addition to using a validated instrument, the researchers reported its reliability in previous studies and its strong internal consistency in their study. The researchers also mentioned testing the data for normality before using a parametric analysis, the *t*-test, to compare the groups' outcomes.

One of the limitations noted by the researchers was that women with metastasis were excluded from the study, thereby limiting the findings' generalizability to that group. Another threat to external validity is that the study was conducted in Iran with women receiving care at two hospitals affiliated with a major university. Overall, threats to design validity were minimal, and the study had several strengths.

EXPERIMENTAL DESIGNS

Experimental designs are included in studies with a precise, consistent intervention (the independent variable) that is implemented in a controlled environment, and changes in the dependent variable are measured using reliable, valid instruments. The participants who meet specific inclusion and exclusion criteria and consent to participate are randomly assigned to receive the intervention or be in the control group. Some intervention studies are relatively simple designs and others are very complex. In some cases, researchers may combine characteristics of more than one design to determine whether the evidence supports the hypothesis. Names of designs vary from one text to another. Because of the similarities between quasi-experimental and experimental designs, researchers may implement what you might consider to be a quasi-experimental study and call it an experimental study. The reverse can also happen. The researchers' control over the environment and intervention is higher in an experiment than in a quasi-experimental study, and the participants are randomly assigned to the intervention or control group.

Multiple groups (both intervention and control) can be used to great advantage in experimental designs. Among persons newly diagnosed with bipolar disorder, one group (the control group) might receive no education other than what they seek for themselves; another group might receive standard care, including brochures; another group might receive a single session of enhanced digital education; and the final group might receive the enhanced digital education initially with a booster session a month later. Each one of multiple experimental groups can receive a variation of the intervention, such as a different frequency, intensity, or duration of nursing care actions, but all experimental groups need to have intervention fidelity (Bonar et al., 2020). These additions greatly increase the generalizability of study findings when the sample is representative of the target population and the sample size is strong.

When reading and critically appraising a published study, determine the researcher's name for the design and/or read the description of the design to determine the type of design used in the study. Some researchers describe the components of the study and do not label the design. In this chapter, we describe the classic experiment with pretest and posttest, posttest-only experiment, and RCTs. More details about specific designs are available from other sources (Gray & Grove, 2021; Kazdin, 2017; Shadish et al., 2002).

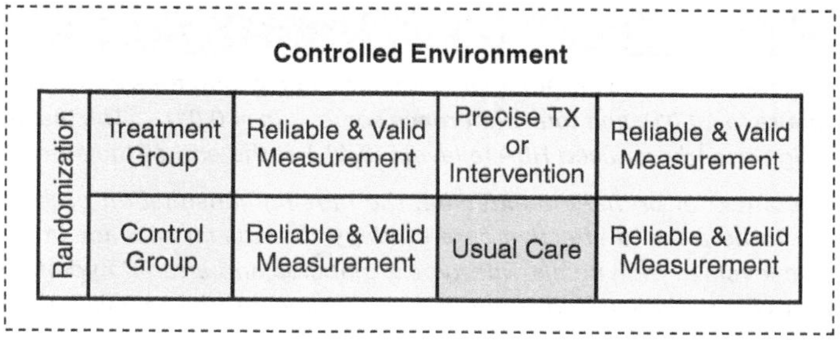

FIG. 8.11 Classic Pretest and Posttest With Experimental and Control Groups. *TX*, Treatment.

Classic Pretest and Posttest Designs With Experimental and Control Groups

A common experimental design used in healthcare studies is the pretest/posttest design with experimental and control groups. The design in Fig. 8.11 is basically the same as the design shown in Fig. 8.10. There are important differences, however. One of the differences is that the experimental study is more tightly controlled in the areas of intervention, setting, measurement, and/or extraneous variables, resulting in fewer threats to design validity. The experimental design is stronger if the initial sample is randomly selected; however, most healthcare studies do not include a random sample but do randomly assign participants to the experimental and control groups. Most studies in nursing use the quasi-experimental designs because of the inability to control extraneous and environmental variables.

Steffen et al. (2021) conducted a pretest and posttest design study in Brazil. The 174 participants who had type 2 diabetes mellitus and arterial hypertension were randomized into experimental and control groups. The participants in the experimental (treatment) group received nurse consultations in which the nurses used motivational interviewing to promote healthy lifestyle changes. The control group received a placebo intervention of nurse consultations on the same topic but without the use of motivational interviewing. Research Example 8.7 provides excerpts from the abstract of the study.

RESEARCH EXAMPLE 8.7

Pretest and Posttest Experimental and Control Group Design

Research/Study Excerpt

Introduction: Motivational interviewing is an effective style of collaborative communication for the promotion of lifestyle changes in the management of Type 2 diabetes and arterial hypertension. This study evaluates the effectiveness of motivational interviewing in the management of these conditions in primary health care.

Intervention: ... The test/motivational interviewing group received the nursing consultation intervention on the basis of motivational interviewing conducted by professionals with 20 hours of training, and the usual-care group received conventional nursing consultation.

Main outcome measures: The main outcome measure was the mean difference in HbA1c. The secondary outcome measures were the mean differences in blood pressure and adherence levels.

Results: After a mean follow-up of 6 months, 174 participants completed the study (usual-care group = 80; test/motivational interviewing group = 94). There were statistically significant differences between the

Continued

RESEARCH EXAMPLE 8.7—cont'd

groups, with improvement in the test/motivational interviewing group for systolic blood pressure (p<0.01), diastolic blood pressure (p<0.01), and total adherence score...(p = 0.01). ...The test/motivational interviewing group showed significantly reduced HbA1c levels (0.4%) at the end of the study (p<0.01).

Conclusions: *In the context of primary health care, the nursing consultation based on motivational interviewing was shown to be a more effective care strategy than usual care for improving blood pressure levels and adherence levels in individuals with type 2 diabetes and arterial hypertension. Moreover, motivational interviewing was demonstrated to be useful in reducing HbA1c levels in diabetes management.* (Steffen et al., 2021, p. e203).

Critical Appraisal

Steffen et al. (2021) implemented an experimental design study that included measurements of hemoglobin A1c (HbA1c), blood pressure, medication adherence, and depression before and after the intervention. The HbA1c level was measured through the outpatient labs using standard techniques. Blood pressure was measured by technicians in the clinics who were blinded to group assignments and followed their technical guidelines for consistent measurement. The measure for adherence had been developed in Cuba but had been previously adapted to be used in Brazil. Steffen et al. (2021) ensured that laboratory technicians, community health workers who did recruitment, and members of the research team were blinded to group assignment to minimize bias in measurement. Information was lacking on the conceptual definitions and scale validity, which was a threat to construct validity.

Participants were randomly assigned by a person who was not on the research team. However, the randomization was done before recruitment on all patients in the facilities' databases who had the documented diagnoses. Of these 421 potential participants, only 189 were found in the community, met the inclusion and exclusion criteria, and agreed to participate. The experimental and control group were unequal in size (*n* = 101 and *n* = 88, respectively), but had low attrition once the study began (174 completed; 92% retention). Being unable to find the person, which meant they were not invited to participate, was the main cause of the discrepancy in the number of those who were eligible and those who participated (35%). Selection was a threat, but other steps were taken to enhance internal validity.

Related to statistical conclusion validity, reliability findings on previous studies, as well as the current study, were not included in the study report. The eight nurses who provided the intervention received 20 hours of interactive training, and their skills and confidence were measured after the training. Once the study began, however, there was no ongoing assessment of intervention fidelity. The researchers acknowledged intervention fidelity to be the major limitation of the study. The statistical analyses conducted were appropriate for the data and the study questions. The researchers conducted an a priori power analysis that indicated they needed a sample of 248 participants. Although they did not reach this sample size, the study did have statistically significant findings. The researchers noted, however, the sample size along with other limitations may have "reduced the effect of the intervention" (Steffen et al., 2021, p. e210).

The external validity of the study was threatened by a possible interaction between selection, setting, and the intervention. The study was conducted in an international setting, which is significantly different from the US health system. Because of the selection threat to internal validity and the intervention fidelity threat to statistical conclusion validity, generalization to other populations would not be appropriate. The study findings still contribute to the literature by providing an example of the challenges of implementing intervention studies in natural settings.

RESEARCH/EBP TIP

Designs with pretest measurements allow researchers to establish whether groups were similar before an intervention. Using pretests enhances the internal validity of a study and increases confidence in the findings.

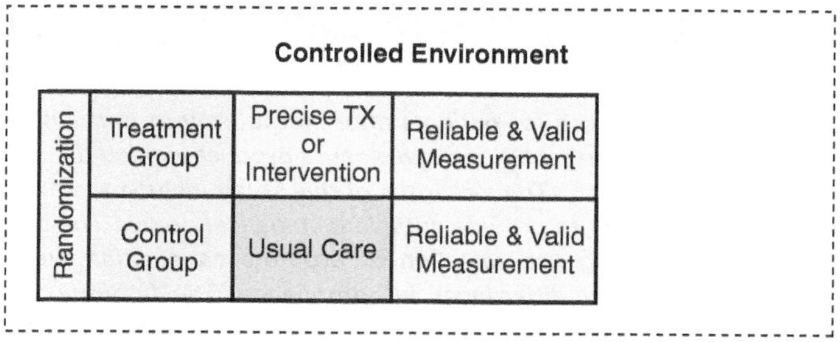

FIG. 8.12 Posttest Only With Control Group.
TX, Treatment.

Posttest-Only With Control Group Design

The experimental posttest-only control group design is also frequently used in healthcare studies when a pretest is not possible or appropriate (Fig. 8.12). To enhance the validity of the study findings, researchers usually measure key variables examined at the start of the study to ensure that the groups are similar. The lack of a pretest in this design increases the potential for error that might affect the findings. Additional research is recommended before generalization of findings.

Bolling et al. (2021) conducted an experiment among women with large breasts (cup size C and higher) who underwent cardiac surgery that involved a sternotomy. Without support, breast movement after surgery can lead to increased pain and interfere with sternum healing. The study was designed to identify which of three bra styles had the highest patient satisfaction and wear compliance. The participants agreed to wear the bra 20 hours each 24-hour period.

Because a pretest would have been of no value, the researchers implemented a posttest-only experimental design with 60 women (Bolling et al., 2021). All three bra styles had front closures because the arm movements needed to secure a back closure would stress the sternum. The styles included the hook-loop closure (like Velcro) bra that was standard of care, a zipper closure bra, and a hook-eye closure bra. Women who were undergoing nonemergent cardiac surgery were recruited and randomized to the intervention or control group. If a woman was randomized to a type of bra that was unavailable in her size, she was removed from the study and received the standard-of-care bra. One of the researchers delivered the appropriate bra to the operating room the day of surgery so that the bra could be placed on the women immediately after surgery (Bolling et al., 2021). More information about the instruments and findings is presented in Research Example 8.8.

RESEARCH EXAMPLE 8.8

Experimental Posttest-Only Control Group Design

Research/Study Excerpt

Instruments

Satisfaction with the bra before discharge was measured on postoperative day 4 or 5 by using a question about satisfaction (self-report); results ranged from 1 to 10 (1 = completely dissatisfied, 10 = completely satisfied). The survey after discharge included the same satisfaction item, a question about whether the participant would recommend the bra to other women undergoing sternotomy (rating scale, 1 = definitely would not recommend to 5 = definitely would recommend), a question about the amount of time the bra was worn after discharge (compliance), and an opportunity to provide any comments about the product.
(Bolling et al., 2021, p. 23)

Continued

RESEARCH EXAMPLE 8.8—cont'd

Discussion

This study aimed to identify the best bra for patients after sternotomy in terms of satisfaction and wear compliance. ...[W]e have determined that the hook-eye closure product yielded the most satisfaction...and greatest wear compliance in this study.... The strengths of this study include the experimental design and the sample size, which is large enough to provide sufficient statistical power. The study contributes to the limited knowledge available regarding bra selection to promote satisfaction and wear compliance.... The study was not powered to detect differences in compliance. The findings supported a change in practice: the hook-eye bra is now the product used as the standard of care for this patient population at the study site. (Bolling et al., 2021, p. 25)

Critical Appraisal

One threat to construct validity of the posttest-only experimental study was the use of researcher-developed, self-report instruments that did not capture variations in patient satisfaction or willingness to recommend the product (Bolling et al., 2021). No information was provided about validation of the instruments. It is likely that one of the researchers collected the data before discharge and at the first postoperative visit (experimenter expectancy). The participants were randomly assigned to the groups, a procedure that strengthened internal validity. However, the flow diagram for study enrollment indicated that three women were randomly assigned to a style that did not come in their size and were removed from the study. Six participants were lost to follow-up due to being ventilated/sedated after surgery. Of the 69 women who were randomly assigned, 20 in each group completed the study, and their data were analyzed (attrition was <20%; Bolling et al., 2021).

Statistical conclusion validity was threatened in that, after discharge, four women did not wear their assigned bras at all (intervention fidelity). Because the data were not normally distributed, the researchers appropriately reported medians and used nonparametric statistical analyses (see Chapter 11). Although the sample size was adequate to identify statically significant differences in satisfaction and willingness to recommend style to other women, it was underpowered for the analysis of differences in compliance. External validity was threatened by the study being conducted in one location (interaction of intervention and setting) and not including women with smaller breast sizes (interaction of intervention and sample). Despite the researchers' efforts to control the intervention and setting, some would argue that the study lacked the valid, reliable instruments; intervention fidelity; and other types of control needed for an experimental study. The findings are questionable because of the threats to design validity that have been identified,

RANDOMIZED CONTROLLED TRIALS

Currently, in nursing and medicine, the randomized controlled trial (RCT) is noted to be the strongest methodology for testing the effectiveness of an intervention because of the elements of the experimental design that limit the potential for bias and error. Participants are randomized to the intervention and control groups to reduce selection bias. In addition, blinding or withholding of study information from data collectors, participants, and their healthcare providers can reduce the potential for bias. RCTs, when appropriately conducted, are considered the gold standard for determining the effectiveness of healthcare interventions. RCTs may be carried out in a single setting or in multiple geographical locations to increase sample size and obtain a more representative sample.

More nurse researchers are conducting RCTs on significant clinical topics. For example, new mothers with postpartum depression are less likely to breastfeed. Zhao et al. (2021) conducted an RCT to determine whether lactation education with a psychoeducation intervention during pregnancy could increase breastfeeding. Their sample was composed of 182 pregnant women who had depression during the antenatal period. Postpartum, the mothers in the intervention group had a statistically significant higher rate of exclusive breastfeeding than did the mothers in the control group (Zhao et al., 2021). Another group of nurse researchers conducted an RCT to compare the effects of reverse Trendelenburg position (intervention) and semirecumbent position (control) on the respiratory status of 110 obese critically ill patients on mechanical ventilation (Hassan & Baraka, 2021). They found statistically significant improvements in physiological measurements of respiratory effectiveness among the intervention group.

Characteristics of Quality RCTs

Early RCTs were not always well designed, which resulted in biases and threats to validity. To address this issue, an expert panel was convened that produced a standard for reporting RCT results, which has since been revised to be the Consolidated Standards for Reporting Trials (CONSORT). The basic guideline, last revised in 2010, includes a checklist and flow diagram that most journals require to be used when clinical trials are published (CONSORT, 2010). Nurse researchers should follow the CONSORT 2010 statement recommendations in conducting and reporting RCTs. The CONSORT flow diagram in Fig. 8.13 provides the structure and key elements to be included in the reports of RCTs. A CONSORT diagram published as part of a study report provides details you can use to critically appraise refusal rates and attrition rates of RCTs. Since 2010, variations of the CONSORT statement have been published online for RCTs with different designs, interventions, and types of data (http://www.consort-statement.org/extensions). As an example of how specialized the guidelines have become, Ibrahim et al. (2021) recently published CONSORT guidelines for RCTs with interventions that use artificial intelligence.

📄 RESEARCH/EBP TIP

Researchers may use the CONSORT flow diagram even in quasi-experimental designs to provide valuable information about the numbers of participants who were eligible for the study, who refused to participate, who were randomly assigned, and who left the study before it was completed. Quality RCTs have the potential to provide sound evidence for practice.

Following the CONSORT checklist and publishing the flow diagram for the study are two characteristics of quality RCTs. Additional characteristics are listed in Table 8.5. You may read reports of RCTs that have threats to design validity in one or more of these characteristics. Remember that no study is perfect because people are involved as researchers and participants.

Zamenjani et al. (2021, p. 148) conducted an RCT "to compare the effects of inhalation aromatherapy with essential oils of sweet orange and damask rose on pain severity after open abdominal surgeries." The researchers did several things to remove other potential influences. For example, nurses might contend that a patient's pain depends on the length of the surgery, the type of surgery, and the surgeon. In the study conducted by Zamenjani et al. (2021), the participants' surgeries were conducted by the same surgeon. To control for the length of the surgery, they used stratified sampling with each participant placed in a "block" depending on the surgery (appendectomy or other) and length of the surgery (<30 minutes, >30 minutes). Then the participants were randomly assigned so that each block was equally represented in each group. Research Example 8.9 provides more information about this RTC. Notice the detail the researchers provided.

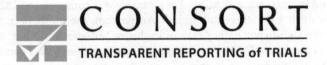

CONSORT 2010 Flow Diagram

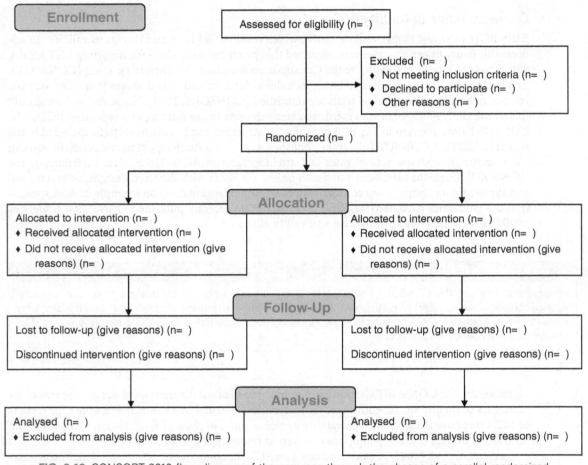

FIG. 8.13 CONSORT 2010 flow diagram of the progress through the phases of a parallel randomized trial of two groups: Enrollment, intervention allocation, follow-up, and data analysis. (Reproduced from CONSORT. [2010]. *The CONSORT flow diagram.* Retrieved from http://www.consort-statement.org/consort-statement/flow-diagram.)

TABLE 8.5 CHARACTERISTICS OF HIGH-QUALITY RANDOMIZED CONTROL TRIALS

STUDY COMPONENT	DESCRIPTION
External review	Study is registered with appropriate agency or group, such as ClinicalTrials.gov. Study is reviewed and approved by an ethical board. Adequate external funding was received to implement a rigorous design and recruit an adequate number of participants to test the hypothesis.
Design	Study is developed and implemented to meet criteria of an experimental study. Threats to validity are minimized by planning and having detailed procedures for each aspect of the study. Researchers, data collectors, caregivers, and/or patients are blinded to group assignment to minimize bias. After recruitment, baseline measurements are followed by random assignment to groups.
Hypothesis	The research hypothesis is that the intervention changes the defined dependent variable. Study is designed to test the hypothesis. Study is designed to either test alternative hypotheses or rule them out.
Setting	The study is conducted in a clinical setting, instead of a laboratory. Researchers control the setting so that alternative causes of the effect are eliminated.
Sample	The sample is selected to meet clearly defined inclusion and exclusion sampling criteria. The sample is recruited from the reference population. The reasons potential participants refused to be in the study are identified. The reasons participants were lost to follow-up are identified. Sample attrition is discussed as possible study limitation and threat to internal validity.
Intervention or independent variable	The intervention is clearly described so that it can be repeated by other researchers and, if effective, used in clinical care. The interventionists are trained, and their knowledge and skill are evaluated related to the intervention. There may be a manual or script for delivering the intervention. The intervention is consistently implemented. During the study, the fidelity of the intervention is evaluated on an ongoing basis.
Dependent variable	The dependent variable is measured with reliable and valid scales or precise and accurate physiological measures.

RESEARCH EXAMPLE 8.9

Randomized Controlled Trial

Research/Study Excerpt

This is a randomized double-blinded, parallel-group controlled trial. ... One hundred twenty patients, who underwent open abdominal surgeries...participated....In all three groups, similar preoperative care was provided by staff blinded to the study. ...all patients in the three groups received intravenous morphine (5 mg) and/or intramuscular pethidine (25 mg) at certain intervals, if necessary. ...When the patient regained

Continued

RESEARCH EXAMPLE 8.9—cont'd

full consciousness...a 10 × 10 cm² gauze impregnated with four drops of either distilled water or essential oils of sweet orange or damask rose was attached to the collar of the patients at a distance of 20 cm from their nose. The patients were then asked to inhale the aroma through normal breathing for 30 minutes. ...Pain severity at the operative site was evaluated and recorded using the VAS [visual analog scale] before the intervention (baseline pain severity) and 4, 8, and 12 hours after the intervention by a nurse blinded to the type of intervention. (Zamenjani et al., 2021, p. 148)

There were no significant differences between groups in terms of demographic and clinical information. ... No differences were observed between the three groups in terms of analgesics consumption during the intervention period. (Zamenjani et al., 2021, p. 149)

The pain-reducing effect of inhalation aromatherapy with sweet orange was significantly greater than with the placebo at 8 hours (− 1.42 ± 0.42; $p = 0.006$) and 12 hours (12.47 ± 0.50; $p < 0.001$). ...A significant difference in the mean pain severity score was also observed between the sweet orange and damask rose groups at 12 hours after the intervention (− 1.52 ± 0.50; $p = 0.009$). (Zamenjani et al., 2021, p. 150)

The limitations of our study are as follows: The safety evaluation using laboratory parameters was not planned for recording the side effects of interventions because of the short-term intervention period. The patients were not genuinely blinded to the intervention and control groups so that each participant was aware of the type of aroma used for him and/or her, and the placebo effect might influence outcomes. However, the patients of each group were intervened on separately in a different room so as to not smell the other oil or placebo. (Zamenjani et al., 2021, p. 151)

Critical Appraisal

This RCT was conducted in a clinical setting with three randomly assigned groups. Data collectors were blinded to group assignment, which is a strength related to construct validity. VASs have been documented to be valid instruments for measuring pain in surgery patients and provide more variation in responses compared with verbal responses to assessing pain on a scale of 1 to 10. One threat to construct validity is using only one means to measure pain. Related to internal validity, the researchers used stratified random assignment to control for the possible threats of surgeon and length and types of surgery. According to the article and CONSORT flow diagram, four possible participants who met the sampling criteria refused to participate, which is a very low refusal rate. After that point, all the participants completed the study. The study lasted only 12 hours, so maturation was not an issue. One factor, the total amount of opioid narcotic pain medications, was equal across groups, but the timing of doses in regard to the pain assessment was not reported. Not including the timing of pain medications and pain assessments was a major threat to design validity.

As noted previously, the VAS has been documented to be a quality method of measurement (Waltz et al., 2017). The essential oils and placebo liquid were prepared in identical containers, and the person delivering the intervention was blinded to which oil/placebo was being delivered until differences in the smells became evident. The intervention was implemented with precision, including number of drops, size of gauze, and location from the participant's nose. The sample and groups were adequate in size to identify statistically significant differences. The external validity is somewhat limited by a possible interaction between the Iranian culture and the intervention. This unknown is a potential threat to external validity. Further indications of the validity of the study design are that the researchers received funding from the Arak University of Medical Sciences. The study was reviewed by the hospital's ethics board and registered with the Iranian Registry of Clinical Trials. Replicating this study in other hospitals and countries will enhance the study's generalizability.

KEY POINTS

- A research design is a blueprint for conducting a quantitative study that maximizes control over factors that could interfere with the validity of the findings.
- The concepts important in understanding quantitative research designs include causality, multicausality, probability, bias, prospective, retrospective, control, and manipulation.
- Study validity is a measure of the truth or accuracy of the findings obtained from a study. Four types of validity are covered in this chapter: construct, internal, external, and statistical conclusion.
- Research designs can be categorized by whether an intervention is implemented.
- Descriptive and correlational designs, called nonexperimental or noninterventional designs, focus on the description and examination of relationships among variables.
- The descriptive designs in this chapter are simple descriptive and comparative descriptive.
- The two types of correlational designs described in the chapter are (1) descriptive correlational, in which the researcher seeks to describe relationships among variables; and (2) predictive correlational, in which the researcher measures independent variables and conducts regression analysis to predict the value of a dependent variable.
- Studies may have a time element, such as being cross-sectional or longitudinal.
- Interventions or treatments are implemented in quasi-experimental and experimental studies to determine their effect on selected dependent variables. Interventions may be physiological, psychosocial, educational, or a combination of these.
- The essential elements of experimental research are (1) the random assignment of participants to groups; (2) the researcher's manipulation of the independent variable; and (3) the researcher's control of the experimental situation and setting, including a control or comparison group.
- Critically appraising a design involves examining the study setting, sample, intervention, measurement of variables, and data collection procedures.
- RCT design is noted to be the strongest methodology for testing the effectiveness of an intervention because the elements of the design limit the potential for bias and threats to design validity.

REFERENCES

Bolling, K., Long, T., Jennings, C., Dane, F., & Carter, M. (2021). Bras for breast support after sternomoty: Patient satisfaction and wear compliance. *American Journal of Critical Care Nursing, 30*(1), 21–26. https://doi.org/10.4037/ajcc2021687

Bonar, J. R. M., Wright, S., Yadrich, D. M., Werkowitch, M., Ridder, L., Spaulding, R., & Smith, C. E. (2020). Maintaining intervention fidelity when using technology delivery across studies. *Computers, Informatics, Nursing, 38*(8), 393–401. https://doi.org/10.1097/CIN.0000000000000625

Bova, C., Jaffarian, C., Crawford, S., Quintos, J. B., Lee, M., & Sullivan-Bolyal, S. (2017). Intervention fidelity: Monitoring drift, providing feedback, and assessing the control condition. *Nursing Research, 66*(1), 54–59. http://doi.org/10.1097/NNR.0000000000000194

Bridi, A., da Silva, R., de Farias, C., Franco, A., & dos Santos, V. (2014). Reaction time of a health care team to monitoring alarms in the intensive care unit: Implications for the safety of seriously ill patients. *Revista Brasileira De Terapia Intensiva, 26*(1), 28–35. https://doi.org/10.5935/0103-507X.20140005

CONSORT. (2010). *CONSORT 2010*. Retrieved from http://www.consort-statement.org/consort-2010

Creswell, J. W., & Creswell, D. (2018). *Research design: Qualitative, quantitative and mixed methods approaches* (5th ed.). Sage.

Fard, N., Keikhaei, A., Rahdar, M., & Razaee, N. (2021). The effect of hope therapy-based training on the happiness of women with breast cancer: A quasi-experimental study. *Medical Surgical Nursing Journal, 9*(4), e113501. https://doi.org/10.5812/msnj.113501

Grainger, A., (2021). Critiquing a published healthcare research paper. *British Journal of Nursing, 30*(6), 354–358. https://doi.org/10.12968/bjon.2021.30.6.354

Gravetter, F., & Forzano, L. A. (2018). *Research methods for the behavioral sciences.* Cengage.

Gray, J. R., & Grove, S. K. (2021). *The practice of nursing research: Appraisal, synthesis, and generation of evidence* (9th ed.). Elsevier.

Grove, S. K., & Cipher, D. J. (2020). *Statistics for nursing research: A workbook for evidence-based practice* (3rd ed.). Elsevier.

Han, K., Kim, Y. H., Lee, H., & Lim, S. (2020). Novice nurses' sleep disturbance trajectories within the first 2 years of work and actual turnover: A prospective longitudinal study. *International Journal of Nursing Studies, 112,* 103575. https://doi.org/10.1016/j.ijnurstu.2020.103575

Hassan, E., & Baraka, A. (2021). The effect of reverse Trendelenburg position versus semi-recumbent position on respiratory parameters of obese critically ill patients: A randomised controlled trial. *Journal of Clinical Nursing, 30,* 995–1002. https://doi.org/10.1111/jocn.15645

Hasson, R., Beemer, L., Ajibewa, T., & Eisman, A. (2021). Adapting the InPACT Intervention to enhance implementation flexibility and fidelity. *Prevention Science, 22,* 324–333. https://doi.org/10.1007/s11121-020-01199-z

Holtrop, K., Miller, D., Durtschi, J., & Forgatch, M. (2021). Development and evaluation of a component level implementation fidelity rating system for the GenerationPMTO Intervention. *Prevention Science, 22,* 288–298. https://doi.org/10.1007/s11121-020-01177-5

Ibrahim, H., Liu, X., Rivera, S., Moher, D., Chan, A. W., Sydes, M., Calvert, M., & Denniston, A. (2021). Reporting guidelines for clinical trials of artificial intelligence interventions: The SPIR IT-AI and CONSORT-AI guidelines. *Trials, 22,* 11. https://doi.org/10.1186/s13063-020-04951-6

Kaplow, R., & Zellinger, M. (2021). Nurses' perceptions of telemedicine adoption in the intensive care unit. *American Journal of Critical Care, 30*(2), 122–127. https://doi.org/10.4037/ajcc2021205

Kazdin, A. (2017). *Research design in clinical psychology* (5th ed.). Pearson.

Kerlinger, F. N., & Lee, H. B. (2000). *Foundations of behavioral research* (4th ed.). Harcourt College Publishers.

Kim, M., Mallory, C., & Valerio, T. (2022). *Statistics for evidence-based practice in nursing* (3rd ed.). Jones & Barlett.

Papermaster, A., & Champion, J. (2021). Curbside consultation: A means to promote quality patient care. *Applied Nursing Research, 57,* 151350. https://doi.org/10.1016/j.apnr.2020.151350

Petursdottir, A., Sigurdardottir, V., Rayens, M., & Svavarsdottir, E. (2020). The impact of receiving a family-oriented therapeutic conversation intervention before and during bereavement among family cancer caregivers. *Journal of Hospice & Palliative Nursing, 22*(5), 383–391. https://doi.org/10.1097/NJH.0000000000000679

Pole, J., & Bondy, S. (2012). Prospective study. In N. J. Salkind (Ed.), *Encyclopedia of research design* (pp. 1131–1132). Sage. https://dx.doi.org/10.4135/9781412961288

Reaves, C., & Angosta, A. (2021). The relaxation response: Influence on psychological and physiological responses in patients with COPD. *Applied Nursing Research, 57,* 151351. https://doi.org/10.1016/j.apnr.2020.151351

Shadish, W. R., Cook, T. D., & Campbell, D. T. (2002). *Experimental and quasi-experimental designs for generalized causal inference.* Rand McNally.

Shajrawi, A., Al-Smadi, A., Al-Shawabkeh, G., Aljribeea, H., & Khalil, H, (2019). Impacts of treatment modalities on physical activity after first acute myocardial infarction in Jordan. *Dimensions of Critical Care Nursing, 38*(6), 284–292. https://doi.org/10.1097/DCC.0000000000000382

Steffen, P., Mendonca, C., Meyer, E., & Faustina-Silva, D. (2021). Motivational interviewing in management of Type 2 diabetes mellitus and arterial hypertension in primary care: An RCT. *American Journal of Preventive Medicine, 60*(5), e203–e212. https://doi.org/10.1016/j.amepre.2020.12.015

Stone, J., Glass, K., Clark, J. Munn, Z., Tugwell, P., & Doi, S. (2019). A unified framework for bias assessment in clinical research. *International Journal of Evidence-Based Health Care, 17*(2), 106–120. DOI: 10.1097/XEB.0000000000000165

Storm, J., & Chen, H. (2021). The relationships among alarm fatigue, compassion fatigue, burnout and compassion satisfaction in critical care and step-down nurses. *Journal of Clinical Nursing, 30,* 443–453. https://doi.org/10.1111/jocn.15555

Unal, N., Tosun, B., Aslan, O., & Tunay, S. (2021). Effects of vapocoolant spray prior to SC LMWH injection: An experimental study. *Clinical Nursing Research, 30*(2), 127–134. https://doi.org/10.1177/1054773818825486

Waltz, C. F., Strickland, O. L., & Lenz, E. R. (2017). *Measurement in nursing and health research* (5th ed.). Springer Publishing Company.

Watson, J. (2011). *Human caring science*. Jones & Bartlett.

Westland, H., Schuurmans, M., Bos-Touwen, I., de Bruin-van Leersum, M., Monninkhof, E., Schröder, C., de Vette, D., & Trappenburg, J. (2020). Effectiveness of the Activate intervention in patients at risk for cardiovascular disease in primary care: A cluster-randomised controlled trial. *European Journal of Cardiovascular Nursing, 19*(8), 721–731. https://doi.org/10.1177/1474515120919547

York, R. (2021). *Social work research methods: Learning by doing*. Sage. https://dx.doi.org/10.4135/9781506387215

Zamenjani, M., Farahani, M., Amirmohseni, L., Pourandish, Y., Shamsikhani, S., Heydari, A., & Harorani, M. (2021). The effects of inhalation aromatherapy on postoperative abdominal pain: A three-arm randomized controlled clinical trial. *Journal of PeriAnesthesia Nursing, 36*, 147–152. https://doi.org/10.1016/j.jopan.2020.07.001

Zhao, Y., Lin, Q., & Wang, J. (2021). An evaluation of a prenatal individualised mixed management intervention addressing breastfeeding outcomes and postpartum depression: A randomised controlled trial. *Journal of Clinical Nursing, 30*, 1347–1359. https://doi.org/10.1111/jocn.15684

CHAPTER

9

Examining Populations and Samples in Research

Susan K. Grove

LEARNING OUTCOMES

After completing this chapter, you should be able to:

1. Describe sampling theory with its relevant concepts.
2. Critically appraise the sampling criteria, refusal rates, and attrition rates in studies.
3. Critically appraise the type(s) of probability and nonprobability sampling methods implemented in quantitative, qualitative, mixed methods, and outcomes research.
4. Describe the aspects of power analysis used to determine sample size in selected studies.
5. Critically appraise the sampling processes implemented in quantitative, qualitative, mixed methods, and outcomes studies.
6. Critically appraise the common settings used in nursing studies.

Many of us have preconceived notions about samples and sampling, which we acquired from television commercials, polls of public opinion, internet surveys, and reports of research findings. The advertiser boasts that four of five doctors recommend a particular medication, a newscaster predicts John Jones will win his senate seat by a 5% majority, an online survey identifies patient satisfaction is high with nurses, and researchers conclude that aggressive treatment of high blood pressure significantly reduces the risk for coronary artery disease.

All these examples include a sampling technique or method. Some of the outcomes from these sampling methods are more valid than others, based on the sampling method used and the sample size achieved. This chapter was developed to assist you in understanding and critically appraising the sampling processes implemented in quantitative, qualitative, mixed methods, and outcomes studies. Initially, the concepts of sampling theory are introduced, followed by a description of nonprobability and probability sampling methods commonly used in nursing studies. The sample sizes for quantitative and outcomes studies are detailed, and the sampling processes in qualitative and mixed methods studies are explained. The chapter concludes with a discussion of the types of setting used in nursing research.

UNDERSTANDING THE KEY CONCEPTS OF SAMPLING THEORY

Sampling involves selecting a group of people, events, objects, or other elements with which to conduct a study. A sampling method or plan defines the selection process, and the sample defines the selected group of people (or elements). A sample selected in a study should represent an identified population. The population might be people who have heart failure (HF), patients who were hospitalized with coronavirus disease 2019 (COVID-19), or persons who received care from a registered nurse (RN). In most cases, however, it would be impossible for researchers to study an entire population. Sampling theory was developed to determine the most effective way to acquire a sample that accurately reflects the population under study. The key concepts of sampling theory are described in the following sections, including relevant examples from published studies.

Populations and Elements

The population is a particular group of individuals or elements, such as patients with type 2 diabetes or intravenous catheters, to be studied. The target population is the entire set of individuals or elements who meet the sampling criteria (defined in the next section), such as adult men, 50 years of age or older, diagnosed with type 2 diabetes, and hospitalized with a lower extremity infection. An accessible population is the portion of the target population to which the researcher has reasonable access. Fig. 9.1 demonstrates the link of the population, target population, and accessible population in a study. The accessible population might include individuals within a state, city, hospital, or nursing units, such as patients with diabetes who are in an acute care hospital in Dallas, Texas. Researchers obtain the sample from the accessible population by using a particular sampling method or plan, such as simple random sampling. The individual units of the population and sample are called elements. An element can be a person, situation, or any other single unit of study. When elements in a study are persons, they are referred to as participants or subjects. However, the term *participant* is more commonly used in all types of nursing study.

Generalization From the Sample to Population

Generalization extends the findings from the sample under study to the larger population. In quantitative and outcomes studies, researchers obtain a sample from the accessible population with the goal of generalizing the findings from the sample to the accessible population and then, more abstractly, to the target population (see Fig. 9.1). The quality of the study design and the consistency of the study's findings with those from previous research in this area influence the extent of the generalization (Kazdin, 2017). If a study has a strong design and findings consistent

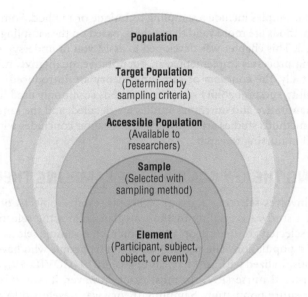

FIG. 9.1 Linking Population, Sample, and Element in a Study.

with previous research, then researchers can be more confident in generalizing their findings to the target population and using the findings in practice. For example, the findings from the study of male patients, diagnosed with type 2 diabetes, and hospitalized with an infection in Dallas, may be generalized to the target population of male patients with type 2 diabetes hospitalized in Texas urban hospitals or, more broadly, to urban hospitals in the southern United States.

📄 **RESEARCH/EBP TIP**

The generalization of quality findings enables you to decide whether to use this evidence in caring for the same type of patients in your practice, with the goal of moving toward evidence-based practice (EBP) (Melnyk & Fineout-Overholt, 2019).

Sampling Criteria

Sampling criteria include the list of characteristics for eligibility in or exclusion from membership in the target population. Inclusion sampling criteria are the characteristics that the study participant or element must possess to be part of the target population. For example, researchers may choose to study the effect of an internet-based early ambulation program on the length of hospital stay for older adults having knee joint replacement surgery. In this example, the inclusion criteria are 60 years or older, able to speak and read English, and undergoing an initial surgical replacement of one knee joint. Exclusion sampling criteria are those characteristics that excluded or eliminate potential participants from the target population for safety reasons or specific characteristics that might alter their responses. For example, any study participant with a history of previous joint replacement surgery, diagnosis of dementia, or a debilitating chronic muscle disease would be excluded from this example study. Researchers should state a sample criterion only once and should not include it as both an inclusion and an exclusion criterion. For example, researchers should *not* have an inclusion criterion of no diagnosis of dementia *and* an exclusion criterion of diagnosis of dementia.

When a quantitative study is completed, the goal is to generalize findings from the sample to the target population, designated by the sampling criteria (Gray & Grove, 2021). Researchers may narrowly define the sampling criteria to make the sample as homogeneous (or similar) as possible to control for extraneous variables. Conversely, the researcher may broadly define the criteria to ensure that the study sample is heterogeneous, with a broad range of values or scores on the variables being studied. If the sampling criteria are narrow and restrictive, the generalization of the findings is to a limited group of individuals. When critically appraising a study, examine the sample inclusion and exclusion criteria to determine to whom the study findings can be appropriately generalized.

Representativeness of a Sample

Representativeness means that the sample, accessible population, and target population are alike in as many ways as possible (see Fig. 9.1). The representativeness of a sample might be evaluated in terms of the setting, characteristics of the participants, and number of participants in a study. Persons seeking care in a particular setting may be different from those who seek care for the same problem in another setting or those who choose to use self-care to manage their problems. In addition, people who do not have access to health care are excluded from most studies. Sample characteristics are used to provide a picture of the sample, and these characteristics need to be reasonably representative of those in the population. In studies testing the effects of interventions, the participants in the experimental and control groups need to have similar demographic characteristics to reduce the potential for errors (see Chapters 5 and 11). A larger sample size usually results in a sample that is more representative of the population (Gray & Grove, 2021; Kazdin, 2017).

📄 RESEARCH/EBP TIP

Researchers who gather data from several participants across a variety of settings have a more representative sample of the population than those limiting their study to a single setting. However, a large sample size does not guarantee accurate study findings (Aberson, 2019).

Acceptance and Refusal Rates in Studies

The probability of sampling error increases when the sampling process is not random. Even in a random sample, however, bias or error can occur when a large number of the potential participants decline participation. As the number of individuals declining participation increases, the possibility of sampling error also increases. In published studies, researchers may identify a refusal rate, which is the percentage of individuals who declined to participate in the study, and their reasons for not participating (Grove & Cipher, 2020). The formula for calculating the refusal rate in a study is as follows:

$$\textbf{Refusal rate} = (\text{number refusing participation} \div$$
$$\text{number meeting sampling criteria approached}) \times 100\%$$

For example, the researcher approaches 80 potential participants who meet the sampling criteria to participate in a hypothetical study about the effects of early ambulation education on the length of hospital stay. Four patients refuse to participate, resulting in the following refusal rate:

Refusal rate $= (4 \div 80) \times 100\% = 0.05 \times 100\% = 5\%$

Some researchers report an acceptance rate, which is the percentage of participants meeting sampling criteria who consent to be in a study. However, researchers should report either the refusal or acceptance rate, but not both. The formula for calculating the acceptance rate in a study is as follows:

Acceptance rate = (number accepting participation ÷ number meeting sampling criteria approached) × 100%

In the hypothetical study, 4 of 80 potential participants refused to participate, so $80 - 4 = 76$ accepted. Plugging the following numbers into the stated formula gives the following:

Acceptance rate $= (76 \div 80) \times 100\% = 0.95 \times 100\% = 95\%$

You can also calculate the acceptance and refusal rates as follows:

Acceptance rate = 100% − *refusal* rate

or

Refusal rate = 100% − *acceptance* rate

In this example, the acceptance rate was 100% − 5% (refusal rate) = 95%, which is a study strength. When researchers report a high acceptance rate, or low refusal rate, for a study, there is less chance for sampling error and the sample is more likely to be representative of the target population. Researchers usually report the refusal rate, and it is best to provide rationales for the individuals who refuse to participate. In addition, the characteristics of those refusing to participate should be compared with those who participated to determine whether they differed in some way.

Sample Attrition and Retention Rates in Studies

Sampling error also may occur in studies with high sample attrition. Sample attrition is the withdrawal or loss of participants from a study and can be expressed as either a number or a percentage. The percentage is the sample attrition rate, and it is best if researchers include both the number of participants withdrawing and the attrition rate. The formula for calculating the sample attrition rate in a study is as follows:

Sample attrition rate = (number of participants withdrawing from a study ÷ sample size of study) × 100%

For example, in the hypothetical study of early ambulation education ($n = 76$), 31 participants (12 from the intervention group and 19 from the comparison group) withdrew for various reasons. Loss of 31 participants means a 41% attrition rate:

Sample attrition rate $= (31 \div 76) \times 100\% = 0.408 \times 100\% = 40.8\% = 41\%$

In this example, the overall sample attrition rate was high (41%) and would be considered a study weakness. Also, the rates differed for the intervention and comparison groups. You can also calculate the attrition rates for the groups. If the two groups were equal at the start of the study with 38 participants, then the attrition rate for the intervention group was (12 ÷ 38) × 100% = 0.316 × 100% = 31.6% = 32%. The attrition for the comparison group was (19 ÷ 38) × 100% = 0.50 × 100% = 50%. The potential for sampling error is greatest when a large number of participants withdraw from the study before data collection is completed or when a large number of participants withdraw from one group but not the other(s) in the study. Researchers must ask whether the participants who withdrew were different in some way and whether the remaining participants represent the target population. In studies involving an intervention, participants in the comparison group, who do not receive the intervention, may be more likely to withdraw from the study. However, sometimes the attrition is higher for the intervention group if the intervention is complex and/or time-consuming (Gray & Grove, 2021). In this example with the early ambulation program, there is a strong potential for sampling error because the sample attrition rate was large (41%), and the attrition rate in the comparison group (50%) was larger than the attrition rate in the intervention group (32%). High refusal and attrition rates (>10–15%) increase the potential for sampling error, which may affect the credibility of the study results and findings (Gray & Grove, 2021; Kazdin, 2017).

The opposite of sample attrition is sample retention, which is the number of participants who remain in and complete a study. You can calculate the sample retention rate in two ways:

Sample retention rate = (number of participants completing study ÷ sample size) × 100%

or

Sample retention rate = 100% − sample attrition rate

In the early ambulation study, 45 participants were retained in the study that had an original sample of 76 participants:

Sample retention rate = (45 ÷ 76) × 100% = 0.592 × 100% = 59.2% = 59%

or

Sample retention rate = 100% − 41% = 59%

The higher the retention rate the more representative the sample is of the target population and the more likely the study results are an accurate reflection of reality. Researchers should identify either the attrition or retention rate, but not both. It is best to provide a rate, as well as the number of participants withdrawing from a study. In addition, researchers need to provide rationales for the participants withdrawing to determine the effect on the study findings. For example, did the study participants have a common reason for withdrawing, such as severe complication, change in work schedule, or moved out of state.

RESEARCH/EBP TIP

Researchers strive to have a sample that is representative of the target population. When the sample in a study has a high acceptance rate (>90%) and a low attrition rate (<10–15%), the potential for sampling error is less, resulting in more credible findings.

? CRITICAL APPRAISAL GUIDELINES

Adequacy of the Populations, Sampling Criteria, Refusal Rates, and Attrition Rates in Quantitative and Outcomes Studies

When conducting an initial critical appraisal of the sampling process in quantitative and outcomes studies, you need to address the following questions:

1. Did the researchers define the target and accessible populations for the study?
2. Are the sampling inclusion and/or exclusion criteria clearly identified and appropriate for the study?
3. Is the sample refusal or acceptance rate identified? Are reasons provided for individuals refusing to participate?
4. Is the sample attrition or retention rate identified? Are reasons provided for individuals withdrawing from a study?
5. If the refusal rate is high and the retention rate is low, did the researcher discuss these limitations and the possible effect they might have on study findings?

Bang and Park (2020) conducted a randomized controlled trial (RCT) to determine the effects of acupressure on the quality of sleep and anxiety in patients undergoing cardiac surgery. These researchers provided a description of their study sampling criteria and documented the participants enrolled in their study using a flow diagram (Fig. 9.2). This flow diagram is based on the CONsolidated Standards of Reporting Trials (CONSORT) Statement that is the international standard for reporting the sampling process in RCTs (CONSORT Group, 2010). The population, inclusion and exclusion sampling criteria, refusal and attrition rates, and representativeness of this sample are described in Research Example 9.1. Particular aspects of the sample, not identified in the original study, have been added in [brackets] for clarity.

◢ RESEARCH EXAMPLE 9.1

Sampling Process in Quantitative Studies

Research/Study Excerpt

Cardiac surgery patients [population] *who were transferred from the ICU* [intensive care unit] *to general wards after recovering from cardiac surgery... were included in the present study. The inclusion criteria were as follows: (1) over 19 years of age; (2) undergone cardiac surgery under general anesthesia, with an unremarkable past medical history regarding psychological diseases such as insomnia, anxiety disorders, and similar conditions; and (3) a Mini-Mental State Examination-Korean (MMSE-K) score greater than or equal to 24. Exclusion criteria included: (1) patients with ongoing complementary therapy (e.g. aroma therapy, massage therapy, foot reflexology, yoga, and taichi); (2) patients with ear lesions (ulcer, eczema, urticaria, etc.); and (3) patients who developed severe complications, presented delirium, or were administered sedatives after cardiac surgery.... Considering the dropout rate, a total of 60 patients* [sample size]—*30 patients in the experimental and 30 in the control group* [group sizes]—*were recruited for this study. Participants were randomly assigned to one of the two groups using the Random Allocation Software program (Version 2.0.0). Some participants dropped out of the study due to severe complications (Experimental = 3, Control = 2); postoperative delirium (Experimental = 2, Control = 3); and discomfort at the site of acupressure (Experimental = 4, Control = 4)* [attrition]. *Finally, 21 patients in each group were included in the study analysis (Fig. 9.2). (Bang & Park, 2020, Methods)*

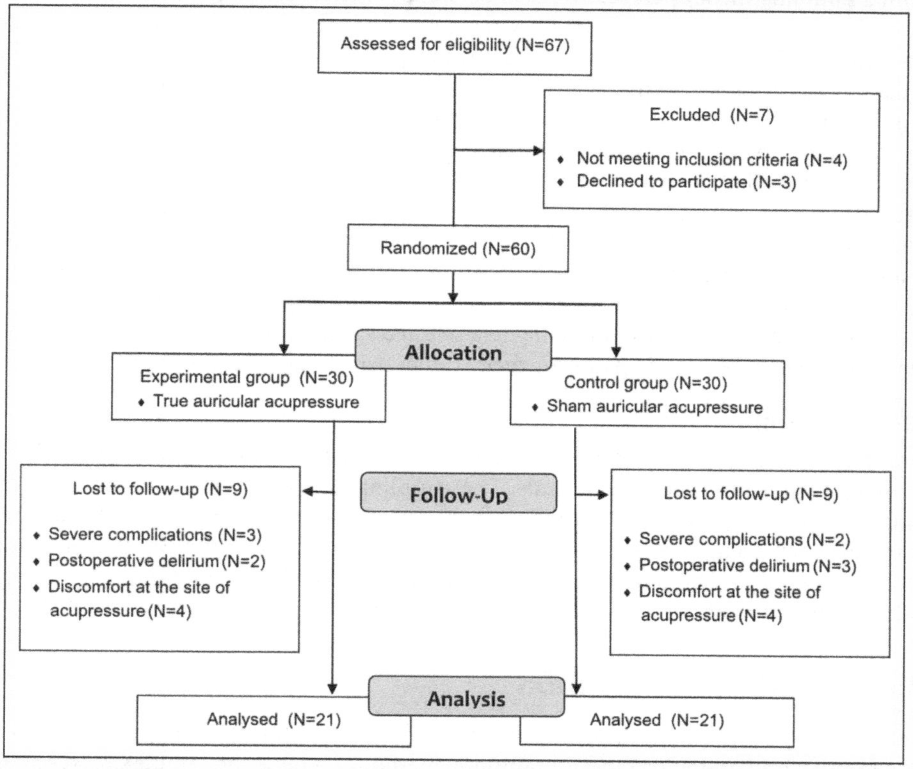

FIG. 9.2 **Flow Chart.** CONsolidated Standards of Reporting Trials (CONSORT) table for screening and enrolment in randomized clinical trials. (From Bang, Y. Y., & Park, H. [2020]. Effects of auricular acupressure on the quality of sleep and anxiety in patients undergoing cardiac surgery: A single-blind, randomized controlled trial. *Applied Nursing Research, 53*, 151269, Methods section. https://doi.org/10.1016/j.apnr.2020.151269)

Critical Appraisal
Bang and Park (2020) clearly identified the inclusion and exclusion sampling criteria used to determine their study target population. A total of 63 (67 − 4 = 63) cardiac surgery patients met these criteria. The sampling criteria were appropriate for the purpose of this study to reduce the effects of possible extraneous variables that might have had an effect on the patients' sleep quality and anxiety. The increased controls imposed by the sampling criteria strengthened the likelihood that the study results were caused by the auricular acupressure (AA) intervention and not by extraneous variables or sampling error.

The refusal rate was limited ($3 \div 63 \times 100\% = 0.0476 \times 1005 = 4.8\%$); however, the researchers provided no rationale for why these patients declined to participate in the study. The final sample included 60 cardiac surgery patients who were randomized into either the experimental ($n = 30$) or control group ($n = 30$); see Fig. 9.1). A total of 18 individuals (9 from each group) withdrew from the study, for a 30% attrition rate ($9 \div 30 \times 100\% = 30\%$). This high attrition rate increases the potential for sampling error and decreases the representativeness of the sample. However, the reasons for the attrition were logical and fairly equal for the groups (see Fig. 9.2). The final experimental and control group sizes were equal at $n = 21$. Bang and Park (2020) found that acupressure significantly improved the sleep and sleep satisfaction scores for the experimental group. However, there were no significant differences between the two groups for anxiety. The nonsignificant findings for anxiety might be the result of the small sample size (Grove & Cipher, 2020).

Sampling Frames

From a sampling theory perspective, each person or element in the population should have an opportunity to be selected for the sample. One method of providing this opportunity is referred to as random sampling. For everyone in the accessible population to have an opportunity for selection in the sample, each person in the population must be identified. To accomplish this, the researcher must acquire a list of every member of the population, using the sampling criteria to define eligibility. This list is referred to as the sampling frame. In some studies, the complete sampling frame cannot be identified because it is not possible to list all members of the population. The Health Insurance Portability and Accountability Act has made it difficult to obtain a complete sampling frame for some studies because of its requirement to protect individuals' health information (see Chapter 4). For some studies, a sampling frame could be identified through licensing boards or certification organizations. For example, a sample of RNs might be randomly selected from a list of RNs recognized by the board of nursing in a selected state. Once a sampling frame has been identified, researchers select participants for their studies using a sampling plan or method.

Sampling Methods or Plans

Sampling methods or plans outline strategies used to obtain samples for studies. Like a design, a sampling plan is not specific to a study. The sampling plan may include probability (random) or nonprobability (nonrandom) sampling methods. Probability sampling methods are designed to increase representativeness and decrease bias or error in quantitative and outcomes studies. Specific types of probability sampling methods are discussed next followed by types of nonprobability sampling methods commonly used in nursing.

PROBABILITY SAMPLING METHODS

In probability sampling, each person or element in a population has an opportunity to be selected for a sample. Probability or random sampling methods increase the sample's representativeness of the target population. All the subsets of the population, which may differ from each other, have a chance to be represented in the sample. To represent a wide range of people in a population, all the subsets need to be included. The opportunity for sampling error is less when participants are selected randomly, but it still can occur (Kazdin, 2017).

With nonrandom sampling strategies, researchers might (consciously or unconsciously) select individuals whose conditions or behaviors are consistent with the study hypotheses. For example, researchers may exclude participants because they are too sick, too healthy, coping too well, not coping adequately, uncooperative, or noncompliant. By using random sampling, researchers leave the selection to chance, thereby increasing the validity of their study findings.

The probability sampling methods included in this text are simple random sampling, stratified random sampling, cluster sampling, and systematic sampling. Table 9.1 identifies the common probability sampling methods used in nursing studies, their applications, and their representativeness of the population. Probability sampling methods are commonly used in quantitative and outcomes studies (Gray & Grove, 2021; Kazdin, 2017; Moorhead et al., 2018).

Simple Random Sampling

Simple random sampling is the most basic of the probability sampling plans. It is achieved by randomly selecting elements from the sampling frame. Researchers can accomplish random selection in a variety of ways; it is limited only by the imagination of the researcher. If the sampling frame is small, researchers can write names on slips of paper, place them into a container, mix them well, and then draw them out one at a time until they have reached the desired sample size.

TABLE 9.1 **PROBABILITY SAMPLING METHODS, COMMON APPLICATIONS, AND SAMPLE REPRESENTATIVENESS IN NURSING RESEARCH**

SAMPLING METHOD	COMMON APPLICATION(S)	SAMPLE REPRESENTATIVENESS
Simple random sampling	Quantitative and outcomes research	Provides strong representativeness of the target population that increases with sample size.
Stratified random sampling	Quantitative and outcomes research	Provides strong representativeness of the target population that increases with control of stratified variable(s).
Cluster sampling	Quantitative and outcomes research	Is less representative of the target population than simple random sampling and stratified random sampling, but representativeness increases with sample size.
Systematic sampling	Quantitative and outcomes research	Is less representative of the target population than simple random sampling and stratified random sampling methods, but representativeness increases with sample size.

A computer program is the most common method for randomly selecting study participants. The researcher can enter the sampling frame (list of potential participants) into a computer, which randomly selects participants until the desired sample size is achieved.

Another method for randomly selecting a study sample is to list potential participants and use a random number generator online. Tables of random numbers can be created online with an option to select a random sample from the table using a program such as QuickCalcs (see http://graphpad.com/quickcalcs/randomN2/).

Edraki and colleagues (2020) conducted an RCT to determine the effects of a peer educational program on the glycosylated hemoglobin (HbA1c) and self-care behaviors of adolescents with type 1 diabetes. A total of 110 adolescents were screened for this study, but 10 were excluded because their HbA1c was less than 7.5%. In addition, four adolescents were unwilling to participate. Thus the final sample size was 96 patients who were randomly assigned to the control ($n = 48$) and intervention ($n = 48$) groups. The researchers' sampling method is described in Research Example 9.2.

RESEARCH EXAMPLE 9.2

Simple Random Sampling

Research/Study Excerpt

The subjects were selected based on the simple random sampling method (selected from a random number table) among all 350 records of the diabetic patients available at the time of the present study in the diabetes center. The patients interested in participating in the research gave their written informed consent. (Edraki et al., 2020, p. 211)

Critical Appraisal

Edraki et al. (2020) clearly identified the sampling method used to select study participants. The sampling frame of the 350 adolescent records from a diabetic clinic seemed appropriate and provided an adequate sample ($N = 96$) for this study. The random numbers table was an easy way to select adolescents for this study. Only four individuals refused to participate, indicating a low refusal rate ($4 \div 110 \times 100\% = 3.6\%$). The strong sampling method and low refusal rate reduced the potential for sampling error in this study (Gray & Grove, 2021). Edraki et al. (2020) found that the peer educational program significantly improved the HbA1c and self-care behaviors of the adolescents in their study.

Stratified Random Sampling

Stratified random sampling is used in situations in which the researcher knows some of the variables in the population that are critical for achieving representativeness. Variables commonly used for stratification include age, gender, race/ethnicity, geographical region, and health status. For example, previous studies (hypothetically) have indicated college athletes have better exercise habits than other college students. Your study is designed to test the efficacy of a smartphone app to increase exercise among college students. The app rewards the number of steps taken each day with access to an online game. You may want to stratify your sampling frame by athletes/nonathlete. Stratification ensures that all levels of the identified variables are adequately represented in the sample by randomly selecting from each stratum. With stratification, researchers can use a smaller sample size to achieve the same degree of representativeness that is derived from using a larger sample selected through simple random sampling (see Table 9.1; Gray & Grove, 2021; Kazdin, 2017).

When stratified random sampling is used, researchers should define the categories (strata) of the variables selected for stratification in the research report. For example, using race/ethnicity for stratification, the researcher may define four strata: white non-Hispanic, black non-Hispanic, Hispanic, and other. The population may be 60% white non-Hispanic, 20% black non-Hispanic, 15% Hispanic, and 5% other. Researchers may select a random sample for each stratum equivalent to the target population proportions of that stratum. Thus a sample of 100 participants would need to include approximately 60 white non-Hispanic, 20 black non-Hispanic, 15 Hispanic, and 5 other. Alternatively, equal numbers of study participants may be randomly selected for each stratum. For example, if age is used to stratify a sample of 100 adult participants, the researcher may obtain 25 subjects 18 to 34 years old, 25 subjects 35 to 50 years old, 25 subjects 51 to 66 years old, and 25 subjects older than 66 years. With equal numbers of study participants in each group, the smaller groups are overrepresented, which can create error (Gray & Grove, 2021; Kazdin, 2017).

Lee and colleagues (2021, Abstract section) conducted a correlational study "to investigate the changes in safe patient handling programs in hospitals, and nurses' perceptions, work practices, and musculoskeletal symptoms by hospital characteristics after the passage of California's safe patient handling legislation." Data were collected using two cross-sectional surveys. This study included a stratified random sampling method that is described in Research Example 9.3.

RESEARCH EXAMPLE 9.3

Stratified Random Sampling

Research/Study Excerpt

We analyzed data from two statewide cross-sectional surveys of California registered nurses conducted in 2013 and 2016. The survey samples were randomly selected from the California Board of Registered Nursing's (BRN) up-to-date list at the time. The sampling was stratified by region (Northern counties, Sacramento region, Central 5-county San Francisco Bay Area, remainder of the San Francisco Bay Area, Central Valley and Sierra, Central Coast, Los Angeles, Inland Empire, and Border counties) (Spetz et al., 2011). The sampling within each stratum was proportional to the population size of the registered nurses in the region... The final sample for data analysis included 254 participants in 2013 and 281 participants in 2016. (Lee et al., 2021, Design and sample section)

Critical Appraisal

Lee et al. (2021) clearly identified their population, sampling frame, and sampling method. RNs were randomly selected from the California BRN current list, which provided a quality sampling frame. However, the process for randomly selecting the RNs was not provided but was probably done by computer. The researchers used proportional stratification to ensure the geographical areas in California were represented according to population size. However, the response rates to the surveys for both 2013 and 2016 were extremely low (<25%). The sampling method was strong, but the low survey response rate could have affected the quality of the findings.

Lee et al. (2021, Abstract section) reported "overall improvements of safe patient handling programs in California hospitals after the passage of safe patient handling legislation...However, greater positive changes in safe patient handling programs shown in certain hospital characteristics were not necessarily linked to more improvements in nurses' safe work practices and experiences of musculoskeletal symptoms or injuries." This study addressed the Quality and Safety Education for Nurses (QSEN, 2020) competency to promote students and practicing nurses providing safe, evidence-based care.

Cluster Sampling

In cluster sampling, a researcher develops a sampling frame that includes a list of all the states, cities, institutions, or units with which elements of the identified population can be linked. A randomized sample of these states, cities, or institutions can then be used in the study. In some cases, this randomized selection continues through several stages and is then referred to as multistage sampling. For example, the researcher may first randomly select states and then randomly select cities within the sampled states. Next, the researcher may randomly select hospitals within the randomly selected cities. Within the hospitals, nursing units may be randomly selected. At this level, all patients on the nursing unit who fit the criteria for the study may be included, or patients can be randomly selected.

Cluster sampling is commonly used in two types of research situation. In the first type of situation, the researcher considers it necessary to obtain a geographically dispersed sample but recognizes that obtaining a simple random sample will require too much travel time and/or expense. In the second, the researcher cannot identify the individual elements making up the population and therefore cannot develop a sampling frame. For example, a complete list of all people in the United States who have had open heart surgery does not exist. Nevertheless, it is often possible to obtain lists of institutions or organizations with which the elements of interest are associated—in this example, perhaps large medical centers, university hospitals with cardiac surgery departments, and large cardiac surgery practices—and then randomly select institutions from which the researcher can acquire study participants.

Obradors-Rial and colleagues (2020) conducted a predictive correlational study to determine whether school and town factors were predictive of risky alcohol consumption among rural and urban 10th-grade adolescents. The researchers obtained their sample using cluster and stratified random sampling methods. The data were collected using a computerized survey that had an 88.4% response rate. The details of their sampling methods are provided in Research Example 9.4, with aspects of the sample identified in [brackets].

RESEARCH EXAMPLE 9.4

Cluster Sampling

Research/Study Excerpt

The study population comprised 15-17-year-old 10th-grade adolescents in secondary education, surveyed during the 2011-2012 academic year....Cluster sampling [sampling method] with the class as the sampling unit was used. A random sampling was conducted to select the classrooms, using stratification [sampling method] by type of school (private/subsidized or public), township size (fewer than 2000 inhabitants classified as rural, 2001 to 10,000 inhabitants as intermediate, and more than 10,000 inhabitants as urban) [strata]...When a classroom of a high school was selected, all classrooms of that high school were included

Continued

RESEARCH EXAMPLE 9.4—cont'd

in the study, so they had the same strata characteristics. High schools refusing to participate were replaced by another high school with similar characteristics based on the strata, until we obtained the sample size needed to be representative....A sample of 1,268 students [sample size] nested in 26 high schools [settings] was finally obtained. (Obradors-Rial et al., 2020, p. 72)

Critical Appraisal

Obradors-Rial et al. (2020) provided detailed information about the cluster and stratified sampling methods used in their study. Multistage cluster sampling included the elements of rural and urban settings, high schools within these settings, and the classrooms in the selected high schools. The formation of representative strata (type of school and township size) were described. The large sample size and the 88.4% return rate for computerized questionnaires increased the representativeness of the sample and the credibility of the findings.

Obradors-Rial et al. (2020) found that the town environment (rural or urban), number of bars, and unemployment rate were not significant predictors of risky alcohol consumption. However, "the individual factors, such as the influence of drinking patterns of siblings and friends, and more alcohol access opportunities, are associated with adolescents' risky alcohol consumption" (Obradors-Rial et al., 2020, p. 71).

Systematic Sampling

Systematic sampling is used when an ordered list of all members of the population is available. The process involves selecting every kth individual on the list, using a starting point selected randomly. If the initial starting point is not random, the sample is a nonprobability or nonrandom sample. To use this design, the researcher must know the number of elements in the population and the size of the sample desired. The population size is divided by the desired sample size, giving k, the size of the gap between elements selected from the list. The formula is:

$$k = \text{population size} \div \text{desired sample size.}$$

For example, if the population size is $N = 1200$ and the desired sample size is $n = 100$, then $k = 12$. Thus the researcher would include every 12th person on the list in the sample. Some have argued that this procedure does not actually give each element of a population an opportunity to be included in the sample and does not provide as representative a sample as simple random sampling and stratified random sampling. Systematic sampling provides a random, but not equal, chance for inclusion of participants in a study (see Table 9.1; Gray & Grove, 2021; Kazdin, 2017).

Momeni and colleagues (2020) conducted a cross-sectional descriptive study to identify the factors that influence married women to obtain a pap smear screening in South Iran. The researchers noted that women in Iran did not take pap smear screening seriously, which influenced the incidence of cervical cancer. Research Example 9.5 describes the systematic sampling method implemented in this study.

RESEARCH EXAMPLE 9.5

Systematic Sampling

Research/Study Excerpt

Accordingly, 202 women who had electronic health records were selected through the systematic random sampling method from two health centers. The sample size was calculated considering the formula of estimating the sample size in descriptive studies...Two health centers of the city were included in the study...the subjects were randomly selected from women with electronic health records. Samples were

> ### ⚡ RESEARCH EXAMPLE 9.5—cont'd
>
> *selected by alternate (i.e. first person selected, second`no, third yes, fourth no, etc.) and continued until the desired sample size was reached.* (Momeni et al., 2020, Methods section)
>
> **Critical Appraisal**
> Momeni et al. (2020) clearly identified their sampling frame as women with electronic health records. A probability sampling method was used to select 202 women who appeared to be representative of the clinic population. However, the systematic sampling plan involved asking every other woman to participate in the study, which increased the potential for error. The researchers needed to provide more details on how they implemented the systematic sampling method to ensure that (1) the start of the sampling process was random and that (2) k was appropriately determined (Gray & Grove, 2021). Momeni et al. (2020) found that more than 50% of the 202 women in their study had never had a pap smear test, and only 14.8% had repeat tests at a standard interval.

> ### 📄 RESEARCH/EBP TIP
>
> Probability sampling methods were developed to reduce potential errors and achieve a sample that is representative of the population. Multiple studies with strong sampling methods have the potential to produce credible findings for use in practice.

NONPROBABILITY SAMPLING METHODS COMMONLY USED IN QUANTITATIVE AND OUTCOMES RESEARCH

In nonprobability sampling, not every element of a population has an opportunity to be selected for a study sample. Although this approach decreases a sample's representativeness of the target population, it is commonly used in nursing studies because a limited number of study participants are available (Grove & Cipher, 2020). You need to be able to identify the common nonprobability sampling methods used in nursing studies, which include convenience, quota, purposive or purposeful, network, and theoretical sampling. Convenience sampling is the most frequently used sampling method for all types of studies conducted in nursing. Quota sampling is occasionally used in quantitative and outcomes studies. Purposive, network, and theoretical sampling are used more frequently in qualitative and mixed methods research. Table 9.2 provides a list of the common applications of nonprobability sampling methods in nursing, the representativeness achieved in quantitative and outcomes studies, and the depth and richness of findings and understanding gained in qualitative and mixed methods studies.

Convenience Sampling

Convenience sampling, also called accidental sampling, is a relatively weak approach because it provides little opportunity to control for biases; participants are included in a study because they happen to be in the right place at the right time (Gray & Grove, 2021). A classroom of students, patients attending a selected clinic, individuals in a support group, and patients hospitalized with a specific diagnosis, such as COVID-19, are examples of convenience samples. The researcher simply enters available participants into the study until the desired sample size is reached. Biases exist in the sample, some of which may be subtle and unrecognized. However, convenience sampling is considered acceptable when it is used with reasonable knowledge and care in implementing a study (Kazdin, 2017).

TABLE 9.2   NONPROBABILITY SAMPLING METHODS, COMMON APPLICATIONS, AND SAMPLE REPRESENTATIVENESS IN NURSING RESEARCH

SAMPLING METHOD	COMMON APPLICATION(S)	REPRESENTATIVENESS, INSIGHT, UNDERSTANDING
Convenience sampling	Quantitative, qualitative, mixed methods, and outcomes research	There is questionable representativeness of the target population, which improves with increasing sample size for quantitative and outcomes research. This method is used in qualitative and mixed methods research to identify participants who are likely to have experience with the research topic.
Quota sampling	Quantitative and outcomes research; rarely, mixed methods research	Use of stratification for selected variables in quantitative and outcomes research makes the sample more representative than convenience sampling. In mixed methods research, participants of different ages, ethnic groups, or severity of illness may be selected to increase the depth and richness of the study findings.
Purposeful or purposive sampling	Qualitative and mixed methods research; rarely quantitative research	Focus is on insight, description, and understanding of a phenomenon, situation, process, or cultural element with specially selected participants who can provide quality data to address the study purpose.
Network or snowball sampling	Qualitative and mixed methods research; rarely quantitative research	Focus is on insight, description, and understanding of a phenomenon, situation, process, or cultural element in a difficult-to-access population. Intent is to identify additional participants who contribute to the study focus.
Theoretical sampling	Qualitative research	Focus is on obtaining quality participants with different perspectives, of an adequate number for developing a relevant framework, model, or theory in a selected area of study.

Convenience samples are inexpensive, accessible, and usually less time-consuming to obtain than other types of samples. This type of sampling provides a means to conduct studies on nursing interventions when researchers cannot obtain a random sample and/or the pool of potential participants is limited. Researchers often think it best to include all individuals who meet sample criteria to increase the sample size.

Many nurses and other healthcare researchers conduct quasi-experimental studies and RCTs with convenience samples. The study design is strengthened when the participants obtained by convenience sampling are randomly assigned to groups (see Chapter 8). However, random assignment to intervention and comparison groups is a *design strategy*, not a sampling method.

The random group assignment helps strengthen the equivalence of the study groups. For RCTs, researchers usually increase the sample size to strengthen the sample's representativeness (Tam et al., 2020).

Brauneis et al. (2021) conducted a quasi-experimental study to examine the effects of low-fidelity simulation-based experiences (SBEs) on medication administration confidence and medication safety knowledge. The SBE was implemented in a class for graduate prelicensure nursing students. These students had degrees in other disciplines and were seeking preparation as RNs. Research Example 9.6 addresses the sampling method used in this study.

RESEARCH EXAMPLE 9.6

Convenience Sampling

Research/Study Excerpt

Participants were a convenience sample of graduate prelicensure nursing students in a pharmacology course placed in the first quarter of a prelicensure accelerated master entry to registered nursing program in a Catholic University in the Midwest United States. After gaining the instructor's permission... all students enrolled in Basic Pathophysiology and Pharmacology (N = 43) were sent emails for recruitment purposes. Furthermore, a recruitment announcement was placed on the course's learning management system home page... The participants were assigned to an experimental group and a control group based upon the course section they were enrolled in. Section Background (n = 21) of this course served as the experimental group and Section Sample (n = 23) was the control group. (Brauneis et al., 2021, p. 44)

Critical Appraisal

Brauneis et al. (2021) used a variety of recruitment strategies to obtain an adequate sample size for their study. The convenience sampling method was appropriate to address the study purpose. The nonrandom groups were formed by the students' enrolment in a particular class section. In addition, the groups were of unequal size that might have influenced the study findings. The SBE was found to be an effective teaching strategy for these students, with the experimental group having significantly more medication administration confidence and medication safety knowledge.

Quota Sampling

Quota sampling uses a convenience sampling technique with an added feature—a strategy to ensure the inclusion of participant types likely to be underrepresented in the convenience sample, such as minority groups, children, and those with limited access to health care. This technique is similar to that used in stratified random sampling. Quota sampling involves stratification by selected subgroups of a population to improve the representativeness of the sample for the problem being studied. Thus quota sampling offers an improvement in representativeness over using only convenience sampling (see Table 9.2; Kazdin, 2017).

Ashford and colleagues (2020, Abstract section) conducted a correlational study to examine "if recent persistent cough or cytokine levels are related to the Electronic Nicotine Delivery Systems (ENDS) use in college students." The sample includes 61 undergraduate students from the University of Kentucky, who completed an online survey on a secure website and provided an oral salivary sample for analysis of cytokines. The quota sampling process used in this study is presented in Research Example 9.7.

RESEARCH EXAMPLE 9.7

Quota Sampling

Research/Study Excerpt

In April 2019, an IRB [institutional review board] approved cross-sectional study was conducted with a convenience sample of college students attending on-campus meetings. Quota sampling was used to ensure roughly equal numbers of ENDS users/nonusers and males/females, with modest compensation provided to all participants. (Ashford et al., 2020, Methods section)

Critical Appraisal

Ashford et al. (2020) used convenience sampling to address their study purpose. The University of Kentucky college campus provided easy access to an adequate number of study participants. Quota sampling was an effective way to ensure that equal numbers of ENDS users and nonusers and females and males were included in the sample, which increased its representativeness (see Table 9.2). The researchers reported that all ENDS users identified JUUL as their primary product. In addition, the ENDS users were younger, used cigarettes and marijuana, reported a persistent cough, and had altered salivary biomarkers.

SAMPLE SIZE IN QUANTITATIVE AND OUTCOMES STUDIES

A serious question that arises during the critical appraisal of a study is whether the sample size was adequate. If the study was designed to make comparisons and significant differences were found, the sample size, or number of individuals participating in the study, was probably adequate. Questions about the adequacy of the sample size occur when *no* significance is found. When nonsignificant findings occur for at least one of the hypotheses or questions, the authors need to address the adequacy of the study sample size. Is there really no difference? Or was an actual difference not found because of inadequacies in the study design and/or sample size?

Currently, the adequacy of the sample size in quantitative and outcomes studies is evaluated using a power analysis (Aberson, 2019; Grove & Cipher, 2020). Power is the ability of the study to detect differences or relationships that actually exist in the population. Expressed another way, it is the ability to reject a null hypothesis correctly (see Chapter 5). The minimum acceptable level of power for a study is 0.8, or 80% (Aberson, 2019; Cohen, 1988). This power level results in a 20% chance of a Type II error (see Chapter 11), in which the study fails to detect existing effects (differences or relationships). The level of significance or alpha (α) is frequently set at 0.05 in nursing studies. The power analysis conducted to determine a study's sample size should be documented in the Methods section of the report. Researchers also need to perform a power analysis to evaluate the power achieved for nonsignificant findings and report it in the Discussion section (Taylor & Spurlock, 2018).

Tam et al. (2020) searched the nursing literature to determine the adequacy of samples in RCTs. They identified 232 RCTs in 116 nursing journals published from January 2016 to December 2016. Only 143 (64.1%) of these studies indicated how they obtained their sample size. Of these studies, only 15% provided all the necessary information (effect size, power, alpha level, and type of statistical analysis) to recompute the power analysis. Sample size calculation is essential to ensure the RCTs, and other quantitative and outcomes studies have adequate power to detect significant differences or relationships. Researchers need to project the attrition rate in their study and increase their sample size to accommodate it. The final sample size should be equal to or greater than the number determined by the power analysis, with relevant power analysis information reported in the study (Aberson, 2019; Tam et al., 2020).

📄 **RESEARCH/EBP TIP**

Detailed reporting of power analysis (effect size, power, alpha level, and type of statistical analysis) is essential for documenting the sample size in quantitative and outcomes studies. This is an area that requires improvement in nursing to generate sound evidence for practice.

Effect Size

Factors that influence the adequacy of sample size (because they affect power) include effect size, type of quantitative study, sensitivity of the measurement methods, and data analysis techniques. The effect is the presence of the phenomenon examined in a study. The effect size is the extent to which the null or statistical hypothesis is false or, stated another way, the strength of the expected relationship between two variables or differences between two groups. In a study in which the researchers are comparing two populations, the null hypothesis states that the difference between the two populations is zero. However, if the null hypothesis is false, an identifiable effect is present—a difference between the two groups does exist. If the null hypothesis is false, it is false to some degree; this is the effect size (Aberson, 2019). The statistical test tells you whether there is a significant difference between groups, or whether variables are significantly related. The effect size tells you the size of the difference between the groups or the strength of the relationship between two variables (Grove & Cipher, 2020).

When the effect size is large (e.g., considerable difference between groups or a strong relationship between two variables), detecting it is easier and can be done with a smaller sample. When the effect size is small (e.g., only a small difference between groups or a weak relationship between two variables), detecting it is more difficult and requires a larger sample. There are different types of effect size measures, and each corresponds to the type of statistic computed (see Chapter 11). Often the effect size is smaller with a small sample, so effects are more difficult to detect. Increasing the sample size also increases the effect size, making it more likely that the effect will be detected, and the study findings will be significant. When critically appraising a study, determine whether the study sample size was adequate by noting whether a power analysis was conducted and what power was achieved. Also, did the researchers calculate the power level of study results that were not significant (Gray & Grove, 2021)?

Sample Size for Different Types of Quantitative Studies

Descriptive (particularly those using survey questionnaires), correlational, and outcomes studies often require large samples with more than 100 participants. In these studies, researchers may examine multiple variables, and extraneous variables are likely to affect participant responses to the variables studied. Researchers often make statistical comparisons on multiple subgroups in a sample, such as groups formed by gender, age, or severity of illness, requiring that an adequate sample be available for each subgroup being analyzed (Grove & Cipher, 2020). When variables are included in the data analyses to answer the research questions or test the hypotheses, the sample size must be increased to detect differences between groups or relationships among variables. However, analyzing demographic variables to describe the sample does not require an increase in sample size. Quasi-experimental and experimental studies often have smaller samples than descriptive and correlational studies because fewer variables are studied and a controlled intervention is implemented in a structured setting (Kazdin, 2017).

Measurement Sensitivity

Quality physiological instruments measure phenomena with accuracy and precision. A thermometer, for example, measures body temperature accurately and precisely. Tools measuring psychosocial variables tend to be less precise. However, a tool that is reliable and valid measures more precisely than a tool that is less well developed (Bandalos, 2018; Waltz et al., 2017). For example, if you are measuring anxiety, and the actual anxiety score of several participants is 50, you may obtain measures ranging from 30 to 70 with a less well-developed tool. There is more variation from the true score with new or less developed scales. As variance in instrument scores increases, the sample size needed to detect significance increases.

Data Analysis Techniques

Data analysis techniques vary in their capability to detect differences in the data. Statisticians refer to this as the "power of the statistical analysis." An interaction also occurs between the measurement sensitivity and power of the data analysis technique (Leedy & Ormod, 2019). The power of the analysis technique increases as precision in measurement increases. Because of this, techniques for analyzing variables measured at interval and ratio levels are more powerful in detecting relationships and differences than those used to analyze variables measured at nominal and ordinal levels (see Chapter 10 for details on levels of measurement). Larger samples are needed when the power of the planned statistical analysis is weak (Grove & Cipher, 2020).

When groups are being compared related to study variables, you may use statistical procedures, such as the t test and analysis of variance. Equal group sizes maximize the effect size, which improves statistical power. The more unbalanced the group sizes, the smaller the effect size, which means a larger sample is needed to detect significant differences (Kraemer & Blasey, 2016). The chi-square test is the weakest of the statistical tests and requires large sample sizes to achieve acceptable levels of power (see Chapter 11).

⁇ CRITICAL APPRAISAL GUIDELINES

Adequacy of the Sample Size and Sampling Method in Quantitative and Outcomes Studies

The initial critical appraisal guidelines for the sampling process in quantitative and outcomes studies were introduced earlier. This section focuses on questions about the sampling method and the adequacy of sample size, which influence the representativeness of the sample.

1. Is the sampling method probability or nonprobability? Is the specific sampling method(s) used in a study identified and appropriate (see Tables 9.1 and 9.2)?
2. Is the sample size identified? Is a power analysis conducted and accurately reported (Grove & Cipher, 2020; Tam et al., 2020)?
3. Was the sample size adequate, as indicated by the power analysis (Aberson, 2019)?
4. If groups were included in the study, is the sample size for each group approximately equal and adequate (Grove & Cipher, 2020)?
5. Is the sample representative of the accessible and target populations?

Bang and Park (2020) conducted an RCT to determine the effects of acupressure on the quality of sleep and anxiety in patients undergoing cardiac surgery. This study was introduced in Research Example 9.1, where the sample criteria and refusal and attrition rates were critically appraised. The power analysis, sample size, and group sizes in this study are presented in Research Example 9.8.

RESEARCH EXAMPLE 9.8

Quantitative Study Sample Size

Research/Study Excerpt

The sample size was analyzed by the G*Power 3.1 program and was calculated using a repeated measures analysis of variance (ANOVA). Based on a previous study in which sleep disturbance in elderly people was significantly improved by AA [auricular acupressure] intervention (Sok, 2009), the inputs for determining the sample size were: significance level = 0.05, power = 0.90, median effect size = 0.35, number of measurements = 3, and number of groups = 2. Consequently, the output showed that at least 20 subjects were needed in each group. Considering the dropout rate, a total of 60 patients—30 patients in the experimental and 30 in the control group—were recruited for this study.

Participants were randomly assigned to one of the two groups using the Random Allocation Software program (Version 2.0.0). Some participants dropped out of the study due to severe complications (Experimental = 3, Control = 2); postoperative delirium (Experimental = 2, Control = 3); and discomfort at the site of acupressure (Experimental = 4, Control = 4). Finally, 21 patients in each group were included in the study analysis (see Fig. 9.2). (Bang & Park, 2020, Subjects section)

Critical Appraisal

Bang and Park (2020) conducted a power analysis to determine the sample size for their RCT. All elements of power analysis were described, and the authors used a 90% power, rather than the standard 80%, which increased the likelihood that significant differences would be found between the experimental and control groups (Aberson, 2019; Tam et al., 2020). The power of the study was increased by randomly assigning 21 participants to each group. The size of the groups met the minimum power analysis requirement of 20 participants per group. The study results were significant (see Research Example 9.1), supporting the adequacy of the sample size in obtaining credible findings (Grove & Cipher, 2020).

SAMPLING METHODS IN QUALITATIVE AND MIXED METHODS RESEARCH

Qualitative research is conducted to gain insights, discover meaning, and promote understanding about a particular phenomenon, situation, or cultural element (Bryant & Charmaz, 2019; Creswell & Poth, 2018). The intent is an in-depth understanding of a situation or problem from the perspective of selected study participants. The sampling in qualitative and parts of mixed method research focuses on obtaining in-depth data to address the study purpose. In ethnographic studies, researchers often select the setting and site and then the population and topic of interest (Marshall & Rossman, 2016). In a phenomenological study, researchers often select the phenomenon of interest and then identify potential participants. The participants selected need to have experience and be knowledgeable in the area of study and willing to share rich, in-depth information about the phenomenon or situation being studied. For example, if the goal of the study is to describe the phenomenon of living with chronic pain, the researcher will select individuals who are articulate and reflective, have a history of chronic pain, and are willing to share their chronic pain experience (Creswell & Poth, 2018). Common sampling methods used in qualitative and mixed methods studies are purposeful, network, theoretical, and convenience (covered earlier) sampling (see Table 9.2). Researchers need to describe the sampling methods used in their study in enough detail to promote the readers' confidence in the findings.

Purposeful Sampling

With purposeful or purposive sampling, sometimes referred to as judgmental or selective sampling, the researcher consciously selects certain participants or situations to include in the study

(Creswell & Poth, 2018). Researchers may try to include typical or atypical participants or similar or varied situations. Qualitative researchers may select participants who are of various age categories, different levels of disability, or those who received an ineffective rather than an effective treatment for their illness. Often, they conduct observations and interviews over time to expand understanding of a phenomenon. For example, researchers describing grief after the loss of a child might include parents who lost a child in the previous 6, 12, and 24 months, and the children who were lost might be of varying ages (<5, 5–10, and >10 years old). The ultimate goal of purposeful sampling is selecting information-rich cases from which researchers can obtain in-depth information for their studies.

Some have criticized the purposeful sampling method because it is difficult to evaluate the accuracy or relevance of the researcher's judgment. To offset this perception, researchers must report the characteristics that they desire in study participants and provide a rationale for selecting these types of individuals to obtain essential data. In qualitative and mixed methods studies, purposeful sampling seems the best way to gain insights into a new area of study; discover new meaning; and/or obtain in-depth understanding of a complex experience, situation, or event (Creswell & Clark, 2018; Miles et al., 2020).

Mulholland and colleagues (2020, p. 34) conducted a phenomenological study "to better understand the lived experiences of military families and strategies they used to combat stressors of deployment and postdeployment." The researchers identified potential study participants using a combination of purposive and snowball (discussed later) sampling methods. Research Example 9.9 provides a description of the sampling methods used in this study.

RESEARCH EXAMPLE 9.9

Purposeful Sampling

Research/Study Excerpt

Purposeful sampling and snowball sampling were used for recruiting participants in this study. A link to the online survey was posted to the researcher's personal Facebook page…The researchers also invited individuals through direct messages on Facebook, Instagram, and e-mail. These individuals were purposively selected based on known military experience that made them potential candidates to complete the survey. (Mulholland et al., 2020, p. 36)

Critical Appraisal

Mulholland et al. (2020), using purposive sampling, identified relevant military family participants. These participants were recruited in a variety of ways with rationale provided for the sampling methods implemented. Additional information regarding the snowball sampling and the sample size of this study are presented in the next section. Mulholland et al. (2020) identified the unique changes military families experienced before and after deployment. They also identified strategies that could be used to assist families with children prepare for the next parental deployment.

Network Sampling

Network sampling, sometimes referred to as snowball or chain sampling, involves finding a few participants who meet the sampling criteria and asking them for their assistance in finding others with similar characteristics. Network sampling holds promise for locating participants who would be difficult or impossible to obtain in other ways or who had not been previously identified for study (Creswell & Poth, 2018; Marshall & Rossman, 2016). Network sampling takes advantage of social networks and the fact that friends tend to have characteristics in common. This strategy is also particularly useful for finding participants in socially devalued populations, such as persons who are dependent on alcohol, addicted to drugs, abuse children, or commit sexual offenses or criminal acts. These persons rarely make themselves known for study.

Other groups, such as widows, grieving siblings, or persons successful at lifestyle changes, also may be located using network sampling. They are typically outside the existing healthcare system and are otherwise difficult to find. Network sampling is an effective strategy for identifying participants who can provide great insight and essential information about a phenomenon or situation being studied.

Researchers often obtain the first few study participants through a purposeful or convenience sampling method and expand the sample size using network sampling. In qualitative research, sampling continues until saturation occurs. Saturation occurs when newly collected data begin to be like previously collected data and yield no new insights or information. With saturation, concepts are understandable and well described, details of a phenomenon are available, or patterns or themes of a theory emerge (Bryant & Charmaz, 2019).

As discussed earlier in Research Example 9.9, Mulholland et al. (2020) used purposeful and snowball sampling methods to identify military families with children who experienced parental deployment. Research Example 9.10 provides addition information about the snowball sampling and sample size in this study.

RESEARCH EXAMPLE 9.10

Network Sampling

Research/Study Excerpt

A link to the online survey was posted to the researcher's personal Facebook page in which viewers could share the post or tag others to view the post, thus initiating the snowball effect...These individuals were purposively selected based on known military experience that made them potential candidates...or they had known connections to others that would qualify for the study. Sampling was completed once data saturation was achieved with 15 participants. This was determined by the researchers when the data revealed to be consistent without new or emerging themes. The sample size was appropriate due to the qualitative nature of the study. (Mulholland et al., 2020, p. 36)

Critical Appraisal

Mulholland et al. (2020) alternated the use of snowball and purposeful sampling methods to identify quality participants to address the study purpose. Facebook was an effective way to initiate snowball sampling with the tagging of other military families. Multiple types of social media were used to identify participants who had connections with other military families who might qualify for the study. Data saturation was achieved indicating an adequate sample for this study (Creswell & Poth, 2018; Miles et al., 2020).

Theoretical Sampling

Theoretical sampling is mainly implemented in grounded theory research. This study method is designed and implemented to develop a model, framework, or theory. The researcher gathers data from any person or group who is able to provide relevant, varied, and rich information for model or theory generation. The data are considered relevant and rich if they include information that generates, clarifies, and saturates the theoretical codes identified through analysis. The theoretical codes form the basis for framework or theory generation (Bryant & Charmaz, 2019). A code is saturated if it is complete and the researcher can see how it fits in the emerging model or theory.

When a code or concept is unclear, the researcher continues to seek participants and gather data, especially participants with different characteristics. The process continues until the codes are saturated, and the theory evolves from the codes and data. Diversity in the sample is encouraged so that the theory developed covers a wide range of behaviors in varied situations and settings.

Crooks and colleagues (2020, Abstract section) conducted a grounded theory study to investigate "the sociocultural conditions and processes of becoming a sexual Black woman in order to understand the sociocultural drivers of STI/HIV [sexually transmitted infections/human immunodeficiency virus] rates among this group." The sample included 20 Black women aged 19 to 62 years in a Midwestern community. The sampling methods used to recruit study participants are described in Research Example 9.11.

⚓ RESEARCH EXAMPLE 9.11

Theoretical Sampling

Research/Study Excerpt

Purposive and theoretical sampling techniques were used for recruitment to provide conceptual clarity and further exploration of data... We initially recruited a purposive sample of women that had STI, however, after six interviews we made a theoretical sampling decision to include women without STI to allow for more variation in participant experience. (Crooks et al., 2020, Data collection section)

Critical Appraisal

Crooks et al. (2020) detailed their sampling methods. Using purposive sampling, they were able to identify women with varied histories and experiences. Initially the study included Black women with STIs. The researchers realized they needed to include women without STIs to expand their understanding of the relationships of these women. Theoretical sampling continued until data saturation was reached after 20 interviews. Crooks et al. (2020) found that "Black men, silencing Black girls and women, cultural norms and messaging about sexuality, and gendered societal expectations and sexual stereotypes contribute to STI/HIV risk in Black girls and women... Our findings demonstrate how the intersection of social and systemic structures (i.e., history, incarceration, unemployment) shape the context of Black heterosexual relationships." (Crooks et al., 2020, Abstract section)

SAMPLING PROCESS IN QUALITATIVE AND MIXED METHODS STUDIES

Qualitative and mixed methods research focus on the depth and richness of information obtained from the person, situation, or event sampled, rather than on the size of the sample (Creswell & Poth, 2018). The purpose and questions developed to guide the study influence the sampling process. Qualitative researchers may collect and analyze data simultaneously. Thus data collection and analysis are considered complete when researchers believe a phenomenon is understood, a cultural aspect is detailed, a model or theory is developed, or a healthcare problem is addressed. The quality of the data and the results of analyses determine the participants, sites, and artifacts sampled (Miles et al., 2020; see Chapter 3).

As discussed earlier, data collection and analysis continue until saturation is reached, with no new information provided through additional interviews and observations. Important factors that need to be considered in determining the participants included in qualitative and mixed methods studies are (1) scope of the study, (2) nature of the topic, (3) quality of the data, and (4) data collection process (Bryant & Charmaz, 2019; Creswell & Clark, 2018; Creswell & Poth, 2018).

Scope of the Study

If the scope of a study is broad, researchers will need extensive data to address the study purpose, and it will probably require additional interviews or observations to reach saturation. A study that has a concise purpose and provides focused data collection usually has richer, more credible findings. For example, a qualitative study of the experience of living with chronic illness in older adults would require more observations, interviews, and participants because of the broad scope of the problem. In contrast, researchers exploring the lived experience of community-dwelling individuals older than 60 years with HF could obtain credible findings with fewer participants or observations. Sometimes researchers change the scope of their study based on initial data collection and analysis. For example, Crooks et al. (2020) expanded the scope of their study from Black women with STIs to also include Black women without STIs. They reported this allowed for more variation in the participant experience.

Nature of the Topic

If the topic of study is easily discussed by the participants, fewer participants are needed to obtain the essential data. If the topic is difficult to define and awkward for people to discuss, more participants are often needed to achieve data saturation (Creswell & Poth, 2018). Topics such as gender identity, loss of a child, and history of child sexual abuse are sensitive, complex topics to investigate. These types of topics probably will require increased participants and interview time to collect essential data. Researchers need to provide a rationale for the types of participant recruited based on the complexity and sensitivity of the topic studied.

Quality of the Data

The quality of the data obtained from interviews or observations influences the number of participants recruited. When data are rich with content, fewer participants are needed to achieve saturation of the study's topic. Quality data are best obtained from articulate, well-informed, and communicative participants (Creswell & Poth, 2018; Miles et al., 2020). These participants are typically self-aware and insightful, which means they are able to share richer data in a clear, concise manner. In addition, participants who have more time to be interviewed usually provide data with greater depth and breadth. The researchers will continue sampling until saturation and verification of data have been achieved to produce the best study results (Miles et al., 2020).

Data Collection Process

Some studies include an increase in the number of interviews with each participant. When researchers conduct multiple interviews with a person, they probably will collect richer data. For example, a study design that includes an interview before and after an event usually produces richer data than a single-interview data collection process. Participants interviewed more than once have time to consider the topic and might gain additional insights between interviews or be more open with the researcher in subsequent interviews. In addition, interviewing families usually produces richer data than with single-participant interviews (Miles et al., 2020).

⟨?⟩ CRITICAL APPRAISAL GUIDELINES

Adequacy of the Sampling Processes in Qualitative and Mixed Methods Studies

When critically appraising the sampling processes in qualitative and mixed methods studies, you need to address the following questions:

1. Is the sampling plan adequate to address the purpose and questions of the study?
   a. If purposive sampling is used, does the researcher provide a rationale for the participants recruited?
   b. If network or snowball sampling is used, does the researcher identify the networks used to recruit participants?

Continued

CRITICAL APPRAISAL GUIDELINES—cont'd

c. If theoretical sampling is used, does the researcher indicate how participants are selected to promote the generation of a framework, model, or theory?
2. Are the sampling criteria identified and appropriate for the study?
3. Does the researcher identify the study setting and describe the entry into the setting?
4. Does the researcher discuss the quality of the data provided by the study participants? Are the participants articulate, well informed, and willing to share information relevant to the study topic?
5. Are saturation and verification of data achieved in the area of the study?
6. Is the number of interviews, observations, and participants recruited adequate for the study scope, nature of the topic, quality of the data, and the data collection process?

Crooks et al.'s (2020) use of theoretical and snowball sampling methods was presented earlier in Research Example 9.11. The sampling process implemented in this grounded theory study is presented in Research Example 9.12.

RESEARCH EXAMPLE 9.12

Qualitative Study Sample

Research/Study Excerpt

Participants were recruited from community and university settings to increase variation within the sample. Recruitment flyers were posted in clinic examination rooms, various locations on university campuses, and the Midwestern community at large...Purposive and theoretical sampling techniques were used for recruitment to provide conceptual clarity and further exploration of data...Inclusion criteria included: (a) self-identify as a Black female, (b) be 18 years or older and (c) fluent in speaking and reading the English language. In this study, we defined Black as anyone having African ancestry, inclusive of Black women from other countries and Black mixed race...

Sampling continued until saturation was reached; a point where no new categories are identified in the data, which occurred at 20 interviews...Saturation helps researchers recognize the importance of a topic, for example, many women shared the experience of protecting Black men, therefore once we kept hearing this concept being repeated in the data, we knew it had been saturated. Each participant was interviewed once. Interviews ranged from 28 to 95 min and averaged 55 min. Interviews were conducted at a convenient time and private location per participant choice. (Crooks et al., 2020, Data collection section)

Critical Appraisal

Crooks et al.'s (2020) study has many sampling strengths, including quality sampling methods (theoretical and snowball), information-rich participants, and extensive interview data. The study topic and scope were clearly addressed and provided a relevant study focus. The recruitment process was varied because of the sensitive nature of the study topic and the need to include Black women of varying ages, education, social status, and experiences with and without STI/HIV. The researchers provided rationale for their sampling methods and presented a detailed explanation of how data saturation were achieved to support the sample size of the study. The study would have been strengthened by knowing how many study participants were obtained by each of the sampling methods.

RESEARCH SETTINGS

The research setting is the site or location used to conduct a study. Three common settings are used in nursing studies: natural, partially controlled, and highly controlled (Gray & Grove, 2021). Chapter 2 initially introduced the types of setting for quantitative research. Some studies are strengthened by having more than one setting, making the sample more representative of the target population (Kazdin, 2017; Tam et al., 2020). The selection of a research setting is based on the study purpose, accessibility of the setting or data collection sites, and number and types of participant available in the setting. The setting needs to be clearly described in the research report, with a rationale for selecting it. If the setting is partially or highly controlled, researchers should include a discussion of how the control was achieved. The following sections describe and provide an example of the common research settings used in nursing research.

Natural Setting

A natural or field setting is an uncontrolled, real-life situation or environment. Conducting a study in a natural setting means that the researcher does not manipulate or change the environment for the study. Many nursing studies are conducted in natural settings, especially qualitative and mixed methods studies (Creswell & Poth, 2018). Descriptive and correlational quantitative studies are usually conducted in natural settings (Gray & Grove, 2021). Ashford et al. (2020) used a natural setting to examine the relationships of e-cigarette use on persistent cough and salivary biomarkers of college students. This study's sampling methods (convenience and quota) were introduced in Research Example 9.7, and the study setting is discussed in Research Example 9.13.

---

⑤ RESEARCH EXAMPLE 9.13

Natural Setting

Research/Study Excerpt

In April 2019, an IRB approved cross-sectional study was conducted with a convenience sample of college students attending on-campus meetings...Eligibility criteria included: between the ages of 18–25 years old, currently enrolled as an undergraduate student at the University of Kentucky...After informed consent, 61 participants completed a 10-minute survey stored on REDCap, a secure web-based data management system; each also provided an oral salivary sample for analysis of cytokines. (Ashford et al., 2020, Design and sample section)

Critical Appraisal

A college campus was an appropriate setting for recruiting potential participants for the Ashford et al. (2020) study. Available students were asked to participate, ensuring that both users and nonusers of e-cigarettes were included in the sample. Data collection took place on campus with a Web-based survey and collection of a salivary sample. The sample size was adequate to find significant differences between the groups. There is no indication that the setting was controlled or manipulated during data collection.

Partially Controlled Setting

A partially controlled setting is an environment that is manipulated or modified in some way by the researcher. An increasing number of nursing studies, usually quasi-experimental and experimental studies, are conducted in partially controlled settings. When interventions are tested in a study, often the setting for delivering the intervention and collecting data are controlled to some extent. Nursing research has expanded in large healthcare settings, which are usually partially controlled (Siedlecki & Albert, 2020). Control is used to reduce the effects of extraneous variables on study outcomes (Kazdin, 2017).

Bang and Park (2020) conducted an RCT in a partially controlled setting to examine the effects of AA on cardiac surgical patients' sleep and anxiety. This study was introduced earlier in Research Examples 9.1 (sampling criteria) and 9.8 (sample size in quantitative research). The study included

61 participants recruited from a general hospital. Research Example 9.14 provides a discussion of the study setting.

Partially Controlled Setting

Research/Study Excerpt

Cardiac surgery patients who were transferred from the ICU to general wards after recovering from cardiac surgery at "K" tertiary general hospital in Seoul, Korea were included in the present study... The intervention was performed six days a week for two weeks by alternately affixing vaccaria seeds to the ears to prevent skin damage from continuous application of pressure on one ear. Patients were instructed to stimulate the affixed points four times a day (three times in the morning and one time before bedtime) for 1 min with firm pressure... The participants were informed that treatments (medication, other complementary therapy) other than AA were not allowed, to prevent the influence of exogenous variables. (Bang & Park, 2020, Methods section)

Critical Appraisal

This partially controlled hospital environment made it possible for the AA treatment to be administered and the dependent variables to be measured with less potential for error. Only participants with improved health conditions, transferred out of the ICU, were enrolled in the study to promote group similarity. The setting was controlled to ensure consistent implementation of the AA and measurement of the dependent variables. The AA was implemented for 2 weeks, which means it was probably started in the hospital and continued by the patients at home. Additional detail is needed to understand how the intervention (AA) was implemented in the home, and the dependent variables were consistently measured.

Highly Controlled Setting

A highly controlled setting is an environment structured for the purpose of conducting research. Laboratories, research or experimental centers, and training units in hospitals or other healthcare facilities are examples of highly controlled environments. This type of setting reduces the influence of extraneous variables, which enables researchers to accurately examine the effects of independent variables on dependent variables. Highly controlled settings are used infrequently in nursing studies.

Cheung and colleagues (2020) investigated the effects of healthcare simulation, provided in a laboratory or on a clinical unit, on the personal strengths of healthcare workers (HCWs) during the COVID-19 pandemic. A total of 1415 HCWs were trained in this study: 1167 nurses (82%), 163 doctors (12%), and 85 patient care assistants (6%). The clinical sites included emergency department, ICU, and general wards. The study setting is discussed in Research Example 9.15.

Highly Controlled Setting

Research/Study Excerpt

Healthcare simulation training replicates any clinical scenarios in a safe environment, bridging between immersive experience, acquired skills, and insights from the training and clinical practice. Not only had technical (e.g., cognitive and psychomotor skills in donning and doffing procedures of Personal Protective Equipment [PPE] in designated clean and dirty zone with buddy system) and nontechnical skills (e.g., teamwork,

RESEARCH EXAMPLE 9.15—cont'd

leadership and communication among HCWs) enhanced, simulation training, either "Lab-based" in simula-
tion training center or 'Insitu' in genuine clinical environment with highest environmental fidelity, could
strengthen personal qualities critical in healthcare industries…

 This crisis served as a precious opportunity for our center to preliminarily investigate whether in-situ
simulation would outweigh lab-based simulation in rating of personal strengths…To examine the study
hypothesis, participants were stratified into two groups: i) in-situ and ii) lab-based. (Cheung et al., 2020,
Healthcare simulation training section)

Critical Appraisal
Cheung et al. (2020) examined the effects of a highly controlled simulation laboratory versus clinical sites on
the HCWs personal strengths (knowledge and skills) in safely managing patients with COVID-19. A large
sample of different types of HCW were included in this study. Determining the best site for training HCWs is
important for improving clinical outcomes during the COVID-19 pandemic. The researchers found no significant
differences between lab-based and clinical sites for simulation training in safely caring for patients with
COVID-19. Thus both sites are effective for training HCWs.

KEY POINTS

- Sampling involves selecting a group of people, situations, behaviors, or other elements to study.
- Sampling theory was developed to determine the most effective way of acquiring a sample that accurately reflects the population being studied.
- Important sampling theory concepts described are population, sampling criteria, target population, accessible population, study elements, representativeness, randomization, sampling frame, and sampling method or plan.
- In quantitative and outcomes research, a sampling plan is developed to increase the representativeness of the target population and decrease sampling error or bias.
- The common probability sampling methods used in quantitative and outcomes research include simple random sampling, stratified random sampling, cluster sampling, and systematic sampling (see Table 9.1).
- Power analysis is an effective way to determine an adequate sample size for quantitative and outcomes studies. In power analysis, effect size, alpha ($\alpha = 0.05$), standard power (0.8 or 80%), and data analysis techniques are used to determine sample size.
- The nonprobability sampling methods discussed include convenience, quota, purposeful, network, and theoretical sampling (see Table 9.2).
- In qualitative and mixed methods research, a sampling plan is developed to increase the depth and richness of the findings related to the phenomenon, situation, processes, or cultural elements being studied.
- Purposeful, network, and theoretical sampling are used more often in qualitative research and the qualitative part of mixed methods studies.
- The number of participants in a qualitative study is adequate when saturation and verification of data are achieved for the study purpose and question.
- Three common settings for conducting nursing research are natural, partially controlled, and highly controlled.

REFERENCES

Aberson, C. L. (2019). *Applied analysis for the behavioral sciences* (2nd ed.). Routledge Taylor & Francis Group.

Ashford, K., McCubbin, A., Rayens, M. K., Wiggins, A., Dougherty, K., Sturgill, J., & Ickes, M. (2020). ENDS use among college students: Salivary biomarkers and persistent cough. *Addictive Behaviors, 108*, 106462. https://doi.org/10.1016/j.addbeh.2020.106462

Bandalos, D. L. (2018). *Measurement theory and applications for the social sciences.* The Guilford Press.

Bang, Y. Y., & Park, H. (2020). Effects of auricular acupressure on the quality of sleep and anxiety in patients undergoing cardiac surgery: A single-blind, randomized controlled trial. *Applied Nursing Research, 53*, 151269. https://doi.org/10.1016/j.apnr.2020.151269

Brauneis, L., Badowski, D., Maturin, L., & Simonovich, S. (2021). Impact of low-fidelity simulation-based experiences in a pharmacology classroom setting in prelicensure graduate nursing education. *Clinical Simulation in Nursing, 50*, 43–47. https://doi.org/10.1016/j.ecns.2020.10.002

Bryant, A., & Charmaz, K. (2019). *The Sage handbook of current developments of grounded theory.* Sage.

Cheung, V. K., So, E. H., Ng, G. W., So, S., Hung, J. L., & Chia, N. (2020). Investigating effects of healthcare simulation on personal strengths and organizational impacts for healthcare workers during COVID-19 pandemic: A cross-sectional study. *Integrative Medicine Research, 19*, 100476. https://doi.org/10.1016/j.imr.2020.100476

Cohen, J. (1988). *Statistical power analysis for the behavioral sciences* (2nd ed.). Academic Press.

CONSORT Group. (2010). *Welcome to the CONSORT website.* Retrieved from http://www.consort-statement.org

Creswell, J. W., & Clark, V. L. P. (2018). *Designing and conducting mixed methods research* (3rd ed.). Sage.

Creswell, J. W., & Poth, C. N. (2018). *Qualitative inquiry & research design: Choosing among five approaches* (4th ed.). Sage.

Crooks, N., Wise, A., & Frazier, T. (2020). Addressing sexually transmitted infections in the sociocultural context of black heterosexual relationships in the United States. *Social Science Medicine, 263*, 113303. https://doi.org/10.1016/j.socscimed.2020.113303

Edraki, M., Zarei, A., Soltanian, M., & Moravej, H. (2020). The effect of peer education on self-care behaviors and the mean of glycosylated hemoglobin in adolescents with type 1 diabetes: A randomized controlled clinical trial. *International Journal of Community Based Nursing and Midwifery, 8*(3), 209–219. https://doi.org/10.30476/ijcbnm.2020.82296.1051

Gray, J. R., & Grove, S. K. (2021). *The practice of nursing research: Appraisal, synthesis, and generation of evidence* (9th ed.). Elsevier.

Grove, S. K., & Cipher, D. J. (2020). *Statistics for nursing research: A workbook for evidence-based practice* (3rd ed.). Elsevier.

Kazdin, A. E. (2017). *Research design in clinical psychology* (5th ed.). Pearson.

Kraemer, H. C., & Blasey, C. (2016). *How many subjects? Statistical power analysis in research* (2nd ed.). Sage.

Lee, S. J., Kang, K. J., & Lee, J. H. (2021). Safe patient handling legislation and changes in programs, practices, perceptions, and experience of musculoskeletal disorders, by hospital characteristics: A repeated cross-sectional survey study. *International Journal of Nursing Studies, 113*, 103791. https://doi.org/10.1016/j.ijnurstu.2020.103791

Leedy, P. D., & Ormrod, J. E. (2019). *Practical research: Planning and design* (12th ed.) Pearson.

Marshall, C., & Rossman, G. B. (2016). *Designing qualitative research* (6th ed.). Sage.

Melnyk, B. M., & Fineout-Overholt, E. (2019). *Evidence-based practice in nursing & healthcare: A guide to best practice* (4th ed.). Wolters Kluwer.

Miles, M. B., Huberman, A. M., & Saldaña, J. (2020). *Qualitative data analysis: A methods sourcebook* (4th ed.). Sage.

Momeni, R., Hosseini, Z., Aghamolaei, T., & Ghanbarnejad, A. (2020). Determinant factors to Pap smear screening among married women in a city of South Iran: Applying the BASNEF model. *BMC Women's Health, 20*, 237. https://doi.org/10.1186/s12905-020-01102-6

Moorhead, S., Swanson, E., Johnson, M., & Maas, M. L. (2018). *Nursing Outcomes Classification (NOC): Measurement of health outcomes* (6th ed.). Elsevier.

Mulholland, E., Dahlberg, D., & McDowell, L. (2020). A two-front war: Exploring military families' battle with parental deployment. *Journal of Pediatric Nursing, 54*(1), 34–41. https://doi.org/10.1016/j.pedn.2020.05.019

Obradors-Rial, N., Ariza, C., Continente, X., & Muntaner, C. (2020). School and town factors associated with risky alcohol consumption among Catalan adolescents. *Alcohol, 82*, 71–79. https://doi.org/10.1016/j.alcohol.2019.04.005

Quality and Safety Education for Nurses (QSEN). (2020). *QSEN competencies: Prelicensure knowledge, skills, and attitudes (KSAs).* Retrieved from https://qsen.org/competencies/prelicensure-ksas/

Siedlecki, S. L., & Albert, N. M. (2020). The growth of nursing research within a large healthcare system. *Applied Nursing Research, 55*, 151291. https://doi.org/10.1016/j.apnr.2020.151291

Sok, S. (2009). A comparative study on the applied effects of auricular acupressure therapy on insomnia in the elderly by sasangin constitution: Based on tae yin in, so Yang in, and so yin in. *Journal of Korean Academy of Community Health Nursing, 20*, 327–334. http://dx.doi.org/10.12799/jkachn.2009.20.3.327

Spetz, J., Keane, D., & Herrera, C. (2011). *California Board of Registered Nursing 2010 Survey of Registered Nurses*. Retrieved from https://www.rn.ca.gov/pdfs/forms/survey2010npcnm.pdf

Tam, W., Lo, K., & Woo, B. (2020). Reporting sample size calculations for randomized controlled trials published in nursing journals: A cross-sectional study. *International Journal of Nursing Studies, 102*, 103450. https://doi.org/10.1016/j.ijnurstu.2019.103450

Taylor, J., & Spurlock, D. (2018). Methodology corner: Statistical power in nursing education research. *Journal of Nursing Education, 57*(5), 262–264. https://doi.org/10.3928/01484834-20180420-02

Waltz, C. F., Strickland, O. L., & Lenz, E. R. (2017). *Measurement in nursing and health research* (5th ed.). Springer Publishing Company.

CHAPTER

10

Clarifying Measurement and Data Collection in Quantitative Research

Susan K. Grove

LEARNING OUTCOMES

After completing this chapter, you should be able to:

1. Describe measurement theory and its relevant concepts of directness of measurement, levels of measurement, measurement error, reliability, and validity.
2. Determine the levels of measurement—nominal, ordinal, interval, and ratio—achieved by measurement methods in studies.
3. Critically appraise the reliability and validity of scales and questionnaires used in studies.
4. Critically appraise the accuracy, precision, and error of physiological measures in studies.

5. Critically appraise the sensitivity, specificity, negative predictive value, and likelihood ratios of screening tests used in research and clinical practice.
6. Critically appraise the measurement strategies—physiological measures, observations, interviews, questionnaires, and scales—used in quantitative and outcomes studies.
7. Critically appraise the data collection section in quantitative and outcomes studies.

Quality measurement of human functions, emotions, and behavior is essential in research and clinical practice. Measurement is the process of assigning numbers or values to concepts, behaviors, or situations using a set of rules. The rules of measurement established for research are similar to those used in nursing practice. For example, a patient's blood pressure (BP) is measured with physiological instruments (e.g., stethoscope, cuff, sphygmomanometer). Measuring a BP requires that the patient be allowed to rest for 5 minutes and then sit with his or her legs uncrossed and arm relaxed on a table at heart level. The BP cuff must be of accurate size and placed correctly on the upper arm that is free of restrictive clothing. In addition, the stethoscope must be correctly placed over the brachial artery at the elbow (Todkar et al., 2021; Weber et al., 2014). Following these rules ensures that the patient's BP is accurately and precisely measured, and that any change in the BP reading can be attributed to a change in BP, rather than to an inadvertent error in the measurement technique. In research, variables should be measured with the highest quality measurement method available to produce trustworthy data for statistical analysis. Quality results from data analyses produce credible research findings to guide nursing practice (Grove & Cipher, 2020; Melnyk & Fineout-Overholt, 2019).

Understanding the logic of measurement is important for critically appraising the adequacy of measurement methods in nursing studies. This chapter includes a discussion of the key concepts of measurement theory, with examples from nursing studies. The critical appraisal guidelines for the reliability and validity of scales and the accuracy, precision, and errors of physiological measures are applied to current studies. The sensitivity, specificity, and likelihood ratios (LRs) of screening tests are also addressed. The most common measurement methods or strategies used in nursing research are briefly described. The chapter concludes with guidelines for critically appraising the data collection process in nursing studies.

CONCEPTS OF MEASUREMENT THEORY

Measurement theory was developed many years ago by mathematicians, statisticians, and other scholars to guide the measurement process (Kaplan, 1963). The rules of measurement promote consistency in individuals' performance of measurements, so that an instrument used by one person will consistently produce similar results when used by another person. This section discusses some of the basic concepts and rules of measurement theory, including directness of measurement, levels of measurement, and measurement error. The concepts' reliability and validity will be covered in a separate section because of their complexity.

Directness of Measurement

Researchers must first identify the behavior, characteristic, or situation to be measured in their study. In some cases, identifying the characteristic to be measured and determining how to measure it are obvious, such as measuring a person's weight and height. These are referred to as direct measures. Direct measures involve determining the value of objective variables, such as waist circumference, temperature, heart rate (HR), and BP. Technology is available to measure many bodily functions, biological indicators, and chemical characteristics (Stone & Frazier, 2017). In these cases, the goal is to ensure the accuracy of the measurement method and the precision of the measurement process. If a patient's BP is to be accurate, it must be measured with quality equipment using a precise or consistent protocol, as discussed earlier. In research, three BP measurements are usually taken and averaged to determine the most accurate and precise BP reading (Todkar et al., 2021). Nurse researchers are also experienced in gathering direct measures of demographic variables, such as age, educational level, and days of hospitalization.

Often in nursing, the focus is on measuring abstract ideas, such as pain, depression, or adherence. Researchers cannot directly measure an abstract idea, but they can capture some of its elements in their measurements, which are referred to as indirect measures or indicators of the concept. Rarely, if ever, can a single measurement strategy capture all aspects of an abstract concept. Therefore multiple measurement methods or indicators are needed, and even then, they cannot be expected to measure all elements of an abstract concept (Bandalos, 2018). For example, multiple measurement methods might be used to describe pain in a study, which decreases the measurement error and increases the understanding of pain. The measurement methods of pain

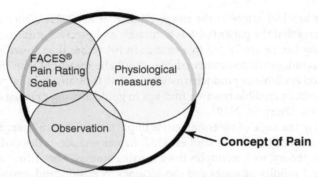

FIG. 10.1 Multiple Measures of the Concept of Pain.

may include the FACES® Pain Rating Scale (presented later); observation (rubbing and/or guarding the area that hurts, facial grimacing, and crying); and physiological measures, such as pulse, BP, and respiration.

Fig. 10.1 demonstrates how multiple measures of pain increase the understanding of the concept. The bold, black-rimmed largest circle represents the concept of pain, and the colored smaller circles represent the measurement methods. The physiological measures (pulse, BP, and respirations) are identified in a larger circle, representing the objective measures of pain. Even with three different types of measurement method used, the entire concept of pain is not measured, as indicated by the white areas within the black-rimmed circle (Gray & Grove, 2021).

Levels of Measurement

Various scales and physiological measures produce data that are at different levels of measurement. The traditional levels of measurement were developed by Stevens (1946), who organized the rules for assigning numbers to objects, so that a hierarchy in measurement was established. The levels of measurement, from low to high, are nominal, ordinal, interval, and ratio. The rules for these levels of measurement are summarized in Fig. 10.2.

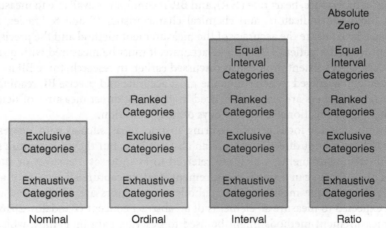

FIG. 10.2 Summary of the Rules for Levels of Measurement.

Nominal-Level Measurement

Nominal-level measurement, sometimes referred to as categorical data, is the lowest of the four measurement categories. With categorical data, the values are names or labels. The numbers are used as labels for each category. Gender, ethnicity/race, marital status, and diagnoses are common types of nominal data analyzed in research. Nominal data can be organized into categories of a defined property, but the categories cannot be rank-ordered. For example, researchers sometimes categorize study participants by medical diagnosis, such as diabetes, hypertension, and dyslipidemia. However, the category of diabetes cannot be rated or ranked as more serious than the category of hypertension; similarly, across categories, dyslipidemia is no more important than diabetes or hypertension. Some variables include only two values and are called dichotomous, such as the disease is present or not present in a patient. Table 10.1 includes some of the terms used in the literature to describe aspects of measurement.

With dichotomous and nominal data, the categories differ in quality, but not quantity, and follow selected rules. It is not possible to say that study participant A possesses more of the property being categorized than participant B. (**RULE:** The categories cannot be rank-ordered.) Categories must be established in such a way that each datum will fit into only one of the categories. (**RULE:** The categories must be exclusive.) For example, a study participant may have been widowed in the past but has remarried. If the demographic questionnaire included *Martial Status* and the categories of *Widowed* and *Married*, which would the individual select? In this situation, the researcher would need to redefine the variable to be *Current Marital Status* so that the categories are exclusive.

All the data must fit into the established categories (see Fig. 10.2). (**RULE:** The categories must be exhaustive.) The demographic questionnaire may include a variable called *Cardiac Diagnoses*, with the options of *Hypertension*, *Heart Failure*, and *Myocardial Infarction*. These options are not exhaustive because individuals with cardiomyopathy would not know what to mark. Researchers might add an *Other* category, making the *Cardiac Diagnoses* options exhaustive, but these data are difficult to analyze and interpret.

Ordinal-Level Measurement

With ordinal-level measurement, data are assigned to categories that can logically be put in order. (**RULE:** The categories can be ranked.) To rank data, one category is judged to be (or is ranked) higher or lower, or better or worse, than another category. With ordinal data, the quantity can be identified, as well as the categories being exclusive and exhaustive (see Fig. 10.2; Stevens, 1946). If you are measuring pain intensity, you could develop categories that rank these different levels of pain, such as no pain, mild, moderate, severe, or excruciating pain. However, in using categories of

TABLE 10.1   TERMS PERTAINING TO MEASUREMENT

TYPE OF VARIABLE	OTHER NAME	DESCRIPTION
Dichotomous	Binary	The variable has only two possible values.
Nominal[a]	Categorical	Numeric values are names or labels, not real numbers.
Continuous Discrete	Interval and Ratio Levels of Data Ordinal level data	Values use the real number scale, including the values between numerals. Numeric values that are not continuous.

[a]From the Latin *nomina*, which means "name."

BOX 10.1   SCALE FOR RATING DYSPNEA WITH ACTIVITIES OF DAILY LIVING

Rate your level of dyspnea in performing activities of daily living (ADLs) using the following scale:
0 = no shortness of breath with ADLs
1 = minimal shortness of breath with ADLs
2 = moderate shortness of breath with ADLs
3 = extreme shortness of breath with ADLs
4 = severe shortness of breath, person is unable to perform ADLs without assistance

---

ordinal measurement, you cannot know with certainty that the intervals between the ranked categories are equal. A greater difference may exist between severe and excruciating pain, for example, than between mild and moderate pain. This means the intervals between ordinal categories are unequal (Grove & Cipher, 2020).

Many scales and questionnaires used in nursing research produce ordinal-level data (Waltz et al., 2017). For example, it is possible to rank levels of mobility, ability to provide self-care, or levels of dyspnea on an ordinal scale. A scale for measuring dyspnea experienced with activities of daily living is presented in Box 10.1. As stated earlier, the measurement is ordinal because it is not possible to claim that equal distances exist between the rankings. A smaller difference may exist between the ranks of 1 and 2 than between the ranks of 3 and 4.

Interval-Level Measurement

Interval-level measurement exists when scales have equal numerical distances between the intervals. These scales follow the rules of mutually exclusive, exhaustive, and ranked categories and are assumed to represent a continuum of values (see Fig. 10.2). (**RULE:** The categories must have equal intervals between them.) Therefore the magnitude of the attribute can be more precisely defined. However, it is not possible to provide the absolute amount of the attribute because the interval scale lacks a zero point. Temperature is the most common example of an interval measure. The difference between the temperatures of 70° F and 80° F is 10° F and is the same as the difference between the temperatures of 30° F and 40° F. Changes in temperature can be measured precisely. However, a temperature of 0° F does not indicate the absence of temperature. Multi-item scales, such as a Likert scale to measure anxiety, also provide interval-level data (Waltz et al., 2017). These types of scale are discussed later in this chapter.

Ratio-Level Measurement

Ratio-level measurement is the highest form of measurement and meets all the rules of other forms of measurement: mutually exclusive categories, exhaustive categories, ordered ranks, equally spaced intervals, and a continuum of values. Interval- and ratio-level data are also referred to as continuous data because the data can be added, subtracted, multiplied, and divided because of the equal intervals and continuum of values (see Table 10.1). In addition, ratio-level measures have an absolute zero value, where a zero value indicates the absence of the property being measured. (**RULE:** The data must have an absolute zero [see Fig. 10.2].) Weight, height, and hemoglobin are examples of ratio measures with an absolute zero value. Because of the absolute zero value, such statements as "Participant A weighs 25 more pounds than participant B" or "Medication container A holds twice as much as container B" can be justified (Stevens, 1946). In addition, interval and ratio data can be analyzed with statistical techniques of greater power to determine significant relationships and differences in studies (Grove & Cipher, 2020; Leedy & Ormrod, 2019). In critically appraising a study, you need to determine the level of measurement achieved for each measurement method.

> **RESEARCH/EBP TIP**
>
> When measuring concepts or variables in research or clinical practice, the strongest measurement method should be used to achieve the highest level of measurement. Variables measured at the interval or ratio levels provide quality data for determining research results and making decisions in clinical practice.

Measurement Error

The ideal or perfect measure is referred to as the true measure or score. However, some error is always present in any measurement strategy. Measurement error is the difference between the actual true measure and what is measured (Gray & Grove, 2021). The amount of error in a measurement method varies from considerable error in one method to minimal in another. Direct measures, which generally are expected to be highly accurate, are subject to error. For example, a weight scale may be inaccurate by 0.5 pound, precisely calibrated BP equipment might decrease in accuracy with use, or a tape measure for measuring the waist of a patient may not be held at the same tension each time. A study participant may be 65 years old but may write illegibly on the demographic form, resulting in an inaccurate age being entered into the database.

With indirect measures, the element being measured cannot be seen directly. For example, you cannot see pain. You may observe behaviors or hear words that you think represent pain, but pain is a sensation that is not always clearly recognized or expressed by the person experiencing it. The measurement of pain is usually conducted with a scale but can also include observation and physiological measures. Sometimes measures may identify some aspects of the concept but may include other elements that are not part of the concept. In Fig. 10.1, the measurement methods of scale, observation, and physiological measures include factors other than pain, as indicated by the parts of the colored circles that are outside the black-rimmed circle of the concept pain. For example, the instruments used for measuring pain might be capturing aspects of anxiety and fear in addition to pain. However, measuring a concept with multiple methods usually decreases measurement error and increases the understanding of the concept.

Two types of error are of concern in measurement: random error and systematic error. The difference between random and systematic error is in the direction of the error. In random measurement error, the difference between the measured value and the true value is without pattern or direction (random). In one measurement, the value obtained may be lower than the true value, whereas in the next measurement, the value obtained may be higher than the true value. A number of chance situations or factors can occur during the measurement process that can result in random error (Waltz et al., 2017). For example, the person taking the measurements may not use the same procedure every time, a study participant completing a scale may accidentally mark the wrong column, or the person entering the data into a computer may punch the wrong key. The purpose of measuring is to estimate the true value, usually by combining several measurements and calculating an average. An average value, such as the mean, is a closer estimate of the true measurement. As the number of random errors increases, the precision of the estimate decreases.

Measurement error that is not random is referred to as systematic error. In systematic measurement error, the variation in measurement values from the calculated average is primarily in the same direction. For example, most of the variation may be higher or lower than the average that was calculated. Systematic error occurs because something else is being measured in addition to the concept. For example, a rating scale designed to measure hope may actually also be measuring perceived support. When measuring participants' weights, a scale that shows weights that are 1 pound over the true weights include systematic error. All the measured weights will be higher than the true weight, and as a result the mean will be higher than if an accurate weight scale had been used.

In critically appraising a study, you will not be able to judge the extent of measurement error directly. However, you may find clues about the amount of measurement error in the published report. For example, if the researchers have described the method of measurement in great detail and have provided evidence of accuracy and precision of the measurement, then the probability of error typically is reduced. The measurement errors for BP readings can be minimized by checking the BP sphygmomanometer for accuracy and recalibrating it periodically during data collection, obtaining three BP readings and averaging them to determine one BP reading for each participant, and having a trained nurse using a protocol to take the BP readings. If a checklist of pain behaviors is developed for observation, less error occurs than if the observations for pain are unstructured. Measurement will also be more precise if researchers describe using a reliable and valid scale, such as the FACES® Pain Rating Scale, instead of developing a new pain scale for their study. You need to critically appraise the steps researchers have taken to decrease measurement error in their studies (Bandalos, 2018; Waltz et al., 2017).

RELIABILITY AND VALIDITY OF SCALES AND QUESTIONNAIRES

The Methods section of a research report identifies the scales or questionnaires used in a study. When using scales or questionnaires to measure variables, researchers need to report the scoring process, reliability, and validity for each scale. The scoring process for a scale is unique to each scale, and if a scale is revised, its scoring process must also be updated. Review the discussion of each scale and determine whether the scoring process and the meaning of the scores are clearly presented. The Center for Epidemiologic Studies Depression Scale (CES-D) is presented in Fig. 10.3, which includes the instructions for completing the scale and the scoring process. "The CES-D includes 20 depressive symptoms that are to be rated on a 4-point Likert scale (0–3): 0—*rarely or none of the time,* 1—*some or a little of the time,* 2—*occasionally or a moderate amount of time,* 3—*all of the time.* The range of the total score is between 0 and 60, with higher scores indicating greater levels of depression. A CES-D score ≥16 has been identified as an indicator of depression (Radloff, 1977)" (Cosco et al., 2017, p. 478).

When describing the instruments used in a study, researchers also need to document the reliability and validity of the instrument based on previous studies and the current study. The following sections present the different types of reliability and validity often reported for scales in nursing studies. The readability of items on a scale is also covered, because participants must be able to read and understand a scale for it to be reliable and valid in a study.

Reliability

Reliability focuses on the consistency of a measurement method. A scale must be reliable to obtain consistent measures of concepts or variables in research and clinical practice. For example, if you use a multiple-item scale to measure depression, the scale should indicate similar depression scores each time an individual completes it within a limit timeframe (Bandalos, 2018; Waltz et al., 2017). For example, the CES-D was developed through extensive research to diagnose depression in mental health patients (Radloff, 1977). Although CES-D was developed for research purposes, this scale is frequently used to screen individuals at risk for clinical depression (Cosco et al., 2017; Jiang et al.,

Center for Epidemiologic Studies Depression Scale DEPA

THESE QUESTIONS ARE ABOUT HOW YOU HAVE BEEN FEELING LATELY.
AS I READ THE FOLLOWING STATEMENTS, PLEASE TELL ME HOW OFTEN YOU FELT OR BEHAVED THIS WAY
IN THE **LAST WEEK**. [*Hand card*]. **FOR EACH STATEMENT, DID YOU FEEL THIS WAY:**
[Interviewer: You may help respondent focus on the whichever "style" answer is easier]
        0 = **R**arely or none of the time (or less than 1 day)?
        1 = **S**ome or a little of the time (or 1–2 days)?
        2 = **O**ccasionally or a moderate amount of time (or 3–4 days)?
        3 = **M**ost or all of the time (or 5–7 days)?

	R	S	O	M	NR
1. I WAS BOTHERED BY THINGS THAT USUALLY DON'T BOTHER ME.	0	1	2	3	--
2. I DID NOT FEEL LIKE EATING; MY APPETITE WAS POOR.	0	1	2	3	--
3. I FELT THAT I COULD NOT SHAKE OFF THE BLUES EVEN WITH HELP FROM MY FAMILY AND FRIENDS.	0	1	2	3	--
4. I FELT THAT I WAS JUST AS GOOD AS OTHER PEOPLE.	0	1	2	3	--
5. I HAD TROUBLE KEEPING MY MIND ON WHAT I WAS DOING.	0	1	2	3	--
6. I FELT DEPRESSED.	0	1	2	3	--
7. I FELT THAT EVERYTHING I DID WAS AN EFFORT.	0	1	2	3	--
8. I FELT HOPEFUL ABOUT THE FUTURE.	0	1	2	3	--
9. I THOUGHT MY LIFE HAD BEEN A FAILURE.	0	1	2	3	--
10. I FELT FEARFUL.	0	1	2	3	--
11. MY SLEEP WAS RESTLESS.	0	1	2	3	--
12. I WAS HAPPY.	0	1	2	3	--
13. I TALKED LESS THAN USUAL.	0	1	2	3	--
14. I FELT LONELY.	0	1	2	3	--
15. PEOPLE WERE UNFRIENDLY.	0	1	2	3	--
16. I ENJOYED LIFE.	0	1	2	3	--
17. I HAD CRYING SPELLS.	0	1	2	3	--
18. I FELT SAD.	0	1	2	3	--
19. I FELT PEOPLE DISLIKED ME.	0	1	2	3	--
20. I COULD NOT GET GOING.	0	1	2	3	--

FIG. 10.3 Center for Epidemiologic Studies Depression Scale (CES-D). (Adapted from Radloff, L. S. [1977]. The CES-D scale: A self-report depression scale for research in the general population. *Applied Psychological Measurement, 1*[3], 385394.)

2019; Kagee et al., 2020). The CES-D has been used nationally and internationally to measure depression in adults and has been revised (CES-R) to include 10 items for measuring depression in children, adolescents, and elderly adults. If the items on this scale consistently measure what they were developed to measure (depression), then this scale is considered to be both reliable and valid. The types of reliability and validity testing outlined in Table 10.2 are discussed in the following sections, and the CES-D is used as an example.

TABLE 10.2   EXAMINING THE RELIABILITY AND VALIDITY OF SCALES AND QUESTIONNAIRES

QUALITY INDICATOR	DESCRIPTION
Reliability	**Stability reliability:** Focused on the reproducibility of scores with repeated measures of the same concept with an instrument over time. Stability is usually examined with **test-retest reliability.**
	Equivalence reliability: Consistency of observers and alternate forms in measuring selected concepts. Includes interrater reliability and alternate forms of reliability.
	Interrater reliability: Comparison of two observers or raters in a study to determine their equivalence in making observations or rating situations.
	Alternate forms reliability: Correlation between different forms of the same instrument to determine their equivalence in measuring a concept.
	Internal consistency: Degree of homogeneity or consistency of the items within a multi-item scale. Each item on a scale is correlated with all other items to determine the consistency of an instrument in measuring a concept. Cronbach alpha coefficient is the statistic frequently reported for internal consistency of a multi-item scale.
Validity	**Content validity:** Examines the extent to which an instrument includes all the major elements relevant to the construct being measured.
	Face validity: Verifies that an instrument looks like it is valid or gives the appearance of measuring the construct for which it was developed.
	Construct validity: Focuses on determining whether the instrument actually measures the theoretical construct that it purports to measure, which involves examining the fit between the conceptual and operational definitions of a variable.
	Validity from contrasting (known) groups: Instrument or scale given to two groups expected to have opposite or contrasting scores; one group scores high on the scale and the other scores low.
	Convergent validity: Two scales measuring the same concept are administered to a group at the same time, and the participants' scores on the scales should be positively correlated. For example, participants completing two scales to measure depression should have positively correlated scores.
	Divergent validity: Two scales that measure opposite concepts, such as hope and hopelessness, are administered to participants at the same time and should result in negatively correlated scores on the scales.
	Validity from factor analysis: Analysis techniques conducted to identify the various dimensions or subconcepts of the construct being measured that are represented as subscales in the scale.
	Criterion-related validity: Validity that is strengthened when a study participant's score on an instrument can be used to infer his or her performance on another variable or criterion.
	Predictive validity: Extent to which an individual's score on a scale or instrument can be used to predict future performance or behavior on a criterion.
	Concurrent validity: Focuses on the extent to which an individual's score on an instrument or scale can be used to estimate his or her present or concurrent performance on another variable or criterion.
Readability	**Readability level:** Approximate level of education required to comprehend a given piece of text. Researchers need to report the level of education needed to read the items on an instrument used in a study. Readability must be appropriate to promote the reliability and validity of an instrument in a population.

Reliability Testing

Reliability testing determines the measurement error in an instrument used in a study (Waltz et al., 2017). Because all measurement methods contain some error, reliability exists in degrees and is usually expressed as a correlation coefficient. *Estimates of reliability are specific to the sample being tested.* High reliability values reported for an established instrument do not guarantee that reliability will be satisfactory in another sample or with a different population. Researchers need to perform reliability testing on each instrument used in a study to ensure that it is reliable for that study population (Bialocerkowski et al., 2010; Waltz et al., 2017). Reliability testing focuses on the stability, equivalence, and internal consistency of scales used in research (see Table 10.2).

Stability Reliability

Stability reliability is concerned with the reproducibility of scores with repeated measures of the same concept or attribute with a scale over time. Basically, does the instrument measure the concept consistently over time? Instrument stability is usually determined using test-retest reliability. An assumption of test-retest reliability is that the attribute to be measured remains fairly stable from one testing time to another. A well-constructed scale can yield high test-retest or stability with values of 0.60 to 0.70. However, the values vary based on the participants and the length of time between administering the scale. A stability value ≥ 0.50 is relatively low but is considered acceptable by many researchers (Bandalos, 2018). For example, the CES-D (see Fig. 10.3) has demonstrated stability reliability values ranging from $r = 0.45$ to $r = 0.70$ in 2- to 8-week intervals. These values indicate that the CES-D is consistently measuring a phenomenon with repeat testing, recognizing that participants' levels of depression vary somewhat over time (Armenta et al., 2014; Cosco et al., 2017). You need to review the Methods section of published studies to ensure stability values from previous studies and possibly the current study are reported for the scales used.

Equivalence Reliability

Reliability testing also includes equivalence, which involves the comparison of two versions of an instrument or of two observers measuring the same behavior or event. Comparison of two observers or judges in a study is referred to as interrater reliability (Waltz et al., 2017). Do multiple raters measure the same concept consistently in a study? Studies that include collecting observational data or the making of judgments by two or more data collectors require the reporting of interrater reliability. There is no absolute value below which interrater reliability is unacceptable (Bialocerkowski et al., 2010). However, any value less than 0.80 should generate serious concern about the reliability of the data, data collectors, or both. The interrater reliability value is best at a value of 0.90 or higher, which means that the data collectors are 90% equivalent during the study (Gray & Grove, 2021).

Comparison of two instruments or scales measuring the same concept is referred to as alternate or equivalent forms reliability. You need to question whether the concept is measured consistently across alternate forms. Alternative forms of instruments are important in the development of normative knowledge testing, such as the Scholastic Aptitude Test (SAT) that is often used as a college entrance requirement. The SAT has been used for decades, and there are many forms of this test, with a variety of items included on each. These alternate forms of the SAT were developed to measure students' knowledge consistently and to protect the integrity of the test. The coefficients of equivalence for standardized tests should be at least 0.80, with strong values approaching ≥ 0.90 (Bandalos, 2018).

Internal Consistency

Internal consistency, also known as homogeneity reliability testing, is used primarily with multi-item scales, in which each item on a scale is correlated with all other items on the scale to determine consistency (see Table 10.2). The principle is that each item should be consistently measuring a concept and, therefore, should be highly correlated with the other items on the scale. The Cronbach alpha coefficient is most commonly calculated to determine the internal reliability for scales with multiple items. This alpha coefficient can be calculated only for interval- and ratio-level data. A coefficient of 1.00 indicates perfect reliability, and a coefficient of 0.00 indicates no reliability (Bandalos, 2018). The stronger correlation coefficients that are closer to 1.0 indicate less random error and a more reliable scale. A reliability of 0.80 is usually considered a strong coefficient for a scale that has been used in a variety of studies. For relatively new scales, a reliability of 0.70 is considered acceptable because the scale is being examined as it is used with different samples (Kerlinger & Lee, 2000). The CES-D has strong internal consistency, with Cronbach alpha coefficients ranging from 0.85 to 0.90 in field studies of adults (Jiang et al., 2019; Locke & Putnam, 2002). Cosco et al. (2017) examined the reliability of the CES-D scale in a population of 1233 middle-aged U.S. adults and found the Cronbach coefficient to be 0.90.

If the data are dichotomous (yes or no responses), the Kuder-Richardson formula (KR-20) is used to estimate internal consistency. The closer the KR-20 reliability value is to 1 the stronger the reliability, but a score ≥ 0.50 is considered acceptable; however, values vary based on the scales used (Bandalos, 2018; Kerlinger & Lee, 2000). A research report should include the results from stability, equivalence, and/or internal consistency reliability testing conducted on a scale from *previous research* and in the *present study.*

Validity

The validity of an instrument indicates how well it measures the abstract concept it was developed to measure. Validity, like reliability, is not an all-or-nothing phenomenon; it is measured on a continuum. No instrument is completely valid, so researchers determine the degree of validity of an instrument rather than whether validity exists (Waltz et al., 2017). Validity will vary from one sample to another and one situation to another; therefore validity testing evaluates the use of an instrument for a population or purpose, rather than the instrument itself. An instrument may be valid in one situation but not another. For example, the original CES-D was developed to measure the depression of patients in mental health settings. Will the same scale be valid as a measure of depression in healthy adults? Researchers examined the validity of the CES-D in different populations and found it to be strong. In addition, different versions of the CES-D were developed and found to be valid in measuring depression in young children (4–6 years of age), school-age children, adolescents, and older adults (Armenta et al., 2014; Cosco et al., 2017; Jiang et al., 2019; Locke & Putnam, 2002).

The validity of measurement methods has been determined using a variety of techniques; however, this chapter will focus on those most commonly reported in nursing studies. Therefore content validity, construct validity, and criterion validity are described (see Table 10.2; Bandalos, 2018; Waltz et al., 2017). Content validity examines the extent to which the measurement method includes all the major elements or items relevant to the construct or concept being measured. The evidence for content validity of a scale includes: (1) how well the items of the scale reflect the description of the concept in the literature (face validity), (2) the content experts' evaluation of the relevance of items on the scale that might be reported as an index, and (3) the study participants' responses to scale items (Bandalos, 2018). Face validity is part of content validity and verifies that an instrument looks like it is valid or gives the appearance of measuring the construct for which it was developed. Face validity is a subjective judgment that might be made by researchers, expert clinicians, or even potential study participants. Face validity is considered the weakest form of validity but is useful in determining participants' willingness to complete a scale. To obtain a content validity index score, researchers send the scale to experts on the topic and ask them to rate each item on the scale for relevance and to make suggestions for changes in wording. Researchers can calculate a content validity index score based on the experts' input. Gray and Grove (2021) provide formulas for calculating these indexes.

Construct Validity

Construct validity focuses on determining whether the instrument actually measures the theoretical construct it purports to measure, which involves examining the fit between the conceptual and operational definitions of a variable (see Chapter 5). Four common types of construct validity presented in nursing studies include evidence of validity from (1) contrasting groups, (2) convergence, (3) divergence, and (4) factor analysis. An instrument's evidence of validity from contrasting groups can be tested by identifying groups that are expected (or known) to have contrasting scores on an instrument. For example, researchers select samples from a group of individuals with a diagnosis of depression and from a group that does not have this diagnosis. You would expect these two groups of individuals to have contrasting scores on the CES-D. The greater the score for a person completing the CES-D the more severe is the person's depression. Therefore the group with the diagnosis of depression would be expected to have higher scores (≥ 16) than those without the depression diagnosis.

Evidence of validity from convergence is determined when a relatively new or revised instrument is compared with an existing instrument(s) that measures the same construct. The two instruments are administered to a sample at the same time, and the results are evaluated with correlational analyses. If the scales have strong positive correlation values, the validity of each instrument is strengthened. For example, the CES-D has shown positive correlations ranging from 0.40 to 0.80 with the Hamilton Rating Scale for Depression (Sharp & Lipsky, 2002). Jiang et al. (2019) correlated the responses of 2068 university student responses on a 14-item CES-D with those on the Beck Depression Inventory-II and found a convergent validity value of 0.744. Thus the CES-D has documented convergent validity with the Hamilton Scale for Depression and the Beck Depression Inventory-II.

Sometimes instruments can be located that measure a concept opposite to the concept measured by an existing instrument. For example, if an instrument was developed to measure hope, you could search for an instrument that measures hopelessness or despair. Having study participants complete these scales, which measure opposite concepts, at the same time is a way to examine evidence of validity from divergence. Correlational procedures are performed with the measures of the two concepts. If the divergent measure (hopelessness scale) is negatively correlated (e.g., -0.4 to -0.8) with the other instrument (hope scale), the construct validity of both scales is supported (Waltz et al., 2017).

Validity from factor analysis is a type of construct validity that involves the use of statistical techniques to determine the various dimensions or subcomponents of a construct of interest. To use factor analysis, the instrument must be administered to a large, representative sample of participants at one time. Usually the data are initially analyzed with exploratory factor analysis to examine relationships among the various items of the instrument (Bandalos, 2018; Waltz et al., 2017). Scale items that are closely related are clustered into a factor. Determining and naming the factors identified through exploratory factor analysis require detailed work on the part of the researcher. Researchers can validate the number of factors or subcomponents in the instrument through the use of confirmatory factor analysis (CFA). The factors confirmed through CFA are the subconcepts of a scale that can be examined in a study. Cosco et al. (2017) conducted a CFA of the 20-item CES-D scale and found it to include four subconcepts: (1) depressed affect, (2) somatic/vegetative factors, (3) positive affect, and (4) interpersonal. This four-factor structure is consistent with the original work conducted by Radloff (1977).

Criterion-Related Validity

Criterion-related validity is strengthened when a study participant's score on an instrument can be used to infer his or her performance or status on another variable or criterion. The two types of criterion-related validity are predictive and concurrent validity (see Table 10.2). Predictive validity is the extent to which an individual's score on a scale or instrument can be used to predict future performance or behavior on a criterion (Bandalos, 2018; Waltz et al., 2017). For example, nurse researchers might want to determine the ability of a scale developed to measure health promotion nutrition behaviors to predict individuals' future body mass index.

Concurrent validity focuses on the extent to which an individual's score on an instrument or scale can be used to estimate his or her present or concurrent performance on another variable or criterion. For example, concurrent validity could be examined if you measured individuals' self-esteem scores and correlated them with current coping behaviors used to manage their type 2 diabetes. Individuals with high scores on a self-esteem scale would be expected to have more coping behaviors. The difference between concurrent validity and predictive validity is the timing of the measurement of the other criterion. Concurrent validity is examined within a short period, and predictive validity is examined in terms of future performance.

As discussed earlier, the evidence of an instrument's validity from previous research and the current study should be included in the research report. In some studies, researchers simply state that the scale or questionnaire has acceptable validity based on previous research. This statement provides insufficient information for you to judge the validity of an instrument. Specific information about validity must be provided for you to critically appraise the measurement methods used in a study. In addition, you cannot consider validity apart from reliability (see Table 10.2). If an instrument does not have acceptable reliability, then it is not valid.

📄 **RESEARCH/EBP TIP**

Scales and questionnaires developed through research are often used to screen individuals for clinical conditions, such as anxiety, stress, and depression. The scales used in clinical practice should have strong reliability values (0.85–0.95) and quality validity to ensure consistent, accurate assessment, diagnosis, and management of conditions in patients.

Readability Level of Measurement Methods

Readability level is the approximate educational level required to comprehend written information. Researchers need to report the educational level needed for participants to read and understand the items on an instrument used in a study. Assessing the level of readability of an instrument is relatively simple and takes about 10 to 15 minutes. Readability formulas use counts of language elements, such as the number of syllabi per word and the number of words per sentence, to provide an index of the probable degree of difficulty of comprehending the items on a scale (Gray & Grove, 2021). Readability formulas are now a standard part of word processing software, so researchers could easily determine and report the readability levels of the scales and questionnaires used in their studies. For example, Misra et al. (2021) examined the readability level of the caregiver education for tracheostomy and home mechanical ventilation provided through a website. The National Institutes of Health and the American Medical Association recommend a fourth- to sixth-grade reading level for patient education materials.

? CRITICAL APPRAISAL GUIDELINES

Reliability and Validity of Scales and Questionnaires

In most studies, the Methods section includes a discussion of measurement methods, and you can use the following questions to critically appraise them:
1. What measurement method(s) were used to measure each study variable?
2. Was the type of measurement direct or indirect?
3. What level of measurement was achieved for each of the study variables (see Fig. 10.1)?
4. Was the process for obtaining, scoring, and/or recording data described? Was the meaning of the scores on each instrument addressed?
5. Was reliability information provided from previous studies and for this study (see Table 10.2)?
6. Was the validity of each instrument adequately described (see Table 10.2)?
7. Was the readability level of the scale used in the study discussed? Was the level appropriate for the study population?

Rapp and colleagues (2021) conducted a longitudinal study to predict the effect of parental criticism on adolescent depression. They "hypothesized that high perceived parental criticism would be associated with more severe depression over 18-months of follow-up" (Rapp et al., 2021, p. 46). The scales used to measure depression and distress in this study are described in Research Example 10.1.

RESEARCH EXAMPLE 10.1

Scoring, Reliability, and Validity of Scales

Research/Study Excerpt
Depression

The CES-D (Radloff, 1977) is a 20-item self-report measure rating depression symptoms during the past week with strong internal consistency in the present sample (Cronbach's α = 0.89 to 0.90, across all three follow-up time points). CES-D scores were available at posttreatment (six months from baseline), 12-month follow-up, and 18-month follow-up. Consistent with prior reports on the YPIC [Youth Partners in Care] trial (Asarnow et al., 2009), continuous CES-D scores were dichotomized using established criteria such that CES-D scores ≥ 24 were considered to represent severe depression (Robert et al., 1991). This was the primary outcome for the present study.

Distress

The Mental Health Index-5 (MHI-5) ... is an established measure consisting of the five items that best reproduced the summary score for the 38-item Mental Health Inventory used in the Medical Outcomes Study. The five items ask about the frequency with which the youth feels: calm and peaceful; downhearted and blue; very nervous; happy; and so down in the dumps that nothing can cheer them up. Items are rated on a scale from 1 ('All of the Time') to 6 ('None of the Time'), resulting in lower scores reflecting greater

Continued

RESEARCH EXAMPLE 10.1—cont'd

emotional distress and higher scores reflecting greater levels of emotional well-being. As expected, given that three of the five items assess depressive symptoms, the MHI-5 and CES-D scores were highly correlated in the present sample (r = −0.73 to −0.79, p < 0.001, across all three follow-up time points). The MHI-5 was administered at all study time points and demonstrated strong internal consistency in the present sample (α = 0.77 to 0.80, across all four time points [baseline and three follow-up assessments]). (Rapp et al., 2021, p. 48)

Critical Appraisal

Rapp et al. (2021) detailed the scoring process and the meaning of the scores for both the CES-D and MHI-5 scales used in their study. The CES-D was an indirect, multi-item scale used to measure depression that produced interval-level data (Bandalos, 2018). The internal reliability of this scale was strong in this study, but additional information is needed about the reliability and validity of this scale from previous research. The researchers identified that a score ≥24 was a criterion for diagnosing *severe depression*, which provides a basis for assessing *severe depression* in clinical practice (criterion-related validity).

The researchers identified the content covered by the MHI-5, supporting the scale's content validity. Three of the items from the MHI-5 focused on depression and were significantly correlated with the CES-D scores (r = −0.73 to −0.79, p < 0.001). These strong negative correlation values indicate that as the CES-D depression scores increased the MHI-5 scores decreased based on how the items were scored. The correlation of the scores from these two scales added to the convergent validity of both scales that measured aspects of depression. The MHI-5 also had internal consistency reliability across the four points of measurement. The CES-D and MHI-5 were reliable and valid scales for measuring the variables in the study. However, the measurement section of the study would have been strengthened by providing information about the scales from previous research. Rapp et al. (2021) found that parental criticism was a strong predictor of youth depression over the 18 months of their study. The researchers recommended clinicians assess adolescents for depression (CES-D scores ≥16 or severe depression ≥24) so treatments might be implemented early.

ACCURACY, PRECISION, AND ERROR OF PHYSIOLOGICAL MEASURES

Physiological measures are instruments used to quantify the level of functioning of human beings (Ryan-Wenger, 2017). Laboratory tests and biomedical devices are used to measure biophysical constructs, such as oxygen saturation in research and practice. Physiological measures usually produce ratio-level data. The precision, accuracy, and error of physiological and biochemical measures often are not reported or are minimally covered in published studies. These routine physiological measures are assumed to be accurate and precise, an assumption that is not always correct. Some of the most common physiological measures used in nursing studies include BP, oxygen saturation, temperature, and laboratory values. Sometimes researchers obtain these measures from patients' records with no consideration given to their accuracy. For example, how many times have you heard a nurse ask a patient his or her height or weight, rather than measuring or weighing the patient? Researchers using physiological measures should provide evidence of the measure's accuracy, precision, and potential for error (Table 10.3; Connor, 2021; Ryan-Wenger, 2017).

Accuracy

Accuracy is comparable with validity in that it addresses the extent to which the instrument measures what it is supposed to measure in a study (Ryan-Wenger, 2017). For example, oxygen saturation measurements with pulse oximetry are considered comparable with measures of oxygen

TABLE 10.3	DETERMINING THE QUALITY OF PHYSIOLOGICAL MEASURES
QUALITY INDICATOR	**DESCRIPTION**
Accuracy	Addresses the extent to which the physiological instrument or equipment measures what it is supposed to in a study. The focus is on the agreement between the measured value and the true or actual value of a physiological variable. Often compared with a criterion or gold standard measurement.
Precision	Degree of consistency or reproducibility of the measurements made with physiological instruments or equipment on the same variables under specified conditions. The smaller the change sensed in the instrument the greater is the precision of the instrument.
Error	Sources of error in physiological measures can be grouped into the following five categories: (1) environment, (2) user, (3) study participant, (4) equipment, and (5) interpretation.

saturation with arterial blood gases. Because pulse oximetry is an accurate measure of oxygen saturation, it has been used in studies because it is easier, less expensive, less painful, and less invasive for study participants. Researchers need to document that previous research has been conducted to determine the accuracy of pulse oximetry for the measurement of an individual's oxygen saturation level. Pulse oximeter also is used frequently in clinical practice to document a patients' oxygen saturation in a variety of healthcare settings.

Precision

Precision is the degree of consistency or reproducibility of measurements made with physiological instruments. The precision of most physiological equipment depends on following the manufacturer's instructions for care and routine testing of the equipment. Test-retest reliability is appropriate for measuring physiological variables that have minimal fluctuations, such as lipid levels, bone mineral density, or weight of adults (Connor, 2021; Ryan-Wenger, 2017). Test-retest reliability can be inappropriate if the variables' values frequently fluctuate with various activities, such as with pulse, respirations, and BP. However, test-retest is a good measure of precision if the measurements are taken in rapid succession. As discussed earlier, national BP guidelines encourage taking three BP readings 1 to 2 minutes apart and then averaging them to obtain the most precise and accurate measure of BP (Todkar et al., 2021).

Error

Sources of error in physiological measures can be grouped into the five categories: environment, user, study participant, equipment, and interpretation (see Table 10.3). The environment affects the equipment and study participant. Environmental factors may include temperature, barometric pressure, and static electricity. User errors are caused by the person using the equipment and may be associated with variations by the same user, different users, or changes in supplies or procedures used to operate the equipment. Participant errors occur when the individual alters the equipment or the equipment alters the individual. For example, inserting an arterial line in a patient alters the pressure in a patient's artery. In some cases, the equipment may not be used to its full capacity because of lack of knowledge. Equipment error may be related to calibration or the stability of the equipment. Signals transmitted from the equipment are also a source of error and can result in misinterpretation. Researchers need to report the protocols followed or steps taken to prevent errors in their use of physiological and biochemical measures in their studies (Ryan-Wenger, 2017; Stone & Frazier, 2017).

❓ CRITICAL APPRAISAL GUIDELINES

Accuracy, Precision, and Error of Physiological Measures

The Methods section includes a discussion of the physiological measure(s) used in a study, and you can use the following questions to evaluate them.

1. What instrument(s) were used to measure physiological variables?
2. What level of measurement was achieved when measuring each of the physiological variables?
3. Did the researchers address the accuracy of each physiological measure based on manufacturers' data and previous research?
4. Did the researchers address the precision of each physiological measure based on manufacturers' data and previous research?
5. Was the process for obtaining, scoring, and/or recording data described?
6. Did the researchers provide an adequate description of the measurement methods to judge the extent of measurement error?

Low vitamin D levels, measured by serum 25-hydroxyvitamin D [(25-OH)D], has been associated with depression, but research among minorities is limited in this area. Therefore Sahasrabudhe and colleagues (2020) conducted a correlational study to examine the association between serum 25(OH)D values and reported depressive symptoms, measured by CES-D, among Puerto Rican adults residing in Massachusetts. The measurement of serum 25(OH)D in this study is described in Research Example 10.2.

🔍 RESEARCH EXAMPLE 10.2

Accuracy, Precision, and Error of Physiological Measures

Research/Study Excerpt

Vitamin D [serum 25(OH)D] measures

Serum concentration of 25(OH)D (in nanograms per milliliter) was assessed in fasting blood samples at baseline. Fasting blood samples were processed and transported on ice, within 3 hours, to the Nutrition Evaluation Laboratory, Jean Mayer USDA [US Department of Agriculture] Human Nutrition Research Center on Aging at Tufts University. 25(OH)D was measured with an I-125 RIA kit (DiaSorin Inc.) as per manufacturer's specifications (68100E). The RIA has been shown to have similar sensitivity and specificity to LC/MS-MS [another measure of vitamin D] and was chosen due to its availability when this measurement was performed. The intra- and interassay ... for these measurements were 10.8% and 9.4%, respectively. We used serum 25(OH)D cut-off points suggested by the Food and Nutrition Board (FNB) at the National Academies of Science, Engineering and Medicine, classifying concentration 20 ng/mL (≥50 nmol/L) as sufficient, <12ng/mL (<30 nmol/L) as deficient, and 12 to <20 ng/mL (30 to <50 nmol/L) as insufficient. (Sahasrabudhe et al., 2020, pp. 3232–3233)

Critical Appraisal

Sahasrabudhe et al. (2020) provided a detail description of how the 25(OH)D serum samples were obtained, transported, and analyzed according to national standards. These detailed descriptions support the accuracy

> **$\boxed{\mathsf{S}}$ RESEARCH EXAMPLE 10.2—cont'd**
>
> and precision of the 25(OH)D values obtained in this study and reduced the potential for error. The researchers provided the values for classifying the serum 25(HO)D concentrations as sufficient, deficient, and insufficient. These classifications also were based on national standards.
>
>   Sahasrabudhe et al. (2020) did not find a significant association between the serum 25(HO)D values and depressive symptoms reported by Puerto Ricans from the Boston area over 5 years. However, they did indicate that their findings should not "alter the public health and clinical recommendation regarding the importance of maintaining sufficient vitamin D status for general health. Further studies are needed on the role for vitamin D in depression in diverse populations" (Sahasrabudhe et al., 2020, p. 3238).

SENSITIVITY, SPECIFICITY, AND LIKELIHOOD RATIOS

An important part of evidence-based practice (EBP) is the use of quality diagnostic tests or screening tools to determine the presence or absence of disease (Straus et al., 2019). You need to know which laboratory test or imaging study is best for diagnosing specific diseases or predicting an outcome (Connor, 2021). When a screening tool is used or a test conducted, are the results accurate? The accuracy of a screening test is evaluated in terms of its ability to predict or confirm the presence or absence of a condition correctly compared with the criterion or gold standard. The criterion standard is the most accurate means of currently predicting or diagnosing a particular condition or current best practice (Umberger et al., 2017). This standard serves as a basis for comparison with newly developed screening tests or the use of existing tests for diagnosing a new condition. If the test is positive, what is the probability that the disease or condition is present? If the test is negative, what is the probability that the condition is not present? When nurses, nurse practitioners, and physicians talk to their patients about the results of their tests, how sure are they that the patient does or does not have a disease? Sensitivity and specificity are terms commonly used to describe the accuracy of a screening test (Grove & Cipher, 2020). You will see these terms used in studies and other healthcare literature, and we want you to be able to understand them and their usefulness for practice and research.

The possible outcomes of a screening test for a disease include (a) true positive, which is an accurate identification of the presence of a disease; (b) false positive, which indicates that a disease is present when it is not; (c) false negative, which indicates that a disease is not present when it is; or (d) true negative, which indicates accurately that a disease is not present. Table 10.4 is

TABLE 10.4	**RESULTS OF SENSITIVITY AND SPECIFICITY OF SCREENING TESTS**		
DIAGNOSTIC TEST RESULT	**DISEASE PRESENT**	**DISEASE NOT PRESENT**	**TOTAL**
Positive test	a (true positive)	b (false positive)	a + b
Negative test	c (false negative)	d (true negative)	c + d
Total	a + c	b + d	a + b + c + d

a, Number of people who have the disease and the test is positive (*true positive*); b, number of people who do not have the disease and the test is positive (*false positive*); c, number of people who have the disease and the test is negative (*false negative*); d, number of people who do not have the disease and the test is negative (*true negative*). From Grove, S. K., & Cipher, D. J. (2020). *Statistics for nursing research: A workbook for evidence-based practice* (3rd ed., p. 427). Elsevier.

commonly used to visualize these four outcomes, which are used to determine a screening test's sensitivity and specificity (Straus et al., 2019).

Sensitivity is the proportion of patients with the condition or disease who have a positive test result, or true-positive rate. The CES-D (see Fig. 10.3) with a score ≥15 has 89% sensitivity for diagnosing depression in adults and 92% sensitivity in older adults. The researcher or clinician might refer to the test sensitivity in the following ways:

- A highly sensitive test is accurate for identifying the disease or a condition in a patient.
- If a test is highly sensitive, it has a low percentage of false negatives, which vary based on the focus of the test and participants' scores on the test.

Specificity is the proportion of patients without the disease who have a negative test result, or true-negative rate. You need to know that as a test becomes more sensitive, it usually becomes less specific (Straus et al., 2019; Umberger et al., 2017). The CES-D with a score ≥15 has 70% specificity for diagnosing depression in adults and 87% specificity in older adults (Cosco et al., 2017; Locke & Putnam, 2002). The researcher or clinician might refer to the test specificity in the following ways:

- A highly specific test is accurate in identifying the patients without a disease or condition.
- If a test is highly specific, it has a low percentage of false positives.

You can calculate sensitivity and specificity based on research findings and clinical practice outcomes to determine the most accurate screening test to use when identifying the presence or absence of a condition for a population. The formulas for calculating sensitivity and specificity are as follows:

$$\textbf{Sensitivity calculation} = \text{probability of disease} = \frac{a}{(a + c)} \times 100\% = \text{true-positive rate}$$

$$\textbf{Specificity calculation} = \text{probability of no disease} = \frac{d}{(b + d)} \times 100\% = \text{true-negative rate}$$

More recently, Umberger et al. (2017, p. 22) recommended calculating the negative predictive value (NPV) for "preventing, detecting, and ruling out disease, where the positive predictive value (PPV) may not be relevant for that purpose." A high NPV test means that the patient probably does not have the disease, which reduces the number of uncomfortable, costly tests and treatments that the patient might have to undergo. The formulas for calculating NPV and PPV are as follows:

$$\textbf{NPV} = \text{percentage of true-negatives among all who test negative}$$
$$= d/(c + d) \times 100\%$$

$$\textbf{PPV} = \text{percentage of true-positives among all who test positive}$$
$$= a/(a + b) \times 100\%$$

Likelihood Ratios

Likelihood ratios (LRs) are additional calculations that can help researchers determine the accuracy of screening tests, which are based on the sensitivity and specificity results. The LRs are calculated to determine the likelihood that a positive test result is a true positive, and that a negative test result is a true negative. The ratio of the true-positive results to false-positive results is known as the positive LR (Straus et al., 2019). The negative LR is the ratio of true-negative results to false-negative results. The positive LR and negative LR are calculated as follows:

$$\textbf{Positive LR} = \text{sensitivity} \div (100\% - \text{specificity})$$
$$\textbf{Negative LR} = (100\% - \text{sensitivity}) \div \text{specificity}$$

The high LRs (or those that are >10) rule in the disease or indicate that the patient has the disease. The low LRs (or those that are <0.1) almost rule out the chance that the patient has the disease. Understanding sensitivity, specificity, NPV, and LR increase your ability to read clinical studies and determine the most accurate screening test to use in clinical practice (Straus et al., 2019; Umberger et al., 2017).

? CRITICAL APPRAISAL GUIDELINES

Sensitivity, Specificity, and Likelihood Ratios

When critically appraising a study, you need to judge the sensitivity, specificity, NPV, and LRs of the screening tests used in a study.
1. Was a screening test used in a study?
2. Are sensitivity values provided for the screening test from previous studies and for this study's population (Grove & Cipher, 2020)? What does the sensitivity value for the current study mean?
3. Are the specificity values provided for the screening test from previous studies and for this study's population? What does the specificity value for the current study mean?
4. Did the researchers discuss the NPV and PPV and what they mean for the accuracy of the test (Umberger et al., 2017)?
5. Were LRs provided in the study, and were their meanings discussed?

Waters and colleagues (2020) reported that less than half of the women with gestational diabetes mellitus (GDM) are screened for type 2 diabetes postpartum because of poor attendance at postpartum visits. Therefore the researchers examined the performance of the oral glucose tolerance test (OGTT) administered during-delivery hospitalization compared with the OGTT at 4- to 12-week postpartum visits. The assessment of OGTTs during-delivery hospitalization was identified as postpartum 1 (PP1) and the OGTT at 4 to 12 weeks was identified as postpartum 2 (PP2). The sample included 319 women from four centers, including six clinical sites. The study's sensitivity, specificity, and LRs are presented in Research Example 10.3.

⚡ RESEARCH EXAMPLE 10.3

Sensitivity, Specificity, and Likelihood Ratios

Research/Study Excerpts

In total, 319 women completed a PP1 screening, with 152 (47.6%) lost to follow-up for the PP2 oral glucose tolerance test [OGTT]. None of the women with a normal PP1 oral glucose tolerance test (n = 73) later tested as having type 2 diabetes at PP2. Overall, 12.6% of subjects (n = 21) had a change from normal to impaired fasting glucose/impaired glucose tolerance or a change from impaired fasting glucose/impaired glucose tolerance to type 2 diabetes. The PP1 oral glucose tolerance test had 50% sensitivity (11.8 to 88.2%), 95.7% specificity (91.3 to 98.2%) with a 98.1% (94.5 to 99.6%) negative predictive value [NPV] and a 30% (95% confidence interval, 6.7 to 65.3) positive predictive value [PPV] for type 2 diabetes vs normal/ impaired fasting glucose/impaired glucose tolerance result. The negative predictive value of having type 2 diabetes at PP2 compared with a normal oral glucose tolerance test ... at PP1 was 100% (95% confidence interval, 93.5 to 100) with a specificity of 96.5% (95% confidence interval, 87.9 to 99.6). (Waters et al., 2020, p. 73.e1)

Continued

RESEARCH EXAMPLE 10.3—cont'd

Critical Appraisal

Waters et al. (2020) addressed the importance of conducting OGTT on women with GDM after their delivery because almost 50% of the women did not return for postpartum visits. Waters et al. (2020) provided a detailed discussion of the sensitivity, specificity, and NPV. Women having a normal OGTT after delivery (PP1) could virtually be ruled out for development of diabetes mellitus at PP2 (NPV = 100%). Remember a high NPV rules out the potential for a disease or condition (true negative when testing negative; Straus et al., 2019). The specificity of OGTT after delivery was also extremely strong (98.1%) in identifying the women who did not have diabetes mellitus (true negative). The sensitivity (true positive) was not strong (50%) in this study, indicating the importance of OGTT screening at postpartum visits for women with impaired fasting blood sugars and impaired OGTT tests at PP1. This study built on the findings from previous research that examined the utility of OGTT of women with GDM before hospital discharge because of the large number of women who were lost to follow-up.

RESEARCH/EBP TIP

Knowledge of sensitivity (patient with disease has a positive test), specificity (patient without the disease has negative test), and NPV (percent of true negative among all those with negative tests) enable you to determine which screening tests are most effective in clinical practice. Quality measurements methods are essential for examining outcomes for EBP.

MEASUREMENT STRATEGIES IN NURSING

Because nursing research examines a wide variety of phenomena, an extensive array of measurement methods is needed to conduct these studies. Some nursing phenomena have not been adequately examined because of the limited measurement methods. For example, the outcomes from health promotion behaviors are difficult to define and measure. This section describes some of the most common measurement methods used in nursing research, including physiological measures, observational measurements, interviews, questionnaires, and scales.

Physiological Measures

Nurse researchers use a variety of approaches to obtain physiological data. Physiological measures include two categories, biophysical and biochemical. Biophysical measures are devices, equipment, or methods used to measure physiological and pathological variables, such as the stethoscope and sphygmomanometer to measure BP. Biophysical measures can be acquired in a variety of ways from instruments within the body (in vivo), such as a reading from an arterial line, or from application of an instrument on the outside of an individual (in vitro), such as a BP cuff (Stone & Frazier, 2017). A biochemical measure determines microchemical values, such as laboratory tests for determining cholesterol values. Physiological variables can be measured either directly or indirectly. Direct measures are used to count and quantify the variable itself and are considered objective with limited influence from judgment issues. They are also specific to that particular variable, such as the 25(OH)D serum laboratory value to test for vitamin D levels (Sahasrabudhe et al., 2020). Indirect measures are obtained to represent the quantity of a variable by measuring one or more characteristics or properties that are related to it. They are often more subjective than are direct measures and may be affected by judgment or experience in administration (Ryan-Wenger,

2017). For example, some physiological measures are obtained by using self-report with diaries, scales, or observation checklists, and other physiological measures are obtained using laboratory tests and electronic monitoring.

The availability of electronic monitoring equipment has greatly increased the possibilities of physiological measurement in nursing studies, particularly in critical care environments (Stone & Frazier, 2017). Electronic monitoring requires placing sensors on or within the study participant, such as electrocardiographic leads and arterial lines. The sensors measure changes in bodily functions as electrical energy. Electronic equipment often provides simultaneous recording of multiple physiological measures that are displayed on a monitor, such as equipment that records the pulse, heart rhythm, and arterial pressure. The equipment is often linked to a computer, which allows retrieval, review, and analysis of the complex data.

Breteler and colleagues (2020) conducted a study to examine the capabilities of wireless monitoring systems in detecting adverse events of high-risk surgical patients. The physiological variables recorded by the sensors in this study were HR, respiratory rate (RR), and oxygen saturation (SpO_2). Research Example 10.4 describes the monitoring systems and their measurement of the study physiological variables. This measurement section was critically appraised using the guidelines presented earlier.

RESEARCH EXAMPLE 10.4

Physiological Measures

Research/Study Excerpt

A subset of patients developed adverse events during these vital signs recordings. In this study, vital sign trend patterns of patients with adverse events are described in more detail and compared to vital sign recordings of patients without occurrence of adverse events.

Heart rate and respiratory rate were continuously recorded in high-risk surgical patients with two wearable patch sensors (SensiumVitals: Sensium Healthcare Ltd, Oxford, UK, and HealthPatch: VitalConnect, California San Jose, CA), a bed-based mattress sensor (EarlySense; EarlySense Ltd, Ramat Gan, Israel), and a patient-worn monitor (Masimo Radius-7: Masimo Corporation, Irvine, CA, USA) simultaneously during the initial days of recovery at a surgical step-down unit (SDU) and subsequent stay on the traumatology or surgical oncology ward of the University Medical center. ...Besides heart and respiratory rate, oxygen saturation was continuously recorded with a SpO_2 finger probe (Masimo Radius-7). No alarms were generated and sent to nurses. A description and image of each sensor is shown in Table 10.5 and Fig. 10.4, respectively. (Breteler et al., 2020, p. S98)

TABLE 10.5 **Overview of Wireless Monitoring Solutions**

Sensor (Manufacturer)	Sensor Type	Vital Signs Measured	Update Rate Vital Signs
Masimo Radius-7 (Masimo Corporation, Irvine, CA, USA)	Patient-worn monitor connected to a pulse oximeter and acoustic adhesive sensor in the neck	Heart rate (pulse rate) Respiration rate Saturation	Every 2 s (storage)
SensiumVitals (Sensium Healthcare Ltd, Oxford, UK)[a]	Wireless adhesive patch sensor on chest	Heart rate Respiration rate	Every 120 s

Continued

RESEARCH EXAMPLE 10.4—cont'd

TABLE 10.5   Overview of Wireless Monitoring Solutions—cont'd

Sensor (Manufacturer)	Sensor Type	Vital Signs Measured	Update Rate Vital Signs
HealthPatch MD (VitalConnect, San Jose, CA, USA)[b]	Wireless adhesive patch sensor on chest	Heart rate Respiration rate	Every 4 s
EarlySense system (EarlySense Ltd, Ramat Gan, Israel)	Contactless piezoelectric sensor under the patient's mattress	Heart rate Respiration rate	Every 60 s

[a]The Sensium system measures axillary temperature as well.
[b]The HealthPatch MD measures skin temperature as well.
From Breteler, M. J. M., Kleinjan, E., Numan, L., Ruurda, J. P., Van Hillegersberg, R., Leenen, L. P., ... Blokhuis, T. J. (2020). Are current wireless monitoring systems capable of detecting adverse events in high-risk surgical patients? A descriptive study. *Injury, 51*(Suppl. 2), S100. https://doi.org/10.1016/j.injury.2019.11.018

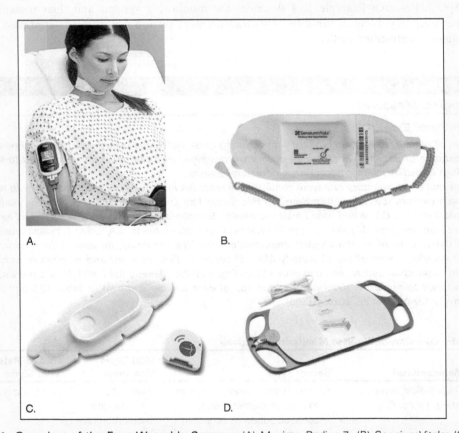

A.

B.

C.

D.

FIG. 10.4   Overview of the Four Wearable Sensors: (A) Masimo Radius-7; (B) SensiumVitals; (C) Health-Patch MD; and (D) Early Sense system. (From Breteler, M. J. M., Kleinjan, E., Numan, L., Ruurda, J. P., Van Hillegersberg, R., Leenen, L. P., ... Blokhuis, T. J. [2020]. Are current wireless monitoring systems capable of detecting adverse events in high-risk surgical patients? A descriptive study. *Injury, 51*[Suppl. 2], S99. https://doi.org/10.1016/j.injury.2019.11.018)

> ### ⟨⟩ RESEARCH EXAMPLE 10.4—cont'd
>
> **Critical Appraisal**
>
> Breteler et al. (2020) provided a clear, concise description of the four monitoring systems examined in their study. These sensors were direct measures of the participants' HR, RR, and SpO_2. The names, manufactures, and types of sensor were summarized in the research report (see Table 10.5). The pictures of the sensors in Fig. 10.4 enable readers to understand how the vital signs were measured and recorded. The sensors were accurate and precise in measuring the physiological variables in this study and in detecting adverse events in high-risk surgical patients.
>
> Breteler et al. (2020) reported 20 adverse events that occurred with 11 of the 31 study participants. The remote wireless patient monitoring systems detected the abnormalities in vital sign patterns in patients. Atrial fibrillation was the most common (20%) adverse event that was recognized with an increased HR by all the sensors. Respiratory insufficiency was detected by an increase in RR and a decrease in SpO_2. "Remote patient monitoring may have potential to improve patient safety by generating early warnings for deterioration to nursing staff" (Breteler et al., 2020, p. S97).

Observational Measurement

Observational measurement involves an interaction between the study participants and observer(s), in which the observer has the opportunity to watch the participant perform in a specific setting (Waltz et al., 2017). Observations are of two types, unstructured and structured. Unstructured observation involves spontaneously watching and recording what is seen in words. Unstructured observation is often used to collect data in qualitative and mixed methods studies (see Chapter 3; Creswell & Clark, 2018; Creswell & Poth, 2018). The analysis of unstructured observation data may lead to a more structured observation and the development of an observational checklist (Bandalos, 2018; Miles et al., 2020). In structured observational measurement, the researcher carefully defines what was observed, who conducted the observations, and how the observations were made, recorded, and coded as numbers (Waltz et al., 2017). For observations to be structured, researchers will develop a category system for organizing and sorting the behaviors or events being observed. Checklists are often used to indicate whether a behavior occurred. Rating scales allow the observer to rate the behavior or event. This provides more information for analysis than dichotomous data, which indicate only whether the behavior occurred. Because observation tends to be more subjective than other types of measurement, it is often considered less credible in quantitative and outcomes studies. However, observation may be the only approach for obtaining important data for nursing knowledge. As with any means of measurement, consistency is very important. As a result, reporting interrater reliability of those doing the observations is essential (see Table 10.2).

？ CRITICAL APPRAISAL GUIDELINES

Observational Measurement

When critically appraising observational measures, consider the following questions:
1. Is the object of observation clearly identified and defined?
2. Are the techniques for recording observations described?
3. Is interrater reliability for the observers described? Is an acceptable interrater reliability value of ≥0.90 (90%) achieved in the study?

McLellan and colleagues (2017) conducted a study to validate the newly developed Children's Hospital Early Warning Score (CHEWS) with the previously validated Brighton Pediatric Early Warning Score (PEWS). The PEWS was originally developed for early detection of critical deterioration of all noncardiac pediatric patients. The CHEWS was a modified version of the PEWS observational tool that was developed to identify pediatric cardiac patients at risk for critical deterioration, enabling clinicians to intervene early and prevent further deterioration. Research Example 10.5 includes part of the researchers' description of their observational tool's validity and reliability.

◢ RESEARCH EXAMPLE 10.5

Observational Measurement

Research/Study Excerpt

The final revised tool (Fig. 10.5, called the Cardiac Children's Hospital Early Warning Score (C-CHEWS) … was successfully piloted, fully implemented and then formally validated (… sensitivity 95.3%, specificity 76.2%) in the pediatric cardiac population in a previous study (McLellan et al., 2014). In this study, the tool demonstrated excellent discrimination in identifying critical deterioration in children with cardiac disease and performed significantly better than the PEWS in identifying critical deterioration (McLellan et al., 2014). To optimize safety and to improve clarity, the hospital leadership decided to implement the cardiac tool throughout all inpatients area rather than having similar but different tools operating in the same institution. The C-CHEWS was renamed the Children's Hospital Early Warning Score (CHEWS) and incorporated into the electronic health record. … Interrater reliability between staff nurses of all experience levels had previously been established for the CHEWS tool (100% score $\geq$ 3, kappa statistic 1.00) during the initial validation study and was not repeated. (McLellan et al., 2017, pp. 53–54)

Children's Hospital Early Warning Score					
	0	**1**	**2**	**3**	**Score**
Behavior/Neuro	• Playing/sleeping appropriately • Alert, at patient's baseline	• Sleepy, somnolent when not disturbed	• Irritable, difficult to console • Increase in patient's baseline seizure activity	• Lethargic, confused, floppy • Reduced response to pain • Prolonged or frequent seizures • Pupils asymmetric or sluggish	
Cardiovascular	• Skin tone appropriate for patient • Capillary refill ≤2 seconds	• Pale • Capillary refill 3–4 seconds • Mild* tachycardia • Intermittent ectopy or irregular HR (not new)	• Grey • Capillary refill 4–5 seconds • Moderate* tachycardia	• Grey and mottled • Capillary refill >5 seconds • Severe* tachycardia • New onset bradycardia • New onset/increase in ectopy, irregular HR or heart block	
Respiratory	• Within normal parameters • No retractions	• Mild* tachypnea/ increased WOB (flaring, retracting) • Up to 40% supplemental oxygen • Up to 1L NC > patient's baseline need • Mild desaturations < patient's baseline • Intermittent apnea self-resolving	• Moderate* tachypnea/increased WOB (flaring, retracting, grunting, use of accessory muscles) • 40–60% oxygen via mask • 1–2 L NC > patient's baseline need • Nebs q 1–2 hr • Moderate desaturations < patient's baseline • Apnea requiring repositioning or stimulation	• Severe* tachypnea • RR < normal for age • Severe increased WOB (i.e. head bobbing, paradoxical breathing) • >60% oxygen via mask • >2 L NC > patient's baseline need • Nebs q 30 minutes – 1 hr • Severe desaturations < patient's baseline • Apnea requiring interventions other than repositioning or stimulation	
Staff Concern		Concerned			
Family Concern		Concerned or absent			
					Total

	Mild*	**Moderate***	**Severe***	
Infant	≥10% ↑ for age	≥15% ↑ for age	≥25% ↑ for age	
Toddler and Older	≥10% ↑ for age	≥25% ↑ for age	≥50% ↑ for age	

FIG. 10.5 The Children's Hospital Early Warning Score. *HR,* Heart rate; *L,* liters; *NC,* nasal cannula; *RR,* respiratory rate; *WOB,* work of breathing. (From McLellan, M. C., Gauvreau, K., & Connor, J. A. [2017]. Validation of the Children's Hospital Early Warning System for critical deterioration recognition. *Journal of Pediatric Nursing, 32*[1], 54.)

RESEARCH EXAMPLE 10.5—cont'd

Sensitivity for scores ≥ 3 was 91.4% for CHEWS and 73.6% for PEWS with specificity of 67.8% for CHEWS and 88.5% for PEWS. Sensitivity scores ≥ 5 was 75.6% for CHEWS and 38.9% for PEWS with specificity of 88.5% for CHEWS and 93.9% for PEWS. The early warning time from critical score (≥ 5) to critical deterioration was 3.8 h for CHEWS versus 0.6 h for PEWS (p < 0.001) ... The CHEWS system demonstrated higher discrimination, higher sensitivity, and longer early warning time than the PEWS for identifying children at risk for critical deterioration. (McLellan et al., 2017, p. 52)

Critical Appraisal

McLellan and colleagues (2017) provided extensive information about the development of the CHEWS from the PEWS instruments. Fig. 10.5 details the behaviors to be observed, the scoring process, and the critical score indicating potential deterioration. The validity and interrater reliability of the CHEWS from previous research (McLellan et al., 2014) were strong. However, the interrater reliability needed to be provided for this study because many staff nurses of different levels were involved in the data collection process.

The CHEWS was found to be a significantly stronger instrument for use in clinical practice than the PEWS, demonstrating content and construct validity. The CHEWS also provided earlier prediction of critical deterioration in children than the PEWS, indicating predictive criterion validity. The CHEWS had extremely strong sensitivity for identifying children at risk for critical deterioration and acceptable specificity in determining children who were not at risk for deterioration (Grove & Cipher, 2020; Straus et al., 2019).

Interviews

An interview involves verbal communication between the researcher and the study participant, during which information is provided to the researcher. Although this data collection strategy is most commonly used in qualitative and descriptive studies, it also can be used in other types of quantitative studies. You can use a variety of approaches to conduct an interview, ranging from a totally unstructured interview (see Chapter 3), in which the content is controlled by the study participant (Creswell & Poth, 2018), to a structured interview, in which the content is similar to that of a questionnaire, with the possible responses to questions carefully designed by the researcher (Dillman et al., 2014; Waltz et al., 2017). Interviews might also be semi-structured or partially structured based on the purpose of the study. Usually, researchers ask specific questions in a designated order and enter the participants' responses onto a structured form or rating scale in quantitative and outcomes research. For example, researchers could use an in-person or telephone interview to obtain and record responses to questions, or they might enter responses into an electronic database.

Because nurses frequently use interviewing techniques in nursing assessment, the dynamics of interviewing are familiar. However, using this technique for measurement in research requires greater sophistication and needs to be discussed in the study's Methods section. The response rate for interviews is higher than for questionnaires, which usually allows a more representative sample to be obtained. Interviewing also allows collection of data from participants who are unable or unlikely to complete questionnaires, such as those who are very ill or may have limited ability to read, write, and express themselves. Interviews are a form of self-report, and it must be assumed that the information provided is accurate. Because of time and cost, sample size is usually limited. Participant bias is always a threat to the validity of the findings, as is inconsistency in data collection from one participant to another (Dillman et al., 2014).

CRITICAL APPRAISAL GUIDELINES

Semistructured and Structured Interviews

When critically appraising interviews conducted in studies, you need to consider the following questions:
1. For semistructured and structured interviews, what guided the interview process?
2. Are the interview questions relevant for the research purpose?
3. Is the process for conducting the interviews described?
4. If multiple interviewers are used to gather data, how were these individuals trained, to what extent, and was consistency achieved for the interview process?
5. If the interview questions were included in the research report, did they seem free from bias?

Chidume (2021) conducted a quasi-experimental study to examine the effects of fall prevention toolkits (FPTs), such as fall risk screenings and fall prevention education (FPE), on the fall incidence of adults 65 years and older living in the community. A semistructured follow-up interview was conducted to examine outcomes related to the FPTs. Research Example 10.6 describes the interview process used in this study.

RESEARCH EXAMPLE 10.6

Semistructured Interview

Research/Study Excerpt

The project-specific, five-question follow-up survey was developed by the nurse with input from colleagues. The survey was completed during the follow-up phone call with participants. The follow-up questions requested additional information concerning possible changes the participants made after the FPT implementation, if they had fallen since the FPE, as well as their evaluation of the FPE provided. The last question on the survey, "Is there anything else you would like for me to know," allowed for participants to express additional feelings and concerns regarding fall prevention awareness, safety, and knowledge. (Chidume, 2021, Instruments)

Critical Appraisal

Chidume (2021) identified the focus of the follow-up interview and the questions asked of the study participants. The interview questions revolved around the changes participants made after the implementation of the FPE. These questions did not appear to be biased and were appropriate for addressing the study purpose. However, the survey was developed for this study and only content validity was addressed. Chidume conducted the interviews consistently by telephone with all 30 study participants. The majority of participants (*n* = 28) had not fallen since they received the FPE. Chidume (2021, Abstract) recommended a longer follow-up period "to fortify FPE and keep participants engaged in fall prevention safety."

Questionnaires

A **questionnaire** is a self-report form designed to elicit information through written, verbal, or electronic responses of the study participant. Questionnaires may be printed and distributed in person, mailed, provided on a computer, or accessed online. Questionnaires are sometimes referred to as surveys, and a study using a questionnaire may be referred to as survey research (Dillman et al., 2014). The information obtained from questionnaires is similar to that obtained by an interview, but the questions tend to have less depth. Study participants are not permitted to elaborate on responses or asked for clarification of comments, and the data collector cannot use probing strategies. However, questions are presented in a consistent manner to each participant, and the opportunity for bias is less than in an interview.

Questionnaires often are used in descriptive studies to gather a broad spectrum of information from participants, such as facts about the participant or facts about persons, events, or situations known by the participant. It is also used to gather information about beliefs, attitudes, opinions, knowledge, or intentions of the study participants. Questionnaires are often developed for a particular study to enable researchers to gather data from a selected population in a new area of study. Like interviews, questionnaires can have various structures. Some questionnaires have open-ended questions, which require written responses (qualitative data) from the participant. Other questionnaires have closed-ended questions, which have limited options from which participants can select their answers (Gray & Grove, 2021).

Although you can distribute questionnaires to large samples face to face, through the mail, or via the internet, the response rate for questionnaires generally is lower than that for other forms of self-report, particularly if the questionnaires are mailed. If the response rate is lower than 50%, the representativeness of the sample is in question (Dillman et al., 2014). The response rate for mailed questionnaires is often small (25%–40%), so researchers frequently are unable to obtain a representative sample, even with random sampling methods. Questionnaires distributed via the internet are more convenient for study participants, which may result in a higher response rate than for mailed questionnaires. Many researchers are choosing the internet format if they have access to the potential participants' e-mail addresses.

Some respondents fail to mark responses to all the questions, especially on long questionnaires. The incomplete nature of the data can threaten the validity of the instrument. Therefore researchers need to describe how missing data were managed in their research report. With most questionnaires, researchers analyze data at the level of individual items, rather than adding the items together and analyzing the total scores as with scales. Responses to items are usually measured at the nominal or ordinal level.

? CRITICAL APPRAISAL GUIDELINES
Questionnaires

When critically appraising a questionnaire in a published study, consider the following questions:
1. Does the questionnaire address the focus of the study outlined in the study purpose and/or objective, questions, or hypotheses?
2. Examine the description of the contents of the questionnaire in the measurement section of the study. Does the study provide information on content-related validity for the questionnaire?
3. Was the questionnaire pilot-tested or used in previous studies? What type of validity and reliability information was provided related to the questionnaire?
4. Was the questionnaire implemented consistently from one study participant to another?

Wentland and Hinderer (2020, Purpose) conducted an outcomes study "to describe the structure and outcomes related to a Nursing Research and EBP Fellowship Program in a Magnet®-designated pediatric medical center and to explore fellowship program participant's perceptions of knowledge, skills, and barriers to finding and reviewing evidence and changing practice." Surveys were administered before the fellowship program (time 1), directly after the program (time 2), and 1 year after the completion of the program. Research Example 10.7 describes the survey used to collect data in this study.

⚙ RESEARCH EXAMPLE 10.7

Questionnaires

Research/Study Excerpt

Descriptive information regarding the fellowship program participants, project details, and project outcomes were extracted from the Institute for Nursing Research and EBP Database. The survey included demographic data questions (gender, age, race, education, hours per week, usual shift) and the Developing Evidence-Based Practice Questionnaire (DEBP). The DEBP is a 49-question multiple-choice survey used to evaluate knowledge and skills related to EBP (Gerrish et al., 2007; Gerrish et al., 2008). The DEBP is not interpreted as a single scale. There are five subscales that use Likert-Style (1 to 5) scoring: (1) Bases of Practice Knowledge; (2) Barriers to Finding and Reviewing Evidence; (3) Barriers to Changing Practice on the Basis of Evidence; (4) Facilitation and Support in Changing Practice; and (5) Skills in Finding and Reviewing Evidence. Reported Cronbach's alpha for the overall survey was 0.874 (Gerrish et al., 2007). The Cronbach's alpha for the entire instrument for the current study was 0.864, 0.924, and 0.862 for Time 1, Time 2, and Time 3, respectively. (Wentland & Hinderer, 2020, Measures)

Critical Appraisal

Wentland and Hinderer (2020) collected data using a survey that was e-mailed to participants at three points in time. This survey included demographic questions and a questionnaire (DEBP) that addressed the purpose of this study. The DEBP was identified as a questionnaire, but the items on the instrument were typical of a Likert scale. The instrument would have been more accurately described as a 49-item Likert scale with five subscales (DeVellis, 2017). Readers are often confused by the interchangeable use of the terms *survey*, *questionnaire*, and *scale*. The content and use of scales are discussed in detail in the next section. The DEBP had been used in previous research (Gerrish et al., 2007; Gerrish et al., 2008) with reported strong reliability (Cronbach alpha = 0.87). The DEBP also had strong reliability in this study for the three repeated measures. The DEBP has construct validity as evidenced by the conduct of factor analysis used to identify the five subscales (see Table 10.2). However, additional discussion of the validity of the DEBP would have strengthened the measurement section of this study.

Wentland and Hinderer (2020) found that the fellowship program was effective in building and sustaining a passion for clinical research and promoting EBP that are required for Magnet status. DEBP has reliability and validity for measuring the knowledge, skills, and barriers to achieving EBP.

📄 RESEARCH/EBP TIP

EBP is the goal of healthcare professionals and agencies and is essential for obtaining and maintaining Magnet status in hospitals. The DEBP appears to be a valuable scale for measuring EBP in clinical practice.

Scales

A scale is a self-report form of measurement composed of several items designed to measure a construct that is more precise than a questionnaire. Most scales are developed to measure psychosocial variables, but researchers also use scaling techniques to obtain self-reports on physiological variables, such as pain, nausea, or dyspnea. The various items on most scales are summed to obtain a single score. These are termed *summated scales*. Fewer random and systematic errors occur when the total score of a scale is used (DeVellis, 2017). The various items in a scale increase the dimensions of the construct that are measured by the instrument. The scales commonly used in nursing research include rating, Likert, and visual analog.

Rating Scales

Rating scales are the crudest form of measurement involving scaling techniques. A rating scale includes an ordered series of categories of a variable that are assumed to be based on an underlying

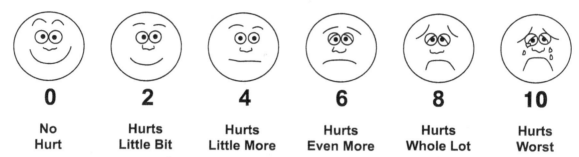

FIG. 10.6 Wong-Baker FACES® Pain Rating Scale. Point to each face using the words to describe the pain intensity. Ask the child to choose the face that best describes the child's own pain and record the appropriate number. (From Wong-Baker FACES Foundation. [2016]. *Wong-Baker FACES® Pain Rating Scale.* Retrieved from https://wongbakerfaces.org)

continuum. A numerical value is assigned to each category, and the fineness of the distinctions between categories varies with the scale. Rating scales are commonly used by the general public. In conversations, one can hear statements such as "On a scale of 1 to 10, I would rank that…" Rating scales are fairly easy to develop, but researchers need to be careful to avoid end statements that are so extreme that no study participant will select them. You can use a rating scale to rate patients' adherence to their medication or the value placed by a study participant on nurse–patient interactions. Rating scales are also used in observational measurement to guide data collection (see Fig. 10.5 of the Children's Hospital Early Warning Score developed by McLellan et al., 2017).

Some rating scales are more valid than others because they were constructed in a structured way and used in a variety of studies with different populations. For example, the Wong-Baker FACES® Pain Rating Scale has documented reliability and validity through extensive previous research and is commonly used to assess the pain of children in clinical practice (Fig. 10.6; Wong-Baker FACES Foundation, 2016). Nurses often assess pain in adults with a numeric rating scale (NRS), similar to the one in Fig. 10.7. Using the NRS is more valid and reliable than asking a patient to rate his or her pain on a scale from 1 to 10. FACES and NRS are also used to measure pain in research.

Likert Scale

The Likert scale is designed to determine the opinions, perceptions, or attitudes of study participants. This scale contains a number of declarative statements, with a scale after each statement. The Likert scale is the most commonly used of the scaling techniques in nursing research. The original version of the scale included five response categories. Each response category was assigned a value, with a value of 0 or 1 given to the most negative response and a value of 4 or 5 given to the most positive response (DeVellis, 2017; Ho, 2017). Response choices in a Likert scale usually address agreement, evaluation, or frequency. Agreement options may include statements such as *strongly disagree, disagree, neutral, agree,* and *strongly agree.* Evaluation responses ask the respondent for an

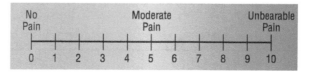

FIG. 10.7 Numeric Rating Scale.

evaluative rating along a bad–good dimension, such as negative to positive or terrible to excellent. Frequency responses may include statements such as *never, rarely, sometimes, frequently,* and *all the time.* The terms used are versatile and are selected based on the content of the questions or items in the scale. For example, an item such as "Describe the nursing care you received during your hospitalization" could have a response scale of *unsatisfactory, below average, average, above average,* and *excellent.*

Sometimes seven options are given on a response scale, sometimes only four. When the response scale has an odd number of options, the middle option is usually an uncertain or neutral category. Using a response scale with an odd number of options is controversial because it allows the study participant to avoid making a clear choice of positive or negative statements. To avoid this, researchers may choose to provide only four or six options, with no middle point or uncertain category. This type of scale is termed a *forced choice version.* Ho (2017) provided an excellent description of the strengths and limitations of Likert scales.

A Likert scale usually consists of 10 to 20 items, with each addressing an element of the concept being measured. The values obtained from each item in the instrument are summed to obtain a single score for each participant. Although the values of each item are technically ordinal-level data, the summed score is often analyzed as interval-level data. The CES-D is a Likert scale (see Fig. 10.3) that is used to assess the level of depression in patients in clinical practice and research. Rapp et al. (2021) used the CES-D in their study presented earlier in Research Example 10.1. The instructions given to participants are presented at the top of the scale in Fig. 10.3 (Radloff, 1977). The Likert scale responses ranged from a low of 0 (rarely or none of the time) to 3 (most or all of the time). As discussed previously, the scores on the 20-item scale can range from 0 to 60, with the higher scores indicating more depressive symptoms. A score of 16 is the cutoff point for depression, and a score ≥24 indicates severe depression. The scale has strong reliability, validity, sensitivity, and specificity (Armenta et al., 2014; Cosco et al., 2017; Jiang et al., 2019; Locke & Putnam, 2002; Siddaway et al., 2017).

Visual Analog Scales

The visual analog scale (VAS) is typically used to measure strength, magnitude, or intensity of individuals' subjective feelings, sensations, or attitudes about symptoms or situations. The VAS is a line that is 100 mm (10 cm) long, with *right angle stops* at either end. Researchers can present the line horizontally or vertically, with bipolar anchors or descriptors beyond either end of the line (DeVellis, 2017). These end anchors must include the entire range of sensations possible for the phenomenon being measured (e.g., all and none, best and worst, no pain and unbearable pain). An example of a VAS for measuring pain is presented in Fig. 10.8. The VAS is a line of continuous values and is potentially extremely sensitive in measuring a sensation or perception before and after an intervention in a study. Another advantage of the VAS is it can be repeated over time, and participants cannot remember their past responses precisely; therefore they give a more valid response to a symptom or situation (Bandalos, 2018; DeVellis, 2017).

Participants are asked to place a mark through the line to indicate the intensity of the sensation or feeling. Then researchers use a ruler to measure the distance between the left end of the line (on a horizontal scale) and the participant's mark. This measure is the value of the sensation. The VAS has been used to measure pain, alertness, craving for cigarettes, quality of sleep, and severity of

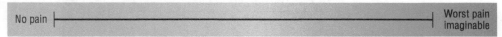

No pain ├───┤ Worst pain imaginable

FIG. 10.8 Example of a Visual Analog Scale.

clinical symptoms. The reliability of the VAS is usually determined by the test-retest method. The correlations between the two administrations of the scale need to be moderate or strong to support the reliability of the scale. Because these scales are used to measure phenomena that are dynamic or changing over time, test-retest reliability is sometimes not appropriate because the low correlation is caused by the change in sensation versus a problem with the scale. Because the VAS contains a single item, other methods of determining reliability, such as internal consistency, cannot be used. The validity of the VAS is usually determined by correlating the VAS scores with other measures, such as rating or Likert scales, that measure the same phenomenon, such as pain (DeVellis, 2017). Arikan and Esenay (2020) conducted an RCT to examine the effect of distraction on children's pain during a venous blood draw. A VAS was used to measure pain for children aged 3 to 18 years, and the 10-cm-long line ranged from "no pain" on the left-hand side to "unbearable pain" on the right-hand side. The distraction group had significantly lower pain as measured by the VAS.

? CRITICAL APPRAISAL GUIDELINES

Scales

When critically appraising a rating scale, Likert scale, or VAS in a study, ask the following questions:
1. Is the rating scale, Likert scale, or VAS clearly described in the research report?
2. Are the techniques used to administer and score the scale provided?
3. Is information about the validity and reliability of the scale described from previous studies and for this study?

Faulkner and colleagues (2020) conducted a secondary analysis of data from five studies completed at an academic medical center in the Pacific Northwest that included 449 participants. The focus of this study was to identify the "unique profiles of perceived dyspnea burden in heart failure" patients (Faulkner et al., 2020, p. 488). The measurement methods for dyspnea symptom perception and depressive symptoms are presented in Research Example 10.8.

🔍 RESEARCH EXAMPLE 10.8

Scales

Research/Study Excerpt

Dyspnea symptom perception

The dyspnea subscale of the Heart Failure Somatic Perception Scale (HFSPS) was used to measure patient-reported dyspnea. The HFSPS dyspnea subscale consists of six items. Participants are asked to rate how bothersome each symptom was during the previous week rated on a scale of 0 to 5 with 0 indicating that they did not have the symptom and 5 indicating the symptom was extremely bothersome. Dyspnea subscale scores are the sum of the responses for each individual item with higher scores indicating greater dyspnea burden (range 0 to 30). The HFSPS dyspnea subscale correlates well with the Physical Limitations subscale of the Kansas City Cardiomyopathy Questionnaire ($r = -0.529$, $p < 0.0001$), and demonstrated good internal consistency using the combined data in the current study (Cronbach's $a = 0.88$)....

Depressive symptoms

Depressive symptoms were evaluated using the 9-item Patient Health Questionnaire (PHQ-9). Each item asks respondents to rate how much they were bothered by a particular symptom in the preceding two

Continued

RESEARCH EXAMPLE 10.8—cont'd

weeks with answers ranging from 0 to 3 with higher scores indicating worse depressive symptoms. Scores for each item are summed to create a PHQ-9 total score ranging from 0 to 30. The PHQ-9 demonstrated good internal consistency in the current study (Cronbach's a = 0.81) and demonstrates high sensitivity and specificity for major depression (88% for both). (Faulkner et al., 2020, p. 489)

Critical Appraisal

Faulkner et al. (2020) described the origin, scoring process, and meaning for the scores for the dyspnea subscale from the HFSPS. In addition, the dyspnea subscale had strong internal consistency ($\alpha = 0.88$) in this study, but reliability from previous research was not addressed. The HFSPS dyspnea subscale had construct validity, as indicated by the strong correlation with the Kansas City Cardiomyopathy Questionnaire, but no other validity information was provided.

The PHQ-9 was a reliable Likert scale for measuring depression in this population. The scoring process and the meaning of the summed scores from this scale were described. This scale has sensitivity and specificity for determining major depression from previous research, but the validity of this scale was not addressed. Both the HFSPS dyspnea subscale and the PHQ-9 seemed appropriate for measuring the variables in this study. However, addition reliability and validity information about these scales would have strengthened the measurement section.

RESEARCH/EBP TIP

Scales usually provide the most reliable and valid way to measure outcomes (Moorhead et al., 2018) in research and practice, which is essential for achieving EBP.

DATA COLLECTION PROCESS

Data collection is the process of acquiring study participants from whom essential data are gathered to address the research purpose. The actual steps of collecting data are specific to each study and depend on the research design, sample, and measurement techniques. During the data collection process, researchers initially train the data collectors, recruit study participants, implement the study intervention (if applicable), collect data in a consistent way, and protect the integrity (or validity) of the study.

The data collection process should be clearly and concisely covered in the research report. Often, the data collection process is addressed in the Methods section of the report in a subsection entitled "Procedures or Data Collection." The strategies used to approach potential participants who meet the sampling criteria (see Chapter 9) should be included in the study report. The number and characteristics of individuals who decline to participate in the study should also be reported. If the study includes an intervention, the details about the intervention and how it was implemented should be addressed (see Chapter 8). The approaches used to perform measurements and the time and setting for the measurements also need to be described. The desired result is a step-by-step description of exactly how, where, and in what sequence the study data are collected. The following sections discuss some of the common data collections tasks described in research reports, including recruitment of study participants, consistency of data collection, and control in implementing the study design. Nurse researchers are also conducting studies using data from existing databases, and it is important to critically appraise data obtained from these databases.

Recruitment of Study Participants

Study participants may be recruited only at the initiation of data collection or may be recruited throughout the data collection period. The design of the study determines the method of selecting the participants. Recruiting the number of participants originally planned is critical because data analysis and interpretation of findings depend on having an adequate sample size (see Chapter 9; Aberson, 2019).

Consistency in Data Collection

Consistency involves maintaining the data collection pattern for each collection event as it was developed in the research plan. A good plan will facilitate consistency and maintain the validity of the study. Researchers should note deviations, even if they are minor, and report their effect on the interpretation of the findings in their final report. If a study uses data collectors, researchers need to report the training process and the interrater reliability achieved during training and data collection (Kazdin, 2017; Waltz et al., 2017).

Control in the Study Design

Researchers build controls into their study plan to minimize the influence of intervening forces on the findings. Control is especially important in quasi-experimental and experimental studies to ensure that the intervention is consistently implemented (see Chapter 8; Kazdin, 2017; Shadish et al., 2002). The research report needs to reflect the controls implemented in a study and any problems that needed to be managed during the study. In addition to maintaining the controls identified in the plan, researchers continually look for previously unidentified, extraneous variables that might have an effect on the data being collected. Extraneous variables are usually specific to a study and identified before the study is conducted. However, some extraneous variables become apparent during the data collection, data analysis, or interpretation of the findings and should be discussed in the research report.

Obtaining Data From Existing Databases

Nurse researchers are using a variety of existing databases to address the research problem and purpose for their study. The reasons for obtaining data from existing databases for a study are varied. With the computerization of healthcare information, more databases have been developed internationally, nationally, regionally, and within clinical agencies. These databases include large amounts of information that have relevance in developing research evidence needed for practice (Melnyk et al., 2017). The costs and technology for storage of data have improved over the past 10–15 years, making these databases more reliable and accessible. Using existing databases makes it possible to conduct complex analyses to expand our understanding of healthcare outcomes (Moorhead et al., 2018). Another reason is that the primary collection of data in a study is limited by the availability of research participants and expense of the data collection process. By using existing databases, researchers can have larger samples, conduct more longitudinal studies, reduce costs during the data collection process, and limit the burdens placed on the study participants (Gray & Grove, 2021; Johantgen, 2010).

The existing healthcare data commonly used in research include secondary and administrative. Data collected for a particular study are considered primary data. Data collected from previous research and stored in a database are considered secondary data when used by other researchers to address their study purpose. Because these data were collected as part of research, details can be obtained about the data collection and storage processes, including any previous publications based on the data. Researchers usually indicate when they used secondary data analyses in the

Methodology section of their study. For example, Faulkner et al. (2020) conducted a secondary data analysis to profile the perceived dyspnea burden experienced by patients with heart failure (see Research Example 10.8).

Data collected for reasons other than research are considered administrative data. Administrative data are collected within clinical agencies; obtained by national, state, and local professional organizations; and maintained by federal, state, and local agencies. The processes for collection and storage of administrative data are more complex and often more unclear than the data collection process for research. The data in administrative databases are collected by different people in different sites using different methods. However, the data elements collected for most administrative databases include demographics, organizational characteristics, clinical diagnosis and treatment, and geographical information. These database elements have been standardized by the Health Insurance Portability and Accountability Act, which has improved the quality of the databases (see Chapter 4). Outcomes studies are often conducted with data from administrative databases (see Chapter 14). When researchers obtain data from an existing database, the data must focus on the study purpose and the objectives, questions, or hypotheses. The validity and reliability of the data from these databases should be described in the research report.

⑦ CRITICAL APPRAISAL GUIDELINES

Data Collection

When critically appraising the data collection process, consider the following questions:
1. Were the study controls maintained as indicated by the design?
2. Were the recruitment and selection of study participants clearly described and appropriate?
3. Did the design include an intervention that was consistently implemented?
4. Were the data collected in a consistent way?
5. Was the integrity of the study protected, and how were any problems resolved?
6. Did the researchers obtain data from an existing database? If so, did the data obtained address the study purpose and objectives, questions, or hypotheses? Were the reliability and validity of the database addressed in the research report?

Chidume's (2021) study (presented earlier in Research Example 10.6) examined the effects of fall prevention education (FPE) on the incidence of falls in adults 65 and older living in the community. Data were collected from elderly individuals attending a mobile community clinic. The clinic services were provided in a variety of settings, including low-income housing communities, community centers, assisted living facilities, and other rural settings. The key elements of the data collection process are presented in Research Example 10.9.

⑤ RESEARCH EXAMPLE 10.9

Data Collection

Research/Study Excerpt
Data collection

All data were collected by the nurse. Data and forms were transported by the nurse in a locked travel bag. No identifiable information was included during the data analysis. All data were systematically logged on paper forms, tabulated, and evaluated using descriptive statistics and parametric analysis (interviews and

RESEARCH EXAMPLE 10.9—cont'd

questionnaires). The data were entered in the Statistical Package for the Social Sciences (SPSS) version 24. Completed surveys and informed consent were placed in a locked file cabinet where they will be retained and accessible only by the nurse for five years.

The MAHC-10 [Missouri Alliance for Home Care 10-question survey] assessment tool was administered upon recruitment and obtained consent from older adult participants. The MAHC-10 fall risk assessment requested information such as the patient's age, medical, and fall history. Points were assigned for each assessment question. The numerical total of the points for each MAHC-10 assessment was the baseline fall risk assessment score. The numerical total of the points for each Stay Independent checklist, was the baseline FPE score.

After one month, follow-up phone communication with participants occurred ... Participants were queried by reassessing the MAHC-10 fall risk and the Stay Independent self-reported checklist. Scripted follow-up questions were also asked. Over the six-week project period, 33 participants were obtained for the initial assessment and FPE. Of the 33 initial participants, 30 were available for the reassessment and follow-up questions. (Chidume, 2021; Data collection)

Critical Appraisal

Chidume (2021) provided a clear, concise description of the data collection process in her study. She recruited all study participants and collected and analyzed the research data, which promoted consistency of the data collection process. The community mobile clinic provided services to many underserved individuals in a variety of settings who were appropriate participants for this study. However, the researcher noted the sample size was small because of the low turnout rates for the clinic. The intervention was provided consistently by Chidume and included a fall risk assessment and FPE. The FPE focused on the needs identified in the fall risk assessment and were personalized to the participants. The MAHC-10 is an extremely strong instrument used in several large studies and has been "validated as a single tool to assess fall risk" (Chidume, 2021, Instrument). In summary, the description of the data collection process included limited information about the recruitment of study participants but included a quality intervention and reliable and valid instruments that addressed the study purpose.

KEY POINTS

- The purpose of measurement is to obtain trustworthy data that can be used to address the quantitative and outcomes study purpose and objectives, questions, or hypotheses.
- The rules of measurement ensure that the assignment of values or categories is performed consistently from one study participant (or situation) to another and, eventually, if the measurement strategy is found to be meaningful, from one study to another.
- The levels of measurement from low to high are nominal, ordinal, interval, and ratio.
- Reliability in measurement is concerned with the consistency of the measurement technique; reliability testing focuses on stability, equivalence, and internal consistency.
- The validity of an instrument is the extent to which the instrument reflects the abstract construct being examined. Content, construct, and criterion validity are addressed.
- Readability level focuses on the study participants' ability to read and comprehend the content of an instrument.
- Physiological measures are examined for precision, accuracy, and error in research.
- Diagnostic tools and screening tests are examined for sensitivity, specificity, NPV, and LRs.

- Common measurement approaches used in nursing research include physiological measures, observation, interviews, questionnaires, and scales.
- Rating scales, Likert scale, and VAS are described for use in research and practice.
- The data collection tasks that should be critically appraised in a study include (1) recruitment of study participants, (2) consistency of data collection, and (3) maintenance of controls in the study design.

REFERENCES

Aberson, C. L. (2019). *Applied analysis for the behavioral sciences* (2nd ed.). Routledge Taylor & Francis Group.

Arikan, A., & Esenay, F. I. (2020). Active and passive distraction interventions in a pediatric emergency department to reduce the pain and anxiety during venous blood sampling: A randomized clinical trial. *Journal of Emergency Nursing, 46,* 779–790. https://doi.org/10.1016/j.jen.2020.05.004

Armenta, B. E., Hartshorn, K. J., Whitbeck, L. B., Crawford, D. M., & Hoyt, D. R. (2014). A longitudinal examination of the measurement properties and predictive utility of the Center for Epidemiologic Studies Depression Scale among North American indigenous adolescents. *Psychological Assessment, 26*(4), 1347–1355. https://doi.org/10.1037/a0037608

Asarnow, J. R., Jaycox, L. H., Tang, L., Duan, N., LaBorde, A. P., Zeldon, L. R., & Wells, K. (2009). Long-tern benefits of short-term quality improvement interventions for depressed youths in primary care. *American Journal of Psychiatry, 166,* 1002–1010. https://doi.org/10.1016/j.jad.2020.09.028

Bandalos, D. L. (2018). *Measurement theory and applications for the social sciences.* The Guilford Press.

Bialocerkowski, A., Klupp, N., & Bragge, P. (2010). Research methodology series: How to read and critically appraise a reliability article. *International Journal of Therapy and Rehabilitation, 17*(3), 114–120. https://doi.org/10.12968/ijtr.2010.17.3.46743

Breteler, M. J. M., Kleinjan, E., Numan, L., Ruurda, J. P., Van Hillegersberg, R., Leenen, L. P., ... Blokhuis, T. J. (2020). Are current wireless monitoring systems capable of detecting adverse events in high-risk surgical patients? A descriptive study. *Injury, 51*(Suppl. 2), S97-S105. https://doi.org/10.1016/j.injury.2019.11.018

Chidume, T. (2021). Promoting older adult fall prevention education and awareness in a community setting: A nurse-led intervention. *Applied Nursing Research, 57,* 151392. https://doi.org/10.1016/j.apnr.2020.151392

Connor, G. J. (2021). *Lab values interpretation: The ultimate laboratory tests manual of reference ranges and what they mean.* Author.

Cosco, T. D., Prina, M., Stubbs, B., & Wu, Y. T. (2017). Reliability and validity of the Center for Epidemiologic Studies Depression Scale in a population-based cohort of middle-aged U.S. adults. *Journal of Nursing Measurement, 25*(3), 476–485. https://doi.org/10.1891/1061-3749.25.3.476

Creswell, J. W., & Clark, V. L. P. (2018). *Designing and conducting mixed methods research* (3rd ed.). Sage.

Creswell, J. W., & Poth, C. N. (2018). *Qualitative inquiry & research design: Choosing among five approaches* (4th ed.). Sage.

DeVellis, R. F. (2017). *Scale development: Theory and applications* (4th ed.). Sage.

Dillman, D. A., Smyth, J. D., & Christian, L. M. (2014). *Internet, phone, mail, and mixed-mode surveys: The tailored design methods* (4th ed.). Wiley.

Faulkner, K. M., Jurgens, C. Y., Denfeld, Q. E., Lyons, K. S., Thompson, J. H., & Lee, C. S. (2020). Identifying unique profiles of perceived dyspnea burden in heart failure. *Heart & Lung, 49*(5), 488–494. https://doi.org/10.1016/j.hrtlng.2020.03.026

Gerrish, K., Ashworth, P., Lacey, A., & Bailey, J. (2008). Developing evidence-based practice: Experiences of senior and junior clinical nurses. *Journal of Advanced Nursing, 62*(1), 62–73. https://doi.org/10.1111/j.1365-2648.2007.04579.x

Gerrish, K., Ashworth, P., Lacey, A., Bailey, J., Cooke, J., Kendall, S., & McNeilly, E. (2007). Factors influencing the development of evidence-based practice: A research tool. *Journal of Advanced Nursing, 57*(3), 328–338. https://doi.org/10.1111/j.1365-2648.2006.04112.x

Gray, J. R., & Grove, S. K. (2021). *The practice of nursing research: Appraisal, synthesis, and generation of evidence* (9th ed.). Elsevier.

Grove, S. K., & Cipher, D. J. (2020). *Statistics for nursing research: A workbook for evidence-based practice* (3rd ed.). Elsevier.

Ho, G. W. K. (2017). Examining perceptions and attitudes: A review of Likert-type scales versus Q-methodology. *Western Journal of Nursing Research, 39*(5), 674–689.

Jiang, L., Wang, Y., Zhang, Y., Li, R., Wu, H., Le, C., & Wu, Y. (2019). The reliability and validity of the Center for Epidemiologic Studies Depression Scale (CES-D) for Chinese university students. *Frontiers in Psychiatry, 10*, 315. https://doi.org/10.3389/fpsyt.2019.00315

Johantgen, M. (2010). Using existing administrative and national databases. In C. F. Waltz, O. L. Strickland, & E. R. Lenz (Eds.), *Measurement in nursing and health research.* (4th ed., pp. 241–250). Springer.

Kagee, A., Bantijes, J., Saal, W., & Sterley, A. (2020). Predicting caseness of major depressive disorder using the Center for Epidemiological Studies Depression Scale (CESD-R) among patients receiving HIV care. *General Hospital Psychiatry, 67*, 70–76. https://doi.org/10.1016/j.genhosppsych.2020.09.005

Kaplan, A. (1963). *The conduct of inquiry: Methodology for behavioral science.* Harper & Row.

Kazdin, A. E. (2017). *Research design in clinical psychology* (5th ed.). Pearson.

Kerlinger, F. N., & Lee, H. B. (2000). *Foundations of behavioral research* (4th ed.). Harcourt College Publishers.

Leedy, P. D., & Ormrod, J. E. (2019). *Practical research: Planning and design* (12th ed.) Pearson.

Locke, B. Z., & Putnam, P. (2002). *Center for Epidemiologic Studies Depression Scale (CES-D Scale).* Bethesda, MD: National Institute of Mental Health.

McLellan, M. C., Gauvreau, K., & Connor, J. A. (2014). Validation of the Cardiac Children's Hospital Early Warning Score: An early warning scoring tool to prevent cardiopulmonary arrests in children with heart disease. *Congenital Heart Disease, 9*(3), 194–202. https://doi.org/10.1111/chd.12132

McLellan, M. C., Gauvreau, K., & Connor, J. A. (2017). Validation of the Children's Hospital Early Warning System for critical deterioration recognition. *Journal of Pediatric Nursing, 32*(1), 52–58. https://doi.org/10.1016/j.pedn.2016.10.005

Melnyk, B. M., & Fineout-Overholt, E. (2019). *Evidence-based practice in nursing & healthcare: A guide to best practice* (4th ed.). Wolters Kluwer.

Melnyk, B. M., Gallagher-Ford, E., & Fineout-Overholt E. (2017). *Implementing evidence-based practice competencies in healthcare: A practical guide for improving quality, safety, & outcomes.* Sigma Theta Tau International.

Miles, M. B., Huberman, A. M., & Saldaña, J. (2020). *Qualitative data analysis: A methods sourcebook* (4th ed.). Sage.

Misra, A. R., Oermann, M. H., Teague, M. S., & Ledbetter, L. S. (2021). An evaluation of websites offering caregiver education for tracheostomy and home mechanical ventilation. *Journal of Pediatric Nursing, 56*, 64–69. https://doi.org/10.1016/j.pedn.2020.09.014

Moorhead, S., Swanson, E., Johnson, M., & Maas, M. L. (2018). *Nursing outcomes classification (NOC): Measurement of health outcomes* (6th ed.). Elsevier.

Radloff, L. S. (1977). The CES-D scale: A self-report depression scale for research in the general population. *Applied Psychological Measurement, 1*, 385–394.

Rapp, A. M., Chavira, D. A., Sugar, C. A., & Asarnow, J. R. (2021). Incorporating family factors into treatment planning for adolescent depression: Perceived parental criticism predicts longitudinal symptom trajectory in the Youth Partners in Care Trial. *Journal of Affective Disorders, 278*, 46–53. https://doi.org/10.1016/j.jad.2020.09.028

Robert, R. E., Lewinsohn, P. M., & Seeley, J. R. (1991). Screening for adolescent depression: A comparison of depression scales. *Journal of the American Academy of Child and Adolescent Psychiatry, 30*, 58–66.

Ryan-Wenger, N. A. (2017). Precision, accuracy, and uncertainty of biophysical measurements for research and practice. In C. F. Waltz, O. L. Strickland, & E. R. Lenz (Eds.), *Measurement in nursing and health research* (5th ed., pp. 427–445). Springer.

Sahasrabudhe, N., Lee, J. S., Scotte, T. M., Punnett, L., Tucker, K. L., & Palacios, N. (2020). Serum vitamin D and depressive symptomatology among Boston-Area Puerto Ricans. *Journal of Nutrition, 150*(12), 3231–3240. https://doi.org/10.1093/jn/nxaa253

Shadish, W. R., Cook, T. D., & Campbell, D. T. (2002). *Experimental and quasi-experimental designs for generalized causal inference.* Rand McNally.

Sharp, L. K., & Lipsky, M. S. (2002). Screening for depression across the lifespan: A review of measures for use in primary care settings. *American Family Physician, 66*(6), 1001–1008.

Siddaway, A. P., Wood, A. M., & Taylor, P. J. (2017). The Center for Epidemiologic Studies-Depression (CES-D) scale measures a continuum from well-being to depression: Testing two key predictions of positive clinical psychology. *Journal of Affective Disorders, 213*, 180–186. https://doi.org/10.1016/j.jad.2017.02.015

Stevens, S. S. (1946). On the theory of scales of measurement. *Science, 103*(2684), 677–680.

Stone, K. S., & Frazier, S. K. (2017). Measurement of physiological variables using biomedical instrumentation. In C. F. Waltz, O. L. Strickland, & E. R. Lenz (Eds.), *Measurement in nursing and health research* (5th ed., (pp. 379–425). Springer.

Straus, S. E., Glasziou, P., Richardson, W. S., & Haynes, R. B. (2019). *Evidence-based medicine: How to practice and teach EBM* (5th ed.). Elsevier.

Todkar, S., Padwal, R., Michaud, A., & Cloutier, L. (2021). Knowledge, perception, and practice of health professionals regarding blood pressure measurement methods: A scoping review. *Journal of Hypertension, 39*(3), 391–399. https://doi.org/10.1097/HJH.0000000000002663

Umberger, R. A., Hatfield, L. A., & Speck, P. M. (2017). Understanding negative predictive value of diagnostic tests used in clinical practice. *Dimensions of Critical care Nursing, 36*(1), 22–29. https://doi.org/10.1097/DCC.0000000000000219

Waltz, C. F., Strickland, O. L., & Lenz, E. R. (2017). *Measurement in nursing and health research* (5th ed.). Springer Publishing Company.

Waters, T. P., Kim, S. Y., Werner, E. Dinglas, C., Carter, E. B., Patel, R., Sharma, A. J., & Catalano, P. (2020). Should women with gestational diabetes be screened at delivery hospitalization for type 2 diabetes? *American Journal of Obstetrics & Gynecology, 222*(1), 73.e1–73.e11. https://doi.org/10.1016/j.ajog.2019.07.035

Weber, M. A., Schiffrin, E. L., White, W. B., Mann, S., Lindholm, L. H., Kenerson, J. G., … Harrap, S. B. (2014). Clinical practice guidelines for the management of hypertension in the community: A statement by the American Society of Hypertension and the International Society of Hypertension. *Journal of Hypertension, 32*(1), 3–15. https://doi.org/10.1111/jch.12237

Wentland, B. A., & Hinderer, K. A. (2020). A nursing research and evidence-based practice fellowship program in a Magnet®–designated pediatric medical center. *Applied Nursing Research, 55*, 151287. https://doi.org/10.1016/j.apnr.2020.151287

Wong-Baker FACES Foundation. (2016). *Wong-Baker FACES® Pain Rating Scale.* Retrieved from https://wongbakerfaces.org/

Understanding Statistics in Research

Susan K. Grove

LEARNING OUTCOMES

After completing this chapter, you should be able to:

1. Describe probability theory and decision theory that guide the statistical analysis of data.
2. Describe the process of inferring from a sample to a population.
3. Compare and contrast Type I and Type II errors that can occur in studies.
4. Discuss the steps of the data analysis process: (a) management of missing data; (b) description of the sample; (c) reliability of the measurement methods; (d) exploratory analysis of the data; and (e) use of inferential statistical analyses guided by study objectives, questions, or hypotheses.
5. Critically appraise the descriptive analyses, frequency distributions, percentages, measures of central tendency, and measures of dispersion conducted to describe the sample and key variables in research reports.
6. Critically appraise the results obtained from the inferential statistical analyses conducted to examine relationships (Pearson product-moment correlation and factor analysis) and make predictions (linear and multiple regression analysis and logistic regression).
7. Critically appraise the results obtained from inferential analyses conducted to examine differences (*t*-test, analysis of variance, analysis of covariance, and chi-square analysis).
8. Describe the five types of results obtained from quasi-experimental and experimental studies that are interpreted within a decision theory framework: (a) significant and predicted results; (b) nonsignificant results; (c) significant and unpredicted results; (d) mixed results; and (e) unexpected results.
9. Compare and contrast the statistical significance and clinical importance of research findings.
10. Critically appraise the findings, generalizations, imitations, nursing implications, suggestions for further research, and conclusions in a published study.

The expectation that nursing practice should be based on research evidence has made it important for students and clinical nurses to acquire skills in reading and evaluating the results from statistical analyses. Nurses probably have more anxiety about data analysis and statistical results than they do about any other aspect of the research process. We hope this chapter will dispel some of that anxiety and facilitate your critical appraisal of the statistical results in research reports. The statistical information in this chapter is provided from the perspective of reading, understanding, and critically appraising the Results sections in quantitative studies, rather than on selecting statistical procedures for data analysis or performing statistical analyses.

Relevant theories and concepts of statistical analysis are described in this chapter to provide a background for understanding the results in research reports. The steps of data analysis are briefly introduced to show how research results are obtained. Some of the common statistical procedures conducted to describe variables, examine relationships among variables, predict outcomes, and test causal hypotheses are discussed. Strategies are provided to determine the appropriateness of statistical analyses conducted to obtain study results. In addition, guidelines are provided for critically appraising the results of studies. This chapter concludes with guidelines for critically appraising the study outcomes presented in the Discussion section of the report. Examples from current studies are provided throughout this chapter to promote your understanding of the content.

UNDERSTANDING THEORIES AND CONCEPTS OF THE STATISTICAL ANALYSIS PROCESS

One reason that nurses tend to avoid statistics is that many were taught only the mathematical procedures for calculating statistical equations, with little or no explanation of the logic behind those procedures or the meaning of the results. Computation is a mechanical process usually performed by a computer, and information about the calculation procedure is not necessary to understand statistical results. We present an approach that will enhance your understanding of the statistical analysis process. You can use this knowledge to critically appraise the analysis techniques, results, and outcomes presented in research reports.

A brief explanation of some of the theories and concepts important in understanding the statistical analysis process is provided. Probability theory and decision theory are discussed, and the concepts of hypothesis testing, level of significance, Type I and Type II errors, inference and generalization, normal curve, tailedness, and degrees of freedom are briefly described. More extensive discussion of these topics can be found in other sources; we recommend our own texts (Gray & Grove, 2021; Grove & Cipher, 2020) and other quality statistical texts (Holmes, 2018; Kim et al., 2022; Knapp, 2017; Leedy & Ormrod, 2019; Pett, 2016).

Probability Theory

Probability theory is used to explain the extent of a relationship, the probability that an event will occur in a given situation, or the probability that selected outcomes will occur in a study. Researchers might want to know the probability that a particular outcome will result from a nursing intervention. For example, researchers want to know how likely is it that the coronavirus disease 2019 (COVID-19) vaccine will reduce the incidence and seriousness of this disease in a community-dwelling elderly population.

Probability is expressed as a lowercase letter p, with values expressed as percentages or as a decimal value, ranging from 0 to 1. For example, if the probability is 0.04, then it is expressed as $p = 0.04$. This means that there is a 4% probability that a particular outcome (e.g., test positive for COVID-19) will occur after vaccination. Probability values also can be stated as less than a specific value, such as 0.05, expressed as $p < 0.05$. A study may indicate the probability that the experimental or intervention group participants were members of the same larger population as the comparison group participants was less than or equal to 5% ($p \leq 0.05$). In other words, it is very unlikely that the comparison and intervention groups are from the same population. There is a 5% chance that the two groups are from the same population, and a 95% chance that they are not from the same population. The inference is that the intervention group is different from the comparison group because of the effect of the intervention in the study. For example, the intervention group, receiving the COVID-19 vaccine, is different from the comparison group, not vaccinated, because of the effect of the intervention, COVID-19 vaccine. Probability values are often stated with the results of inferential statistical analyses (Grove & Cipher, 2020).

Decision Theory, Hypothesis Testing, and Level of Significance

Decision theory assumes that all of the groups in a study (e.g., experimental and comparison) used to test a particular hypothesis are components of the same population relative to the variables under study. This expectation (or assumption) traditionally is expressed as a null hypothesis, which states: *There is no difference between (or among) the groups in a study for the variables expressed in the hypothesis* (see Chapter 5 for more details about hypotheses). It is the decision of the researcher whether to provide evidence for a genuine difference between the groups. For example, researchers may hypothesize that the frequency of positive COVID-19 tests in chronically ill participants who are vaccinated is no different from the frequency of positive tests in those who are not vaccinated. A cutoff point is selected before data collection to test this null hypothesis. The cutoff point, referred to as alpha (α) or level of statistical significance, is the probability level at which the statistical results for relationships or differences are judged to be significant. The level of significance selected for most nursing studies is 0.05. If the p value found in the statistical analysis is ≤ 0.05, the intervention and control groups are considered to be significantly different (members of different populations). In the example about the effectiveness of the COVID-19 vaccine, $p = 0.04$ was less than $\alpha = 0.05$, indicating the experimental and comparison groups were significantly different in this study, and the null hypothesis was rejected.

Decision theory requires that the cutoff point selected for a study be absolute. Absolute means that even if the value obtained is only a fraction above the cutoff point, the samples are considered to be from the same population, and no meaning can be attributed to the differences (Makin & Orban de Xivry, 2019). It is inappropriate when using decision theory to state that the findings approached significance at $p = 0.055$ if the α level was set at 0.05. Using decision theory rules, this finding indicates that the groups tested are not significantly different, and the null hypothesis is accepted. In contrast, once the level of significance has been set at 0.05 by the researcher, if the analysis reveals a significant difference of 0.001, this result is not considered more significant than the $\alpha = 0.05$ originally proposed. The level of significance is dichotomous, which means that the difference is significant or not significant; there are no "degrees" of significance. However, some people, not realizing that their reasoning has shifted from decision theory to probability theory, indicate in their research report that the 0.001 result makes the findings more significant than if they had obtained a value of $p = 0.05$.

From the perspective of probability theory, there is considerable difference in the risk for a Type I error—saying something is significant when it is not—when the probability is between 0.05 and 0.001. If $p = 0.001$, the probability that the two groups are components of the same population is 1 in 1000; if $p = 0.05$, the probability that the groups belong to the same population is 5 in 100. In computer analysis, the probability value obtained from each data analysis (e.g., $p = 0.04$ or $p = 0.07$) frequently is provided on the printout and should be reported in the published study, together with the level of significance that was set before data analysis was conducted.

> 📄 **RESEARCH/EBP TIP**
>
> The level of significance (α) is set before the conduct of a study and is usually set at $\alpha = 0.05$. The α level determines whether the probability (p) value for a particular analysis in a study met the cutoff point for a significant difference between groups or a significant relationship between variables.

Type I and Type II Errors

According to decision theory, Type I and Type II errors can occur when a researcher is deciding what the result of a statistical test means (Table 11.1). A Type I error occurs when the null hypothesis is rejected when it is true (e.g., when the results indicate there is a significant difference, when in reality there is not). The risk for a Type I error is indicated by the level of significance or alpha (α). There is a greater risk for a Type I error with $\alpha = 0.05$ (5 chances for error in 100) than with $\alpha = 0.01$ (1 chance for error in 100).

A Type II error, or beta (β), occurs when the null hypothesis is regarded as true but is in fact false (see Table 11.1). For example, statistical analyses may indicate no significant relationship between variables or difference between groups; but in reality, there is a significant relationship or difference that was not identified by statistical analysis. There is a greater risk for a Type II error when the level of significance is set at 0.01 than when it is set at 0.05. However, Type II errors are often caused by flaws in the research design, sample, and measurement methods. Strong designs (see Chapter 8; Kazdin, 2017) and reliable and valid measurement methods (see Chapter 10; Waltz et al., 2017) increase the power of a study to detect statistically significant relationships and differences in studies. Power analysis is an effective technique for determining adequate sample size for quantitative and outcomes studies (see Chapter 9; Aberson, 2019).

In many nursing situations, multiple variables interact to cause differences within populations. When only a few of the interacting variables are examined, small differences between groups may be overlooked. This leads to nonsignificant study results, which can cause researchers to conclude falsely that there are no differences between the groups when there actually are. Thus the risk for a Type II error is often high in nursing studies (Gray & Grove, 2021). Box 11.1 identifies the common statistical mistakes that are made in nursing and other disciplines that you need to be aware of when reviewing the results of studies.

> 📄 **RESEARCH/EBP TIP**
>
> Studies with minimal Type I and Type II errors usually provide sound results and findings with possible implications for practice. Evidence-based practice (EBP) evolves from a strong body of research evidence.

TABLE 11.1   TYPE I AND TYPE II ERRORS

NULL HYPOTHESIS OUTCOME	DECISION	
	REJECT NULL HYPOTHESIS[a]	ACCEPT NULL HYPOTHESIS[a]
Null[a] hypothesis is true.	Type I error: alpha (α)	Correct decision
Null[a] hypothesis is false.	Correct decision	Type II error: beta (β)

[a]The null hypothesis states that no difference or relationship exists in the study sample.

BOX 11.1 COMMON STATISTICAL MISTAKES TO RECOGNIZE WHEN REVIEWING A RESEARCH REPORT

1. Absence of an adequate control or comparison group
2. Using a small sample not supported by power analysis or arbitrarily selecting a sample size
3. Failing to address participant attrition and missing data or deleting missing data without justification
4. Failing to correct for multiple comparisons, such as conducting multiple *t*-tests in a study
5. Confusing data from independent groups with data from paired groups
6. Selecting inappropriate statistical analysis techniques to address the study purpose and the hypotheses or questions
7. Conducting inappropriate analyses based on the data level of measurement
8. Overinterpreting nonsignificant results
9. Confusing correlation with cause and effect
10. Confusing statistical significance with practical or clinical importance

Information was abstracted from Kim, M., Mallory, C., & Valerio, T. D. (2022). *Statistics for evidence-based practice in nursing* (3rd ed.). Jones & Bartlett Learning; and Makin, T. R., & Orban de Xivry, J. (2019). Ten common statistical mistakes to watch out for when writing or reviewing a manuscript. *eLife, 8,* e48175. https://doi.org/10.7554/eLife.48175

Inference and Generalization

An inference is a conclusion or judgment based on research evidence. Statistical inferences are made with caution and great care. The decision theory rules used to interpret the results of statistical procedures increase the probability that inferences are accurate. A generalization is the application of information that has been acquired from a specific instance to a general situation. Generalizing requires making an inference. An inference is made from a specific case and extended to a general truth, from a part to the whole, from the concrete to the abstract, and from the known to the unknown. In research, an inference is made from the study findings obtained from a specific sample and applied to a more general target population, using the results from statistical analyses. For example, researchers may conclude that a significant difference was found in the depression levels between two samples, one in which the participants received online counseling with standard care and another in which the participants received only standard care. These researchers may conclude that this difference can be expected in all patients who have received online counseling. Thus the findings are generalized from the sample in the study to all patients receiving online counseling.

Statisticians and researchers can never prove something using inference; they can never be certain that their inferences and generalizations are correct. The researchers' generalization about the effectiveness of the counseling may not have been carefully thought out—the findings may have been generalized to a population that was overly broad. It is possible that in the more general population, there is no difference in the depression levels of individuals receiving online counseling. Additional studies in this area with similar results increase the strength of an inference and can expand generalization of the findings. Generalized findings are part of the Discussion section of a research report presented later in this chapter.

Normal Curve

A normal curve is a theoretical frequency distribution of all possible values in a population; however, no real distribution exactly fits the normal curve (Fig. 11.1). The idea of the normal curve was developed by an 18-year-old mathematician, Johann Gauss, in 1795. He found that the results from the analysis of data from variables (e.g., the mean of each sample) determined repeatedly in

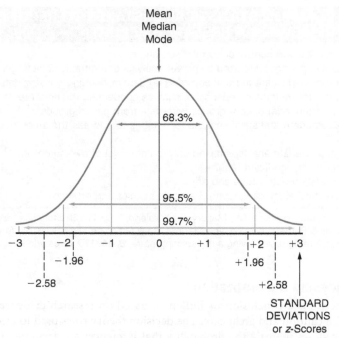

FIG. 11.1 Normal Curve.

many samples from the same population can be combined into one large sample. From this large sample, a more accurate representation can be developed of the pattern of the curve in that population than is possible with only one sample. Surprisingly, in most cases, the curve is similar, regardless of the specific variables examined or the population studied. For example, numerous studies have been conducted to examine the effectiveness of the COVID-19 vaccine, and the means from these studies when combined would form a normal curve.

Levels of significance and probability are based on the logic of the normal curve. The normal curve in Fig. 11.1 shows the distribution of values for a single population. Note that 95.5% of the values are within two standard deviations (*SDs*) of the mean, ranging from −2 to +2 *SDs*. There is approximately a 95% probability that a given measured value (e.g., the mean of a group) would fall within approximately 2 *SDs* of the mean of the population, and there is a 2.5% (2.5% + 2.5% = 5%) probability that the value would fall in either of the tails of the normal curve (Fig. 11.2). The tails are the extreme ends of the normal curve that include less than −2 (−1.96 exactly) *SDs* (2.5%) or greater than +2 (+1.96 exactly) *SDs* (2.5%). If the groups being compared are from the same population (not significantly different), you would expect the values (e.g., the means) of each group to be within the 95% range of values on the normal curve. If the groups are from significantly different populations, you would expect one of the group values to be outside the 95% range of values. An inferential statistical analysis performed to determine differences between groups, using a level of significance (α) set at 0.05, would test that expectation. If the statistical test demonstrates a significant difference (the value of one group does not fall within the 95% range of values), the groups are considered to belong to different populations. However, in 5% of statistical tests, the value of one of the groups can be expected to be outside of the 95% range of values but still belong to the same population (a Type I error).

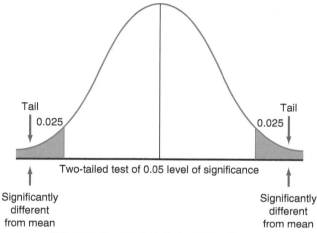

FIG. 11.2 Two-Tailed Test of Significance.

📄 **RESEARCH/EBP TIP**

The normal curve provides a theoretical distribution of all possible values in a population. This curve provides the basis for determining significant differences and relationships when conducting inferential statistics.

Tailedness

With nondirectional hypotheses, researchers assume that an extreme score can occur in either tail of the normal curve (see Fig. 11.2). The analysis of a nondirectional hypothesis is called a two-tailed test of significance, because significance testing is conducted for both tails of the normal curve. In a one-tailed test of significance, the hypothesis is directional, and extreme statistical values that occur in a single tail of the curve are of interest (see Chapter 5 for a discussion of directional and nondirectional hypotheses). The hypothesis might state that the extreme score is greater than that for 95% of the population, indicating that the sample with the extreme score is not a member of the same population. Fig. 11.3 shows a one-tailed test of significance, in which the statistical values considered for significance are in the right tail. In this case, 5% of statistical values that are considered significant will be in one tail (e.g., the right tail in Fig. 11.3), rather than two. Extreme statistical values occurring in the other tail of the curve (e.g., the left tail of Fig. 11.3) are not considered significantly different.

Developing a one-tailed hypothesis requires that researchers have sufficient knowledge of the variables to predict whether the difference will be in the tail above the mean or in the tail below the mean. A one-tailed test is statistically stronger and more likely to identify significant differences or relationships that exist in a sample (Grove & Cipher, 2020). Lerret and colleagues (2020) conducted a quasi-experimental study to examine the effects of the intervention, Engaging Parents in Education for Discharge (ePED) iPad application, on the outcomes of quality of discharge teaching and care coordination. This study included the following directional hypothesis: "Parents exposed to discharge teaching using ePED will have higher quality discharge teaching scores than parents exposed to usual discharge teaching" (Lerret et al., 2020, p. 42). This directional hypothesis predicts that the area of significance is in the right tail of the normal curve as shown in Fig. 11.3.

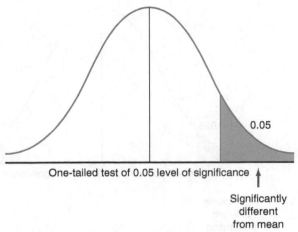

0.05

One-tailed test of 0.05 level of significance

Significantly
different
from mean

FIG. 11.3 One-Tailed Test of Significance.

Lerret et al. (2020) found that the parents receiving *e*PED intervention reported higher discharge teaching scores than the parents exposed to standard discharge teaching. Because the study results were significant, this hypothesis was accepted.

📄 RESEARCH/EBP TIP

One-tailed statistical tests are uniformly more powerful than two-tailed tests in detecting significant differences or relationships in a sample, decreasing the possibility of a Type II error.

Degrees of Freedom

The concept of degrees of freedom (*df*) is important for calculating statistical analyses and interpreting the results. Degrees of freedom involve the freedom of a score value to vary given the other existing scores' values and the established sum of these scores (Gray & Grove, 2021; Kim et al., 2022). Degrees of freedom are usually reported with statistical results, so you may look up the results on statistical tables (see the appendices in Gray & Grove, 2021).

IDENTIFYING THE STEPS OF THE DATA ANALYSIS PROCESS

The data analysis process in quantitative and outcomes research involves the management of numerical data using statistical analyses to produce study results. Statistical analyses are techniques or procedures conducted to examine, consolidate, and give meaning to the numerical data gathered in a study. Statistical techniques are divided into two major categories, descriptive and inferential. Descriptive statistics are summary statistics that allow the researcher to organize data in ways that give meaning and facilitate insight. Descriptive statistics are calculated to describe the sample and major study variables. Inferential statistics are designed to address objectives, questions, and hypotheses in studies to allow inference from the study sample to the target population. Inferential analyses are conducted to examine relationships, make predictions, and determine group differences in studies.

BOX 11.2 STEPS OF THE DATA ANALYSIS PROCESS

1. Management of missing data
2. Description of the sample
3. Examination of the reliability of the measurement methods
4. Exploratory analysis of the data
5. Inferential statistical analyses guided by study purpose, hypotheses, or questions

When critically appraising a study, it is helpful to understand the following steps that researchers implement during data analysis: (1) management of missing data, (2) description of the sample, (3) examination of the reliability of measurement methods, (4) performance of exploratory analyses of data, and (5) performance of inferential analyses guided by the study hypotheses or questions (Box 11.2). Although not all these steps are equally reflected in the final report of the study, they all contribute to the insights that can be gained from analysis of study data.

Management of Missing Data

Missing data points are identified during data entry into the computer or during review of the data. In some cases, study participants must be excluded from an analysis because data considered essential to that analysis are missing. In examining the results of a published study, you might note that the number of participants included in the final analyses is less than the original sample. This could be a result of attrition and/or participants with missing data being excluded from analyses.

Craig et al. (2021) conducted a quasi-experimental study to examine the effects of a structured medication safety enhancement simulation program on Bachelor of Science in Nursing (BSN) students' medication administration knowledge and competence. The researchers reported three students, two in the intervention group and one in the control group, did not complete week 4 of data collection. Craig et al. (2021) reported the attrition of these students but provided no information about their characteristics or reasons for dropping out of the study. This is a common statistical mistake when attrition and management of missing data are not addressed in a research report (see Box 11.1).

RESEARCH/EBP TIP

When critically appraising study results, examine the information provided on participant attrition, missing data, and the management of these in the study.

Description of the Sample

Researchers present as complete a picture of the sample as possible in their research report. Variables relevant to the sample are called demographic variables, which might include age, gender, educational level, and diagnosis. Analysis of demographic variables produces the sample characteristics for the study participants (see Chapter 5). When a study includes more than one group (e.g., intervention and comparison groups), researchers often compare the groups in relation to the demographic variables. For example, it might be important to know whether the group distributions of age and educational level were similar. When demographic variables are similar for the intervention and comparison groups, the study results are more likely to be caused by the intervention than by group differences at the initiation of the study.

Reliability of Measurement Methods

Researchers need to report the reliability of the measurement methods used in their study. The reliability of observational or physiological measures is usually determined during the data collection phase and noted in the research report. If a multi-item scale was used to collect data in a study, the Cronbach's alpha value should be included in the research report (Bandalos, 2018; Waltz et al., 2017). A Cronbach's alpha coefficient value of 0.80 to 0.90 reported by other researchers in previous studies and reported for this study indicates strong instrument reliability. The t-test or Pearson correlation statistics may be used to determine test-retest reliability. If the validity of a measurement method is examined in a study, this content also needs to be included in the research report (see Chapter 10).

In Craig et al.'s (2021) study, the Medication Safety Knowledge Assessment (MSKA) was used to measure the BSN students' knowledge. The MSKA is a 25-item multiple-choice instrument that was shown to have strong reliability (Cronbach's alpha $r = 0.96$) when administered during the study posttest. The MSKA also had established content validity by nurse educators and content experts (content validity index = 0.94). Strong measurement methods increased the power of this study and the credibility to the research results and findings.

📄 RESEARCH/EBP TIP

In critically appraising a study, you need to examine the reliability and validity of the measurement methods and the statistical procedures used to determine these values.

Exploratory Analyses

The next step, exploratory analysis, is used to examine all the data descriptively. This step is discussed in more detail later in this chapter. Data on each study variable are examined using measures of central tendency and dispersion to determine the nature of variation in the data and to identify outliers. Outliers are study data points that have extreme values (values that lie far from the other plotted points on a graph) that seem unlike the rest of the sample. Researchers usually indicate whether outliers are identified during data analysis and how these were managed. In critically appraising a study's results, note any discussion of outliers and how they were managed. Did the outliers have an effect on the study results?

Inferential Statistical Analyses

The final phase of data analysis involves conducting inferential statistical analyses for the purpose of generalizing findings from the study sample to appropriate accessible and target populations. A rigorous research methodology is needed to justify generalization of the results from inferential analyses, including a strong research design (Kazdin, 2017; Shadish et al., 2002), reliable and valid measurement methods (Bandalos, 2018), and an adequate sample size (Aberson, 2019; Cohen, 1988).

Most researchers include a section in their research report that identifies the statistical program and analysis techniques conducted on study data. Statistical analysis programs commonly reported by nurse researchers are Statistical Program for Social Sciences (SPSS) and Statistical Analysis Software (SAS). The discussion of data analyses includes the inferential analysis techniques (e.g., those focused on relationships, prediction, and differences) and sometimes the descriptive analysis techniques conducted in the study. The data analysis techniques conducted in a study are usually presented just before the study's Results section. As introduced earlier, Lerret et al. (2020) conducted a study to determine the effects of the *e*PED intervention on the quality of discharge teaching and coordination of care for parents with hospitalized children. Research Example 11.1 provides a description of the data analyses planned for this study.

RESEARCH EXAMPLE 11.1

Data Analysis Planned for a Study

Research/Study Excerpt

Data Analysis

Descriptive statistics were used to describe the sample and compare between the ePED implementation and non-ePED comparison units [groups]. The Cronbach alpha (α) was used to assess the reliability of the QDTS-D [Quality of Discharge Teaching Scale] and CTM [Care Transition Measure] scales in the study population. ... The significance level was set at p<0.05, t-tests were performed to identify if there was a mean difference in the QDTS-D and the CTM between parents of the children from implementation [group] who received teaching guided by ePED and parents of children from the comparison unit who did not receive teaching guided by the ePED. (Lerret et al., 2020, p. 45)

Critical Appraisal

Lerret et al. (2020) provided a clear, concise description of the analyses conducted in their study. The reliability of the measurement methods was examined to determine any limitations. The descriptive and inferential statistics were appropriate to test the study hypotheses and to analyze the interval data collected in this study.

STATISTICS CONDUCTED TO DESCRIBE VARIABLES

As discussed earlier, descriptive statistics allow researchers to organize numerical data in ways that give meaning and facilitate insight. Initially, numerical data in a study are analyzed with descriptive statistics. For some descriptive studies, researchers limit data analyses to descriptive statistics. For other studies, researchers use descriptive statistics primarily to describe the characteristics of the sample and the dependent or research variables. The descriptive statistics frequency distributions, percentages, measures of central tendency, measures of dispersion, and standardized scores are discussed in the following sections.

Frequency Distributions

Frequency distribution describes the occurrence of scores or categories in a study. For example, the frequency distribution for gender in a study might be 42 males and 58 females. A frequency distribution usually is the first method used to organize the data for examination. There are two types of frequency distributions: ungrouped and grouped.

Ungrouped Frequency Distributions

Most studies have some categorical data that are presented in the form of an ungrouped frequency distribution, in which a table is developed to display all numerical values obtained for a particular variable. This approach is generally used on discrete rather than continuous data. Examples of data commonly organized in this manner are gender, ethnicity/race, and marital status, and values obtained from the measurement of selected research and dependent variables. Table 11.2 is an example table developed for this text; it includes seven different scores obtained by 50 participants. This is an example of ungrouped frequencies because each score is represented in the table with the number of participants receiving this score.

TABLE 11.2   EXAMPLE OF AN UNGROUPED FREQUENCY TABLE (*N* = 50)

SCORE	FREQUENCY	PERCENTAGE	CUMULATIVE FREQUENCY (*f*)	CUMULATIVE PERCENTAGE
1	4	8%	4	8%
3	6	12%	10	20%
4	8	16%	18	36%
5	14	28%	32	64%
7	8	16%	40	80%
8	6	12%	46	92%
9	4	8%	50	100%

Grouped Frequency Distributions

Grouped frequency distributions are used when continuous variables are being examined. Many measures taken during data collection, including age, body temperature, weight, laboratory values, scale scores, and time, are measured using a continuous scale. Any method of grouping results in loss of information. For example, if age is grouped, a breakdown into two groups, those younger than 65 years and those who are 65 years and older, provides less information about the data than groupings of 10-year age spans. As with levels of measurement (see Chapter 10), rules have been established to guide data classification systems. For best results, there should be at least 3 to 4 groups, but not more than 10. The categories established must be exhaustive; each datum must fit into one of the identified categories. The categories must be exclusive; each datum must fit into only one (Grove & Cipher, 2020). A common mistake occurs when the ranges contain overlaps that would allow a datum to fit into more than one category. For example, a researcher may classify age ranges as 20 to 30, 30 to 40, 40 to 50 years, and so on. By this definition, participants aged 30 years, 40 years, and so on can be classified into more than one category. The range of each category must be equivalent. For example, if 10 years is the age range, each age category must include 10 years of ages. This rule is violated in some cases to allow the first and last categories to be open-ended and worded to include all scores greater than or less than a specified point. Income data are usually presented in groups because most people do not want to report their exact income. Table 11.3 presents an example of a grouped frequency distribution for registered nurses' income; the categories are exhaustive and mutually exclusive.

TABLE 11.3   INCOME OF FULL-TIME REGISTERED NURSES IN HOSPITALS (*N* = 100)

INCOME	FREQUENCY, *n* (%)	CUMULATIVE PERCENTAGE
<$70,000	5 (5)	5%
$70,000–$79,999	20 (20)	25%
$80,000–$89,999	35 (35)	60%
$90,000–$100,000	25 (25)	85%
>$100,000	15 (15)	100%

Percentage Distributions

A percentage distribution indicates the percentage of study participants in a sample whose scores fall into a specific group and the number of scores in that group. Percentage distributions are particularly useful for comparing the present data with findings from other studies that have different sample sizes. A cumulative distribution is a type of percentage distribution in which the percentages and frequencies of scores are summed as one moves from the top to the bottom of the table. Consequently, the bottom category would have a cumulative frequency equivalent to the sample size and a cumulative percentage of 100 (see Table 11.2). Frequency distributions are also displayed using graphs (e.g., pie chart, bar chart, line graph). Graphic displays of the frequency distribution of data from Table 11.2 are presented in Fig. 11.4. You might note in the bar and line graphs that the data distribution forms a normal curve.

Measures of Central Tendency

Measures of central tendency are referred to as the midpoint in the data or as an average of the data. These measures are the most concise statement of the nature of the data in a study. The three measures of central tendency that are commonly conducted in statistical analyses are the mode, median, and mean. For a data set that has a perfect normal distribution, these values are equal (see Fig. 11.1); however, data obtained from real samples do not have *perfect* distributions.

Mode

The mode is the numerical value or score that occurs with greatest frequency; it does not necessarily indicate the center of the data set. The mode can be determined by examination of an ungrouped frequency distribution of the data. In Table 11.2, the mode is the score of 5, which occurred 14 times in the data set. The mode can be used to describe the typical study participant or identify the most frequently occurring value on a scale item. The three diagrams in Fig. 11.4 show that 5 is the mode of this distribution. The mode is the appropriate measure of central tendency for nominal data. A data set can have more than one mode. If two modes exist, the data set is referred to as bimodal distribution (Fig. 11.5). A data set with more than two modes is said to be multimodal (Gray & Grove, 2021).

Median

The median is the midpoint or the score at the exact center of the ungrouped frequency distribution—the 50th percentile. The median is obtained by rank-ordering the scores. If the number of scores is uneven, exactly 50% of the scores are greater than the median, and 50% are less than it. If the number of scores is even, the median is the average of the two middle scores; thus the median may not be one of the scores in the data set. Unlike the mean, the median is not affected by extreme scores or outliers in the data. The median is the most appropriate measure of central tendency for ordinal data. The median for the data in Table 11.2 is 5.

Mean

The most commonly conducted measure of central tendency is the mean. The mean is the sum of the scores divided by the number of scores being summed. Like the median, the mean may not be a member of the data set. The mean is the appropriate measure of central tendency for interval- and ratio-level (continuous) data. However, if the study has outliers, the mean is most affected by these, and the median might be the measure of central tendency included in the research report. The mean for the data in Table 11.2 is 5.28. The scores are summed (264) and then divided by the number of study participants ($N = 50$). Thus the mean is calculated as follows: $264 \div 50 = 5.28$.

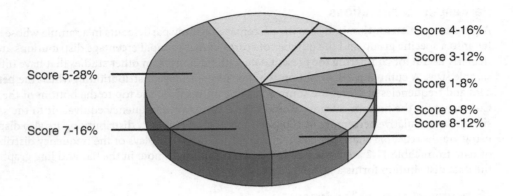

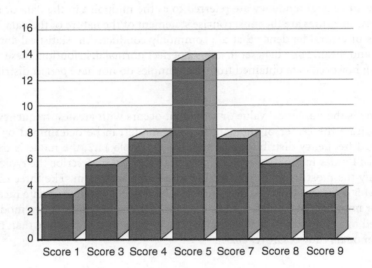

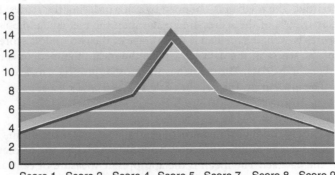

FIG. 11.4 Commonly Used Graphic Displays of Frequency Distributions.

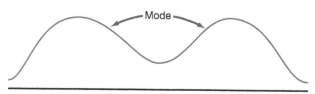

FIG. 11.5 Bimodal Distribution.

Measures of Dispersion

Measures of dispersion, or variability, are measures of individual differences of the members of the sample. They give some indication of how scores in a sample are dispersed or spread around the mean. These measures provide information about the data that are not available from measures of central tendency. The measures of dispersion, such as range, variance, and *SD*, indicate how different the scores are or the extent to which individual scores deviate from one another (Grove & Cipher, 2020). If the individual scores are similar, measures of variability are small, and the sample is relatively homogeneous, or similar, in terms of those scores. A heterogeneous sample has a wide variation in scores. The measures of dispersion generally included in research reports are range and *SD*. Standardized scores (discussed later) also may be used to express measures of dispersion. Scatterplots (discussed later) frequently are used to illustrate or graphically represent the dispersion of data in a study.

Range

The simplest measure of dispersion is the range, which is obtained by subtracting the lowest score from the highest score. The range for the scores in Table 11.2 is calculated as $9 - 1 = 8$. The range is a difference score, which uses only the two extreme scores for the comparison. Despite being a crude measure of dispersion, the range is sensitive to outliers. The range might also be expressed as the lowest to the highest scores. For the data in Table 11.2, the range might also be expressed as the scores from 1 to 9.

Variance

The variance for scores in a study is calculated with a mathematical equation and indicates the spread or dispersion of the scores. The variance can be calculated on data only at the interval or ratio level of measurement (see Grove & Cipher, 2020, for the equation and calculation). The numerical value obtained from the calculation depends on the measurement method used, such as the laboratory measurement of fasting blood glucose values or the scale measurement of weights. Generally, the larger the variance value, the greater is the dispersion of scores. The variance for the data in Table 11.2 is 4.94.

Standard Deviation

The standard deviation (*SD*) is the square root of the variance. Just as the mean is the average value for the center of data, the *SD* is the average difference (deviation) value. The *SD* provides a measure of the average deviation of a value from the mean in that particular sample. It indicates the degree of error that would result if the mean alone were used to interpret the data. In the normal curve, 68% of the values will be within 1 *SD* more than or less than the mean, 95% will be within 1.96 *SD*s greater than or less than the mean, and 99% will be within 2.58 *SD*s greater than or less than the mean (see Fig. 11.1; Grove & Cipher, 2020).

The *SD* for the example data presented in Table 11.2 is 2.22. The mean is 5.28, so the value of a study participant's score 1 *SD* less than the mean would be 5.28 − 2.22, or 3.06. The value of another participant's score might be 1 *SD* greater than the mean, which would be 5.28 + 2.22, or 7.50. Therefore approximately 68% of the sample can be expected to have values in the range of 3.06–7.50, which is expressed as (3.06, 7.50). Extending this calculation further, the value of a participant's score 2 *SDs* below the mean would be 5.28 − 2.22 − 2.22 = 0.84, and the value of a participant's score 2 *SDs* above the mean would be 5.28 + 2.22 + 2.22 = 9.72. The values for 2 *SDs* below and above the mean would be expressed as (0.84, 9.72). Using this strategy, the entire distribution of values can be estimated (Grove & Cipher, 2020). The value of a single individual can be compared with the value calculated for the total sample (e.g., mean, median, mode). *SD* is an important measure, both for understanding dispersion within a distribution and interpreting the relationship of a particular value to the distribution. In a published study, the *SD* is often written as the mean ± (plus or minus) the *SD*—for example, 5.28 ± 2.22.

📄 RESEARCH/EBP TIP

Researchers should include the mean and *SD* for each of the interval/ratio or continuous variables in their study. These values are important for comparing the results from one study with those of previous studies in a selected area. In addition, *SDs* and means are essential for conducting meta-analyses (see Chapter 13) to summarized data from selected studies to determine the effectiveness of an intervention for use in practice.

Confidence Interval

When you analyze data collected on a variable, you may want to know how likely it is that the population's value is near the sample's value. The known probability of including the value of the population within an interval estimate is referred to as a confidence interval (*CI*). *CIs* provide a range of values that have a greater probability of including a population parameter than a point estimate obtained from statistical analysis of a sample's data. Calculating a *CI* involves the use of two formulas to identify the upper and lower ends of the interval (see Grove & Cipher, 2020, for the formulas and calculations).

The *CI* for a study might include a lower value of 15.34 and an upper value of 20.56 and would be expressed as (15.34, 20.56). *CIs* are usually calculated for 95% and 99% intervals. The 95% *CI* indicates that 95% of the time, the population mean would be within this interval. Theoretically, we can produce a *CI* for any population value or parameter of a distribution. It is a generic statistical procedure. For example, *CIs* can also be developed around correlation coefficients and *t*-test values. Estimation can be used for a single population or for multiple populations. Researchers have increased their reporting of *CIs* for the key results of their studies. The range of values in a *CI* increases the probability that the population parameter is identified and provides a margin for error (Grove & Cipher, 2020; Kim et al., 2022).

Standardized Scores

Because of differences in the characteristics of various distributions, comparing a value in one distribution with a value in another is difficult. For example, perhaps you want to compare test scores from two classroom examinations. The highest possible score on one test is 100 and on the other it is 70, making the scores difficult to compare. To facilitate this comparison, a mechanism was developed to transform raw scores into standardized scores using the means and *SDs* for a variable. Numbers that make sense only within the framework of measurements used within a specific study are transformed into numbers (standardized scores) that have a more general meaning. Transformation into standardized scores allows an easy conceptual grasp of the meaning of the score. A common standardized score is the z-score. It expresses deviations from the mean (difference scores) in terms of *SD* units (see Fig. 11.1). A score that is greater than the mean will have a positive z-score, whereas a score that is less than the mean will have a negative z-score. The mean expressed as a z-score is zero. The *SD* is equal to the z-score. Thus a z-score of 2 indicates that the score from which it was obtained is 2 *SD*s above the mean. A z-score of −0.5 indicates that the score is 0.5 *SD* below the mean. A table of complete z-scores can be found in Appendix A of Gray and Grove's (2021) graduate research text.

Scatterplots

A scatterplot has two scales: horizontal and vertical. Each scale is referred to as an axis. The vertical scale is called the *y*-axis; the horizontal scale is the *x*-axis. A scatterplot can be used to illustrate the dispersion of values on a variable. In this case the *x*-axis represents the possible values of the variable. The *y*-axis represents the number of times each value of the variable occurred in the sample. Scatterplots also can be used to illustrate the relationship between values on one variable and values on another. Then each axis will represent one variable. For example, if a graph is developed to illustrate the relationship between study participants' anxiety and depression scores measured with Likert scales, the horizontal axis could represent anxiety and the vertical axis could represent depression. For each unit or participant, there is a value for *x* and a value for *y*. The point at which the values of *x* and *y* for a single participant intersect is plotted on the graph. Fig. 11.6 provides the structure for a scatterplot that was developed to graph the relationship between anxiety (on the *x*-axis) and depression (on the *y*-axis) in a group of study participants. In this example scatterplot, the values for *x*(5) and *y*(1) are plotted for one unit or study participant (see Fig. 11.6). When the values for each participant in the sample have been plotted, the degree of relationship between the variables is revealed (Fig. 11.7). If the scatterplot in Fig. 11.7 was an

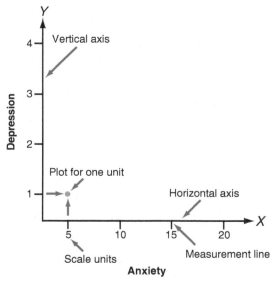

FIG. 11.6 Structure of a Plot.

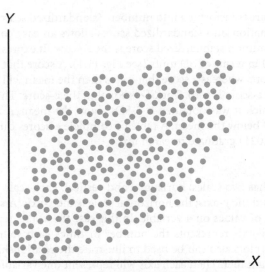

FIG. 11.7 Example of a Scatterplot.

example of the relationship between anxiety and depression, the plot is positive and indicates that as anxiety increases, so does depression in the study participants. The plotted points in a positive relationship extend from the lower left to the upper right corners of the scatterplot, as in Fig. 11.7. With a negative relationship, the plotted points extend from the upper left to lower right corners of the plot. The closer the plotted points are to a straight line, the stronger the relationship between the two variables. Grove and Cipher (2020) provide different types of scatterplots in their text and guidelines for critically appraising scatterplots in published studies.

Understanding Descriptive Statistical Results

Descriptive statistics are conducted to describe the sample and study variables. The descriptive statistical values are presented in tables and the narrative of a study's Results section (American Psychological Association [APA], 2020). Measures of central tendency (mode, median, and mean) and measures of dispersion (range and *SD*) are usually calculated to describe study variables. For example, you can review a table in a research report to identify that the mean age of the study participants was 41.8 years (*SD* = 4.3). Also, descriptive and inferential statistics might be presented together to describe differences or similarities between groups at the beginning of a study. When a team of researchers want to know whether a study intervention given to one group has made a difference, they first must know whether the groups were different at the beginning of the study. If the groups are different from the beginning, the effect of the intervention on the outcome may be exaggerated or attenuated. Inferential statistical procedures often used for this purpose include the chi-square (X^2) test for nominal-level data and the *t*-test for interval- and ratio-level data. From a perspective of descriptive analyses, the purpose is not to test for causality, but rather to describe the differences or similarities between or among the groups in a study.

Ding et al. (2020) conducted a quasi-experimental study to examine the effectiveness of an empathy clinical educational program on the empathy and communication skills of nursing students caring for children. Both the experimental and control groups of nursing students were provided the standard internship. The experimental group also received an intervention, the knowledge, simulation, and sharing module. The group assignments for the 250 participants were made based on convenience, with the first 125 students registering for the course being placed into the control group and the last 125 students registering being assigned to the experimental group. The demographic variables and the empathy scores (dependent variable) for the intervention and control groups were described and examined for differences before the internship, as presented in Research Example 11.2.

RESEARCH EXAMPLE 11.2
Description of Study Variables

Research/Study Excerpt
Results

In total, 250 participants were included in the study, with 125 students in the experimental group and 125 in the control group. There was no loss to follow-up in the 9-month internship period. ... No differences were observed at baseline between the two groups in terms of gender, age, education, educational system, only child status, and birth location (Table 11.4). ... The experimental group had lower empathy scores than the control group at the beginning of the internship. (Ding et al., 2020, Results section)

However, these scores were not significantly different with $p = 0.672$ (Table 11.5).

Critical Appraisal

Ding and colleagues (2020) provided a clear, concise presentation of the demographic variables and dependent variable empathy using tables and narrative. Most of the demographic variables were measured at the nominal level and were appropriately described with frequencies and percentages. Age was measured at the ratio level and was described with a mean and *SD* (see Table 11.4). Empathy was measured using a Likert scale that produces interval-level data, which was described using mean and *SD* (Waltz et al., 2017). The descriptive analyses conducted were appropriate; however, including the range for the age and empathy variables would have indicated if outliers existed in the data.

Differences between the groups were appropriately analyzed with x^2 or independent samples *t*-tests based on each variable's level of measurement (see Tables 11.4 and 11.5). The participants were not randomly assigned to groups, so there is a potential for bias. However, because the intervention and control groups had no significant differences for the demographic or dependent variables at the beginning of the study, these groups were considered similar for these variables. In addition, the study had no attrition of participants. Because the groups were similar at the beginning of the study, the significant differences noted at the end of the study are more likely to be a result of the study intervention than from error. Additional results from this study are presented later in the *t*-tests section.

TABLE 11.4 Demographic Characteristics of Participants

Variables	Control Group, *n* (%)	Experimental Group, *n* (%)	x^2/t	*p*-value
Gender			0.278	0.598
Male	5 (4.0)	6 (4.8)		
Female	120 (96.0)	119 (95.2)		
Age, yr	20.04 ± 1.41	20.31 ± 1.26	−1.608	0.109
Education			0.130	0.719
Diploma	108 (86.4)	106 (84.8)		
Bachelor	17 (13.6)	19 (15.2)		

Continued

RESEARCH EXAMPLE 11.2—cont'd

TABLE 11.4   Demographic Characteristics of Participants—cont'd

Variables	Control Group, n (%)	Experimental Group, n (%)	X^2/t	p-value
Education System			0.177	0.915
3-year diploma	83 (66.4)	80 (64.0)		
4-year BSc	7 (5.6)	8 (6.4)		
5-year diploma	35 (28.0)	37 (29.6)		
One child in family			0.161	0.688
Yes	13 (10.4)	15 (12.0)		
No	112 (89.6)	110 (88.0)		
Birth location			0.110	0.740
Rural	104 (83.2)	102 (81.6)		
City	21 (16.8)	23 (18.4)		

Adapted from Results section of Ding, X., Wang, L., Sun, J., Li, D., Zheng, B., He, S., ... Latour, J. M. (2020). Effectiveness of empathy clinical education for children's nursing students: A quasi-experimental study. *Nurse Education Today, 85*, 104260. https://doi.org/10.1016/j.nedt.2019.104260

TABLE 11.5   Empathy Scores in the Two Groups before the Standard Internship Education and the Knowledge, Simulation, Sharing Module

	n	Preinternship Mean (*SD*)
Control group	125	109.06 (12.12)
Experimental group	125	108.39 (12.62)
Mean difference (95% *CI*)		−0.664 (−3.745, 2.417)
p- Value		0.672

Empathy scores are scores of the Jefferson Scale of Empathy-Health Profession-Students Questionnaire. *SD*, Standard deviation.
Data are abstracted from Table 3 in Ding, X., Wang, L., Sun, J., Li, D., Zheng, B., He, S., ... Latour, J. M. (2020). Effectiveness of empathy clinical education for children's nursing students: A quasi-experimental study. *Nurse Education Today, 85*, 104260. https://doi.org/10.1016/j.nedt.2019.104260

DETERMINING THE APPROPRIATENESS OF INFERENTIAL STATISTICS IN STUDIES

Multiple factors are involved in determining the appropriateness or suitability of inferential statistical techniques conducted in a study. Inferential statistics are conducted to examine relationships, make predictions, and determine causality or differences in studies. Evaluating statistical procedures requires that you make a number of judgments about the nature of the data and what the researcher wanted to know. You need to determine (1) the nature of the research question or hypothesis; (2) whether the data for analysis were treated as nominal, ordinal, or interval/ratio (see

Fig. 10.2 in Chapter 10); (3) how many groups were in the study; and (4) whether the groups were paired (dependent) or independent.

You might see analysis techniques identified as parametric or nonparametric, based on the level of measurement of the study variables. If the variables are measured at the nominal and ordinal levels, nonparametric analyses are conducted (Pett, 2016). If variables are at the interval or ratio levels of measurement, and the values of the study participants for the variable are normally distributed, parametric analyses are conducted. Interval/ratio levels of data are often included together because the analysis techniques are the same whether the data are at the interval or ratio level of measurement. Researchers should run a computer program to determine whether the data for variables are normally distributed before conducting inferential statistics and include the results in their research report. If the interval/ratio data are not normally distributed (skewed), then nonparametric analyses need to be conducted on the data. Grove and Cipher (2020) provide instructions for examining the distribution of data in a study and interpreting the findings.

In independent groups, the selection of one study participant is unrelated to the selection of other participants. For example, if participants are randomly assigned to the intervention and control groups, the groups are independent. In paired groups, participants or observations selected for data collection are related in some way to the selection of other participants or observations. For example, study participants may serve as their own control with the outcome variable measured before and after the intervention. The pretest is considered the control group, and the posttest is the experimental group. The measurements (and therefore the groups) are paired. Also, if matched pairs of participants are used for the intervention and control groups, the observations are paired (see Chapter 8). Researchers sometimes match groups according to age and severity of illness to control the effects of these demographic variables in a study. Obtaining repeated measures of a dependent variable in a group of participants over time results in paired groups. The analysis technique conducted varies for independent versus paired groups; therefore researchers should not confuse the types of group used in their studies (see Box 11.1).

One approach for judging the appropriateness of an analysis technique in a study is to use a decision tree or algorithm. As you make a choice at each decision point about the study and the data, the algorithm gradually narrows the number of appropriate analysis techniques. The algorithm in Fig. 11.8 identifies four factors related to the appropriateness of an analysis technique: nature of the research question or hypothesis, level of measurement of the dependent and research variables, number of groups in the study, and research design. To use the algorithm in Fig. 11.8, you would:

1. determine whether the research question or hypothesis is focused on differences or associations (relationships);
2. determine the level of measurement (nominal, ordinal, or interval/ratio) of the study variables;
3. select the number of groups that are included in the study; and
4. determine the design, with independent or paired samples, that most closely fits the study you are critically appraising.

The lines on the algorithm are followed through each selection to identify the appropriate analysis technique that is listed at the far right of the figure. The algorithm in Fig. 11.8 might be used to determine the appropriateness of the independent samples t-test conducted by Ding et al. (2020) to examine the difference between empathy scores for the experimental and control groups at the beginning of their study (see Table 11.5). Empathy was measured with a Likert scale that produced interval-level data. The study included two independent groups that were formed based on student registration time. According to Fig. 11.8, the independent samples t-test is the appropriate analysis technique to conduct in this study (Grove & Cipher, 2020).

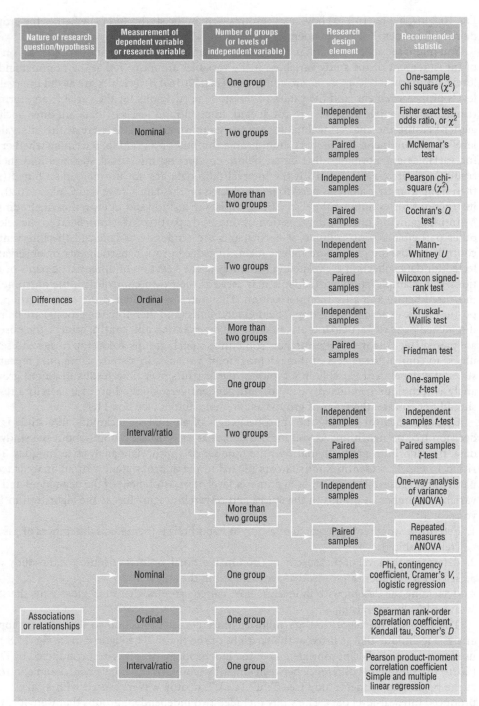

FIG. 11.8 Algorithm or Decision Tree for Determining Appropriate Statistical Techniques for Nursing Studies. (From Cipher, D. J. [2020]. Algorithm or decision tree for determining appropriate statistical techniques for nursing studies. In S. K. Grove & D. J. Cipher. *Statistics for nursing research: A workbook for evidence-based practice* [3rd ed. p. 126]. Elsevier.)

RESEARCH/EBP TIP

An algorithm, such as Fig. 11.8, can be extremely valuable to students in determining the appropriateness of the inferential analyses reported in studies. The credibility of study results depends on correct statistics being calculated and accurate results being reported.

Critical Appraisal Guidelines for the Results Section in Studies

To critically appraise the Results section of quantitative and outcomes studies, you need to identify the analyses conducted and determine their appropriateness. In addition to appraising the results reported in a study, you need to compare the statistical techniques with others that could have been conducted, perhaps to greater advantage.

CRITICAL APPRAISAL GUIDELINES

Results Presented in Studies

The appraisals of analysis techniques presented later in this chapter are guided by the following questions:
1. Was the focus of the study on examining relationships, making predictions, and/or determining group differences?
2. Were appropriate analyses performed to address the study purpose and/or objectives, questions, or hypotheses?
3. Was the analysis technique appropriate for the level of measurement of the data (nominal, ordinal, or interval/ratio), number of groups, and study design (independent or paired groups (see Fig. 11.8)?
4. Were the results from the analyses clearly presented in figures, tables, and narrative (APA, 2020; Grove & Cipher, 2020)?
5. Did the researchers identify the level of significance or α used in the study? Were the results statistically significant?
6. Were the results clinically important?
7. Were the results appropriately interpreted?
8. Were the effect size and power presented for nonsignificant findings? Was the power adequate for the study, at least 0.80 or stronger, or was there a potential for a Type II error (see Table 11.1)?
9. Were any common statistical mistakes identified in Box 11.1 noted in the study?
10. Should additional analyses have been conducted? Provide a rationale for your answer (Gray & Grove, 2021; Grove & Cipher, 2020; Holmes, 2018; Kim et al., 2022; Leedy & Ormrod, 2019; Pett, 2016).

STATISTICS CONDUCTED TO EXAMINE RELATIONSHIPS

Researchers conduct correlational analyses to describe relationships between variables, clarify the relationships among theoretical concepts, or assist in identifying possible causal relationships by examining group differences. In correlational analysis, the data from variables must be from a single population. Variables measured at the interval/ratio level provide the best information on the nature of a relationship. However, correlational analysis procedures are available for nominal- and ordinal-level data (see Fig. 11.8). Data for correlational analysis also need to span the full range of possible values on each variable included in the analysis. For example, if values for a particular variable can range from a low of 1 to a high of 9, each of the values from 1 to 9 will probably be found in the data set. If all or most of the values are in the middle of that scoring range (4, 5, and 6), and few or none has extreme values, a full understanding of the relationship cannot be obtained from the analysis. Therefore large samples with diverse scores are desirable for correlational analyses (Grove & Cipher, 2020; Kim et al., 2022).

Pearson Product-Moment Correlation

The Pearson product-moment correlation is an inferential analysis technique conducted to examine bivariate correlations in studies. Bivariate correlation measures the extent of the relationship between two variables. Data are collected from a single sample, and measures of the two variables to be examined must be available for each study participant in the data set. Less commonly, data are obtained from two related participants, such as breast cancer incidence in mothers and daughters. Correlational analysis provides two pieces of information about the data—the nature of a relationship (positive or negative) between the two variables and the magnitude (or strength) of the relationship. Scatterplots sometimes are presented to illustrate the relationship graphically (see Fig. 11.7). The outcomes of correlational analyses are symmetrical, rather than asymmetrical. Symmetrical means that the variables are related to each other but the analysis gives no indication of the direction of the relationship. It is not possible to establish from correlational analysis whether variable A leads to or causes variable B, or that B causes A. For example, anxiety is related to depression, but being anxious does not cause depression.

📄 RESEARCH/EBP TIP

The focus of correlational analysis techniques is *examining relationships, not determining cause and effect* (Kazdin, 2017). Relationships (positive or negative) of varying strength identified through research increase nurses' understanding of patient needs and values (Straus et al., 2019).

Interpreting Pearson Product-Moment Correlation Analysis Results

The result of the Pearson correlation analysis is a correlation coefficient (r) with a value between -1 and $+1$. This r value indicates the degree of relationship between the two variables. A value of 0 indicates no relationship. A value of $r = -1$ indicates a perfect negative (inverse) correlation. In a negative relationship, a high score on one variable is correlated with a low score on the other variable. For example, a person's number of smoking pack-years (number of packs of cigarettes smoked per day multiplied by the number of years the person smoked) is negatively related to a person's forced expiratory volume in 1 second (FEV_1). Thus individuals with a high number of smoking pack-years usually have a lower FEV_1. Patients' FEV_1 is used to determine the severity of their chronic obstructive pulmonary disease.

A value of $r = +1$ indicates a perfect positive relationship. In a positive relationship, a high score on one variable is correlated with a high score on another variable. A positive correlation also exists when a low score on one variable is correlated with a low score on another variable. For example, research has shown that anxiety and depression are related, with depression increasing as anxiety increases. A decrease in anxiety is related to a decrease in depression. Thus the variables (anxiety and depression in this example) vary or change in the same direction, either increasing or decreasing together. As the negative or positive values of r approach 0, the strength of the relationship decreases.

Traditionally, an r value of less than 0.3 or -0.3 is considered a weak relationship, and a value between 0.3 and 0.5 or -0.3 and -0.5 indicates a moderate relationship; if the r value is greater than 0.5 or -0.5, it is considered a strong relationship (Gray & Grove, 2021). Box 11.2 summarizes

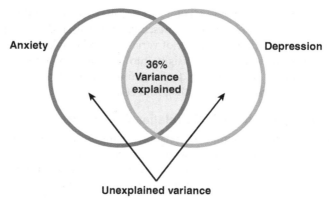

FIG. 11.9 Explained and Unexplained Variances Between Anxiety and Depression.

BOX 11.3 PEARSON CORRELATIONAL VALUES FOR SMALL, MODERATE, AND STRONG RELATIONSHIPS

Small relationships: $r < 0.3$ or $r < -0.3$
Moderate relationships: $r = 0.3–0.5$ or $r = -0.3$ to -0.5
Strong relationships: $r > 0.5$ or $r > -0.5$

the values for weak, moderate, and strong associations for positive and negative relationships. The interpretation of the r value depends to a great extent on the variables being examined and the situation in which they were measured. Therefore interpretation requires some judgment on the part of the researcher (Gray & Grove, 2021; Leedy & Ormrod, 2019).

When a Pearson correlation coefficient is squared (r^2), the resulting number is the percentage of variance explained by the relationship. For example, researchers may state that the relationship of the two variables anxiety and depression in their study was $r = 0.6$ and $r^2 = 0.36 \times 100\% = 36\%$. The explained variance (r^2) is provided by the relationship between two variables, anxiety and depression, in this example (Fig. 11.9). This means that the patients' anxiety scores can explain 36% of the variance in their depression scores. Even when two variables are strongly related, the values of the two variables will not be a perfect match ($r = 1$ or $r = -1$). This variation is the result of factors other than the relationship and is called unexplained variance. In the example provided in Fig. 11.9, $100\% - 36\%$ (explained variance) $= 64\%$ unexplained variance. The unexplained variance is a result of something other than the relationship studied, perhaps variables that were not examined in the study.

A strong correlation has more explained variance than a weak correlation (Box 11.3). Thus nursing researchers have had the tendency to disregard weak correlations in their studies. This approach can result in overlooking a relationship that may actually have some meaning within nursing knowledge if the relationship is examined in the context of other variables. The common reasons for this situation include the following: (1) Nursing measurements are not powerful enough to detect fine discriminations. Some instruments may not detect extreme scores, and a relationship may be stronger than that indicated by the crude measures available. (2) Correlational studies must have a wide range of scores for relationships to be detected. If the study scores are homogeneous or the sample is small, relationships that exist in the population may not show up as clearly in the sample. (3) In many cases, bivariate analysis does not provide a clear picture of the dynamics in the situation. A number of variables can be linked through weak correlations, which together may provide increased insight into situations of interest. Statistical procedures (e.g., regression analysis) are available for examining the relationships among multiple variables simultaneously (Grove & Cipher, 2020; Kim et al., 2022).

Testing the Significance of a Correlation Coefficient

Before inferring that the sample correlation coefficient applies to the population from which the sample was taken, statistical analysis must be performed to determine whether the coefficient is significantly different from zero (no correlation). With a small sample, a strong correlation coefficient can be nonsignificant. With a large sample, the correlation coefficient can be statistically significant when the degree of association is too small to be clinically important. The significance of a correlation coefficient is usually determined by conducting a t-test. Therefore in judging the significance of the coefficient, both the size of the coefficient and its statistical significance need to be considered.

McKay and colleagues (2020, p. 572) conducted a correlational study "to explore whether frailty, fear of falling, and depression are associated with an increased risk for falls in the Program for All-Inclusive Care (PACE) participants." The variables frailty, fear of falling, depression, and risk for falls were measured with multiple-items scales that provided interval-level data (Waltz et al., 2017). The scales used to measure these variables were described in detail in the research report and had acceptable to strong reliability according to the Cronbach's alpha coefficients reported. The data from these scales were analyzed with the Pearson product-moment correlational statistic, and the results are presented in Research Example 11.3.

RESEARCH EXAMPLE 11.3

Pearson Product-Moment Correlation Results

Research/Study Excerpt
Statistical Analysis

Data were analyzed with SPSS (Version 24.0, Armonk, NY: IBM Corp.). Descriptive statistics, specifically mean, standard deviation, skewness, kurtosis and range were used to examine survey results, demographic, and background data. ... Correlational statistics were used to determine if frailty, fear of falling, and depression are related to the risk for falls. (McKay et al., 2020, p. 573)

Results

Pearson correlation coefficients were presented in Table 11.6. Frailty, fear of falling, and depression were significantly associated with the risk for falls in the study sample. Frailty had a significant positive association with the risk for falls (r (82) = 0.565, p < 0.001). Fear of falling also had a significant positive association with the risk for falls (r (82) = 0.608, p <0 .001). The presence of frailty and fear of falling explained 31.9% [0.565² × 100%= 31.92%] and 39.4% [0.608² × 100% = 39.4%] of the variance in the risk for falls, respectively. There was a significant positive association between depression scores and the risk for falls (r (82) = 0.454, p = 0.001), but explained only 20.6% of the variance in the risk for falls which is notably less than frailty and fear of falling. (McKay et al., 2020, p. 574)

RESEARCH EXAMPLE 11.3—cont'd

TABLE 11.6 Pearson Correlations for Frailty, Fear of Falling, and Depression with the Risk for Falls

Variable	Risk for Falls
Frailty	0.565***
Fear of Falling	0.608***
Depression	0.454***

***$p < 0.001$, two tailed; **$p < 0.01$, two tailed.
Table 3, p. 574, of McKay, M. A., Todd-Magel, C., & Copel, L. (2020). Factors associated with the risk for falls in PACE participants. *Geriatric Nursing, 41*(5), 571–578. https://doi.org/10.1016/j.gerinurse.2020.03.002

Critical Appraisal
McKay et al. (2020) provided a detailed discussion of the planned data analyses and the results obtained for their study. The study data were examined for skewness and were found to be normally distributed. The scales had acceptable reliability as indicated earlier. The variables had moderate to wide ranges of scores, which enabled accurate relationships to be identified among them. Pearson r was the appropriate statistic for correlating the variables measured by multi-item scales (see Fig. 11.8). The strength of each relationship was appropriately described. The bivariate correlation values were clearly presented in a table, with the significance of the p values identified using asterisks (***$p < 0.001$, two tailed). The correlation values were examined for significance in both tails of the normal curve using two-tailed t-tests (see Fig. 11.2). The variances explained for risk for falls by frailty (31.9%) and depression (20.6%) were accurately reported, but the variance of risk for falls explained by fear of falling should have been 37% ($0.608^2 \times 100\% = 0.3697 \times 100\% = 37\%$). In summary, the correlational values and their significance were clearly presented in Table 11.6 and discussed in the study narrative.

Factor Analysis

This section briefly introduces you to factor analysis so you might recognize it in research reports. Factor analysis is commonly conducted to examine the interrelationships among large numbers of items on a scale and disentangles those relationships to identify clusters of items that are most intricately linked. Intellectually, you might do this by identifying categories and sorting the items according to your judgment into the most appropriate category. The accuracy of your judgments can be examined using factor analysis to sort scale items into categories according to how closely related they are to the other items in a category. Closely related items are grouped together into a factor. Several factors may be identified within a data set. Once the factors have been identified mathematically, the researcher must interpret the results by explaining why the analysis grouped the items in a specific way. Statistical results will indicate the amount of variance in the data set that can be explained by a particular factor and the amount of variance in the factor that can be explained by a particular item.

Factor analysis is frequently used in the process of developing measurement instruments, particularly those related to psychological variables, such as attitudes, beliefs, values, and opinions (Kim et al., 2022; Waltz et al., 2017). Factor analysis aids in the identification of theoretical constructs; it is also conducted to confirm the accuracy of a theoretically developed construct. For example, a theorist may state that the concept of "hope" consists of the following elements: (1) anticipation of the future, (2) belief in positive outcomes, and (3) optimism. Ways to measure these three elements can be developed, usually with a multi-item scale. The scale operationalizes the theoretical concept, such as hope, with items on it linked to one of the three subscales that measure the elements of hope. A factor analysis can be conducted on the data to determine whether the participants' responses clustered into these three factors or subscales for the concept of hope. In this way, factor analysis is being conducted to examine the construct validity of a scale for the population studied (see Chapter 10).

STATISTICS CONDUCTED TO PREDICT OUTCOMES

The ability to predict future events is becoming increasingly more important worldwide. People are interested in predicting who will win the football game, what the weather will be like next week, or which stocks are likely to increase in value in the near future. In nursing practice, as in the rest of society, the ability to predict is essential. For example, nurse researchers would like to predict the responses of patients with a variety of characteristics (e.g., age, sex, level of education) to nursing interventions. Nurses need to know which variables play an important role in predicting health outcomes in patients and families. For example, variables of hours of sleep per night, minutes of exercise per week, calories consumed per day, and body mass index might be used to predict individuals' risk for diabetes. Predictive analyses are based on probability theory, not on decision theory (see earlier discussion). Prediction is one approach for identifying hypotheses that might be examined in quasi-experimental and experimental research (Grove & Cipher, 2020; Kazdin, 2017).

Regression Analysis

Regression analysis is used to predict the value of one variable when the value of one or more other variables is known. The variable to be predicted in a regression analysis is referred to as the *dependent* or *outcome variable*. The dependent variable is usually measured at the interval/ratio level. The goal of the analysis is to explain as much of the variance in the dependent variable as possible. In regression analysis, variables used to predict values of the dependent variable are referred to as *independent variables*. Simple linear regression is conducted when one independent variable is used to predict one dependent variable. For example, researchers might conduct simple linear regression to predict depression (dependent variable) by examining the influence of average hours of sleep per week (independent variable).

Multiple regression is conducted to analyze study data that include two or more independent variables. Using multiple regression analysis, researchers might measure the influence of average hours of sleep per week, perceived social support, and family history of depression (independent variables) on depression. In regression analysis, the symbol for the dependent variable is y, and the symbol for the independent variable(s) is x. Scatterplots and a bivariate correlation matrix are often developed before regression analysis is performed to examine the relationships that exist among the variables. The purpose of regression analysis is to develop a line of best fit that reflects the values on the scatterplot. The line of best fit is often illustrated as an overlay on the scatterplot (Fig. 11.10). Different types of regression analysis have been developed to analyze data, such as logistic regression conducted to predict values of a dependent variable measured at the nominal level (Grove & Cipher, 2020; Kim et al., 2022).

Interpreting Regression Analysis Results

The result of regression analysis is the regression coefficient, R. When R is squared (R^2), it indicates the amount of variance in the data that is explained by the equation. When more than one independent variable is being used to predict values of the dependent variable, R^2 is sometimes referred to as the coefficient of multiple determination. The test statistic used to determine the significance of a regression coefficient may be t (from t-test) or F (from the analysis of variance

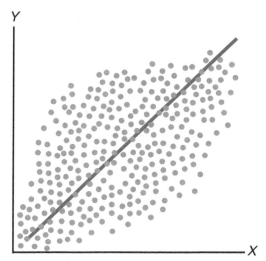

FIG. 11.10 Overlay of Scatterplot and Best-Fit Line.

[ANOVA]). Small sample sizes decrease the possibility of obtaining statistical significance. Values for R^2 and t or F are reported with the results of regression analysis. Many studies using regression analysis are complex, including multiple independent variables and involving more than one regression procedure. Understanding the discussion of complex results requires reading each sentence carefully for comprehension, looking up unfamiliar terms, and determining the statistical significance of the results.

McKay et al. (2020) conducted a multiple regression analysis to predict the risk for falls in 84 elderly adults. This study was introduced earlier in Research Example 11.3. The correlational results in Table 11.6 provided direction for the variables included in the regression analysis. The independent variables, frailty, fear of falling, and depression, were used to predict the dependent variable risk for falls in community-dwelling older adults. The results of the multiple regression analysis are presented in Research Example 11.4.

RESEARCH EXAMPLE 11.4

Regression Analysis

Research/Study Excerpt

A multiple linear regression was conducted to determine which variables predict the risk for falls. The results are illustrated in Table 11.7. A significant regression equation was found (F (3, 80) = 25.333, p <0.001) with an R^2 of 0.487. Thus, almost 50% of the variance in the risk for falls was explained by frailty, fear of falling, and depression. However, tests of individual beta weights indicated that, when controlling for other predictors in the equation, only frailty (β = 0.378, p < 0.001) and fear of falling (β = 0.450, p < 0.001) remained significantly predictive of the risk for falls, while depression was not a significant predictor of the risk for falls in this model. (McKay et al., 2020, pp. 574–575)

Continued

RESEARCH EXAMPLE 11.4—cont'd

TABLE 11.7   Summary of the Multiple Regression Analyses for Risk for Falls

Variables	B	SE	β	t	p
Constant	0.07	0.969		0.073	0.942
Frailty	0.447	0.121	0.378	3.698	<0.001***
Fear of falling	0.138	0.029	0.450	4.804	<0.001***
Depression	0.001	0.110	0.001	0.006	0.995

***$p < 0.001$; **$p < 0.01$; *$p < 0.05$.
B, Unstandardized coefficient; β, standardized coefficient; *p*, probability; *SE*, standard error; *t*, *t*-test value.
Table 4, p. 575, from McKay, M. A., Todd-Magel, C., & Copel, L. (2020). Factors associated with the risk for falls in PACE participants. *Geriatric Nursing, 41*(5), 571–578. https://doi.org/10.1016/j.gerinurse.2020.03.002

Critical Appraisal

McKay et al. (2020) appropriately conducted multiple regression analysis to answer the second aim of their study, to determine whether frailty, fear of falling, and depression in combination predict the risk for falls. The significant Pearson correlation values presented in Table 11.6 supported including all three of the independent variables (frailty, fear of falling, and depression) to predict the dependent variable risk for falls. The results of the multiple regression analysis were concisely presented in Table 11.7 and discussed in the research report. The researchers did additional analyses to control for other predictors, such as number of falls in the previous 6 months, incontinence, and psychiatric illness. The researchers correctly concluded that frailty and fear of falling remained significant predictors of fall risk, but not depression. McKay et al. (2020) appropriately conducted *t*-tests to determine the significance of individual predictors (see Table 11.7). An ANOVA was the correct analysis conducted to determine the significance of the regression model. The regression results were strong, explaining 48.7% of the variance in the risk for falls for older adults. McKay et al. (2020) recommended using these results to increase the assessments and identify interventions to decrease the risk for falls in these elderly adults.

Odds Ratio and Logistic Regression

Logistic regression is used when the dependent variable is dichotomous, that is, has two values, such as yes or no. For example, you might analyze the variables that could predict a surgical infection. The patients either had or did not have an infection (dependent variable). Independent variables might include the patients' diabetic status, glucose control, and surgery complexity. The odds ratio (*OR*) is defined as the ratio of the odds of an event occurring in one group versus another group (see Chapter 10; Grove & Cipher, 2020). When both the predictor and the dependent variables are dichotomous, the *OR* is the commonly used statistic to obtain an indication of association. Therefore the *OR* is a way of comparing whether the odds of a certain event is the same for two groups. For example, it was noted that veterans taking an angiotensin-converting enzyme inhibitor for hypertension had fewer adenomatous colon polyps. If the *OR* was 0.63, this indicates that angiotensin-converting enzyme inhibitor use was associated with a lower likelihood of the development of adenomatous colon polyps in veterans.

The *OR* can also be computed when the dependent variable is dichotomous and the predictor is continuous (interval/ratio level of data) and would be computed by performing logistic regression analysis. Logistic regression tests a predictor (or set of predictors) with a dichotomous dependent variable. The output yields an adjusted *OR*, meaning that each predictor's *OR* represents the relationship between that predictor and the dependent variable, after adjusting for the presence of the other predictors in the model (Kim et al., 2022; Pett, 2016). As is the case with multiple linear regression, each predictor serves as a covariate to every other predictor in the model.

The Lerret et al. (2020) study, used in Research Examples 11.1 and 11.5, examined the effects of the *e*PED iPad intervention on the parents' experience of the quality of discharge teaching and care coordination. The sample size (*N* = 395) was strong, with 211 parent–child dyads in the *e*PED intervention group and 184 parent–child dyads in the comparison group. Discharge teaching was measured with the QDTS-D, and care coordination was measured with the CTM, which provided interval-level data. These researchers also collected dichotomous data about a child having a chronic illness or not and whether the child was readmitted within 30 days of discharge. Lerret et al. (2020) used logistic regression to determine whether QDTS-D, CTM, and child with chronic condition were significant predictors for the 30-day readmission of the child. The results of this analysis are presented in Research Example 11.5.

RESEARCH EXAMPLE 11.5

Logistic Regression

Research/Study Excerpt

Logistic regression was used to evaluate QDTS-D, CTM and chronic condition as predictors for one or more readmission for each ePED and non-ePED groups separately (Table 11.8). For the ePED group, controlling for other predictors in the model, the strongest and only significant predictor of readmission was the CTM score. As CTM increases by one point (on a 4-point scale), the chance of having at least one readmission decreases by 55% (OR = 0.45). None of the three predictor variables made a unique statistically significant contribution to the model for readmission in the non-ePED group. (Lerret et al., 2020, p. 45)

Critical Appraisal

Lerret et al. (2020) clearly presented the results of their logistic regression analysis in Table 11.8. In their narrative, the researchers discussed that only CTM was a significant predictor of 30-day readmission. The sample size of this study was strong, and the group sizes were adequate. However, the intervention group included 27 more participants than the comparison group. Lerret et al. (2020) described the limitations of the study and

TABLE 11.8   Logistic Regression of 30-Day Readmission on QDTS-D, CTM, and Chronic Condition for *e*PED and Non-*e*PED Parent Groups

Implementation Group	Predictors	*p* value	*OR* (95% *CI*)
*e*PED	(Intercept)	0.83	0.35 (0.00, 506.8)
	QDTS-D	0.88	1.08 (0.51, 3.67)
	CTM	0.01	0.45 (0.24, 0.89)
	Chronic condition	0.29	1.99 (0.56, 7.98)
Non-*e*PED	(Intercept)	0.05	0.0008 (0.00, 0.37)
	QDTS-D	0.32	1.43 (0.79, 3.30)
	CTM	0.80	1.17 (0.43, 5.80)
	Chronic condition	0.09	3.65 (0.98, 23.88)

CI, Confidence interval; CTM, care transition measure; *OR*, odds ratio; *p*, probability; QDTS-D, Quality of Discharge Teaching Scale Delivery.
Adapted from table 4 in Lerret, S. M., Johnson, N. L., Polfuaa, M., Weiss, M., Gralton, K.,...Sawin, K. (2020). Using the Engaging Parents in Education for Discharge (*e*PED) iPad Application to improve parent discharge experience. *Journal of Pediatric Nursing, 52*, 47. https://doi.org/10.1016/j.pedn.2020.02.041

Continued

RESEARCH EXAMPLE 11.5—cont'd

concluded: "Enhancements are needed to better understand the role of the *e*PED app used by nurses during discharge education with families. Refinement of the *e*PED app needs to clearly address teaching needs related to care coordination. The concept of care coordination should be explored further to focus on populations with complex and/or chronic conditions" (Lerret et al., 2020, p. 47).

RESEARCH/EBP TIP

Regression analysis and logistic regression are appropriate techniques for predicting outcomes in research that ultimately might be applied to practice.

STATISTICS CONDUCTED TO EXAMINE DIFFERENCES

Inferential statistics are used to examine differences between groups, such as examining differences between the intervention and control groups on selected demographic variables (see Table 11.4 in Research Example 11.2). Statistical techniques conducted to examine differences are also used to determine causality of the independent variable on the dependent variable. Causality (cause and effect) is a way of knowing that one event leads to or causes another. Analysis techniques conducted to examine causality determine the effects of interventions on patient and family outcomes. Causality is determined by testing for significant differences in outcomes between the intervention and control groups. The common statistical techniques conducted to examine differences are the *t*-test, ANOVA, analysis of covariance (ANCOVA), and χ^2 test of independent samples. The *t*-test is conducted to examine differences between two groups, and the ANOVA, ANCOVA, and χ^2 tests can be conducted to examine differences among three or more groups. The *t*-test, ANOVA, and ANCOVA are conducted to analyze interval/ratio levels of data, and the χ^2 test is conducted to analyze nominal or ordinal levels of data (Grove & Cipher, 2020; Kim et al., 2022; Pett, 2016).

t-Test

One of the most common analyses conducted to test for significant differences between two samples when variables are measured at the interval or ratio level is the *t*-test. Different *t*-tests are conducted for various types of sample. For example, when independent groups are being compared, the *t*-test for independent samples is conducted. For paired groups, the *t*-test for paired samples is conducted (see Fig. 11.8). A common statistical mistake is not differentiating between independent and paired samples when conducting analyses (see Box 11.1).

Sometimes researchers misuse the *t*-test by conducting multiple *t*-tests to examine differences in various aspects of data collected in a study. Conducting multiple *t*-tests can increase the risk for a Type I error—that is, saying that something is significant when it is not (Makin & Orban de Xivry, 2019). The Bonferroni procedure, which controls for the escalation of significance, may be used when multiple *t*-tests must be performed on different aspects of the same data set (Gray & Grove, 2021). This procedure makes the significance level more stringent based on the number of comparisons conducted. For example, if five *t*-tests were conducted, the level of significance would need to be set at 0.01 ($0.05 \div 5 = 0.01$).

Interpreting *t*-Test Results

The result of the *t*-test analysis is a *t* statistic, and the value and significance of this result are reported in a study. The *t*-test results in published studies can be validated by comparing them with the critical or significant *t* values in a statistical table (see Appendix A in Grove & Cipher, 2020). If the computed *t* statistic is greater than or equal to the critical value in the table, the groups are significantly different.

In the Lerret et al. (2020) study used in Research Examples 11.1 and 11.5, the effects of *e*PED intervention on quality of discharge teaching (QDTS-D) and care coordination (CTM) were examined for parent–child dyads preparing for hospital discharge. The *e*PED group QDTS-D and CTM scores were compared with those of the non-*e*PED group using *t*-tests. The groups were considered independent because participants were obtained from two different units in a pediatric medical center. Participants from the surgical unit were entered into the intervention group, and those from a medical care unit were included in the comparison group. Lerret et al. (2020) conducted one-tailed (see Fig. 11.3), independent samples *t*-tests to determine differences between the *e*PED and the non-*e*PED groups. The results of the *t*-tests are presented in Research Example 11.6.

◢ RESEARCH EXAMPLE 11.6

t-Test Results

Research/Study Excerpt

Testing of the primary hypotheses evaluated differences between parents exposed to ePED and parents receiving usual discharge teaching on the parent's discharge experience, specifically their perceptions of the quality of discharge teaching (hypothesis 1) and care coordination (hypothesis 2). QDTS-D scores were significantly higher for parents exposed to the ePED app (mean = 9.59, SD = 0.65) than parents not exposed to the app (mean = 9.33, SD = 1.0, p = 0.002), though effect size (Cohen d) was small (d = 0.32). CTM scores were not statistically different between parent groups (mean = 3.77, SD = 0.60 for ePED, and mean = 3.74, SD = 0.49 for non-ePED parents). t-Test results are provided in Table 11.9. (Lerret et al., 2020, p. 45)

Critical Appraisal

Lerret et al. (2020) were testing directional hypotheses in their study; therefore differences were examined by conducting one-tailed *t*-tests for independent samples (see Fig. 11.8). The groups were not significantly different for care coordination. These nonsignificant results might have been influenced by the participants being selected from two different hospital units (surgical and medical) and the *e*PED and non-*e*PED groups being of unequal size. However, the effect size (Cohen *d*) was small, indicating that the results were probably an accurate reflection of reality and that the *e*PED intervention had a limited effect on care coordination.

TABLE 11.9 Comparison of Parent Experience Outcomes for *e*PED and Non-*e*PED Parent Groups

	*e*PED Group Mean (*SD*), Range	Non-*e*PED Group Mean (*SD*), Range	Test Statistics (*t*-test): *t, df, p, d*
CDTS-D	9.59 (0.65), 4.0–10	9.33 (1.0), 4.8–10	−3.09, 306.1, 0.002, 0.32
TCM	3.77 (0.60), 1–4	3.74 (0.49), 1–4	−0.58, 385.4, 0.56, 0.05

CTM, Care transition measure; *d*, Cohn *d* (effect size); *df*, degrees of freedom; *p*, probability; QDTS-D, Quality of Discharge Teaching Scale Delivery; *SD*, standard deviation; *t*, statistic for *t*-test.
Adapted from Table 2 in Lerret, S. M., Johnson, N. L., Polfuaa, M., Weiss, M., Gralton, K., . . . Sawin, K. (2020). Using the Engaging Parents in Education for Discharge (*e*PED) iPad Application to improve parent discharge experience. *Journal of Pediatric Nursing, 52*, 46. https://doi.org/10.1016/j.pedn.2020.02.041

Analysis of Variance

Analysis of variance (ANOVA) is a parametric statistical technique conducted to examine differences among three or more groups. Because this is a parametric analysis, the variables must be measured at the interval/ratio level. There are many types of ANOVA, which are conducted to analyze data from complex experimental designs (Grove & Cipher, 2020). The repeated measures ANOVA is conducted when the dependent variables are measured repeatedly over time (Kim et al., 2022). As discussed earlier, ANOVA is the appropriate analysis when a study includes three or more groups, but also when the dependent variables are measured repeatedly over time.

Rather than focusing just on differences between means, ANOVA tests for differences in variance. One source of variance is the variance within each group because individual scores in the group will vary from the group mean. This variance is referred to as the within-group variance. Another source of variance is the variation of the group means around the grand mean, referred to as the between-group variance. The assumption is that if all the samples are taken from the same population, these two sources of variance will exhibit little difference. When these two types of variance are combined, they are referred to as the total variance.

ANOVA indicates significant differences among the groups but does not specify which groups are different. When significant differences are found among three or more groups, post hoc analyses are conducted to determine which of the groups are significantly different. For example, a study might have examined three groups of nurses (home health nurses, clinic nurses, and hospital-based nurses) regarding smoking and determined that they were significantly different. Post hoc analyses are needed to identify which groups are significantly different.

Interpreting Analysis of Variance Results

The results of an ANOVA are reported as an F statistic. The F distribution table can be used to validate the significance of the F values reported in studies (see Appendix C in Grove & Cipher, 2020). If the F value is equal to or greater than the critical F value identified in the table, there is a statistically significant difference between the groups. If only two groups are being examined, the location of a significant difference is clear. As discussed earlier, post hoc analyses are conducted to determine the location of the differences among three or more groups. The frequently used post hoc tests are the Bonferroni correction, Newman–Keuls, Tukey honestly significant difference, Scheffé, and Dunnett tests (Kim et al., 2022).

Yektatalab and colleagues (2017) conducted an RCT to determine the effectiveness of a counseling intervention based on the Bowen System Theory of marital conflict of couples in a family nursing practice. Marital conflict was measured with a 42-item Likert scale that had a Cronbach's alpha = 0.95 for this study. The couples were sorted into either the intervention or the control group using a table of random numbers. The intervention group received the eight sessions of family counseling, and the control group received standard care. The design included measurement of marital conflict at pretest and two posttests, one immediately after the intervention and the other 1 month later. Power analysis indicated that a sample of 24 couples was needed, but the researchers used 42 couples because of possible high attrition during the study. One couple was lost from both the intervention and control groups, resulting in a sample of 40 couples (80 participants). Research Example 11.7 includes the study results.

RESEARCH EXAMPLE 11.7
ANOVA

Research/Study Excerpt
Results
Conflict

> The study results revealed no statistically significant differences between the study groups regarding the total marital conflict scores (t = 2.8, p = .93)... before the intervention (p > .05). However, a significant difference was observed between the two groups in this regard immediately and one month after the intervention (p < .05). ... Repeated measures [ANOVA] test was used to investigate the changes in the couples' mean scores of conflict in three successive stages. The results demonstrated a significant difference between the intervention and control groups regarding the conflict scores... during the three study periods and groups (p < .001) (Table 11.10). Thus, the results supported the study hypothesis. (Yektatalab et al., 2017, p. 257)

Critical Appraisal

Yektatalab and colleagues (2017) conducted a longitudinal study to determine the differences between the intervention and the control group at three points in time (pretest, posttest, and 1-month follow-up). Marital conflict was measured with a Likert scale that had strong reliability in this study. The final sample of 40 couples was strong based on the power analysis results. Attrition was only 5%, losing one couple from each group, which resulted in equal groups for analysis. Data were collected by the research assistant, who was blinded to the intervention. Repeated measures ANOVA is the appropriate analysis technique for two or more study groups with repeated measures and variables measured at least at the interval level. They clearly presented their ANOVA results in table format and discussed their results in the article. In summary, this study had a strong design, sample size, and data collection process, with significant results that support the effectiveness of the counseling intervention on marital conflict. These researchers recommended additional studies with larger samples and longer follow-up periods. The implications for practice include ensuring that couples with marital conflict obtain family counseling.

TABLE 11.10 Comparison of Couples' Mean Marital Conflict Score[a]

Marital Conflict	MEAN ± SD			RM-ANOVA, *F, p*		
	Pretest	**Posttest**	**Follow-up**	**Time**	**Group**	**Time-group**
Intervention	126.40 ± 5.79	106.55 ± 11.12	103.17 ± 12.48	$F = 45.78$	$F = 45.03$	$F = 79.43$
Control	126.55 ± 5.75	128.45 ± 7.68	130.25 ± 7.40	$p < 0.001$	$p < 0.001$	$p < 0.001$
p value	$p = 0.930$	$p < 0.001$	$p < 0.001$			
t-test[b]	$t = 2.80$	$t = 0.86$	$t = 0.75$			

[a]Before, after, and 1 month after the end of the intervention in both groups and between the groups under testing.
[b]Independent *t*-test.
RM-ANOVA, Repeated measures of analysis of variance; *SD*, standard deviation.
From Yektatalab, S., Oskouee, S., & Sodani, M. (2017). Efficacy of Bowen theory on marital conflict in the family nursing practice: A randomized controlled trial. *Issues in Mental Health Nursing, 38*(3), 258. https://doi.org/10.1080/01612840.2016.1261210

Analysis of Covariance

Analysis of covariance (ANCOVA) allows the researcher to examine the effect of a treatment apart from the effect of one or more potentially confounding variables (see Chapter 5). Potentially confounding variables that are generally of concern include pretest scores, age, education, income, and anxiety level. If the confounding variables are measured, their effects on study variables can be statistically removed by performing regression analysis before the ANOVA is carried out. Once this effect is removed, the effect of the treatment can be examined more precisely. This technique sometimes is used as a method of statistical control when it is not possible to design the study so that potentially confounding variables are controlled. However, control through careful planning of the design is more effective than statistical control.

ANCOVA may be used in pretest-posttest designs in which differences occur in groups on the pretest. For example, people who achieve low scores on a pretest tend to have lower scores on the posttest than those whose pretest scores were higher, even if the treatment had a significant effect on posttest scores. Conversely, if a person achieves a high pretest score, it is doubtful that the posttest will indicate a strong change as a result of the treatment. ANCOVA maximizes the capability to detect differences in such cases (Kim et al., 2022; Plichta & Kelvin, 2013). This information was provided to help you understand why ANCOVA is conducted and identify the confounding variables in a study.

χ^2 Test of Independence

The chi-square (χ^2) test of independence determines whether two variables are independent or related; the test can be used with nominal or ordinal data. The procedure examines the frequencies of observed values and compares them with the frequencies that would be expected if the data categories were independent of each other. The analysis has limited power; thus the risk for a Type II error is high—the outcome of the study is nonsignificant when significant differences actually exist. Large sample sizes are needed to decrease the risk for a Type II error (Grove & Cipher, 2020; Kim et al., 2022). Most studies using this analysis place little importance on results in which no differences are found. Researchers might perform multiple χ^2 tests in a sample but include only the results for significant χ^2 values.

Interpreting χ^2 Results

Sentences with statistical results include a great deal of information in a small amount of space. For example, in the results $\chi^2(1) = 18.10$, $p = 0.001$, the author is using χ^2 analysis to compare two groups on a selected variable, such as the presence or absence of COVID-19. The author provides the degrees of freedom ($df = 1$) so that the reader can validate the accuracy of the results using a statistical χ^2 table (see Appendix D in Grove & Cipher, 2020). The numerical value 18.10 is the χ^2 value obtained from calculating the χ^2 equation (frequently using a computer). As noted earlier, the symbol p is the abbreviation for probability. The groups were significantly different because $p = 0.001$, which is less than the level of significance set at $\alpha = 0.05$. The groups are reported as significantly different because there is only 1 chance in 1000 that the study results are an error. If a study variable has only two categories, such as the presence or absence of COVID-19, the researchers know what is significantly different. With three or more categories, post hoc analyses are conducted to identify the categories in which the significant differences occur.

Akkayaoğlu and Çelik (2020) conducted a comparative descriptive study to examine the eating attitudes, perceptions of body image, and quality of life of patients before and after bariatric surgery. The study sample size ($N = 50$) was determined using power analysis. Data were collected using the Three-Factor Eating Questionnaire to describe eating attitudes and the Body Image

Perception Questionnaire to describe perceptions of body image. X^2 analyses were conducted to examine differences in the patients' eating attitudes and perceptions of body image preoperatively and postoperatively at 1, 3, and 6 months after surgery. The study results are presented in Research Example 11.8.

RESEARCH EXAMPLE 11.8

Chi-Square (X^2)

Research/Study Excerpt

Statistically significant differences were found between the mean factor scores of the patients from the Three-Factor Eating Questionnaire before and after the surgery (p = 0.001). It was determined that the mean scores of the patients for uncontrolled eating behavior, degree of emotional eating and hunger sensitivity were the highest before the surgery and the lowest at the 6th postoperative month. It was also seen that the patients' negative eating attitudes decreased following the surgery. As seen in the same table, the patients' mean score of limiting food intake consciously was calculated as the lowest before the surgery and the highest at 6 months following the surgery, and it was determined that they improved their behavior of limiting food intake consciously (Table 11.11).

It was found that the difference between the mean scores of the Body Image Perception Questionnaire in the preoperative and postoperative periods was statistically significant (p = 0.001). The body image perceptions of the patients at six months following bariatric surgery were found to be significantly higher than their perceptions before the surgery (p = 0.001). It was found that low body image perceptions before the operation were enhanced from three months following the surgery (Table 11.11). (Akkayaoğlu & Çelik, 2020, Results section)

TABLE 11.11   Mean Three-Factor Eating Questionnaire and Body Image Perception Questionnaire Scores of the Patients Undergoing Bariatric Surgery During Preoperative and Postoperative Periods

Three-Factor Questionnaire	Preoperative Period, Mean (SD)	POSTOPERATIVE PERIOD			Chi-Square (X^2)	p
		1st Month, Mean (SD)	3rd Month, Mean (SD)	6th Month, Mean (SD)		
Uncontrolled eating	15.28 (2.48)	10.52 (2.67)	9.50 (2.02)	8.52 (2.01)	92.364	0.001*
Emotional eating levels	9.80 (2.30)	5.56 (2.43)	5.34 (1.12)	4.32 (1.28)	92.707	0.001*
Limiting food intake consciously	10.12 (2.86)	19.28 (3.76)	19.50 (2.13)	20.68 (2.01)	89.469	0.001*
Hunger sensitivity	13.50 (2.23)	9.18 (2.51)	7.06 (1.27)	5.64 (1.47)	116.56	0.001*
The Body Image Perception Questionnaire	88.10 (23.98)	109.82 (16.47)	147.78 (12.01)	171.56 (14.57)	144.097	0.001*

*$p < 0.001$.
SD, Standard deviation.
From Results section of Akkayaoğlu, H., & Çelik, S. (2020). Eating attitudes, perceptions of body image and patient quality of life before and after bariatric surgery. *Applied Nursing Research, 53*, 151270. https://doi.org/10.1016/j.apnr.2020.151270

Continued

> **RESEARCH EXAMPLE 11.8—cont'd**
>
> **Critical Appraisal**
>
> Akkayaoğlu and Çelik (2020) clearly presented their study results in a table that was concisely discussed in the study narrative (Table 11.11). x^2 analysis is appropriate to examine differences in the patients' eating attitudes and perception of body image over time. All results were significant from the preoperative to the postoperative periods. The authors needed to provide more explanation of the changes that occurred from postoperative periods of 1, 3, and 6 months. Akkayaoğlu and Çelik (2020, Conclusion section) concluded "that nurses should improve the quality of care for obese patients during the preoperative and postoperative periods. They also need to monitor physiological and psychological changes occurring in patients for the long run. This may facilitate patient follow up."

> **RESEARCH/EBP TIP**
>
> Understanding the *t*-test, ANOVA, and chi square analyses will assist you in examining the differences found in a study's Results section.

INTERPRETING RESEARCH OUTCOMES

Interpreting research outcomes involves examining the entire research process for strengths and weaknesses, organizing the meaning of the results, and forecasting the usefulness of the findings for evidence-based nursing practice (Gray & Grove, 2021; Melnyk et al., 2018). The outcomes in research include the following elements: findings, significance of the findings, generalization of findings, limitations, implications for nursing, recommendations for further research, and conclusions. These elements are included in the Discussion section at the end of a research report.

Types of Results

Interpretation of results from quasi-experimental and experimental studies has been traditionally based on decision theory, with five possible results: (1) significant results that agree with those predicted by the researcher, (2) nonsignificant results, (3) significant results that are opposite from those predicted by the researcher, (4) mixed results, and (5) unexpected results (Gray & Grove, 2021; Shadish et al., 2002). In critically appraising a study, you need to identify which types of results are presented.

Significant and Predicted Results

Significant results agree with those predicted by the researcher and support the logical links developed by the researcher among the purpose, questions or hypotheses, variables, framework, and measurement tools. In examining the results, however, you must consider the possibility of alternative explanations for the positive findings.

Nonsignificant Results

Nonsignificant (or inconclusive) results, often referred to as "negative" results, may be a true reflection of reality. In that case, the reasoning of the researcher or the theory used by the researcher to develop the hypothesis is in error. If it is, the negative findings are an important addition to the body of knowledge. However, the results may stem from a Type II error resulting from inappropriate methodology, a biased or small sample, threats to design validity (see Chapter 8), inadequate measurement methods, weak statistical techniques, or faulty analyses. In such cases, the reported results could introduce faulty information into the body of knowledge (Angell, 1989). Negative results do not mean that no relationships or differences exist among the variables; they indicate only that the study failed to find any. Nonsignificant results provide no evidence of the truth or falsity of the hypothesis (Shadish et al., 2002).

Significant and Unpredicted Results

Significant and unpredicted results are the opposite of those predicted by the researcher and indicate that flaws are present in the logic of the researcher and theory being tested. If the results are valid, however, they constitute an important addition to the body of knowledge. For example, a researcher may propose that social support and empathy are positively correlated. If a relevant study shows that strong social support is correlated with low empathy, the result is the opposite of that predicted.

Mixed Results

Mixed results are usually the most common outcomes of studies. In this case, one variable may uphold predicted characteristics, whereas another does not, or two dependent measures of the same variable may show different results. These differences may be caused by methodology problems, such as differing reliability and validity of the scales used to measure the variable. The mixed results may also indicate the theory that guided the development of the hypotheses might need to be modified.

Unexpected Results

Unexpected results usually are relationships found between variables that were not hypothesized and not predicted from the study framework. Most researchers examine as many elements of data as possible in addition to those directed by the questions or hypotheses. These findings can be useful in the development of new studies. In addition, unexpected or serendipitous results are important evidence for developing the implications of the study. However, serendipitous results must be interpreted carefully because the study was not designed to examine these results.

Findings

Results in a study are translated and interpreted to become study findings. Although much of the process of developing findings from results occurs in the mind of the researcher, evidence of these thought processes can be found in research reports.

Exploring the Significance of Findings

The significance of a study's findings is associated with the contribution the findings make to nursing's body of knowledge. The significance of study findings is not a dichotomous characteristic (significant or nonsignificant) because studies contribute in varying degrees to the body of knowledge. The study findings' significance may be associated with the amount of variance explained, the degree of control in the study design to eliminate unexplained variance, and/or the ability to detect statistically significant differences or relationships. To the extent possible at the time the study is reported, researchers are expected to clarify the significance of the study findings.

Significant studies can make an important difference in people's lives, such as the development of the 95% effective COVID-19 vaccine. In addition, when a study has a large sample and strong design, the findings can be generalized beyond the study sample to the population (Shadish et al., 2002). The implications of significant studies go beyond concrete facts to abstractions and lead to the generation of theories or revisions of existing theory (Chinn & Kramer, 2018). A significant study often has implications for one or more disciplines in addition to nursing. The study is accepted by others in the discipline and is referenced frequently in the literature. Over time, the significance of a study is measured by the number of additional studies that it generates. For example, the Braden Scale for Predicting Pressure Ulcer Risk has been studied extensively and is currently implemented by many nurses in clinical settings to prevent and manage pressure ulcers.

Clinical Importance of Findings

The strongest findings of a study are those that have both statistical significance and clinical importance. Clinical importance is related to the practical relevance of the findings. There is no common agreement in nursing about how to evaluate the clinical importance of a finding, but the effect size has been relevant in determining clinical importance. For example, one group of patients may have a body temperature 0.1° F higher than that of another group. Data analysis may indicate that the two groups are statistically significantly different, but the findings have no clinical importance. The effect size or differences between two groups is not sufficiently important to warrant changing patient care. In many studies, however, it is difficult to judge how much change would constitute clinical importance (Straus et al., 2019). In studies testing the effectiveness of an intervention, clinical importance may be demonstrated by the proportion of study participants who showed improvement or the extent to which study participants returned to normal functioning. But how much improvement must they demonstrate for the findings to be considered clinically important? Questions also arise regarding who should judge clinical importance—patients and their families, clinicians, researchers, or society at large. At this point in the development of nursing knowledge, clinical importance is ultimately a value judgment (Gray & Grove, 2021; LeFort, 1993).

📄 RESEARCH/EBP TIP

Researchers should document the statistical significance and clinical importance of their study findings in their research report. This information helps clinicians determine how findings might be used in practice.

Limitations

Limitations are restrictions or problems in a study that may decrease the generalizability of the findings. Studies might include construct validity limitations, such as a poorly developed or linked study framework and unclear conceptual definitions of variables. The limited conceptual definitions of the variables might decrease the validity of the operationalization or measurement of the study variables (see Chapter 5). Internal and external validity limitations result from factors such as nonrepresentative samples, weak designs, single setting, limited control over the implementation of the intervention, instruments with limited reliability and validity, and limited control over data collection (see Chapter 8). Threats to statistical conclusion validity can occur with improper use and interpretation of statistical analyses. Study limitations can alter the credibility of the findings and conclusions and restrict the population to which the findings can be generalized. Most researchers identify the limitations of their study and indicate how these might have affected the study findings. Often, they might recommend future studies to overcome the limitations in the current study.

Generalizing Findings

Generalization extends the implications of the findings from the sample studied to a larger population (see earlier Inference and Generalization section). For example, if the study had been conducted on patients with osteoarthritis, it may be possible to generalize the findings from the sample to the larger target population of patients with osteoarthritis or other types of arthritis.

Implications for Nursing

Implications for nursing are the meanings of the findings and conclusions for nursing knowledge, theory, education, and practice (Chinn & Kramer, 2018; Melnyk & Fineout-Overholt, 2019). Implications are based on findings from the current and previous studies, study significance, clinical importance, generalization, and conclusions. Implications provide specific suggestions for implementing the findings in nursing. For example, a researcher might suggest how nursing practice should be modified based on this study's and previous studies' findings. If these studies indicate that a specific solution is effective in decreasing pressure ulcers in hospitalized older patients, the implications will state how the care of older patients needs to be modified to reduce the risk for pressure ulcers.

📄 RESEARCH/EBP TIP

Interventions with extensive research support provide the basis for developing EBP guidelines and ensuring quality, safe, cost-effective nursing practice.

Recommendations for Further Research

In every study the researcher gains knowledge and experience that can be used to design a stronger study the next time. Therefore researchers often make suggestions for further study that emerge logically from the present study. Recommendations for further research may include replications or repeating the design with a different or larger sample, using different measurement methods, or testing a modified or new intervention. Recommendations may also include the formation of hypotheses to further test the framework in use. This section provides other researchers with ideas for further study to develop the knowledge needed for EBP.

Conclusions

Conclusions are a synthesis of the findings. In forming conclusions, the researcher uses logical reasoning, creates a meaningful whole from pieces of information obtained through data analysis and findings from previous studies, and considers alternative explanations of the data. One of the risks in developing conclusions is going beyond the study results or forming conclusions that are not warranted by the findings. However, conclusions accurately developed based on the current study and previous research promote the expansion of nursing knowledge.

❓ CRITICAL APPRAISAL GUIDELINES

Research Outcomes

When critically appraising the outcomes of a study, you need to examine the discussion section of the research report and address the following questions:
1. What were the study findings and were they appropriate, considering the statistical results?
2. Was the significance of the findings addressed?
3. Were the study findings linked to previous research findings?
4. Were the findings clinically important?

Continued

5. What study limitations were identified by the researchers? What other limitations may be present? How might the study limitations have affected the study conclusions?
6. To what population(s) did the researchers generalize the study findings? Were the generalizations appropriate?
7. What implications for nursing knowledge, theory, education, and practice were identified?
8. Were the implications for nursing practice appropriate based on the study findings, findings from previous research, and limitations?
9. Did the researchers make recommendations for further studies? Were these recommendations based on the study results, findings, limitations, and conclusions?
10. Were the conclusions appropriate based on the study results, findings, and limitations?

The research results from the McKay et al. (2020) study were introduced in Research Examples 11.3 and 11.4 (correlational and regression analyses). The purpose of this study was to determine whether frailty, fear of falling, and depression were predictive of the risk for falls in community-dwelling older adults. As identified in Table 11.7, the variables frailty, fear of falling, and depression were significantly related to risk for falls. Frailty and fear of falling were significantly predictive of risk for falls, but depression was not (see Table 11.8). Research Example 11.9 includes information from the Discussion section of the McKay et al. (2020) study; the key elements of this section are identified in brackets.

⤴ RESEARCH EXAMPLE 11.9

Research Outcomes

Research/Study Excerpt
Discussion

The significant relationship between frailty and the risk for falls was consistent with the literature indicating that intermediately frail or frail older adults have a higher risk for experiencing a fall as compared to non-frail community-dwelling older adults (...Ensrud et al., 2009). Fear of falling in older adults is associated with a significant increase in the risk for functional impairment, altered mobility, and experiencing a fall in the following year [Findings] (...Friedman et al., 2002). ...

The results in this group of PACE participants are similar to those reported in which depression was not a significant predictor for the risk for falls when controlling for ADL [activities of daily living] performance, mobility, and depression in older adults. ...In previous studies, fear of falling and decreased ADL and mobility measures are known predictors of experiencing a fall and the progression to physical frailty over time. ...Frailty, fear of falling, and incontinence explained over 82% of the variance in the risk for falls among the study sample. Similar results were reported when accounting for extensive falls risk factors, including those studied here...(Tromp et al. (2001) [Findings]. (McKay et al., 2020, pp. 575–576)

Therefore, proper depression screening and interventions are necessary in a vulnerable nursing home eligible population such as described in this study. ...A simple model that includes frailty, fear of falling, and incontinence, that is able to predict over 80% of the variance in the risk for falls may be useful in falls risk screening measures and could provide a quick snapshot of the health status of vulnerable community-dwelling older adults [Implications for practice]. (McKay et al., 2020, pp. 575–576)

Several limitations are noted in the study. First, the sample size was smaller than expected and required by power analysis for the multiple regression analysis. The required sample size for the correlation statistics

RESEARCH EXAMPLE 11.9—cont'd

was 84, and 114 participants were expected for the multiple regression based on an alpha = 0.05, power = 0.80 and a medium effect size. ... The majority of the participants were female; therefore, males were underrepresented [Limitations]. ...

The older adults who participated in the study were primarily African American and eligible for nursing home admission but chose to live in the community with the support of comprehensive healthcare services. This limits the generalizability of the results to other ethnic groups and community-dwelling older adults who do not receive or require services to live safely in the community. However, minorities are frequently underrepresented in health research. Therefore, the results of this study provide new data regarding nursing home eligible minority older adults living within the community and add to the literature on the relationships of the studied variables [Generalization]. (McKay et al., 2020, p. 576)

Future Research

... Conducting a longitudinal study beginning on admission to the PACE program and at specific follow-up points would indicate whether the support provided by the program effect the prevalence of each variable and relationships among the studied variables. ...Further study of intervention and treatment programs can guide the development and progression of these programs to benefit PACE participants. (McKay et al., 2020, p. 576)

Conclusion

Falls are the leading cause of fatal and non-fatal injuries in older adults with an even greater number of falls occurring in those over 85 years of age. ...This study provides a further understanding of the relationship between frailty, fear of falling, and depression with the risk for falls in vulnerable nursing home eligible community-dwelling older adults as well as provides a model that includes frailty, fear of falling, and incontinence for the prediction of the risk for falls. (McKay et al., 2020, p. 576)

Critical Appraisal

McKay et al. (2020) concisely presented their findings, which were consistent with their study results (see Tables 11.7 and 11.8). The findings were also consistent with those of other studies with comparable samples cited by the researchers. McKay et al. (2020) found that depression was not a significant predictor of risk for falls, which was consistent with the findings of the Kaminska et al. (2015) study. The findings are clinically important because the researchers developed a model that recommended screening the older adults for frailty, fear of falling, and incontinence to determine those most at risk for falls.

McKay et al. (2020) identified their study limitations (small sample size, males underrepresented in the sample, and cognitively impaired adults excluded from the study) that could limit the generalization of findings. In addition, the authors indicated the sample was primarily African American, which also limited generalization of results. The researchers suggested additional relevant studies to strengthen the knowledge regarding the prediction and management of the risk for falls in community-dwelling older adults. McKay et al.'s (2020) conclusions were consistent with the findings of this study and previous studies and provided the basis for future research.

RESEARCH/EBP TIP

Strong, consistent research findings from current and previous studies provide the evidence needed for modifying practice and improving patient and family outcomes.

KEY POINTS

- Probability theory is used to explain a relationship, the probability of an event occurring in a given situation, or the probability of accurately predicting an event.
- Decision theory assumes that all the groups in a study used to test a specific hypothesis are components of the same population in relation to the study variables.
- A Type I error occurs when the null hypothesis is rejected, although it is true. The risk for a Type I error is indicated by the level of significance (α).
- A Type II error occurs when the null hypothesis is accepted when it is actually false; this error often occurs because of flaws in the research methods.
- Quantitative data analysis includes the following steps: (1) management of missing data, (2) description of the study sample, (3) examination of the reliability of measurement methods, (4) performance of exploratory analyses of the data, and (5) conduct of inferential analyses guided by the hypotheses or questions.
- Frequency distributions, percentages, measures of central tendency, measures of dispersion, and scatterplot are descriptive or summary statistics.
- Statistical analyses conducted to examine relationships include Pearson product-moment correlation and factor analysis.
- Regression and logistic analyses are conducted to predict the value of a dependent variable using one or more independent variables.
- Statistical analyses conducted to examine group differences and determine causality include the t-test, ANOVA, ANCOVA, and χ^2 analysis.
- Research outcomes usually include findings, significance of findings, generalization of findings, limitations, implications for nursing, recommendations for further studies, and conclusions.
- In critically appraising a study, you should evaluate the appropriateness and completeness of the researchers' Results and Discussion sections using the guidelines in this chapter.

REFERENCES

Aberson, C. L. (2019). *Applied analysis for the behavioral sciences* (2nd ed.). Routledge Taylor & Francis Group.

Akkayaoğlu, H., & Çelik, S. (2020). Eating attitudes, perceptions of body image and patient quality of life before and after bariatric surgery. *Applied Nursing Research, 53*, 151270. https://doi.org/10.1016/j.apnr.2020.151270

American Psychological Association. (2020). *Publication manual of the American Psychological Association* (7th ed.).

Angell, M. (1989). Negative studies. *New England Journal of Medicine, 321*(7), 464–466. https://doi.org/10.1056/NEJM198908173210708

Bandalos, D. L. (2018). *Measurement theory and applications for the social sciences.* The Guilford Press.

Chinn, P. L., & Kramer, M. K. (2018). *Knowledge development in nursing: Theory and process* (10th ed.). Mosby.

Cipher, D. J. (2020). Algorithm or decision tree for determining appropriate statistical techniques for nursing studies. In S. K. Grove & D. J. Cipher (Eds.), *Statistics for nursing research: A workbook for evidence-based practice* (3rd ed., pp. 257–269). Elsevier.

Cohen, J. (1988). *Statistical power analysis for the behavioral sciences* (2nd ed.). Academic Press.

Craig, S. J., Kastello, J. C., Cieslowski, B. J., & Rovnyak, V. (2021). Simulation strategies to increase nursing student clinical competence in safe medication administration practices: A quasi-experimental study. *Nurse Education Today, 96*, 104605. http://doi.org/10.1016/j.nedt.2020.104605

Ding, X., Wang, L., Sun, J., Li, D., Zheng, B., He, S.... Latour, J. M. (2020). Effectiveness of empathy clinical education for children's nursing students: A quasi-experimental study. *Nurse Education Today, 85*, 104260. https://doi.org/10.1016/j.nedt.2019.104260

Ensrud, K. E., Ewing, S. K., Cawthon, P. M., Fink, H. A., Taylor, B. C., Cauley, J. A., ... Cummings, S. R. (2009). A comparison of frailty indexes for the prediction of falls, disability, fractures, and mortality in older men.

Journal of American Geriatric Society, 57(3), 492–498. https://doi.org/10.1115/1.3071969

Friedman, S. M., Munoz, B., West, S. K., Rubin, G. S., & Fried, L. P. (2002). Falls and fear of falling: Which comes first? A longitudinal prediction model suggests strategies for primary and secondary prevention. *Journal of the American Geriatric Society, 50*(8), 1329–1335. https://doi.org/10.1046/j.1532-5415.2002.50352.x

Gray, J. R., & Grove, S. K. (2021). *The practice of nursing research: Appraisal, synthesis, and generation of evidence* (9th ed.). Elsevier.

Grove, S. K., & Cipher, D. J. (2020). *Statistics for nursing research: A workbook for evidence-based practice* (3rd ed.). Elsevier.

Holmes, L., Jr. (2018). *Applied biostatistical principles and concepts: Clinicians' guide to data analysis and interpretation.* Routledge.

Kaminska, M., Brodowski, J., & Karakiewicz B. (2015). Fall risk factors in community-dwelling elderly depending on their physical function, cognitive status, and symptoms of depression. *International Journal of Environmental Research and Public Health, 12*(4), 3406–3416. https://doi.org/10.3390/ijerph120403406

Kazdin, A. E. (2017). *Research design in clinical psychology* (5th ed.). Pearson.

Kim, M., Mallory, C., & Valerio, T. D. (2022). *Statistics for evidence-based practice in nursing* (3rd ed.). Jones & Bartlett Learning.

Knapp, H. (2017). *Practical statistics for nursing using SPSS.* Sage.

Leedy, P. D., & Ormrod, J. E. (2019). *Practical research: Planning and design* (12th ed.). Pearson.

LeFort, S. M. (1993). The statistical versus clinical significance debate. *Image—The Journal of Nursing Scholarship, 25*(1), 57–62. https://doi.org/10.1111/j.1547-5069.1993.tb00754.x

Lerret, S. M., Johnson, N. L., Polfuaa, M., Weiss, M., Gralton, Klingbeil, C. G.,…Sawin, K. (2020). Using the Engaging Parents in Education for Discharge (ePED) iPad Application to improve parent discharge experience. *Journal of Pediatric Nursing, 52*, 41–48. https://doi.org/10.1016/j.pedn.2020.02.041

Makin, T. R., & Orban de Xivry, J. (2019). Ten common statistical mistakes to watch out for when writing or reviewing a manuscript. *eLife, 8*, e48175. https://doi.org/10.7554/eLife.48175

McKay, M. A., Todd-Magel, C., & Copel, L. (2020). Factors associated with the risk for falls in PACE participants. *Geriatric Nursing, 41*(5), 571–578. https://doi.org/10.1016/j.gerinurse.2020.03.002

Melnyk, B. M., & Fineout-Overholt, E. (2019). *Evidence-based practice in nursing & healthcare: A guide to best practice* (4th ed.). Wolters Kluwer.

Melnyk, B. M., Gallagher-Ford, L., Zellefrow, C., Tudher, S., Van Dromme, L., & Thomas, B. K. (2018). Outcomes from the first Helene Fuld Health Trust National Institute for evidence-based practice in nursing and healthcare invitational expert forum. *Worldviews on Evidence-Based Nursing, 15*(1), 5–15. https://doi.org/10.1111/wvn.12272

Pett, M. A. (2016). *Nonparametric statistics for health care research: Statistics for small samples and unusual distributions* (2nd ed.). Sage.

Plichta, S. B., & Kelvin, E. (2013). *Munro's statistical methods for health care research* (6th ed.). Lippincott Williams & Wilkins.

Shadish, W. R., Cook, T. D., & Campbell, D. T. (2002). *Experimental and quasi-experimental designs for generalized causal inference.* Rand McNally.

Straus, S. E., Glasziou, P., Richardson, W. S., & Haynes, R. B. (2019). *Evidence-based medicine: How to practice and teach EBM* (5th ed.). Churchill Livingstone Elsevier.

Tromp, A. M., Pluijm, S. M. F., Smit, J. H., Deeg, D. J. H., Bouter, L. M., & Lips, P. (2001). Fall-risk screening test: A prospective study on predictors for falls in community dwelling elderly. *Journal of Clinical Epidemiology, 54*(8), 837–844. https://doi.org/10.1016/S0895-4356(01)00349-3

Waltz, C. F., Strickland, O. L., & Lenz, E. R. (2017). *Measurement in nursing and health research* (5th ed.). Springer Publishing Company.

Yektatalab, S., Oskouee, S., & Sodani, M. (2017). Efficacy of Bowen theory on marital conflict in the family nursing practice: A randomized controlled trial. *Issues in Mental Health Nursing, 38*(3), 253–260. https://doi.org/10.1080/01612840.2016.1261210

Critical Appraisal of Quantitative and Qualitative Research for Nursing Practice

Susan K. Grove and Jennifer R. Gray

LEARNING OUTCOMES

After completing this chapter, you should be able to:

1. Discuss the reasons for conducting critical appraisals of healthcare studies.
2. Examine the principles for conducting intellectual critical appraisals of nursing studies.
3. Describe the three steps for critically appraising a study: step 1, identifying the steps or elements of the research process in the study; step 2,

determining study strengths and weaknesses; and step 3, evaluating the credibility and meaning of the study findings.

4. Conduct a critical appraisal of a quantitative research report.
5. Conduct a critical appraisal of a qualitative research report.

The nursing profession continually strives for evidence-based practice (EBP), which includes critically appraising studies, synthesizing the findings, applying the scientific evidence in practice, and determining the practice outcomes (American Association of Colleges of Nursing [AACN], 2021; Gray & Grove, 2021; Jones et al., 2020; Moorhead et al., 2018). Critically appraising studies is an essential step toward basing your practice on current research evidence. The term *critical appraisal* or critique is an examination of the quality of a study to determine the credibility, meaning, and relevance of the findings for nursing knowledge and practice. Critique is often associated with the word *criticize*, which is frequently viewed as negative. In the arts and sciences, however, critique is associated with critical thinking and evaluation—tasks that require carefully developed intellectual skills. This type of critique is referred to as an intellectual critical appraisal that is directed at the product, such as a study, rather than at the creator, and involves the evaluation of the quality of the product.

The idea of the intellectual critical appraisal of research was introduced earlier in this text and has been woven throughout the chapters. As each step of the research process was introduced, guidelines were provided to direct the critical appraisal of that aspect of a research report. This chapter summarizes and builds on previous critical appraisal content and provides direction for conducting critical appraisals of studies. The critical appraisals of studies by nursing students, practicing nurses, nurse educators, and researchers are discussed. The key guidelines for implementing intellectual critical appraisals of studies are described to provide an overview of the critical appraisal process. The steps for critical appraisal of quantitative studies are detailed followed by an example appraisal of a quantitative study. The chapter concludes with the critical appraisal steps for qualitative research with an example critical appraisal of a qualitative study.

REASONS FOR CONDUCTING CRITICAL APPRAISALS OF STUDIES IN NURSING

An intellectual critical appraisal of a study involves a rigorous, complete examination of a study to judge its strengths and weaknesses and to determine the credibility and meaning of the findings. A quality study focuses on a significant problem, demonstrates sound methodology, produces credible findings, indicates implications for practice, and provides a basis for further research (Grainger, 2021; Gray & Grove, 2021). Ultimately, the findings from several quality studies can be synthesized to provide empirical evidence for use in practice (Melnyk & Fineout-Overholt, 2019; Straus et al., 2019). We believe that performing a critical appraisal of a study involves the three essential steps presented in Box 12.1. By critically appraising studies, you will expand your analytic skills, strengthen your knowledge base, and increase your use of research evidence in practice. Research critical appraisals are conducted for class projects, following verbal presentations of studies, after published research reports, selection of abstracts of studies to be presented at conferences, article selection for publication, and evaluation of research proposals for implementation or funding. Therefore nursing students, practicing nurses, nurse educators, and nurse researchers are all involved in the critical appraisal of research.

📄 **RESEARCH/EBP TIP**
Studies are critically appraised to broaden understanding, summarize current nursing knowledge, provide a knowledge base for future research, and determine the research evidence ready for use in practice.

Students' Critical Appraisal of Studies

Students usually acquire basic knowledge of the research process and critical appraisal process in their entry-level professional nursing education (AACN, 2021). Entry-level professional nurses are expected to critique research and determine its applicability to practice. One aspect of learning the

BOX 12.1   **STEPS OF THE CRITICAL APPRAISAL PROCESS IN NURSING**
Step 1: Identifying the steps or elements of the research process in the study
Step 2: Determining the study strengths and weaknesses
Step 3: Evaluating the credibility and meaning of the study findings

research process is being able to read and comprehend published research reports. However, because conducting a critical appraisal of a study is not a basic skill, the content presented in previous chapters is essential for implementing this process. By critically appraising studies, you will expand your analysis skills, strengthen your knowledge base, and increase your use of research evidence in practice. Striving for EBP is one of the competencies identified for associate degree and baccalaureate degree (prelicensure) students by the Quality and Safety Education for Nurses (2021) project, and EBP requires a critical appraisal and synthesis of study findings for practice. More advanced analytic skills are taught at the master's and doctoral levels. Therefore critical appraisal of studies is an important part of your education and your practice as a nurse (AACN, 2021; Gray & Grove, 2021).

Critical Appraisal of Studies by Practicing Nurses, Nurse Educators, and Researchers

Practicing nurses need to critically appraise studies so their practice is based on current research evidence and not on tradition or trial and error. Nursing actions need to be updated in response to current evidence that is generated through research and theory development. It is important for practicing nurses to develop strategies to remain current in their practice areas. Reading research journals and posting or e-mailing current studies at work can increase nurses' awareness of study findings but are not sufficient for critical appraisal to occur. Nurses need to question the quality of the studies, credibility of the findings, and meaning of the findings for practice. For example, nurses might participate in an EBP committee in their agency that critically appraises studies, synthesizes their findings, and plans for the use of the findings in practice (AACN, 2021). EBP is essential in agencies that are seeking or maintaining Magnet status to promote the delivery of quality, evidence-based care (American Nurses Credentialing Center, 2021; Melnyk et al., 2020).

Your faculty members and other nurse educators critically appraise research to expand their clinical knowledge base and to develop and refine the nursing educational process. The careful analysis of current nursing studies provides a basis for updating curriculum content for use in classroom and clinical settings. Faculty members serve as role models for their students by examining new studies, evaluating the information obtained from research, and indicating which research evidence to use in practice. For example, in class, nursing instructors might critically appraise and present the most current evidence about social determinants of health related to hypertension and caring for people with hypertension (Wakefield et al., 2021). Nursing instructors may also role model the management of patients with hypertension in clinical and community settings (Todkar et al., 2021; Whelton et al., 2018).

Nurse researchers critically appraise previous research to plan and implement their next study. Many researchers have a program of research in a selected area, and they update their knowledge base by critically appraising new studies in that selected area. For example, a team of nurse researchers might have a program of research to identify effective interventions for minimizing the effects of social determinants of health (Wakefield et al., 2021), assisting patients in managing their hypertension, and reducing their cardiovascular risk factors (Whelton et al., 2018). As new studies are published on hypertension prevention and management, the researchers appraise the studies and consider the effect of the findings for their own research.

📄 **RESEARCH/EBP TIP**

Skills for critical appraisal of research enable students, practicing nurses, educators, and researchers to determine the quality of studies and to synthesize the most credible, significant, and appropriate evidence for use in their practice.

Critical Appraisal of Research Following Presentations and Publications

When nurses attend research conferences, they note that critical appraisals and questions often follow presentations of studies. These critical appraisals assist researchers in identifying the strengths and weaknesses of their studies and generating ideas for further research. Participants listening to critiques of studies might gain insight into the conduct of research. In addition, experiencing the critical appraisal process may increase the conference participants' ability to evaluate studies and judge the usefulness of the research evidence for practice.

Critical appraisals have also been published after some studies in research journals. For example, the research journals *Scholarly Inquiry for Nursing Practice* and *Western Journal of Nursing Research* include commentaries after the research articles. In these commentaries, other researchers critically appraise the authors' studies, and the authors have a chance to respond to these comments. Published research critical appraisals often increase the reader's understanding of the study and the quality of the study findings. The American Psychological Association (APA, 2020) is a format used in many nursing research journals, and this text provides guidance in developing quality research reports. This content can guide you in critically appraising a published nursing study. A more informal critical appraisal of a published study might appear in the form of a letter to the editor, in which a reader comments on the strengths and weaknesses of published studies by writing to the journal editor.

Critical Appraisal of Research for Presentation and Publication

Planners of professional conferences often invite researchers to submit an abstract of a study they are conducting or have completed for potential presentation at the conference. The amount of information available for review is usually limited because many abstracts are restricted to 100 to 250 words. Nevertheless, reviewers must select the best-designed studies with the most significant outcomes for presentation at nursing conferences. This process requires an experienced researcher who needs few cues to determine the quality of a study. Critical appraisal of an abstract usually addresses the following criteria: (1) appropriateness of the study for the theme and purpose of the conference; (2) completeness of the research project; (3) overall quality of the study problem, purpose, methodology, and results; (4) contribution of the study to the nursing knowledge base; (5) contribution of the study to nursing theory; (6) originality of the work (i.e., not previously published); (7) implication of the study findings for practice; and (8) clarity, conciseness, and completeness of the abstract (APA, 2020; Gray & Grove, 2021).

Some nurse researchers serve as peer reviewers for professional journals to evaluate the quality of research papers submitted for publication. The role of these scientists is to ensure that the studies accepted for publication are well designed and contribute to the body of knowledge. Journals that have their articles critically appraised by expert peer reviewers are called peer-reviewed journals or refereed journals (APA, 2020). The reviewers' comments or summaries of their comments are sent to the researchers to direct their revision of the manuscripts for publication. Refereed journals usually have studies and articles of higher quality that you might review for your practice (see Chapter 6).

Critical Appraisal of Research Proposals

Critical appraisals of research proposals are conducted to approve student research projects; permit data collection in an institution; and select the best studies for funding by local, state, national, and international organizations and agencies. You might be involved in a proposal review if you are participating in collecting data as part of a class project or studies done in your clinical agency.

Research proposals are reviewed for funding from selected government agencies, corporations, and foundations. Corporations and foundations develop their own format for reviewing and funding research projects (Gray & Grove, 2021). The peer review process in federal funding agencies involves a structured, complex critical appraisal. Nurses are involved in this level of research review through national funding agencies, such as the National Institute of Nursing Research (2021) and the Agency for Healthcare Research and Quality (2021).

KEY PRINCIPLES FOR CONDUCTING INTELLECTUAL CRITICAL APPRAISALS OF QUANTITATIVE AND QUALITATIVE STUDIES

Because the major focus of this chapter is conducting critical appraisals of quantitative and qualitative studies, key principles for conducting intellectual critical appraisals of these types of study are summarized in Box 12.2. You need to be rigorous in reading and examining the quality of a research report. A study needs to include a significant and relevant problem that is examined using sound methodology to produce credible findings (Grainger, 2021; Straus et al., 2019). All studies have weaknesses or flaws; if every flawed study were discarded, no scientific evidence would be available for use in practice. In fact, science itself is flawed. Science does not completely or perfectly describe, explain, predict, or control reality. However, improved understanding and an increased ability to predict and control phenomena depend on recognizing the weaknesses or limitations in studies and science. Additional studies can then be planned to minimize the limitations of earlier studies. You also need to recognize a study's strengths to determine the quality of a study and credibility of its findings. When identifying a study's strengths and weaknesses, you need to provide examples and rationale for your judgments that are documented with current sources.

In addition to the principles presented in Box 12.2, we have developed three steps for critically appraising both quantitative and qualitative studies that were introduced earlier (see Box 12.1). The steps provide the organization for detailed appraisal guidelines presented later in this chapter. These guidelines stress the importance of reviewing the entire study, addressing the study's strengths and weaknesses, and evaluating the credibility and meaning of the study findings (Grainger, 2021; Gray & Grove, 2021; Meadows-Oliver, 2019; O'Mathúna & Fineout-Overholt, 2019). The detailed questions in the critical appraisal guidelines are specific to the type of study and provide the criteria for a final evaluation to determine the credibility of the study findings, any implications for practice, and ideas for further research. These guidelines provide a basis for the critical appraisal process of quantitative research discussed in the next section and for qualitative research discussed later.

BOX 12.2   KEY PRINCIPLES FOR CRITICALLY APPRAISING QUANTITATIVE AND QUALITATIVE STUDIES

- **Read and critically appraise the entire study.** A research critical appraisal involves examining the quality of all aspects of the research report.
- **Examine the organization and presentation of the research report.** A well-prepared report is concise, complete, logically organized, and clearly presented. It does not include excessive jargon that is difficult to read. The references need to be current, complete, and presented in a consistent format.
- **Examine the significance of the problem studied for nursing practice.** Nursing studies need to be focused on significant problems if a sound knowledge base is to be developed for evidence-based nursing practice.

BOX 12.2   **KEY PRINCIPLES FOR CRITICALLY APPRAISING QUANTITATIVE AND QUALITATIVE STUDIES—cont'd**

- *Indicate the type of study conducted and identify the steps or elements of the study.* This might be done as an initial critical appraisal of a study, indicating your knowledge of the different types of quantitative and qualitative studies and the elements included in these studies.
- *Identify the strengths and weaknesses of a study.* All studies have strengths and weaknesses. Review the limitations identified by the researchers in a study and how they were managed to ensure the credibility of the findings.
- *Be objective and realistic in identifying the study's strengths and weaknesses.* Be balanced in your critical appraisal of a study. Try not to be overly critical in identifying a study's weaknesses or overly flattering in identifying the strengths. Take the limitations identified by the researchers into consideration but do not repeat these in your critique.
- *Provide specific examples of the strengths and weaknesses of a study.* Examples provide evidence for your critical appraisal of a study's strengths and weaknesses.
- *Provide a rationale for your critical appraisal comments.* Include justifications for your critical appraisal and document your ideas with sources from the current literature.
- *Evaluate the quality of the study.* Describe the credibility of the findings, consistency of the findings with those from previous studies, and appropriateness of the study conclusions.
- *Discuss the usefulness of the findings for practice.* The findings from the study need to be linked to the findings of previous studies and examined for use in clinical practice.

RESEARCH/EBP TIP

When relevant, credible findings from multiple quality studies are synthesized, nurses are able to build a solid base of evidence for practice.

UNDERSTANDING THE QUANTITATIVE RESEARCH CRITICAL APPRAISAL PROCESS

The quantitative research critical appraisal process includes the three basic steps presented in Box 12.1. These steps occur in sequence, vary in depth, and presume accomplishment of the preceding steps. Critical appraisal guidelines are presented with relevant questions for these steps. These questions have been selected as a means for stimulating the logical reasoning and analysis necessary for critically appraising a quantitative study. Because you are new to critical appraisal of research, you will initially focus on step 1 of identifying the elements or steps of the research process. The questions for determining the study strengths and weaknesses are covered together because this process occurs simultaneously in the mind of the person conducting the critical appraisal. Evaluation is covered separately because of the increased expertise needed to perform this step. As you gain critical appraisal experience, you will probably perform two or three of these steps simultaneously.

Step 1: Identifying the Steps of the Research Process in Quantitative Studies

Initial attempts to comprehend research articles are often frustrating because the terminology and stylized manner of the report are unfamiliar. Identifying the steps of the research process in a quantitative study involves understanding the terms and concepts in the report, as well as identifying study steps and grasping the nature, significance, and meaning of these elements. The following guidelines will direct you in critically appraising quantitative nursing studies.

Guidelines for Identifying the Steps of the Research Process in Quantitative Studies

The first step involves reviewing the abstract and reading the study from beginning to end. As you read, think about the following questions about the presentation of the study:

- Was the writing style of the report clear and concise?
- Were relevant terms defined? You might underline the terms you do not understand and determine their meaning from the glossary at the end of this textbook.
- Were the following parts of the research report clearly identified (APA, 2020)?
  - Introduction section with the problem, purpose, literature review, framework, study variables, and objectives, questions, or hypotheses.
  - Methods section with the design, sample, intervention (if applicable), measurement methods, and data collection procedures.
  - Results section with the specific results presented in tables, figures, and narrative.
  - Discussion section with the findings, limitations, implications for practice, suggestions for future research, and conclusions (Gray & Grove, 2021).

Next, we recommend reading the entire study a second time and highlighting or underlining the steps of the quantitative research process that were described previously in Chapter 2. After reading and comprehending the content of the study, you are ready to write your initial critical appraisal of the study. In step 1, you need to identify each step of the research process concisely and respond briefly to the guidelines and questions included in the following Critical Appraisal Guidelines box.

? CRITICAL APPRAISAL GUIDELINES

Step 1: Identifying the Steps of the Study

1. Introduction
   a. Was the article title clear? Does the title indicate the type of study conducted (descriptive, correlational, quasi-experimental, or experimental), variables, and population (Gray & Grove, 2021; Kazdin, 2017; Shadish et al., 2002)?
   b. Did the abstract include the purpose, type of design, sample, and intervention (if applicable) and present key results and conclusions (APA, 2020)?
2. State the problem.
   a. Did the researchers provide the significance of the problem, such as number of people affected, its importance to nursing practice, and cost incurred?
   b. Did the researchers provide the background of the problem?
   c. Was there a clear problem statement (see Chapter 5)?
3. State the purpose.
4. Examine the literature review.
   a. Does the literature review cite previous studies and theory for the framework?
   b. Are the references current? Number and percentage of sources in the last 10 years and in the last 5 years? (see Chapter 6; Jones et al., 2020)
5. Examine the study framework or theoretical perspective.
   a. Is the framework explicitly expressed, or must you extract the framework from statements in the introduction or literature review of the study?
   b. Were the concepts and at least one relationship identified, providing a theoretical basis for the study (Chinn et al., 2022; Smith & Liehr, 2018)?
6. List the research objectives, questions, and/or hypotheses guiding the study.
7. Identify which of the following types of variable were included in the study: independent, dependent, and/or research variables. A study with an independent variable also includes dependent variables. Research variables are commonly included in descriptive and some correlational studies (see Chapter 5).

? CRITICAL APPRAISAL GUIDELINES—cont'd

What were the conceptual and operational definitions of two study variables or concepts that were identified in the objectives, questions, or hypotheses? If these are not stated, you need to identify and define two variables in the study purpose.

8. Identify attribute or demographic variables.
   a. What person-related demographic variables were measured, such as income, age, and marital status?
   b. Were other demographic variables measured, such as diagnosis, time since diagnosis, and prescriptions identified?

9. Identify the research design.
   a. What is the specific design of the study (see Chapter 8; Gray & Grove, 2021; Kazdin, 2017; Shadish et al., 2002)?
   b. Does the study include a treatment or intervention? If so, identify the intervention.
   c. If the study has more than one group, how were participants assigned to groups?

10. Describe the sample and setting.
    a. What were the inclusion and exclusion criteria for the sample (see Chapter 9)?
    b. What specific type of probability or nonprobability sampling method was used to obtain the sample? Did the researchers identify the sampling frame for the study?
    c. What was the sample size? Discuss the refusal rate and percentage, and include the rationale for refusal if presented in the article. Identify if power analysis was used to determine sample size (Aberson, 2019).
    d. What was the attrition of the sample (number and percentage) for the study?
    e. What were the characteristics of the sample?
    f. What was the study setting?

11. Identify the ethical considerations.
    a. Was the study reviewed by an institutional or ethical board?
    b. What was the process for informed consent?

12. Identify at least two measurement strategies used in the study. Include the essential information listed below for a scale or physiological measure in a table format.

Variable Measured	Name of Measurement Method	Type of Method and Level of Measurement	Reliability or Precision	Validity or Accuracy

   a. What were two key variables that were measured?
   b. What was the name of each measurement method, such as the Spiritual Well-Being Scale or adherence questionnaire?
   c. What type of measurement strategy was used (e.g., Likert scale, visual analog scale, physiological measure, or existing database) (Bandalos, 2018; DeVellis, 2017; Waltz et al., 2017)?
   d. What was the level of measurement (nominal, ordinal, interval, or ratio) achieved by the measurement method used in the study (Grove & Cipher, 2020)?
   e. What information was provided about the reliability of each scale based on previous studies and for this study? What information was provided about the precision of each physiological measure (Bandalos, 2018; Bialocerkowski et al., 2010; Ryan-Wenger, 2017; Waltz et al., 2017)?
   f. What information was provided about the validity of each scale (DeVellis, 2017) and the accuracy of physiological measures (Ryan-Wenger, 2017)?

Continued

? CRITICAL APPRAISAL GUIDELINES—cont'd

Example Table of Measurement Methods

Variable Measured	Name of Measurement Method	Type of Method and Level of Measurement	Reliability or Precision	Validity or Accuracy
Depression	Beck Depression Inventory	Likert Scale Interval-level data	Cronbach's alphas of 0.82–0.92 from previous studies and 0.84 for this study. Reading level at sixth grade.	*Content validity* from concept analysis, literature review, and reviews of experts. *Construct validity:* convergent validity of 0.04 with Zung Depression Scale. *Predictive validity* of patients' future depression episodes. *Successive use validity* with previous studies and this study.
Blood pressure (BP)	Omron BP equipment	Physiological measure Ratio-level data	Test-retest values of BPs in previous studies. BP equipment new and recalibrated every 100 BP readings.	Documented accuracy of systolic and diastolic BPs to 1 mm Hg by company developing Omron BP cuff. Designated protocol for taking BP (Whelton et al., 2018). Average three BP readings to determine most accurate BP.

13. Identify the procedures for data collection.
14. Describe the statistical analyses used.
    a. What statistical procedures were conducted to describe the sample?
    b. Was the level of significance or alpha identified? If so, indicate what it was (0.05, 0.01, or 0.001).
    c. Identify the statistical procedures conducted to address the research objectives, questions, or hypotheses (see Chapter 11; Grove & Cipher, 2020; Kim et al., 2022; Leedy & Ormrod, 2019).
    d. Complete a table with the following information from the appraised study: (1) identify the focus (description, relationships, or differences) for each analysis technique, (2) list the statistical technique performed, (3) list the statistic, (4) provide the specific results, and (5) identify the probability (*p*) of the statistical significance achieved by the result (Grove & Cipher, 2020; Kim et al., 2022; Leedy & Ormrod, 2019).

Example Table of Statistical Analyses

Purpose of Analysis	Analysis Technique	Statistic	Results	Probability
Description of subjects' pulse rate	Mean Standard deviation Range	*M* *SD* *Range*	71.52 5.62 58–97	
Difference between adult males and females for oxygen saturation	*t*-test	*t*	3.75	*p* = 0.001
Differences of diet group, exercise group, and comparison group for pounds lost in adolescents	Analysis of variance	*F*	4.27	*p* = 0.04
Relationship of depression and anxiety in the elderly	Pearson correlation coefficient	*r*	0.46	*p* = 0.03

? CRITICAL APPRAISAL GUIDELINES—cont'd

15. What were the findings of the study? Identify two findings discussed by the researchers.
16. What study limitations did the researcher identify?
17. Did the researcher generalize the findings?
18. What were the implications of the findings for nursing practice?
19. What suggestions for further study were identified?
20. What conclusions did the researchers identify?

CRITICAL APPRAISAL EXAMPLE 12.1

Step 1: Identifying the Steps of the Study

This example critical appraisal was conducted on an experimental study by Sarhangi and colleagues (2021). This article can be located in the Research Article Library online for this text. These researchers examined the effects of the intervention, the mother's heartbeat sound on neonate's pain, and other physiological parameters. The steps of this study are identified using the guidelines previously introduced.

1. Introduction
   a. The title of this study was "The Effect of the Mother's Heartbeat Sound on Physiological Parameters and Pain Intensity after Blood Sampling in Neonates in the Intensive Care Unit: A Randomized Controlled Clinical Trial" (Sarhangi et al., 2021). The title clearly identified the experimental study as a randomized controlled trial (RCT). The intervention, the mother's heartbeat sound, was proposed to have a positive effect on the neonates' pain intensity and other physiological variables. The population included neonates in the intensive care unit (ICU) setting and their mothers.
   b. The abstract is concise and clearly covers the essential areas of aims, methods, results, and conclusions.
2. State the problem. The parts of the problem are identified in brackets.

   Invasive procedures conducted by clinical nurses on neonates admitted to the intensive care unit including heel blood sampling, respiratory tract suction, peripheral vein path insertion, gastric tube and urinary catheter insertions are painful. . . . Full-term and preterm neonates can feel pain in response to annoying and painful stimuli and uncontrolled pain can impact on neural development [Significance]. *. . . Painful and stressful stimuli can increase catecholamine release, heart rate, blood pressure and intracranial pressure. . . . Nonpharmacological interventions and the use of alternative and complementary medicines, such as nonnutritive sucking (NNS) with or without sucrose, breast milk or breastfeeding, swaddle. . . have been shown effective for the management of mild to moderate pain in neonates. . . One of the potentially effective methods to relieve pain in neonates is to listen to the mother's heartbeat sound* [Background]. *. . . However, there is a lack of knowledge of the effect of the mother's heartbeat sound alone on the improvement of physiological parameters during and after painful procedures in neonates admitted to neonatal intensive care units* [Problem statement]. (Sarhangi et al., 2021, pp. 123–124)

3. State the purpose.

   Therefore, this study using an experiential design aimed to examine the effect of the mother's heartbeat sound on pain intensity and physiological parameters after blood sampling in neonates in the intensive care unit. (Sarhangi et al., 2021, p. 124)

4. Examine the literature review.
   a. Previous studies, such as Babaei et al. (2016) and Zimmerman et al. (2013), were cited. The theoretical sources cited, such as Hall and Anand (2014) and Sanders and Hall (2018), have physiological and pathological foci.
   b. Are the references current? The sources' publication dates ranged from 1983 to 2018 with six sources published in the last 5 years (20%) and 14 published in the last 10 years (45%). The sources are fairly current, but no new studies were cited 3 years prior to the publication of this article.

Continued

CRITICAL APPRAISAL EXAMPLE 12.1—cont'd

5. Examine the study framework or theoretical perspective.

   The framework for this study is implied, and the concepts and relationships can be identified in the Introduction section. Example theoretical relationships include the following: *Therefore, painful procedures such as neonates' blood sampling cause psychological trauma and stress to neonates and even impacts on the brain structural development (Sanders & Hall, 2018...). Painful and stressful stimuli can increase catecholamine release, heart rate, blood pressure and intracranial pressure* (Sarhangi et al., 2021, p. 123).

6. List the research objectives, questions, and/or hypotheses.

   The study hypothesis was that the mother's heartbeat sound reduced pain intensity and improved physiological parameters after blood sampling in neonates admitted to the intensive care unit. (Sarhangi et al., 2021, p. 124).

7. Identify and define (conceptually and operationally) two of the study variables.

   Sarhangi et al. (2021) study included the independent variable mother's heartbeat and the primary outcome or dependent variable pain intensity. Secondary outcomes examined included oxygen saturation, respiratory rate, heart rate, and mean arterial blood pressure.

   Mother's heartbeat sound (independent variable or intervention)

   Conceptual definition: Nonpharmacological intervention that includes the use of alternative methods to manage pain and physiological parameters.

   Operational definition: *The mother's heartbeat sound was played inside the incubator using two small 200-W speakers (SONY®) placed on either side of the neonate's head, 20 cm from the neonate's ears with the sound threshold about 50 dB set by an audiologist. The sound was played 10 min before blood sampling and was continued until 10 min after it* (Sarhangi et al., 2021, p. 125).

   Pain intensity (dependent variable or outcome)

   Conceptual definition: Traumatic sensation experienced after invasive, stressful stimuli.

   Operational definition: *Data were gathered using the neonatal infant pain scale (NIPS) through recording videos from neonates before, during, and after the arterial blood sampling procedure. The neonates' pain intensity was assessed and scored via the observation of the videos by a research assistant* (Sarhangi et al., 2021, p. 125).

8. Identify attribute or demographic variables.

   The medical and demographic variables of the neonate included: *Age, gender, medical diagnosis, duration of hospitalization, type of maternal delivery, Apgar score at one and 5 min after delivery, weight, maternal pregnancy duration (on a weekly basis). ...These were found in the neonates' medical files and were registered on the researcher-made form by the main researcher* (Sarhangi et al., 2021, p. 125).

9. Identify the research design.

   This experimental study included an RCT design with intervention and control groups. The participants were randomized into a group using the flip of a coin. The intervention (mother's heartbeat sound) was detailed in the study: *The neonates in the intervention group were lying supine during taking blood samples and were in a separate room far from the intensive care unit to avoid noises. The mother's heartbeat sound was played inside the incubator using two small 200-W speakers (SONY®) placed on either side of the neonate's head. ...The intervention duration was approximately 30 min on average.*

   In the control group, neonates received routine care in the intensive care unit except for listening to the mother's heartbeat sounds. In other words, the speaker was placed to the incubator for neonates in the control groups, but no sound was played (Sarhangi et al., 2021, p. 125).

10. Describe the sample and setting [brackets are used to identify the elements of the sample and setting].

   Subjects were 60 full-term neonates [Sample size and population] *admitted to an intensive care unit in a teaching hospital* [Setting]. *They were selected using a convenience sampling method* [Nonprobability sampling method] *and were randomly assigned to the intervention and control groups (n = 30 in each group) through flipping coins* [Assignment to groups]. *Inclusion criteria were full-term neonates with no hearing impairments based on the audiologist's diagnosis, not receiving analgesics at least 3 h before and during blood sampling,*

CRITICAL APPRAISAL EXAMPLE 12.1—cont'd

absence of underlying diseases and not undergoing surgeries causing severe pain, absence of crippling diseases and anatomical abnormalities in limbs, and undergoing the arterial blood sampling procedure for laboratory and diagnostic purposes ordered by the physician. Those neonates who were undergoing ventilation and staff nurses failed to take blood samples in the first attempt were excluded [Sampling criteria]. (Sarhangi et al., 2021, pp. 124–125)

The sampling process for this study is presented in Fig. 12.1. The researchers assessed the eligibility of 60 neonates, and all 60 were included in the study, indicating a 100% acceptance rate. In addition, 60 neonates completed the study, with 30 in each group. Therefore no attrition of neonates occurred during the study, so there was a 100% retention rate in both groups. The sample characteristics are presented in Table 12.1; the control and intervention groups were not significantly different for any of these characteristics, which is expected because the neonates were randomly assigned to the groups.

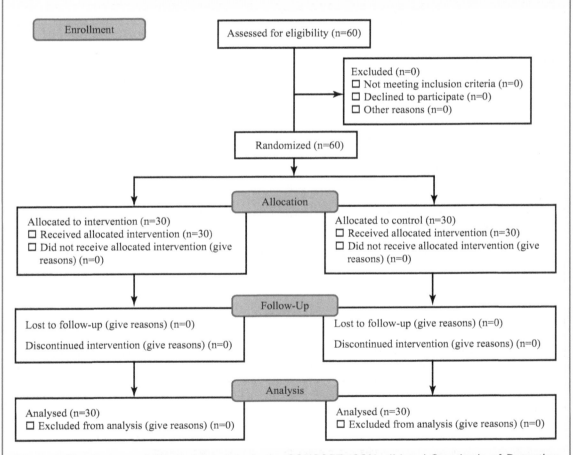

FIG. 12.1 The Process of Study According to the CONSORT (CONsolidated Standards of Reporting Trials) Flow Diagram. (From Sarhangi, F., Azarmnejad, E., Javadi, M., Tadrisi, S. D., Rejeh, N., & Vaismoradi, M. [2021]. The effect of the mother's heartbeat sound on physiological parameters and pain intensity after blood sampling in neonates in the intensive care unit: A randomized controlled clinical trial. *Journal of Neonatal Nursing, 27,* 123–128. https://doi.org/10.1016/j.jnn.2020.07.006)

Continued

CRITICAL APPRAISAL EXAMPLE 12.1—cont'd

TABLE 12.1 Demographic Characteristics of the Neonates in the Groups

Variable	Control ($n = 30$) Mean (*SD*)	Intervention ($n = 30$) Men (*SD*)	*p* Value and Statistics
Age (week)	4.43(2.64)	5.23(2.70)	*$F_{(58)}$ = 023, $t = -1.15$, $p = 0.25$
Length (cm)	47.50(3.55)	46.60(3.63)	*$F_{(58)}$ = 018, $t = 0.97$, $p = 0.33$
Weight (kg)	3.02(0.57)	3.01(0.58)	*$F_{(58)}$ = 0.05, $t = 0.01$, $p = 0.98$
Gestational age (week)	38.07(1.04)	37.97(1.27)	**Mdn = 38, U = 436.500, p= 0.83
APGAR 1 min	8.97(0.18)	8.87(0.51)	**Mdn = 9, U = 434, $p = 0.53$
APGAR 5 min	9.97(0.18)	9.80(0.76)	**Mdn = 10, U = 434, $p = 0.53$
	n(%) (n = 30)	*n(%) (n = 30)*	***p* Value and Statistics**
Gender			
Male	14(46.7)	13(43.3)	Fisher's exact test = 0.99
Female	16(53.3)	17(56.7)	
Delivery method			
NVD	4(13.3)	6(20)	Fisher's exact test = 0.77
C/S	26(86.7)	24(80)	

*p value is calculated by independent t-test and the Fisher's exact test for between-group comparisons. Kolmogorov-Smirnov, $p > 0.5$.
**p value is calculated by Mann–Whitney U test for between-group comparisons. Kolmogorov–Smirnov, $p < 0.5$.
APGAR, Appearance, pulse, grimace, activity, and respiration; *C/S,* cesarean section; *Mdn,* median; *NVD,* normal vaginal delivery.
From Sarhangi, F., Azarmnejad, E., Javadi, M., Tadrisi, S. D., Rejeh, N., & Vaismoradi, M. (2021). The effect of the mother's heartbeat sound on physiological parameters and pain intensity after blood sampling in neonates in the intensive care unit: A randomized controlled clinical trial. *Journal of Neonatal Nursing, 27,* 123–128. https://doi.org/10.1016/j.jnn.2020.07.006.

11. Identify the ethical considerations.

    Informed consent was obtained from the neonates' parents after explaining the process and aim of the study. Also, permission to record videos of the neonates was achieved with the consideration of confidentiality of the neonate's information and recorded videos. The neonates' parents were ensured of the voluntary nature of participation in the study and the possibility of withdrawal from it without having negative effects on the neonates' treatment and care process. Those parents who accepted to participate in the study signed the informed consent form. Since taking blood samples were ordered by the physician on the basis of laboratory and diagnostic purposes and the procedure was performed by the expert staff nurses who followed the standard guideline for blood sampling, no risk of harm for neonates was present. (Sarhangi et al., 2021, p. 125)

CRITICAL APPRAISAL EXAMPLE 12.1—cont'd

12. Identify and describe at least two measurement methods used in this study. The following table includes the critical information about these two methods.

Variable Measured	Name of Measurement Method	Type of Method and Level of Measurement	Reliability or Precision	Validity or Accuracy
Neonatal pain intensity	NIPS	Likert Scale Interval level measurement	Reliability was confirmed for previous studies. Internal consistency reliability: Interclass correlation coefficient >0.9. Interrater reliability for data collectors: Minimum correlation coefficient between raters was reported as 0.868.	*Content validity:* Investigates crying, facial expressions, respiratory pattern, movements of hands and legs, and the state of arousal in newborns. *Construct validity:* Confirmed from previous studies. Convergent validity was supported with a high, significant correlation between the NIPS and the visual analog scale ($r = 0.949$; $p < 0.001$). *Successive use validity:* Scale used frequently in previous studies and in this study.
Physiological parameters: neonates' heart rate, oxygen saturation, mean arterial pressure, and respiratory rate	Portable pulse oximeter device	Physiological measure Ratio level measurement	Precision in physiological measures: *Data were gathered 10 min before as the baseline, immediately after, and 10 min after the blood sampling procedure* (Sarhangi et al., 2021, p. 125).	Documented accuracy: *Portable pulse oximeter device with 2% calibration accuracy* (Sarhangi et al., 2021, p. 125) *Validity of the data collection tools was assessed through content validity by 10 faculty members who were experts in the fields of neonatal nursing care* (Sarhangi et al., 2021, 125).

13. Identify the procedures for data collection.

Data were gathered using the neonatal infant pain scale (NIPS) through recording videos from neonates before, during and after the arterial blood sampling procedure. The neonates' pain intensity was assessed and scored via the observation of the videos by a research assistant. ... The mother's heartbeat sound for each neonate was recorded by the Cool Edit2000 software using the Summit Doppler Sonicade Series L350 (Summit Doppler Company®, USA). ... The weight of the neonates was measured using a digital scale (German vurf model, Beurer company®) with the accuracy of 10 g. ... Moreover, the medical and demographic characteristics of the neonates ... were found in the neonates' medical files and were registered on the researcher-made form by the main researcher. (Sarhangi et al., 2021, p. 125)

Continued

⑤ CRITICAL APPRAISAL EXAMPLE 12.1—cont'd

14. Describe the statistical analyses used.

Demographic and medical variables were presented using frequency, percentage, mean, and standard deviation. The Kolmogorov–Smirnov test was used to assess the normal distribution of data. The independent t-test, the Fisher's exact test and ANOVA test were used for between groups and within group comparisons of demographic and medical variables and physiological parameters [see Table 12.1]. The Mann–Whitney U test and the Friedman test were used for between groups and within group comparisons of pain intensity. p < 0.05 was considered statistically significant. (Sarhangi et al., 2021, p. 125)

Review the Results section of the Sarhangi et al. (2021) study in the Research Article Library for this text. The results are presented in tables and described in the study narrative. The following table includes a few of the many results presented in this study.

Purpose of Analysis	Analysis Technique	Statistic	Results, Baseline/ Immediately After Int./10 min After Int.	Probability
Neonates' pain score for control group ($n = 30$)	Descriptive: mean (standard deviation)	M (SD)	0.33 (0.54)/5.20 (1.06)/5.00 (1.08)	
Neonates' pain score for Int. group ($n = 30$)	Descriptive: mean (standard deviation)	M (SD)	0.20 (0.40)/3.97 (1.67)/3.07 (1.68)	
			Results of Inferential Statistics	
Difference between Int. and control groups for pain intensity at 10 min after Int.	Inferential: Mann–Whitney U test	U	$U = 166$	*$p = 0.001$
Difference between Int. and control groups for heart rate at 10 min after Int.	Inferential: analysis of variance (ANOVA)	F	$F(2,57) = 46.03$	*$p = 0.001$

*p value is significant at < 0.05.
Int., Intervention.

15. Identify two findings discussed by the researchers.

Our findings showed that listening to the mother's heartbeat sound did not affect mean arterial pressure, but it had medium to large effects on oxygen saturation and respiratory rate immediately after and 10 min after the intervention, as well as had a large effect on heart rate immediately after the intervention. Also, statistically significant medium to large effects of the intervention on pain intensity immediately after and 10 min after it were reported. (Sarhangi et al., 2021, p. 127)

16. What study limitations did the researcher identify?

As a limitation, it was impossible to eliminate all noises in the research zone that might have affected the study outcome, but sound levels were monitored by a sound meter throughout the intervention to prevent reaching sound to an unsafe decibel level for the neonates' ears, when it was combined with the intervention sound. (Sarhangi et al., 2021, p. 127)

17. Did the researcher generalize the findings?

The researchers did not indicate that they generalized the findings. However, they did recommend additional clinical trials to examine the effectiveness of the mother's heartbeat sound in reducing neonates' suffering.

18. What were the implications of the findings for nursing practice?

Since the presence of the mother at the neonate's bedside in case of hospitalization in the intensive care unit is not always possible, the use of the mother's heartbeat sound by nurses for reducing pain and sufferings in neonates during painful and invasive procedures is suggested. (Sarhangi et al., 2021, p. 127)

> **⚡ CRITICAL APPRAISAL EXAMPLE 12.1—cont'd**
>
> 19. What suggestions for further study were identified?
>
> *More clinical trials are needed to assess the effect of the mother's heartbeat sound on neonates' physiological and psychological parameters and compare it with other alternative and complementary medicines methods in intensive care units.* (Sarhangi et al., 2021, p. 127)
>
> 20. What conclusions did the researchers identify?
>
> *The present study showed the short-term and long-term effects of the mother's heartbeat sound on the reduction of pain intensity and physiological parameters during the arterial blood sampling procedure.* (Sarhangi et al., 2021, p. 127)

Step 2: Determining the Strengths and Weaknesses of Quantitative Studies

The second step in critically appraising nursing studies requires determining study strengths and weaknesses. To accomplish this, you need to have knowledge of what each step of the research process should be like based on expert sources, such as this textbook and other relevant references (Bandalos, 2018; Bonar et al., 2020; Critical Appraisal Skills Programme, 2020, 2021; Creswell & Creswell, 2018; Grainger, 2021; Gray & Grove, 2021; Grove & Cipher, 2020; Kazdin, 2017; Kim et al., 2022; Leedy & Ormrod, 2019; O'Mathúna & Fineout-Overholt, 2019; Waltz et al., 2017). The ideal ways to conduct the steps of the research process are then compared with the actual study steps. During this comparison, you examine the extent to which the researcher followed the guidelines for an ideal study, noting any strengths and weaknesses.

You also need to examine the logical links or flow of the steps in the study being appraised. For example, the problem needs to provide background and direction for the statement of the purpose. The variables identified in the study purpose need to be consistent with the variables identified in the research objectives, questions, or hypotheses. The variables identified in the research objectives, questions, or hypotheses need to be conceptually defined in light of the study framework. The conceptual definitions should provide the basis for the development of operational definitions. The study design and analyses need to be appropriate for the investigation of the study purpose, as well as for the specific objectives, questions, or hypotheses (Grove & Cipher, 2020). The results should address the purpose or the objectives, questions, or hypotheses and provide a basis for study findings.

> **📄 RESEARCH/EBP TIP**
>
> Examining the quality and logical links among the steps of a study will enable you to determine which steps are strengths and which are weaknesses. This critical appraisal step is essential for identifying knowledge that might be used in practice.

Guidelines for Determining Quantitative Study Strengths and Weaknesses

The following questions were developed to assist you in examining the different aspects of a quantitative study and determining its strengths and weaknesses. *The intent is not to answer each of these questions but to read the questions and then make judgments about the steps in the study.* You need to provide a rationale for your decisions and document from relevant sources, such as those listed in the previous section and in the References at the end of this chapter. For example, you might decide the study purpose is a strength because it addresses the study problem, clarifies the focus of the study, and is feasible to investigate (Gray & Grove, 2021).

? CRITICAL APPRAISAL GUIDELINES

Step 2: Determining Study Strengths and Weaknesses

1. Research problem and purpose
   a. Is the problem significant for nursing (Gallagher-Ford et al., 2020; O'Mathúna & Fineout-Overholt, 2019)?
   b. Does the purpose narrow and clarify the focus of the study?
   c. Was the study feasible to conduct in terms of money commitment; the researchers' expertise; and availability of participants, facilities, and equipment (see Chapter 5)?
2. Review of literature
   a. Is the literature review organized to demonstrate the progressive development of evidence from previous research?
   b. Does the summary of the literature review identify what is known and not known about the research problem and provide direction for the formation of the purpose (Grainger, 2021; Jones et al., 2020)?
3. Study framework
   a. Is the framework presented with clarity? If a model or conceptual map of the framework is present, is it adequate to explain the phenomenon of concern?
   b. If a proposition from a theory is to be tested, is the proposition clearly identified and linked to the study hypotheses (Chinn et al., 2022; Gray & Grove, 2021)?
   c. Is the framework related to the study findings?
4. Research objectives, questions, or hypotheses
   a. Are the objectives, questions, or hypotheses expressed clearly and logically linked to the purpose (Gray & Grove, 2021)?
   b. Are hypotheses stated to direct the conduct of quasi-experimental and experimental research (Kazdin, 2017; Shadish et al., 2002)?
   c. Are the objectives, questions, or hypotheses logically linked to the study results (Grove & Cipher, 2020; Kim et al., 2022)?
5. Variables
   a. Are the variables reflective of the concepts identified in the framework?
   b. Are the variables clearly defined (conceptually and operationally) and based on previous theories and research (Chinn et al., 2022; Smith & Liehr, 2018)?
   c. Is the conceptual definition of a variable consistent with the operational definition?
6. Design
   a. Is the design used in the study the most appropriate design to address the research purpose and to obtain essential data (Gray & Grove, 2021; Kazdin, 2017; Shadish et al., 2002)?
   b. Does the design provide a means to examine all the objectives, questions, or hypotheses?
   c. Is the treatment or intervention clearly described? Is the intervention appropriate for examining the study purpose and hypotheses? Does the study framework explain the links between the intervention (independent variable) and the proposed outcomes (dependent variables)?
   d. Was a protocol developed to promote consistent implementation of the intervention to ensure intervention fidelity (Bonar et al., 2020; Eymard & Altmiller, 2016)? Did the researcher monitor implementation of the intervention to ensure consistency? If the intervention was not consistently implemented, what might be the effect on the findings?
   e. Did the researcher identify the threats to design validity (statistical conclusion validity, internal validity, construct validity, and external validity) and minimize them as much as possible? (see Chapter 8; Gray & Grove, 2021; Kazdin, 2017; Shadish et al., 2002)
   f. If more than one group is used, do the groups appear equivalent?
   g. How were the groups formed? Were the participants randomly assigned to the intervention or control group, or were the groups naturally occurring?
   h. Were the participants in the groups matched?

? CRITICAL APPRAISAL GUIDELINES—cont'd

7. Sample, population, and setting
   a. Is the sampling method adequate to produce a representative sample?
   b. Are any participants excluded from the study because of age, socioeconomic status, or ethnicity without a sound rationale?
   c. Did the sample include an understudied population, such as the young, elderly, or a minority group?
   d. Were the sampling criteria (inclusion and exclusion) appropriate for the type of study conducted (Gray & Grove, 2021; O'Mathúna & Fineout-Overholt, 2019)?
   e. If a power analysis was conducted, were the results of the analysis clearly described and used to determine the final sample size (Aberson, 2019)? If a power analysis was not conducted, how did the researchers determine the sample size?
   f. Was the rate of refusal to participate a problem? If so, how might this weakness have influenced the findings?
   g. Is the setting used in the study appropriate?
   h. Was sample attrition a problem? If so, how might this weakness influence the final sample and the study results and findings (Aberson, 2019; Gray & Grove, 2021)?
8. Ethical considerations
   a. Were the rights of the study participants protected?
   b. Is the study ethical?
9. Measurements
   a. Do the measurement methods selected for the study adequately measure the study variables? Should additional measurement methods have been used to improve the quality of the study outcomes (Bandalos, 2018; Gray & Grove, 2021; Waltz et al., 2017)?
   b. Do the measurement methods used in the study have adequate validity and reliability? What additional reliability or validity testing is needed to improve the quality of the measurement methods (Bandalos, 2018; Bialocerkowski et al., 2010; Waltz et al., 2017)?
   c. Respond to the following questions, which are relevant to the measurement approaches used in the study:
      (1) Scales and questionnaires
         (a) Are the instruments clearly described?
         (b) Are techniques to complete and score the instruments provided?
         (c) Are validity and reliability of the instruments described from previous research?
         (d) Did the researcher examine the reliability of instruments for the present sample?
         (e) If the instrument was developed for the study, is the instrument development process described (Bandalos, 2018; DeVellis, 2017; Waltz et al., 2017)?
      (2) Observation
         (a) Is what is to be observed clearly identified and defined?
         (b) Is interrater reliability described?
         (c) Are the techniques for recording observations described (Waltz et al., 2017)?
      (3) Structured interviews
         (a) Do the interview questions address concerns expressed in the research problem?
         (b) Are the interview questions relevant for the research purpose and objectives, questions, or hypotheses (Dillman et al., 2014; Waltz et al., 2017)?
      (4) Physiological measures
         (a) Are the physiological measures or instruments clearly described (Ryan-Wenger, 2017)? If appropriate, are the brand names, such as Space Labs or Hewlett-Packard, of the instruments identified?
         (b) Are the physiological measures appropriate for the research purpose and objectives, questions, or hypotheses?
         (c) Are the accuracy, precision, and error of the physiological instruments discussed (Ryan-Wenger, 2017)?
         (d) Are the methods for recording data from the physiological measures clearly described? Is the recording of data consistent (Gray & Grove, 2021)?

Continued

> ## ❓ CRITICAL APPRAISAL GUIDELINES—cont'd
>
> 10. Data collection
>   a. Is the data collection process clearly described (Gray & Grove, 2021)?
>   b. Are the forms used to collect data organized to facilitate computerizing the data?
>   c. Is the training of data collectors clearly described and adequate?
>   d. Is the data collection process conducted in a consistent manner?
>   e. Are the data collection methods ethical?
>   f. Do the data collected address the research objectives, questions, or hypotheses?
>   g. Did any adverse events occur during data collection; if so, were these appropriately managed?
> 11. Data analysis
>   a. Are data analysis procedures appropriate for the type of data collected (Grove & Cipher, 2020; Kim et al., 2022; Leedy & Ormrod, 2019)?
>   b. Did the researcher address any problems with missing data and how they were managed?
>   c. Do the data analysis techniques address the study purpose or the research objectives, questions, or hypotheses? Are data analysis procedures clearly described?
>   d. Are the results presented in an understandable way by narrative, tables, or figures, or a combination of methods (APA, 2020)?
>   e. Is the sample size sufficient to detect significant differences or relationships if they are present?
>   f. Was a power analysis conducted for nonsignificant results (Aberson, 2019)?
>   g. Are the results interpreted appropriately?
> 12. Interpretation of findings
>   a. Are findings discussed in relation to each objective, question, or hypothesis?
>   b. Are various explanations for significant and nonsignificant findings examined?
>   c. Are the findings clinically important (O'Mathúna & Fineout-Overholt, 2019)?
>   d. Are the findings linked to the study framework (Smith & Liehr, 2018)?
>   e. Are the findings consistent with the findings of previous studies in this area?
>   f. Does the study have limitations not identified by the researcher?
>   g. Did the researcher generalize the findings appropriately?
>   h. Were the identified implications for practice appropriate based on the study findings and the findings from previous research (Melnyk & Fineout-Overholt, 2019)?
>   i. Were quality suggestions made for future research?
>   j. Do the conclusions fit the findings from this study and previous studies?

Review the Sarhangi et al. (2021) research article and the step 1 Critical Appraisal. You are now ready to determine the strengths and weaknesses of this RCT. The questions identified in the previous section were developed to stimulate your thinking and direct you in writing the step 2 Critical Appraisal. This intellectual critical appraisal is a narrative organized by the major sections of a research report: Introduction, Methods, Results, and Discussion (APA, 2020).

📋 CRITICAL APPRAISAL EXAMPLE 12.2

Step 2: Determining Study Strengths and Weaknesses

Introduction
Sarhangi et al. (2021) identified a significant problem that focused on the physical and emotional trauma experienced by neonates during blood draws. This problem is common for neonates in the ICU and can be detected, managed, and monitored by nurses. The study purpose addressed the research problem and provided a clear, concise focus for this RCT. The variables, population, setting, and type of study are evident in the purpose (Gray & Grove, 2021). The purpose also provided focus to the literature review for this study.

CRITICAL APPRAISAL EXAMPLE 12.2—cont'd

Sarhangi et al. (2021) presented a brief literature review that included very few theoretical sources. The empirical sources cited were relevant but older, with no new studies cited in the 3 years before publication. However, a clear summary of the literature was provided identifying what was known and not known in the area of study (Critical Appraisal Skills Programme, 2020; Grainger, 2021). The statement of what was not known, the problem statement, was followed by the concise, focused purpose statement. The purpose statement provided the basis for the relevant hypothesis that was tested in this study (Kazdin, 2017).

Sarhangi et al. (2021) did not identify a framework for their study. The elements of the framework (concepts and relationships) had to be abstracted from the physiological and psychological statements in the literature review. The focus was on managing the suffering and pain of neonates during invasive procedures. Nonpharmacological interventions were discussed as an effective way of managing neonates' pain and physiological parameters. No proposition was identified for testing in this study, but the hypothesis did focus on the theoretical relationship between nonpharmacological interventions and the outcomes of pain and physiological responses (Chinn et al., 2022). The theoretical concepts were linked to the study variables, such as the nonpharmacological intervention was linked to the mother's heartbeat sound, and suffering and pain were linked to pain intensity. However, no clear conceptual definitions were provided that could be linked to the operations definitions that were detailed in the study.

Methods

The design was clearly identified as an RCT in the study title and the Methods section. The research process for this study was detailed using the CONsolidated Standards of Reporting Trials (CONSORT) Statement (see Fig. 12.1), which is considered the international standard for reporting an RCT (Liberati et al., 2009). The intervention (mother's heartbeat) was discussed in detail and consistently implemented by research assistants according to a structured protocol. Thus intervention fidelity was achieved during the study, strengthening the statistical conclusion validity (Bonar et al., 2020). The study included intervention and control groups, and participants were randomly assigned to a group by the flip of a coin. The research assistants were blinded to the group assignment during the collection of pain intensity and physiological parameters data, which strengthened the external design validity. Internal design validity was strengthened by the quality of the intervention, random assignment of participants to groups, and the 0% participant attrition (Gray & Grove, 2021; Shadish et al., 2002).

The target population of full-term neonates was designated by relevant sampling criteria. This understudied population of neonates in an ICU setting was appropriate for testing the study hypothesis. The sampling method was one of convenience, which increases the potential for bias and decreases generalization. However, convenience sampling is common in RCTs and many healthcare studies due to the limited number of participants available for research (Straus et al., 2019). The sample size was limited ($N = 60$), and no power analysis was addressed to identify the minimum sample size for this study (Aberson, 2019). All outcome variables were significantly different after the intervention except the mean arterial pressure, which might indicate a Type II error. The 0% refusal and attrition rates and equal group sizes increased the representativeness of the sample and supported the credibility of the findings (Gray & Grove, 2021). The ethical discussion in this study was extremely strong, detailing the institutional review board approval, informed consent process, and protection of the participants' rights. For example, the researchers worked with an audiologist to ensure the decibel level of the recording (intervention) did not harm the neonates.

Sarhangi et al. (2021) measured their variables with a reliable Likert scale and highly accurate physiological measures (Ryan-Wenger, 2017). Pain intensity, measured with the NIPS, had an extremely strong internal consistency ($r = 0.9$) for this study (DeVellis, 2017; Waltz et al., 2017). However, the NIPA was reported to have confirmed reliability and validity from previous research, but no specific information was provided. The scoring process for the scale also was missing (Gray & Grove, 2021). The neonates' heart rate, oxygen saturation, mean arterial pressure, and respiratory rate were measured objectively and precisely with a highly accurate portable pulse oximeter.

Continued

CRITICAL APPRAISAL EXAMPLE 12.2—cont'd

Data collection tools were developed for this study, and their content validity was assessed by 10 faculty members with neonatal expertise. The data were collected by research assistants, blinded to group assignment, which reduced the potential bias. In addition, the research assistants had strong interrater reliability (0.868) for the collection of data (Waltz et al., 2017). The data collected were relevant for testing the study hypothesis. Therefore the measurement methods and data collection process reduced the potential for error and supported the credibility of the findings (Gray & Grove, 2021; Shadish et al., 2002).

Results

The descriptive and inferential statistical analysis techniques were clearly identified and appropriate for the study data (Grove & Cipher, 2020). The results were presented in tables and clearly discussed in the study narrative (APA, 2020). The demographic characteristics of the neonates in the intervention and control groups were not significantly different at the start of the study as demonstrated by the nonsignificant findings in Table 12.1. The groups were reported as homogenous with equal numbers of male and females in each group, which suggests the changes in the groups were probably due to the intervention and not error (Grove & Cipher, 2020; Kim et al., 2022). The two groups were not significantly different for pain before the intervention but were significantly different immediately and 10 minutes after the intervention. The pain intensity and physiological parameters except for mean arterial pressure were significantly different in the intervention group compared with the control group. However, a power analysis was not conducted to address the nonsignificant finding that might have been caused by the small sample size (Aberson, 2019). The results were interpreted correctly and supported the use of the mother's heartbeat sound as an effective intervention for managing neonates' trauma after an invasive procedure. The results were considered statistically significant and clinically important, and the research hypothesis was accepted (Grove & Cipher, 2020; Shadish et al., 2002).

Discussion

Sarhangi et al. (2021) briefly described their study findings and reported previous studies that generally supported the effectiveness of listening to the mother's heartbeat and voice on the neonates' pain intensity and physiological responses. The researchers identified only one study limitation, which was the noise in the ICU that might have interfered with the study findings. However, the study lacked a framework, which limited the link of study findings to nursing's body of knowledge. In addition, no power analysis was conducted to determine an adequate sample size, and the NIPS lacked adequate reliability and validity information. The implications for practice were supported by the study findings and had a potential for future use in practice. In addition, this study needs replication with a large sample, and the effectiveness of the mother's heartbeat sound should be compared with other alternative therapies for managing the pain and suffering of neonates in the ICU.

Step 3: Evaluating the Credibility and Meaning of Quantitative Study Findings

Evaluating the credibility and meaning of study findings involves determining the validity, significance, trustworthiness, and contributions of the study by examining the relationships among the steps of the study, study findings, and the findings of previous studies. The steps of the study are evaluated in light of previous studies, such as an evaluation of the present design based on previous designs, present methods of measuring variables based on previous methods of measurement, and present data collection process based on previous data collection processes. The findings of the present study are examined in light of the findings of previous studies. Evaluation builds on conclusions reached during the first two steps of the critical appraisal process so that the credibility and meaning of the study findings can be determined.

Guidelines for Evaluating the Credibility and Meaning of Study Findings

An evaluation of a quantitative study's credibility and meaning involves reviewing steps 1 and 2 of the critical appraisal process discussed earlier. Next, examine the Discussion section of the study, focusing on the findings, limitations, implications for practice, suggestions for further research, and conclusions. Then summarize your thoughts based on the guidelines presented in the following box.

? CRITICAL APPRAISAL GUIDELINES

Step 3: Evaluating the Credibility and Meaning of Quantitative Study Findings

Using the following questions as a guide, summarize your evaluation of the study and document your responses.
1. Do the findings from this study build on the findings of previous studies? Review the Discussion section of the study and read some of the other relevant studies cited by the researchers to address this question.
2. When the findings are examined in light of previous studies, what is now known and not known about the phenomenon under study?
3. Could the limitations of the study have been corrected?
4. Do you believe the study findings are valid? How much confidence can be placed in the study findings (Gray & Grove, 2021)?
5. To what populations can the findings be generalized (Kazdin, 2017; Shadish et al., 2002)?
6. Are the findings ready for use in practice (Melnyk & Fineout-Overholt, 2019)?
7. What is your expert opinion of the study's quality and contribution to nursing knowledge and practice?

⚑ CRITICAL APPRAISAL EXAMPLE 12.3

Step 3: Evaluating the Credibility and Meaning of the Study Findings

Sarhangi et al. (2021) focused on a significant clinical problem and conducted a quality study to address this concern. This study has many strengths and few weaknesses, which leads one to conclude that the findings are trustworthy and an accurate reflection of reality (Gray & Grove, 2021). The findings were as expected and supported the study hypothesis that mother's heartbeat was effective in reducing the neonates' pain and improving their physiological parameters when exposed to an invasive procedure in an ICU. Sarhangi et al. (2021) used a stronger design (RCT) than most of the previous studies. In addition, these researchers used quality measurement methods and a detailed, structured data collection process, which increased the validity of the findings. The limitation of the noise in the ICU was reduced by the researcher and thought to not affect the findings. However, the lack of a study framework, small sample size, and limited reliability and validity information for the scale in this study could have been corrected and need to be addressed in future studies. Correcting these weaknesses will increase the confidence in future study findings.

Sarhangi et al. (2021) recommended that nurses implement the mother's heartbeat intervention for managing neonates' pain and suffering in the ICU. They also recommended additional clinical trials to determine the best alternative therapies for managing neonates' pain and suffering. We believe this study addressed a significant clinical problem using quality methodology and determined the effectiveness of an evidence-based intervention for neonates in ICUs. However, the study's lack of a framework makes the contribution to nursing knowledge less clear. This is an important area of research, and additional studies with larger samples are needed to generalize findings regarding the best alternative therapies to use in caring for neonates.

UNDERSTANDING THE QUALITATIVE RESEARCH CRITICAL APPRAISAL PROCESS

Nurses in every phase and field of practice need experience in critically appraising qualitative and quantitative studies. Although qualitative studies are a "different approach to scholarly inquiry" (Creswell & Creswell, 2018, p. 179), appraisal in both cases has a common purpose: determining the rigor with which the methods were applied and the extent to which the conclusions of the study were trustworthy. Critical appraisal of qualitative studies focuses on how the integrity of the design and methods will affect the credibility and meaningfulness of the findings and their usefulness in clinical practice (Dane, 2018; Straus et al., 2019). Different criteria are used to appraise qualitative studies critically (Creswell & Poth, 2018; Morse, 2018; Munthe-Kaas et al., 2019; Sawatsky et al., 2019). We include a set of criteria synthesized from these published criteria and have organized them into three broad steps, similar to those used for critical appraisal of quantitative studies. Therefore the qualitative research critical appraisal process consists of (1) identifying the components of the qualitative research process in studies, (2) determining study strengths and weaknesses, and (3) evaluating the trustworthiness and meaning of study findings. The questions provided for each step are different from those provided for appraising quantitative studies, because they have been changed to be consistent with qualitative philosophies and standards. As you gain expertise and confidence in your ability to appraise qualitative studies, you may perform two or three steps of this process simultaneously.

📄 RESEARCH/EBP TIP

Qualitative research has different criteria by which it is evaluated. Its unique strength is providing the context and richness of an experience in contrast with the clarity of numerical results.

Step 1: Identifying the Components of the Qualitative Research Process in Studies

In a qualitative critical appraisal, just like in a quantitative critical appraisal, the first step involves reviewing the abstract, reading the study from beginning to end, and highlighting or underlining the elements of the qualitative study. Rereading the article, you might also want to underline the terms that you do not understand and determine their meaning from the glossary at the end of this text. After reading and comprehending the content of the study, you are ready to write your initial critical appraisal of the study.

Ask yourself these questions about the presentation of the study report:
- Was the writing style of the report clear and concise?
- Were the following parts of the research report clearly identified (APA, 2020)?
  - Introduction section with the problem, purpose, literature review, framework or philosophical foundation, study concepts, and research objectives or questions.
  - Methods section with the qualitative design, sample, method of data collection, data management, and analysis.
  - Results section with the specific results presented in tables, figures, and narrative.
  - Discussion section with the findings, limitations, implications for practice, suggestions for future research, and conclusions (Gray & Grove, 2021).

Read the study a second time and label each step of the research process. Now, you are ready to write your critical appraisal of the study. In step 1, you need to identify each step of the research process and respond briefly to the guidelines and questions in the following box.

📄 **RESEARCH/EBP TIP**

Reports of quantitative and qualitative studies frequently have the same major headings. However, qualitative studies have longer Results sections because participant quotations are included to support the themes or major concepts the researchers found.

💡 **CRITICAL APPRAISAL GUIDELINES FOR QUALITATIVE RESEARCH**

Step 1: Guidelines for Identifying the Components of the Qualitative Research Process in Studies

1. Introduction
   a. Was the article title clear?
   b. Does the title indicate the phenomenon of interest and design of the study conducted—phenomenology, grounded theory, ethnography, or exploratory-descriptive qualitative research (APA, 2020; Creswell & Poth, 2018; Gray & Grove, 2021)?
   c. Did the abstract include the purpose, sample, key results, and conclusions (APA, 2020)?
2. State the problem.
   a. Did the researchers describe the significance of the problem and/or its importance to nursing practice?
   b. Did the researchers provide the background of the problem?
   c. Was there a clear problem statement (see Chapter 5)?
3. State the purpose.
   a. Were research objectives used to guide the study?
   b. Was there an overall research question?
4. Examine the literature review.
   a. Does the review include a description of a theory and previous studies?
   b. Are the references current? (Number and percentage of sources in the last 10 years and in the last 5 years?) (see Chapter 6; Jones et al., 2020)
5. Examine the philosophical foundation or theoretical perspective of the study.
   a. Is the philosophy that supports the research design described?
   b. Was a theoretical perspective described?
6. Sampling
   a. Were inclusion and exclusion criteria identified (see Chapter 9)?
   b. How many participants were in the sample?
   c. Did the researchers identify the specific type of sampling that was used, such as purposive, network, convenience, or theoretical sampling (see Chapter 9)? If more than one type of sampling was used, did the researchers identify how many participants were recruited through each type of sampling?
7. Identify the ethical considerations.
   a. Was the study reviewed by an institutional or ethical board?
   b. What was the process for informed consent?

Continued

? **CRITICAL APPRAISAL GUIDELINES FOR QUALITATIVE RESEARCH—cont'd**

8. Data collection
   a. What methods were used to collect data: Interviews, focus groups, observation, or examination of documents?
   b. Did the researchers describe how data were managed and analyzed?
9. Results
   a. How were the participants described—age, marital status, or other relevant demographic variables?
   b. Were the results of the analysis presented as themes, concepts, or a diagram?
10. Discussion
    a. What were the findings of the study? Identify two findings discussed by the researchers.
    b. What study limitations did the researcher identify?
    c. Did the researcher indicate whether the findings might be applicable to other samples?
    d. What were the implications of the findings for nursing practice, if any?
    e. What suggestions for further study were identified?
11. Conclusions
    a. What conclusions did the researchers identify?

Example Critical Appraisal Step 1: Identification of the Components of the Study

Barton et al. (2021) conducted a phenomenological study with fathers of infants hospitalized in the neonatal ICU (NICU). Previous studies had found gender differences between the parents, and fewer studies had been conducted with fathers. Because of this, Barton et al. (2021) focused their study on the fathers. This article can be found in the online Research Article Library for this text. The steps of this study are identified using the guidelines previously introduced.

⚑ **CRITICAL APPRAISAL EXAMPLE 12.4**

1. Introduction
   a. The title of the article was "The Lived Experience of a NICU Father: A Descriptive Phenomenological Study" (Barton, et al., 2021).
   b. The title included the phenomenon of interest [lived experiences of NICU fathers] and the qualitative design [descriptive phenomenology].
   c. The abstract was only 150 words long and included the purpose, sample, five themes, and conclusions (APA, 2020).
2. State the problem.
   a. Barton et al. (2021) noted that the NICU admissions were increasing and were stressful for parents.
      Fathers were found to have higher levels of stress at discharge compared to mothers. . . . Fathers expressed feeling anxious and fearful and having difficulties in paternal role acquisition (Barton et al., 2021, p. 206). Addressing the stress, anxiety, and fears of patient families is a critical aspect of the nursing role. Barriers to acquiring the parental role may affect the father's relationship with the child and his ability to provide emotional support to his wife and child.
   b. In addition to the stress and emotional responses of fathers,
      the role of the father is multifaceted. . . many fathers juggle a variety of responsibilities including employment, supporting their partner, caring for other children, and maintaining the home. . . role demands, a variety of interpersonal, infant-related, and environmental aspects may impact a father's involvement during the infant's stay in the NICU (Barton et al., 2021, p. 206).
   c. *There is limited research regarding the paternal experience internationally, however there is a paucity of research exploring father's experiences in the United States. Paternal experiences may differ in the United States compared to European countries* (Barton et al., 2021, p. 206).

> ## ◢ CRITICAL APPRAISAL EXAMPLE 12.4—cont'd
>
> 3. State the purpose. *This study aims to minimize these gaps in research by exploring the lived experiences of fathers who had a child admitted to the Neonatal Intensive Care Unit* (Barton et al., 2021, p. 206).
>   a. The overall research question was unstated: What is the lived experience of fathers whose infants are admitted to the NICU?
>   b. Barton et al. (2021) did not identify research objectives.
> 4. Examine the literature review.
>   a. The literature cited did not explicitly identify a theory, but the theories of stress, role acquisition, and gender difference were implicit in the research that was cited. In their concise literature review, the researchers cited 11 different studies. The studies supported their argument that most studies had been conducted in other countries or had been conducted with fathers of premature infants.
>   b. Barton et al. (2021) cited 18 references, with 11 (61%) published in the last 10 years. Four of the seven older citations were references related to qualitative methods. Only 2 (11%) of the 18 citations were published in the last 5 years (2016 or later).
> 5. Examine the philosophical foundation or theoretical perspective of the study.
>   a. Phenomenology provides the philosophical foundation for the study. Barton et al. (2021) did not provide any description of the philosophy beyond stating that descriptive phenomenology relied on first-persons accounts of experiences and citing a secondary source.
>   b. No theoretical perspective was described.
> 6. Sampling
>   a. Inclusion *criteria included: 1) Fathers of infants born within the United States [US], 2) English-speaking fathers, 3) Fathers of infants with diagnoses that were not known until birth, 4) Fathers of infants who were in the NICU for longer than a week* (Barton et al., 2021, p. 207). Fathers were excluded if their infants were born outside of the US.
>   b. The sample was comprised of 6 fathers who were 3 weeks to 19 years postdischarge. The time since discharge represented a wide range to capture a more diverse group of experiences. Recruitment continued until the researchers reached data saturation.
>   c. Snowball sampling was used to recruit all the fathers.
> 7. Identify the ethical considerations.
>   a. The study was approved by the institutional review board of the researchers' university prior to data collection.
>   b. *All fathers provided written consent prior to data collection* (Barton et al., 2021, p. 207). No other information was provided about the process of obtaining informed consent.
> 8. Data collection
>   a. *An audio recorded, semi-structured interview, lasting approximately 60 min, was conducted for the purposes of the study...fathers were asked to reflect on their NICU experience* (Barton et al., 2021, p. 207).
>   b. *Audio-recorded interviews were transcribed verbatim. After transcription, all audio recordings were destroyed* (Barton et al., 2021, p. 207). The researchers used *Colaizzi's method that includes seven rigorous steps to ensure trustworthiness. ... Three members of the research team independently familiarized themselves with the data through multiple readings of each transcribed interview. Significant statements of direct relevance to the phenomenon were extracted from each interview. After reviewing the significant statements, formulated meanings were created revolving around the phenomenon as experienced* (Barton et al., 2021, p. 207). Consistent with Colaizzi's method, all fathers could review the researchers' description of their own lived experiences, and two fathers validated the descriptions of their experiences.
> 9. Results
>   a. The results of the quantitative analysis of demographic characteristics were reported in a table, with one column per father. For example, the father represented by the third column was 35 to 44 years old, white,
>
> *Continued*

CRITICAL APPRAISAL EXAMPLE 12.4—cont'd

married, worked between 36 and 50 hours per week, and made between $50,000 and $90,000 per year. He was interviewed 3 weeks after the discharge of his twins. Minimal description was provided by the researchers except for noting the diversity of experiences *from six different NICUs and two NICU transfers in order to receive a higher level of care. The study sample included four fathers with one child in the NICU and two fathers of multiple birth children, a set of twins and a set of triplets* (Barton et al., 2021, p. 207).

   b. The results were presented as themes with supporting quotes from the fathers. *The following themes emerged as a final result of the analysis process: horrible storm, piece by piece, 'I'm the father,' support, and little fighters* (Barton et al., 2021, p. 208).

10. Discussion

   a. *The results of this study support previous work noting that the Neonatal Intensive Care Unit (NICU) experience is traumatic, stressful, and creates fear and anxiety in parents. ...During this horrible storm, fathers experienced a loss of control, fear of the unknown, and continued traumatic memories. ... Fathers identified support from nurses, family, programs, interventions, and God; however, support was lacking from HCPs [healthcare professionals]* (Barton et al., 2021, p. 209).

   b. *A possible limitation was that the research team did not explore the experiences of fathers who anticipated a NICU admission. The participants of this study included only US, English-speaking, heterosexual fathers. ...Another limitation is that all interviews were conducted by a female researcher, which may have impacted fathers' responses* (Barton et al., 2021, p. 209).

   c. The researchers did not note whether the findings were applicable to other samples.

   d. *Support came through multiple sources including spouse, family, healthcare workers, spirituality and God. The support from nurses was seen as a critical element in guiding fathers as they navigated the NICU experience* (Barton et al., 2021, p. 210).

   e. *Future research is needed to explore diverse populations. ...Future studies conducted by male researchers may bring additional information to light* (Barton et al., 2021, p. 209). The recommendations for future studies were directly related to the identified study limitations.

11. Conclusions

   a. *Findings from this study indicate that fathers with a child in the NICU experience a variety of perceptions throughout their child's stay. Their journey is quite extensive, with many unexpected roadblocks and challenges along the way. ...Fathers consistently discussed the NICU experience as a traumatic experience where they felt they had little control and/or access to their own child. Fathers in this study identified support as a major factor in managing the horrible storm that they experienced* (Barton et al., 2021, p. 210).

Step 2: Determining the Strengths and Weaknesses of Qualitative Studies

At this step, the differences in the critical appraisal processes of quantitative and qualitative studies become more obvious. However, the goal of the critical appraisal remains the same: determining the strengths and weaknesses of the study (Morse, 2018). Knowledge of the different qualitative approaches and data collection processes is needed to answer the questions during this step. You may want to refer to Chapter 3 and supplement your knowledge with additional sources, such as other texts and reference books (Creswell & Poth, 2018; Denzin & Lincoln, 2018; Gray & Grove, 2021). The actual methods of a qualitative study are compared with the expectations of experts, especially the original proponents of different qualitative approaches. Because different qualitative experts agree less on the "rules" for implementing qualitative studies, using the guidelines recommended by a specific expert in the methodology used by the researchers in the study is important. The guidelines are based on the underlying philosophy for the different qualitative methodologies and designs. For each step of a study that is being appraised, the areas of consistency with other steps of the study and the expectations of experts are strengths of the study, whereas areas of inconsistency may indicate weaknesses of the study.

You need to appraise the rigor of the study methods by looking for information about the carefulness of data collection and thoroughness of the data analysis (Miles et al., 2020). The questions asked about each component of the study will focus your attention on the rigor of the methods and the logical links among the study elements. Logical links among the study elements are critical to the credibility of the study (Gray & Grove, 2021; Kazdin, 2017). For example:

- Is the purpose of the study consistent with the research questions?
- Are the purpose and research questions appropriate to address the research problem?
- Is the selected qualitative approach the best way to answer the research questions?

Similar to quantitative research, logical inconsistencies and improperly applied methods are common weaknesses of qualitative studies. Because qualitative research has fewer rules, critically appraising qualitative studies can seem daunting. The questions in the critique guidelines that follow provide a structure for you to examine the strengths and weaknesses of each aspect of a qualitative study. Remember to consult other references, as needed, to answer the questions.

📄 RESEARCH/EBP TIP

The report of a qualitative study should document why the topic was important; why a qualitative study needed to be done; how the design, sampling, data collection, and data analysis methods were appropriate for the study purpose; and how the data supported the findings and conclusions.

❓ CRITICAL APPRAISAL GUIDELINES

Step 2: Determining the Strengths and Weaknesses of Qualitative Studies

1. Research problem and purpose
   a. Is the problem significant for nursing (Gallagher-Ford et al., 2020; Meadows-Oliver, 2019)?
   b. Does the purpose fit the research problem (Leedy & Ormond, 2019)?
2. Review of literature
   a. Is the literature review organized to demonstrate the progressive development of evidence from previous research (Creswell & Creswell, 2018; Leedy & Ormond., 2019)?
   b. Does the summary of the literature review identify what is known and not known about the research problem and provide direction for the formation of the purpose (Grainger, 2021)?
3. Study framework: Philosophical and theoretical foundations
   a. Was the philosophical foundation or theory appropriate for the research design (Creswell & Poth, 2018)?
   b. If a theory guided the study, was it appropriate for the phenomenon of interest and study purpose and used to guide the research questions and data analysis (Creswell, & Poth, 2018; Meadows-Oliver, 2019)?

Continued

⚡ CRITICAL APPRAISAL GUIDELINES—cont'd

4. Research objectives, questions, or hypotheses
   a. Were the objectives and questions expressed clearly and consistent with the study design (Gray & Grove, 2021)?
   b. Were the objectives and questions logically linked to the study results (Leedy & Ormrod, 2019; O'Sullivan & Jefferson, 2020)?
5. Design
   a. Was the design consistent with the philosophical foundation of the study (Creswell & Creswell, 2018; Creswell & Poth, 2018)?
   b. Was the design consistent with the purpose and research question (Leedy & Ormrod, 2019)?
6. Sampling and the researcher–participant relationship
   a. Were the participants' characteristics and life experiences appropriate to the qualitative approach (see Chapter 3)?
   b. Was the number of participants adequate to fulfill the purpose of the study (Creswell & Poth, 2018)?
   c. Were the length and depth of the researcher–participant relationships in the study appropriate to the study approach and study purpose (Seidman, 2019)?
7. Ethical considerations
   a. Were the rights of the study participants protected (see Chapter 4)?
   b. Was the data collection conducted in a safe and private setting (Creswell & Creswell, 2018)?
8. Data collection
   For the data collection methods used in the study, answer the following questions:
   a. Interviews
      (1) Do the interview questions address concerns expressed in the research problem?
      (2) Are the interview questions relevant for the research purpose and objectives or questions?
      (3) Were the interviews adequate in length and number to address the research purpose or answer the research question (see Chapter 3; Seidman, 2019)?
   b. Focus groups
      (1) Were the size, composition, and length of the focus group adequate to promote group interaction and to produce robust data (Creswell & Poth, 2018; Kamberelis et al., 2018)?
      (2) Were questions used during the focus group relevant to the study's research purpose and objectives or questions (Gray & Grove, 2021; Seidman, 2019)?
   c. Observation
      (1) Did the researcher provide details about how much time was spent in observation, including at what times of the day, on which days of the week, and the cumulative amount of time spent (Leedy & Ormrod, 2019)?
      (2) Did the researcher describe how notes were made about the observations, such as were notes made during the observation or after the observation (Creswell & Poth, 2018)?
      (3) Were the observations of adequate length and implemented across days and times to provide rich data related to the study purpose (Leedy & Ormrod, 2019)?
   d. Examining documents and media as data
      (1) Were the documents or media materials created specifically for the study, such as participants' textual responses to a series of open-ended questions on a questionnaire?
      (2) For materials not created for the study, were their authenticity and authorship confirmed, such as policy documents and information on websites (Decker et al., 2021)?
9. Data management, analysis, and interpretation
   a. Were data analysis and interpretation consistent with the philosophical orientation, research problem, methodology, research question, and purpose of the study (Creswell & Poth, 2018; Miles et al., 2020)?
   b. Did the researchers describe how they recorded decisions made during analysis and interpretation, usually in the form of an audit trail (Miles et al., 2020)?
   c. Did the researchers link the codes and themes used with participants' quotes?

? **CRITICAL APPRAISAL GUIDELINES—cont'd**

d. Did the researchers provide adequate description of the data analysis and interpretation processes (Miles et al., 2020)?

10. Results
   a. Were the results presented in a way that was consistent with the qualitative design and philosophy (Creswell & Poth, 2018)?
      (1) Phenomenology—rich description of lived experience
      (2) Grounded theory—theoretical description of social processes
      (3) Ethnography—description of a culture, whether race/ethnic or an organization
      (4) Exploratory-descriptive qualitative research—problem-solving answer to the research question
   b. Were the results supported by participant quotes, specific observations, or analysis of the documents (Miles et al., 2020; O'Sullivan & Jefferson, 2020)?

11. Discussion
   a. Are findings discussed in relation to the objectives or questions?
   b. Are the findings linked to the study framework or philosophical foundation (Smith & Liehr, 2018)?
   c. Are the findings consistent with the findings of previous studies in this area (Creswell & Creswell, 2018)?
   d. Does the study have limitations not identified by the researcher?
   e. Were the identified implications for practice appropriate based on the study findings and the findings from previous research (Melnyk & Fineout-Overholt, 2019)?
   f. Were quality suggestions made for future research?
   g. Do the conclusions fit the findings from this study and previous studies?

Example Critical Appraisal Step 2: Determining Study Strengths and Weaknesses

Begin this step by reviewing the Barton et al. (2021) article and its step 1 critical appraisal. The second step focuses on the strengths and weaknesses of this phenomenological study. Use the questions in the previous section to stimulate your thinking as you write a narrative of the strengths and weaknesses of the study. Like the quantitative example, the intellectual critical appraisal is organized by the components of the study: Introduction, Methods, Results, and Discussion (APA, 2020).

🔍 **CRITICAL APPRAISAL EXAMPLE 12.5**

Introduction

Barton et al. (2021) identified the experiences of fathers as being a significant problem for society because of the increased number of infants being admitted to NICUs. The research problem was significant for nurses who play a key role in supporting and educating the parents of pediatric patients. The studies cited by Barton et al. (2021) were organized to identify the gap in knowledge, because existing studies focused on mothers and had not addressed gender differences in stress and coping. In addition, the few studies describing fathers' experiences were conducted internationally and may not be applicable to the United States. The study purpose was logically linked to the research problem (Leedy & Ormrod, 2019).

Methods

The study was identified as being a descriptive phenomenological design. A single-sentence description of the design was provided, but the report lacked information about the underlying philosophy and the characteristics of the design. The researchers assumed that readers knew the underlying philosophy and how descriptive phenomenology is different from other types of phenomenological designs. Consistent with phenomenology,

Continued

CRITICAL APPRAISAL EXAMPLE 12.5—cont'd

a theoretical perspective was not identified. The fathers were recruited by snowball sampling until data satura-tion was reached. The participants were recruited because of their experiences, which was the phenomenon of interest. The fathers gave consent before data collection began. The interviewer met with each participant one time (Barton et al., 2021). After collecting demographic data, the interviews were guided by four prompts to elicit the fathers' descriptions of their NICU-related experiences. The interviews were adequate in length to address the research purpose (Seidman, 2019). Despite the richness of the themes and quotes, the sample size was small and lacked race/ethnic diversity.

Colaizzi's steps were followed, which were consistent with phenomenology and the study's purpose. The researchers worked independently and collaboratively to identify key statements and themes. Rich thick de-scriptions of the experience were developed for each interview, and each father was given the option to review the researchers' description of his experiences (Morse, 2018).

Results
The sample was diverse in that the fathers represented varying age, different hospitals, a wide range of time since the hospitalization, and single and multiple births. The data analysis resulted in five themes that were labeled by phrases from the fathers' interviews. The presentation of the themes comprised two of the article's five pages, including the depth of results. Each theme was supported by multiple quotes selected to help the reader hear the fathers' voices and understand the range of their experiences. The themes and quotes provided a rich description of the phenomenon (Miles et al., 2020).

Discussion
The findings were consistent with the findings of previous studies in the areas of the stressfulness of the NICU experience, including the environment. Barton et al. (2021) inserted additional quotes from the fathers to support the discussion. The researchers identified the lack of diversity of the sample based on the fathers being English-speaking and heterosexual. They did not note the lack of diversity due to the fathers being mar-ried, employed, primarily white, and having incomes greater than $50,000 per year. Although the varying times since the NICU admission represented a wide range, five of the father's children were three or more years old when they were interviewed. The passage of time since the hospitalization and the effect on the child's growth and development may have allowed the fathers to revise their perspectives. The study limitations also should have included the effect of time on the fathers' memories of the experience, or the article title could have been changed to "Fathers' Memories of NICU Experiences." The recommendations for future studies directly re-lated to the identified limitations but might have also included a recommendation to study the mothers and fathers of the same infants to contrast the gender differences. As appropriate for a qualitative study, the im-plications for practice were cautious and focused on nurses recognizing the fathers' need for support (Barton et al., 2021).

Step 3: Evaluating the Trustworthiness and Meaning of Study Findings

The final step in the critical appraisal of qualitative studies is based on the information that you have identified and the conclusions that can be made from the first two steps of the process. Evaluating the trustworthiness of a study involves determining the credibility, transferability, de-pendability, and confirmability of the study findings. The person conducting the critical appraisal evaluates all aspects of a qualitative study and makes a judgment about its trustworthiness. Trustworthiness is a determination that a qualitative study is rigorous and of high quality (Sawatsky et al., 2019). Trustworthiness is the extent to which a qualitative study is dependable, confirmable, credible, and transferable (Amin et al., 2020). A thorough report of a qualitative study should include adequate information so that the reader can assess the report's dependability and confirmability. Dependability and confirmability are like the reliability criteria of measurement in quantitative studies. Dependability is the documentation of steps taken and decisions made during analysis (Stahl & King, 2020). Recall from Chapter 3 that the researchers' record of the analysis process is called an *audit trail*. Confirmability is the extent to which other researchers can review the audit trail and agree that the authors' conclusions are logical (Amin et al., 2020). In addition, the researchers indicate their position related to the phenomenon of interest, which is described as reflexivity.

When a study's findings are appraised to be confirmable and dependable, they have more credibility. Credibility is the confidence of the reader about the extent to which the researchers have produced results that reflect the views of the participants; this is comparable with internal validity in the critical appraisal of quantitative studies (Amin et al., 2020; Stahl & King, 2020). Qualitative findings that are in-depth may transcend the specific sample and be usable with other similar groups. This ability to transcend the sample and be applicable with similar participants is called transferability (Amin et al., 2020). Although these terms can be defined individually, strategies used by the researchers to enhance the dependability of the findings directly affect the credibility and confirmability of the findings.

📄 RESEARCH/EBP TIP

The findings from a qualitative study are transferable (applicable) when the sample is described thoroughly and the reader has confidence in the credibility, dependability, and confirmability of the findings. Thus these findings have a potential to be used in practice.

❓ CRITICAL APPRAISAL GUIDELINES

Step 3: Evaluating the Trustworthiness and Meaning of Qualitative Study Findings

1. Do the study findings accurately portray the perspectives of the participants (Stahl & King, 2020)?
2. Were standards of qualitative research applied during the study, such as the detail built into the design, carefulness of data collection, and thoroughness of analysis (Creswell & Creswell, 2018; Morse, 2018)?
3. Do the findings from this study build on the findings of previous studies?
4. When the findings are integrated with the findings of previous studies, what is now known and not known about the phenomenon under study?
5. Could the limitations of the study have been corrected?
6. Do you believe the study findings are trustworthy and credible? How much confidence can be placed in the study findings (Gray & Grove, 2021; Meadows-Oliver, 2019)?
7. What is your overall evaluation of the study's quality and contribution to nursing knowledge and practice?

Example Critical Appraisal Step 3: Evaluating the Trustworthiness and Meaning of the Study Findings

---

🔍 CRITICAL APPRAISAL EXAMPLE 12.6

Barton et al. (2021) enhanced the trustworthiness of their findings by providing rich descriptions of each theme with several participant quotes. The article lacked some details about length of the interviews and locations where they were held. The use of Colaizzi's method of data analysis and the collaboration among the team members promoted confirmability (Miles et al., 2020). The findings identified by Barton

Continued

> **CRITICAL APPRAISAL EXAMPLE 12.6—cont'd**
>
> et al. (2021) were congruent with the findings of other researchers that the environment prevented bonding, the experience was frightening and anxiety producing, and parents needed to support each other. Barton et al. (2021) also concurred with previous researchers that healthcare professionals' support, or the lack thereof, was critical to the emotions and coping of the parents. The researchers integrated the interpretation of their findings with the findings of the previous studies. The small number of participants contributed to the limited diversity of the sample and could have been prevented by recruiting additional participants whose infants had been more recently discharged and fathers who had lower incomes.
>
> Barton et al. (2021) made an important contribution to nursing knowledge in that their findings reinforce the significance of the NICU experience in the lives of fathers. Fathers who were interviewed several years after their infants were discharged from the NICU had vivid, emotional-laden descriptions of their experiences that had not faded with the passage of time. Although healthcare systems are structurally and culturally different in various countries, the Barton et al. (2021) study highlighted the common elements of NICU stresses and fathers' needs for education and support.

KEY POINTS

- An intellectual critical appraisal of research requires careful examination of all aspects of a study to judge its strengths, weaknesses, credibility, meaning, and usefulness in practice.
- Research is critically appraised to broaden understanding, improve practice, and provide a background for conducting a study.
- A critical appraisal of research includes the following steps: step 1, identifying the steps of the study; step 2, determining the study's strengths and weaknesses; and step 3, evaluating the credibility and meaning of the study findings.
- Strong quantitative studies are guided by a significant problem; clear, concise purpose; and appropriate objectives, questions, and/or hypotheses. The study framework is clearly expressed and linked to the steps of the study.
- Quantitative studies have rigorous methodology that includes a relevant design with minimal threats to validity.
- Quantitative data are collected using a precise plan that includes reliable and valid scales and accurate and precise physiological measures. Data analyses address the study objective, questions, and/or hypotheses.
- Quantitative studies with credible, meaningful findings have a potential to influence nursing knowledge and practice.
- Rigorous qualitative studies have an explicit philosophical orientation that is congruent with the selected qualitative design.
- Building on that foundation, the researcher implements data collection and analysis methods that enhance the study's trustworthiness.
- Detailed guidelines for conducting critical appraisals of quantitative and qualitative studies are described.
- Example critical appraisals are provided for a quantitative study and a qualitative study.

REFERENCES

Aberson, C. L. (2019). *Applied power analysis for the behavioral sciences* (2nd ed.). Routledge Taylor & Francis.

Agency for Healthcare Research and Quality. (2021). *AHRQ: Funding & grants.* Retrieved from https://www.ahrq.gov/funding/index.html

American Association of Colleges of Nursing. (2021). *The essentials: The core competencies of professional nursing.* Author. Retrieved from https://www.aacnnursing.org/Portals/42/AcademicNursing/pdf/Essentials-2021.pdf

American Nurses Credentialing Center. (2021). *Find a Magnet organization.* Retrieved from https://www.nursingworld.org/organizational-programs/magnet/find-a-magnet-organization/

American Psychological Association. (2020). *Publication manual of the American Psychological Association* (7th ed.).

Amin, M., Nørgaard, L., Cavaco, A., Witry, M., Hillman, L., Cernasev, A., & Dessell, S. (2020). Establishing trustworthiness and authenticity in qualitative pharmacy research. *Research in Social and Administrative Pharmacy, 16*, 1472–1482. https://doi.org/10.1016/j.sapharm.2020.02.005

Babaei, K., Alhani, F., & Khaleghipour, M. (2016). Effect of mother's voice on postoperative pain in pediatric tonsillectomy surgery. *Journal of Pediatric Nursing, 3*(2), 51–56. https://doi.org/10.21859/jpen-03027

Bandalos, D. L. (2018). *Measurement theory and applications for the social sciences.* The Guilford Press.

Barton, N., Hall, C., & Risko, J. (2021). The lived experience of a NICU father: A descriptive phenomenological study. *Journal of Neonatal Nursing, 27*, 206–210. https://doi.org/10.1016/j.jnn.2020.09.003

Bialocerkowski, A., Klupp, N., & Bragge, P. (2010). Research methodology series: How to read and critically appraise a reliability article. *International Journal of Therapy and Rehabilitation, 17*(3), 114–120. https://doi.org/10.12968/ijtr.2010.17.3.46743

Bonar, J. R. M., Wright, S., Yadrich, D. M., Werkowitch, M., Ridder, L., Spaulding, R., & Smith, C. E. (2020). Maintaining intervention fidelity when using technology delivery across studies. *Computers, Informatics, Nursing, 38*(8), 393–401. https://doi.org/10.1097/CIN.0000000000000625

Chinn, P. L., Kramer, M. K., & Sitzman, K. (2022). *Integrated theory and knowledge development in nursing* (11th ed.). Elsevier.

Creswell, J. W., & Creswell, J. D. (2018). *Research design: Qualitative, quantitative, and mixed methods approaches* (5th ed.). Sage.

Creswell, J. W., & Poth, C. N. (2018). *Qualitative inquiry & research design: Choosing among five approaches* (4th ed.). Sage.

Critical Appraisal Skills Programme. (2020). *CASP randomised controlled trial standard checklist.* Retrieved from https://casp-uk.b-cdn.net/wp-content/uploads/2020/10/CASP_RCT_Checklist_PDF_Fillable_Form.pdf

Critical Appraisal Skills Programme. (2021). *CASP checklists.* Retrieved from https://casp-uk.net/casp-tools-checklists/

Dane, F. (2018). *Evaluating research: Methodology for people who need to read research* (2nd ed.). Sage.

Decker, S., Hassard, J., & Rowlinson, M. (2021). Rethinking history and memory in organization studies: The case for historiographical reflexivity. *Human Relations, 74*(8), 1123–1155. https://doi.org/10.1177/0018726720927443

Denzin, N. K., & Lincoln, Y. S. (Eds.). (2018). *The Sage handbook of qualitative research* (5th ed.). Sage.

DeVellis, R. F. (2017). *Scale development: Theory and applications* (4th ed.). Sage.

Dillman, D. A., Smyth, J. D., & Christian, L. M. (2014). *Internet, phone, mail, and mixed-mode surveys: The tailored design methods* (4th ed.). Wiley.

Eymard, A. S., & Altmiller, G. (2016). Teaching nursing students the importance of treatment fidelity in intervention research: Students as interventionists. *Journal of Nursing Education, 55*(5), 288–291. https://doi.org/10.3928/01484834-20160414-09

Gallagher-Ford, L., Thomas, B. K., Connor, L., Sinott, L. T., & Melnyk, B. M. (2020). The effects of an intensive evidence-based educational and skills building program on EBP competency and attributes. *Worldviews on Evidence-Based Nursing, 17*(1), 71–81. https://doi.org/10.1111/wvn.12397

Grainger, A. (2021). Critiquing a published healthcare research paper. *British Journal of Nursing, 30*(6), 354–358. https://doi.org/10.12968/bjon.2021.30.6.354

Gray, J. R., & Grove, S. K. (2021). *The practice of nursing research: Appraisal, synthesis, and generation of evidence* (9th ed.). Elsevier.

Grove, S. K., & Cipher, D. J. (2020). *Statistics for nursing research: A workbook for evidence-based practice* (3rd ed.). Elsevier.

Hall, R. W., & Anand, K. J. (2014). Pain management in newborns. *Clinics in Perinatology 41*(4), 895–924. https://doi.org/10.1016/j.clp.2014.08.010

Jones, E. P., Brennan, E. A., & Davis, A. (2020). Evaluation of literature searching and article selection skills of an evidence-based practice team. *Journal of the Medical Library Association, 108*(3), 487–493. https://doi.org/10.5195/jmla.2020.865

Kamberelis, G., Dimitriadis, G., & Welker, A. (2018). Focus group research and/in figured worlds. In N. K. Denzin & Y. S. Lincoln (Eds.), *The Sage handbook of qualitative research* (5th ed., pp. 671–693). Sage.

Kazdin, A. E. (2017). *Research design in clinical psychology* (5th ed.). Pearson.

Kim, M., Mallory, C., & Valerio, T. (2022). *Statistics for evidence-based practice in nursing* (3rd ed.). Jones & Bartlett Learning.

Leedy, P. D., & Ormrod, J. E. (2019). *Practical research: Planning and design* (12th ed.) Pearson.

Liberati, A., Altman, D. G., Tetzlaff, J., Mulrow, C., Gotzsche, P. C., Ioannidis, J. P.,…Moher, D. (2009). The PRISMA Statement for reporting systematic reviews and meta-analyses of studies that evaluate healthcare interventions: Explanation and elaboration. *Annals of Internal Medicine, 151*(4), W-65-94. https://doi.org/10.1371/journal.pmed.1000100

Meadows-Oliver, M. (2019). Critically appraising qualitative evidence for clinical decision making. In B. M. Melnyk & E. Fineout-Overholt (Eds.), *Evidence-based practice in nursing & healthcare: A guide to best practice*. (2nd ed., pp. 189–218). Wolters Kluwer.

Melnyk, B. M., & Fineout-Overholt, E. (2019). *Evidence-based practice in nursing & healthcare: A guide to best practice* (4th ed.). Wolters Kluwer.

Melnyk, B. M., Zellefrow, C., Tan, A., & Hsieh, A. P. (2020). Differences between Magnet and non-Magnet-designated hospitals in nurses' evidence-based practice knowledge, competencies, mentoring, and culture. *Worldviews on Evidence-Based Nursing, 17*(5), 337–347. https://doi.org/10.1111/wvn.12467

Miles, M., Huberman, A., & Saldaña, J. (2020). *Qualitative data analysis: A methods sourcebook* (4th ed.). Sage.

Moorhead, S., Swanson, E., Johnson, M., & Maas, M. L. (2018). *Nursing outcomes classification (NOC): Measurement of health outcomes* (6th ed.). Elsevier.

Morse, J. M. (2018). Reframing rigor in qualitative inquiry. In N. K. Denzin & Y. S. Lincoln (Eds.). *The Sage handbook of qualitative research* (5th ed., pp. 796–817). Sage.

Munthe-Kaas, H., Glenton, C., Booth, A., Noyes, J., & Lewin, S. (2019). Systematic mapping of existing tools to appraise methodological strengths and limitations of qualitative research: First stage in the development of the CAMELOT tool. *BMC Medical Research Methodology, 19*, 113. https://doi.org/10.1186/s12874-019-0728-6

National Institute of Nursing Research. (2021). *Spotlights on nursing research*. Retrieved from https://www.ninr.nih.gov/researchandfunding/spotlights-on-nursing-research

O'Mathúna, D. P., & Fineout-Overholt, E. (2019). Critically appraising quantitative evidence for clinical decision making. In B. M. Melnyk & E. Fineout-Overholt (Eds.), *Evidence-based practice in nursing & healthcare: A guide to best practice* (4th ed., pp. 124–188). Wolters Kluwer.

O'Sullivan, T., & Jefferson, C. (2020). A review of strategies for enhancing clarity and reader accessibility of qualitative research results. *American Journal of Pharmaceutical Education, 84*(1), 7124. https://doi.org/10.5688/ajpe7124

Quality and Safety Education for Nurses Institute. (2021). *Definitions and Pre-licensure knowledge, skills, and attitudes (KSAs)*. Retrieved from http://qsen.org/competencies/pre-licensure-ksas

Ryan-Wenger, N. A. (2017). Precision, accuracy, and uncertainty of biophysical measurements for clinical research and practice. In C. F. Waltz, O. L. Strickland, & E. R. Lenz (Eds.), *Measurement in nursing and health research* (4th ed., pp. 371–383). Springer.

Sanders, M. R., & Hall, S. L. (2018). Trauma-informed care in the newborn intensive care unit: Promoting safety, security and connectedness. *Journal of Perinatology, 38*(1), 3–10. https://doi.org/10.1038/jp.2017.124

Sarhangi, F., Azarmnejad, E., Javadi, M., Tadrisi, S. D., Rejeh, N., & Vaismoradi, M. (2021). The effect of the mother's heartbeat sound on physiological parameters and pain intensity after blood sampling in neonates in the intensive care unit: A randomized controlled clinical trial. *Journal of Neonatal Nursing, 27*, 123–128. https://doi.org/10.1016/j.jnn.2020.07.006

Sawatsky, A., Ratelle, J., & Beckman, T. (2019). Qualitative research methods in medical education. *Anesthesiology, 131*, 14–22. https://doi.org/10.1097/ALN.0000000000002728

Seidman, I. (2019). *Interviewing as qualitative research: A guide for researchers in education and the social sciences.* Teachers College Press.

Shadish, W. R., Cook, T. D., & Campbell, D. T. (2002). *Experimental and quasi-experimental designs for generalized causal inference.* Rand McNally.

Smith, M. J., & Liehr, P. R. (2018). *Middle range theory for nursing* (4th ed.). Springer.

Stahl, N., & King, J. (2020). Expanding approaches for research: Understanding and using trustworthiness in qualitative research. *Journal of Developmental Education, 44*(1), 26–28.

Straus, S. E., Glasziou, P., Richardson, W. S., & Haynes, R. B. (2019). *Evidence-based medicine: How to practice and teach EBM* (5th ed.). Elsevier.

Todkar, S., Padwal, R., Michaud, A., & Cloutier, L. (2021). Knowledge, perception, and practice of health professionals regarding blood pressure measurement methods: A scoping review. *Journal of Hypertension, 39*(3), 391–399. https://doi.org/10.1097/HJH.0000000000002663

Wakefield, M., Williams, D., Le Menestrel, S., & Flaubert, J. (Eds.). (2021). *The future of nursing 2020-2030: Charting a path to achieve health equity.* National Academies Press. https://doi.org/10.17226/25982

Waltz, C. F., Strickland, O. L., & Lenz, E. R. (2017). *Measurement in nursing and health research* (5th ed.). Springer.

Whelton, P. K., Carey, R. M., Aronow, W. S., Casey, D. E., Collins, K. J., Himmelfarb, C. D.,…Wright, J. W. (2018). 2017 guideline for the prevention, detection, evaluation, and management of high blood pressure in adults: Executive summary: A report of the American College of Cardiology/American Heart Association task force on clinical practice guidelines. *Hypertension, 71*(6), 1269–1324. https://doi.org/10.1161/HYP.0000000000000066

Zimmerman, E., Keunen, K., Norton, M., & Lahav, A. (2013). Weight gain velocity in very low-birth-weight infants: Effects of exposure to biological maternal sounds. *American Journal of Perinatology, 30*(10), 863–870. https://doi.org/10.1055/s-0033-1333669

Building an Evidence-Based Nursing Practice

Susan K. Grove

LEARNING OUTCOMES

After completing this chapter, you should be able to:

1. Describe the benefits and challenges related to evidence-based practice in nursing.
2. Use the PICO format to formulate clinical questions to identify evidence for use in practice.
3. Implement research-based protocols, algorithms, guidelines, and policies in your practice.
4. Critically appraise the following research syntheses commonly published in nursing: systematic reviews, meta-analyses, meta-syntheses, and mixed methods research syntheses.

5. Describe the models used to promote evidence-based practice in nursing.
6. Apply the Iowa Model of Evidence-Based Practice to make changes in healthcare agencies.
7. Apply the Grove Model to implement evidence-based guidelines in your practice.
8. Describe the significance of evidence-based practice centers and translational research in developing evidence-based health care.

Research evidence continues to expand at a rapid rate as numerous quality studies in nursing, medicine, and other healthcare disciplines are conducted and disseminated. These studies are commonly communicated via journal publications, the internet, books, conferences, and social media. The expectations of society and the goals of healthcare systems are the delivery of high-quality, safe, cost-effective health care to patients, families, and communities (Straus et al., 2019). The delivery of quality health care requires the use of the best research evidence available in practice. Healthcare systems are emphasizing the delivery of evidence-based care, and nurses and physicians are focused on developing evidence-based practice (EBP) (Ost et al., 2020). For many years, nursing programs have provided education to encourage students and graduates to base their practice on current research. The emphasis on evidence-based nursing practice in educational programs and clinical agencies has improved outcomes for patients, families, nurses, and healthcare agencies, but there are still many areas for improvement (Bell, 2020; Cullen et al., 2018; Gallagher-Ford et al., 2020).

EBP is an important theme in this text; it was defined in Chapter 1 as the conscientious integration of best research evidence with nurses' clinical expertise and patients' circumstances and values in the delivery of quality, safe, cost-effective health care (Quality and Safety Education for Nurses [QSEN] Institute, 2020; Straus et al., 2019). Best research evidence is produced by the conduct and synthesis of numerous high-quality studies in a selected health-related area. This chapter builds on previous EBP discussions in this textbook to provide you with strategies for implementing the best research evidence in your practice and moving the nursing profession toward EBP.

The benefits and challenges associated with EBP are described to increase your understanding of the complex process for implementing EBP. A format is provided for developing clinical questions to direct your searches for current research evidence to use in practice. Guidelines are provided for critically appraising research syntheses (systematic reviews, meta-analyses, meta-syntheses, and mixed methods research syntheses) to determine the knowledge that is ready for use in practice. Two nursing models that have been developed to facilitate EBP in healthcare agencies are introduced. Expert researchers, clinicians, and consumers—through government agencies, professional organizations, universities, and healthcare agencies—have developed an extensive number of evidence-based guidelines. A framework is provided for reviewing the quality of these guidelines and directing their use in practice. This chapter concludes with a discussion of the nationally designated EBP centers and translational research implemented to facilitate evidence-based health care.

BENEFITS AND CHALLENGES RELATED TO EVIDENCE-BASED NURSING PRACTICE

EBP is a goal for the nursing profession and each practicing nurse (National Institute of Nursing Research [NINR], 2021). Currently, some nursing interventions are evidence based, or supported by the best research knowledge available from research syntheses. However, many nursing interventions require additional research to generate essential knowledge for making changes in practice (Duncombe, 2018; Gallagher-Ford et al., 2020). Some healthcare agencies and administrators are supportive of EBP and provide resources to facilitate this process; however, other agencies and chief nurse executives (CNEs) place EBP as a low priority (Duncombe, 2018; Melnyk et al., 2016; Ost et al., 2020). This section describes important benefits and challenges related to EBP to expand your understanding of EBP and the delivery of evidence-based care to your patients.

Benefits of Evidence-Based Nursing Practice

The most important benefit of EBP is improved outcomes for patients, providers, and healthcare agencies (Gorsuch et al., 2020). Government departments, professional organizations, universities, and healthcare agencies have promoted the synthesis of the best research evidence for thousands of healthcare topics by teams of expert researchers, clinicians, and other professionals. Research synthesis is a summary of relevant studies to determine the empirical knowledge in an area that is critical to the advancement of practice, research, and policy development (Higgins & Thomas, 2020; Melnyk & Fineout-Overholt, 2019). Systematic reviews and meta-analyses are the most common research syntheses conducted to provide support for EBP guidelines. These guidelines identify the best treatment plan or gold standard for patient care in a selected health area to promote quality, safe, cost-effective healthcare outcomes (Moorhead et al., 2018).

Individual studies, research syntheses, and evidence-based guidelines assist students, registered nurses (RNs), educators, and advanced practice nurses (APNs) in promoting EBP. Expert APNs, such as nurse practitioners (NPs), clinical nurse specialists, nurse anesthetists, and nurse midwives, are resources to other nurses and facilitate access to research evidence and the conduct of studies focused on practice problems (Bell, 2020; Hickman et al., 2018).

Some CNEs are highly supportive of EBP as indicated by their attitudes and provision of resources to promote EBP. In a national study of CNEs, Melnyk et al. (2016) found that an organization with an EBP culture of conducting and using research evidence in practice had substantial improvements in several patient outcomes. A healthcare agency with an EBP culture includes:

- Making EBP an agency priority;
- Developing organizational policies for EBP;
- Training nurses in research methods and EBP strategies;
- Designating mentors to promote EBP;
- Improving access to research reports, syntheses, and guidelines;
- Supporting and rewarding EBP activities; and
- Providing official time to conduct research and evidence-based projects (Duncombe, 2018; Mackey & Bassendowski, 2017; Ost et al., 2020; Pintz et al., 2018; Wang et al., 2021; Warren et al., 2016).

Leaders in these healthcare agencies recognize that EBP promotes quality patient outcomes, improves nurses' satisfaction, and facilitates achievement of accreditation requirements. The Joint Commission (2021) standards include accreditation criteria that emphasize patient care quality and safety achieved through EBP.

Many CNEs and healthcare systems are trying either to obtain or to maintain Magnet status, which documents the excellence of nursing care in an agency. Approval for Magnet status is obtained through the American Nurses Credentialing Center (ANCC, 2021b), and national and international healthcare agencies that currently have Magnet status can be viewed online (ANCC, 2021a). The Magnet Recognition Program® recognizes EBP as a way to improve the quality of patient care and revitalize the nursing environment. Magnet status requires that healthcare agencies promote the following research activities: critically appraising and using research evidence in practice and policy development; budgeting for research activities; providing a research infrastructure with the help of consultants; supporting nurses as principal investigators with time and money; educating, training, and mentoring nursing staff in research activities and EBP; and tracking research and other scholarly outcomes (ANCC, 2021a). Pintz and colleagues (2018) conducted a national study of Magnet®-designated hospitals and found these hospitals provided the needed research infrastructure and culture supportive of nursing research and EBP.

The QSEN (2020) project, introduced earlier, was implemented to improve prelicensure nurses' "knowledge, skills, and attitudes (KSAs) that are necessary to continuously improve the quality and safety of the healthcare systems within which they work." QSEN competencies were developed in the following six areas essential for students' and RNs' practice: patient-centered care, teamwork and collaboration, EBP, quality improvement, safety, and informatics. EBP is an important area in your prelicensure education where educators are assisting you in achieving the essential EBP competencies presented in Box 13.1.

📄 **RESEARCH/EBP TIP**

Students and RNs are encouraged to embrace the benefits of EBP by critically appraising research evidence, refining agency protocols and policies based on research, and using evidence-based guidelines in practice.

BOX 13.1   EVIDENCE-BASED COMPETENCIES FOR PRELICENSURE STUDENTS

- Participate effectively in appropriate data collection and other research activities.
- Adhere to institutional review board guidelines.
- Base individualized care plan on patient values, clinical expertise, and evidence.
- Read original research and evidence reports related to area of practice.
- Locate evidence reports related to clinical practice topics and guidelines.
- Participate in structuring the work environment to facilitate the integration of new evidence into standards of practice.
- Question rationale for routine approaches to care that result in less-than-desired outcomes or adverse events.
- Consult with clinical experts before deciding to deviate from evidence-based protocols (QSEN Institute, 2020).

Challenges to Evidence-Based Nursing Practice

The challenges to the EBP movement have been both practical and conceptual. Research evidence is strong in the medical management of diseases but limited regarding the effectiveness of many nursing interventions in managing diseases, preventing illnesses, and promoting health (Moore & Tierney, 2019). EBP requires synthesizing research evidence from randomized controlled trials (RCTs) and other types of interventional studies, but these types of studies are still limited in nursing (Duncombe, 2018; Higgins & Thomas, 2020). A recent review of research evidence in high-impact nursing journals (e.g., *Nursing Research*, *Research in Nursing & Health*, *Western Journal of Nursing Research*, *Journal of Nursing Scholarship*, and *Advances in Nursing Science*) indicate that studies are predominately nonexperimental and less than 30% are experimental and quasi-experimental. Quality RCTs, other experimental studies, and quasi-experimental studies are needed to generate evidence regarding the effectiveness of nursing interventions (Gray & Grove, 2021; NINR, 2021). In addition, systematic reviews and meta-analyses conducted in nursing are limited compared with other disciplines, such as medicine and psychology (Cochrane Collaboration, 2021; Cooper, 2017). The nursing discipline requires additional funding to generate the studies and syntheses needed to improve practice (NINR, 2021).

Another challenge is that research evidence is generated based on population data and then is applied in practice to individual patients. Sometimes it is difficult to transfer research knowledge to individual patients, who respond in unique ways or have unique circumstances and values. More work is needed to promote the use of evidence-based guidelines with individual patients (Weiss et al., 2018). In response to this concern, the National Institutes of Health (NIH, 2021a) are supporting translational research (discussed later in this chapter) to improve the use of research evidence with different patient populations in various settings. Patients who have poor outcomes when managed according to an evidence-based guideline need to be reported and, if possible, their circumstances should be published as a case study. Electronic health records (EHRs) make it more feasible to determine patient outcomes when using EBP guidelines.

As mentioned earlier, some healthcare agencies and administrators do not provide the resources or support necessary for nurses to implement EBP. Such CNEs and agencies have the following challenges: (1) inadequate resources for proving access to research journals, research syntheses, and evidence-based guidelines; (2) inadequate numbers of mentors and mentoring programs for implementing EBP; (3) inadequate nursing staff resulting in heavy workloads; (4) limited authority to change patient care based on research findings; (5) limited support from nursing administrators or medical staff to make evidence-based changes in practice; (6) limited funds to support research projects and research-based changes in practice; and (7) minimal rewards provided to nurses who give evidence-based care to patients and families (Duncombe, 2018; Pintz et al., 2018; Wang et al., 2021; Warren et al., 2016). The success of EBP is determined by all involved, including healthcare agencies, administrators, nurses, physicians, and other healthcare professionals.

Many students and RNs have limited knowledge of the EBP competencies, which requires expansion through educational programs and practice areas (Bell, 2020; Gorsuch et al., 2020; Melnyk et al., 2018). Gallagher-Ford et al. (2020) developed a 5-day intensive EBP education and skills building program to expand nurses' EBP competency and attributes. These researchers found that the nurses' EBP attributes significantly improved and were sustained by the intensive EBP immersion program offered by the Fuld Institute. Wang et al. (2021) studied the effectiveness of having EBP mentors for nurses in six hospitals in China. These researchers found that EBP mentors were essential for nurses to achieve the knowledge and skills needed to obtain competency in EBP. However, the number of EBP mentors was limited in some hospitals, and the mentors lacked the time to educate the nurses in EBP. Melnyk et al. (2020, p. 337) conducted an extensive survey of 2344 nurses to examine "differences between Magnet and non-Magnet designated hospitals in nurses' EBP knowledge, competencies, mentoring, and culture." They found that nurses in the Magnet designated hospitals had higher EBP knowledge, perceived EBP culture, and had greater EBP mentoring than the non-Magnet designated hospitals. However, the nurses in Magnet designated agencies did not meet the EBP competencies.

📄 RESEARCH/EBP TIP

Extensive work has been done to promote EBP in nursing, but additional studies and research syntheses are needed to generate the evidence needed to change practice. In addition, educators and healthcare agencies need to provide nursing students and nurses with the knowledge and skills required to achieve EBP competency to promote quality, safe, cost-effective care.

DEVELOPING CLINICAL QUESTIONS TO GUIDE THE SEARCH FOR RESEARCH EVIDENCE

Developing a clinical question in an area of interest and conducting an extensive search of evidence-based sources is an effective way to identify current evidence for use in practice. The clinical question often is developed using the PICO format, outlined as follows:

P: population or participants of interest in your clinical setting
I: intervention needed for practice
C: comparisons of interventions to determine the best intervention for your practice
O: outcomes needed for practice and ways to measure the outcomes in your practice

The PICO format helps you organize the search for research evidence in a variety of databases, websites, policies, and government documents. You can identify research syntheses (systematic reviews, meta-analyses, meta-syntheses, and mixed methods research syntheses); evidence-based guidelines, protocols, and algorithms; and individual studies through searches of electronic databases, national library sites, and EBP organizations and collections. Some of the key resources for EBP are listed in Table 13.1. At least 2500 new systematic reviews are reported in English and indexed in the Medical Literature Analysis and Retrieval System Online (MEDLINE, 2021) each year. The Cochrane Collaboration (2021), a library of systematic reviews, is an excellent resource with more than 11,000 entries relevant to nursing and health care. In 2009 the Cochrane Nursing Care (CNC) Field was developed to support the conduct, dissemination, and use of systematic reviews in nursing. The CNC Field produces the *Cochrane Corner* columns (summaries of *Cochrane Reviews* relevant to nursing care) that are regularly published in collaborating nursing care–related journals (CNC, 2021). The Joanna Briggs Institute (2021) in Australia provides quality resources for locating and conducting research syntheses in nursing. In addition, the Nursing Reference

TABLE 13.1   EVIDENCE-BASED PRACTICE RESOURCES

RESOURCE	DESCRIPTION
Bibliographic or Electronic Databases	
CINAHL (Cumulative Index to Nursing and Allied Health Literature)	CINAHL is an authoritative resource of the English-language journals for nursing and allied health. The database was developed in the United States and includes sources published from 1982 forward. Within EBSCO, you can search for Evidence-Based Care Sheets.
MEDLINE (PubMed—National Library of Medicine)	MEDLINE is the US National Library of Medicine® (NLM) premier bibliographic database that contains more than 25 million references to journal articles in life sciences with a concentration on biomedicine that dates back to the mid-1960s.
MEDLINE with MeSH	Database provides authoritative medical information on medicine, nursing, dentistry, veterinary medicine, the healthcare system, preclinical services, and more.
PsycINFO	Database was developed by the American Psychological Association and includes professional and academic literature for psychology and related disciplines from 1887 forward.
CANCERLIT	Database of information on cancer developed by the US National Cancer Institute.
National Library Sites	
Cochrane Library	The Cochrane Library provides high-quality evidence to inform people providing and receiving health care and people responsible for research, teaching, funding, and administration of health care at all levels. Included in the Cochrane Library is the Cochrane Collaboration, which has many systematic reviews of research. Cochrane Reviews are available at http://www.cochrane.org/evidence/.
National Library of Health (NLH)	NLH is located in the United Kingdom. You can search for evidence-based sources at http://www.evidence.nhs.uk/.
Evidence-Based Practice Organizations	
Cochrane Nursing Care Network	The Cochrane Collaboration includes 11 different fields, one of which is the Cochrane Nursing Care Field (CNCF), which supports the conduct, dissemination, and use of systematic reviews in nursing, which can be searched at http://cncf.cochrane.org/.
National Institute for Health and Clinical Excellence (NICE)	NICE was organized in the United Kingdom to provide access to the evidence-based guidelines that have been developed. These guidelines can be accessed at https://www.nice.org.uk/.
Joanna Briggs Institute	This international evidence-based organization, originating in Australia, has a search website that includes evidence summaries, systematic reviews, systematic review protocols, evidence-based recommendations for practice, critical appraisal tools, outcomes measures, and consumer information sheets. Membership is required to access many of the resources. Search the Joanna Briggs Institute at http://joannabriggs.org/.

Continued

TABLE 13.1	EVIDENCE-BASED PRACTICE RESOURCES—cont'd
RESOURCE	**DESCRIPTION**
Registered Nurses' Association of Ontario	Nurses, nurse practitioners, and nursing students are members of this organization that was formed to develop and implement evidence-based guidelines for this Canadian territory. These resources are available at https://rnao.ca/.
US Preventive Services Task Force	A panel of national experts was formed, as an independent organization, to develop evidence for preventive care with resources that can be accessed at https://www.uspreventiveservicestaskforce.org/.

Center includes evidence-based care sheets for numerous nursing interventions and clinical conditions (see Table 13.1).

EVIDENCE GUIDING INTRAMUSCULAR INJECTIONS FOR PROPHYLACTIC PURPOSES

The accurate, safe, skillful delivery of intramuscular (IM) injections is a current focus of evidence-based knowledge because individuals worldwide are encouraged to obtain the coronavirus disease 2019 (COVID-19) vaccination (Gordon, 2021; Schnyder et al., 2021). The best research evidence reports the COVID-19 vaccine should be given IM in the deltoid site without aspiration to adolescents and adults (Gordon, 2021; Isseven & Midilli, 2020; Schnyder et al., 2021). In general, immunization rates are lower than desired and continue to be a challenge for healthcare personnel (Gordon, 2021; Strohfus et al., 2017). The clinical question for this evidence-based guideline focuses on: *What site is appropriate, and should aspiration be used in giving IM injections for prophylactic purposes?* The PICO format is used to identify the evidence needed for practice.

P: populations: infants, toddlers, children, adolescents, and adults receiving immunizations by IM route for prophylactic purposes;

I: intervention: prophylactic IM injection given without aspiration in the right site based on the age of the patient (Schnyder et al., 2021; Sisson, 2015; Thomas et al., 2016);

C: comparison intervention: IM injection given with 5 to 10 seconds of aspiration in all sites, regardless of patient age (Cocoman & Murray, 2008; Nicoll & Hesby, 2002); and

O: outcome: IM injection of vaccine safely, accurately, and without complications (Gordon, 2021; Schnyder et al., 2021; Sisson, 2015).

Older evidence-based guidelines by Nicoll and Hesby (2002) and Cocoman and Murray (2008) recommended aspiration for 5 to 10 seconds with each IM injection to prevent injecting substances directly into a patient's bloodstream. However, a systematic review by Sisson (2015) recommended no aspiration with IM injections given in the deltoid, ventrogluteal, and vastus lateralis sites. Nurses should only aspirate when giving IM injections in the dorsogluteal site because of the close proximity of the gluteal artery. However, researchers recommend that the dorsogluteal site not be used for IM injections (Gordon, 2021; Sisson, 2015). Schnyder et al. (2021) conducted a systematic review to compare the equivalence of vaccine doses given by IM versus subcutaneous (SQ) route. These authors found that the immunological response was stronger if the vaccines were accurately given IM rather than SQ. Thus the deltoid site is better for delivering IM vaccinations to ensure the vaccine is delivered in the muscle. The current research evidence regarding site selection and aspiration during IM injections is summarized in Box 13.2. Site selection and

BOX 13.2 CLINICAL PRACTICE GUIDELINE: PROPHYLACTIC INTRAMUSCULAR INJECTIONS WITHOUT ASPIRATION

Patient Population
- Infants, toddlers, children, adolescents, and adults receive immunizations by the IM route for prophylactic purposes.

Objective
- Administer IM immunizations accurately and safely into the appropriate site to ensure delivery into the muscle without patient injury or discomfort.

Intervention: Prophylactic IM Injection of Immunizations
- Site selection is based on the age of the patient (Gordon, 2021; Ogston-Tuck, 2014; Schnyder et al., 2021; Sisson, 2015):
- Infants—vastus lateralis is the preferred site
- Toddlers and children—deltoid or vastus lateralis sites
- Adolescents and adults—deltoid site

Medication volume for immunizations
- Small volumes of medication (≤1 mL) may be given in the deltoid site for toddlers, children, adolescents, and adults and in the vastus lateralis for infants (Gordon, 2021; Schnyder et al., 2021; Sisson, 2015).

Aspiration with Injection
- Cleanse the site with alcohol and allow it to dry.
- Insert the needle into the muscle at the appropriate site (Gordon, 2021; Schnyder et al., 2021).
  - There should be *no aspiration* with deltoid, ventrogluteal, and vastus lateralis sites (Gordon, 2021; Sisson, 2015; Thomas et al., 2016).
  - Aspirate for 5–10 seconds when using the dorsogluteal site because of the proximity to the gluteal artery, but current research recommends not to use this site (Gordon, 2021; Sisson, 2015; Schnyder et al., 2021; Thomas et al., 2016).
  - Inject medication slowly.
  - Withdraw needle slowly; apply gentle pressure with a dry sponge.
  - Cover the site with an adhesive bandage.
  - Safely dispose of the equipment used for the injection.
  - Record the type of immunization and the time and date in the EMR.

Outcome
- Assess site for complications, immediately and 2–4 hours later, if possible.
- Record the number of complications and types of complication, such as pain, redness, and/or warmth, in the EMR.

EMR, Electronic medical record; *IM*, intramuscular.

Adapted from Nicoll, L. H., & Hesby, A. (2002). Intramuscular injections: An integrative research review and guideline for evidence-based practice. *Applied Nursing Research, 16*(2), 149–162. https://doi.org/10.1053/apnr.2002.34142; Gordon, C. (2021). COVID-19 vaccination: Intramuscular injection technique. *British Journal of Nursing, 30*(6), 350–353. https://doi.org/10.12968/bjon.2021.30.6.350; Isseven, S. D., & Midilli, T. S. (2020). A comparison of the dorsogluteal and ventrogluteal sites regarding patients' levels of pain intensity and satisfaction following intramuscular injection. *International Journal of Caring Sciences, 13*(3), 2168–2179; Ogston-Tuck, S. (2014). Intramuscular injection technique: An evidence-based approach. *Nursing Standard, 29*(4), 52–59. https://doi.org/10.7748/ns.29.4.52.e9183; Schnyder, J. L., Garrido, H. M. G., De Pijper, C. A., Daams, J. G., Stijnis, C., Goorhuis, A., & Grobusch, M. P. (2021). Comparison of equivalent fractional vaccine doses delivered by intradermal and intramuscular or subcutaneous routes: A systematic review. *Travel Medicine and Infections Disease, 41*, 102007. https://doi.org/10.1016/j.tmaid.2021.102007; Sisson, H. (2015). Aspirating during the intramuscular injection procedure: A systematic literature review. *Journal of Clinical Nursing, 24*(17/18), 2368–2375. https://doi.org/10.1111/jocn.12824; Thomas, C. M., Mraz, M., & Rajcan, L. (2016). Blood aspiration during IM injection. *Clinical Nursing Research, 25*(5), 549–559. https://doi.org/10.1177/1054773815575074.

aspiration are still important areas for education because Thomas et al. (2016) found that 74% of the nurses were still aspirating after IM injections 90% of the time and were sometimes unsure of site selections for injections.

📄 RESEARCH/EBP TIP

Nursing students and RNs require additional education to ensure they are knowledgeable about and use the best research evidence in practice when giving IM injections for prophylactic purposes.

CRITICALLY APPRAISING SYSTEMATIC REVIEWS AND META-ANALYSES

Nursing students and RNs should be able to review research syntheses and determine the evidence to use in practice. This section provides guidelines for understanding and critically appraising systematic reviews and meta-analyses.

Critically Appraising Systematic Reviews

A systematic review is a structured, comprehensive synthesis of the research literature to determine the best research evidence available to address a healthcare question or problem. A systematic review involves identifying, locating, appraising, and synthesizing quality research evidence for clinicians to use in practice (Chowdhury et al., 2020; Cooper, 2017; Page et al., 2021). Systematic reviews are usually conducted by two or more researchers, expert clinicians, and consumers and include rigorous research methodology to promote the accuracy of the findings and minimize the reviewers' bias. Table 13.2 provides a checklist for critically appraising the steps or elements of systematic reviews and meta-analyses. A systematic review often includes a meta-analysis for a smaller group of similar studies that are focused on examining the effectiveness of an intervention (Higgins & Thomas, 2020).

The steps presented in Table 13.2 are based on the Preferred Reporting Items for Systematic Reviews and Meta-Analyses (PRISMA) statement. The PRISMA statement was developed in 2009 by an international group of expert researchers and clinicians to improve the quality of reporting for systematic reviews and meta-analyses (Liberati et al., 2009). The PRISMA statement was updated in 2020 to replace the "2009 statement and includes new reporting guidance that reflects advances in methods to identify, select, appraise, and synthesize studies" (Page et al., 2021, Introduction section). The PRISMA 2020 statement includes 27 items, which can be found at http://prisma-statement.org and are detailed in the article by Page et al. (2021). These items were consolidated into a 22-item checklist to assist you in critically appraising systematic reviews and meta-analyses.

The systematic review conducted by Chua and Shorey (2021) included a meta-analysis, and both are presented as examples. These researchers focused on the effectiveness of educational interventions in improving nursing students' and RNs' attitudes toward death and the care of dying patients. You can find the Chua and Shorey (2021) article in the online Research Article Library developed to support this text. We recommend that you read this article and use the checklist in Table 13.2 to critically appraise this systematic review and compare your findings with the following discussion.

Step 1: Did the Title Indicate a Systematic Review and/or Meta-Analysis Was Conducted?

Chua and Shorey (2021) clearly identified they had conducted both a systematic review and meta-analysis in the title of their report: "Effectiveness of End-of-Life Educational Interventions

TABLE 13.2 CHECKLIST FOR CRITICALLY APPRAISING SYSTEMATIC REVIEWS AND META-ANALYSES

SYSTEMATIC REVIEW STEPS	STEP COMPLETE? (YES OR NO)	COMMENTS: QUALITY AND RATIONALE
1. Did the title indicate that a systematic review, meta-analysis, or both were conducted?		
2. Was an abstract included that provided a structured summary of objectives, question, eligibility criteria, inclusion of studies, risk of bias, study appraisal and synthesis methods, participants, interventions, outcomes, results, and conclusions?		
Introduction		
3. Was a rationale provided for the review based on existing knowledge? Were the objectives of the review addressed?		
4. Was the clinical question clearly expressed and significant? Was the PICOS format (*p*articipants, *i*ntervention, *c*omparative interventions, *o*utcomes, and *s*tudy design) used to develop the question?		
Methods		
5. Were the literature search criteria clearly identified? Were the years covered, language, and publication status of sources identified in the criteria?		
6. Were the information sources specified, including databases, registers, websites, organizations, reference lists, and other sources?		
7. Was a comprehensive, systematic search strategy conducted using the criteria identified in step 5 and the sources included in step 6? Did the search include published studies, grey literature, etc.?		
8. Was the selection process for studies and other sources identified and consistently implemented? Was the collection of data from the sources addressed?		
9. Were the publication biases addressed, such as time lag bias, location bias, duplicate publication bias, citation bias, and language bias? Reporting bias?		
10. Were the synthesis methods detailed?		
Results		
11. Were the results of study selection described and presented in flow diagram?		
12. Were key elements (population, sampling process, design, intervention, outcomes, and results) of each study clearly discussed and presented in a table?		

Continued

	STEP COMPLETE? (YES OR NO)	COMMENTS: QUALITY AND RATIONALE
TABLE 13.2 CHECKLIST FOR CRITICALLY APPRAISING SYSTEMATIC REVIEWS AND META-ANALYSES—cont'd		
SYSTEMATIC REVIEW STEPS		
13. Was a quality critical appraisal of the studies conducted? Was there confidence in the body of evidence for each outcome?		
14. Was a meta-analysis conducted as part of the systematic review? Were the details of the meta-analysis process and results described?		
15. Were the results of the systematic review or meta-analysis clearly described (i.e., in the narrative and tables)? Were study interventions compared and contrasted in a table? Were the outcome variables clearly identified and the quality of the measurement methods addressed?		
Discussion		
16. Did the report conclude with a clear Discussion section?		
a. Were the review findings summarized to identify the current best research evidence?		
b. Were the limitations of the review and how they might have affected the findings addressed?		
c. Were the implications for practice, policy, and future research addressed?		
Other Information		
17. Did the authors of the review develop a clear, concise, quality report for publication? Was the report inclusive of the items identified in the PRISMA statement in this table?		
18. Was registration information for the review provided?		
19. Was financial or nonfinancial support addressed? Competing interests?		

PRISMA, Preferred Reporting Items for Systematic Reviews and Meta-Analyses.
Adapted from Page, M. J., McKenzie, J. E., Bossuyt, P. M., Boutron, I., Hoffmann, T. C., Mulrow, C. D., . . . Moher, D. (2021). The PRISMA 2020 statement: An updated guideline for reporting systematic reviews. *Systematic Reviews, 10,* 89. https://doi.org/10.1186/s13643-021-01626-4.

at Improving Nurses and Nursing Students' Attitude Toward Death and Care of Dying Patients: A Systematic Review and Meta-Analysis." When the type of synthesis is identified in the title, it is much easier for you to locate these sources when searching the literature.

Step 2: Did the Abstract Include a Structured Summary of the Research Synthesis?

Beller et al. and the PRISMA Group for Abstracts (2013) published guidelines to improve the quality and structure of the abstracts included in systematic reviews and meta-analyses. These abstracts should be clear, concise, and complete and organized by the standard areas of background, methods, results, and discussion. The content to be covered in each of these abstract areas was detailed by Beller et al. (2013). In 2020, Jiancheng et al. (2020) conducted a study to determine whether the reporting quality of systematic review abstracts in nursing journals had improved with the release of the PRISMA for Abstract (PRISMA-A) guidelines. They found that the overall abstract compliance with the PRISMA-A had not significantly improved and remains a weakness in reporting systematic reviews and meta-analyses. Chua and Shorey (2021) included additional sections in their abstract (design, data sources, review methods) that were not part of the PRISMA-A. However, they did provide most of the essential content identified by Beller et al. (2013) in their abstract.

Step 3: Was a Rationale Provided for the Review Including the Review Objectives?

Chua and Shorey (2021) addressed the significance of healthcare professionals managing death and dying patients because more than 50% of people in the United States die in hospitals, nursing homes, or long-term care facilities. The current knowledge (what is known and not known) in the area of a systematic review is followed by the objectives or aims developed to guide the synthesis process (Page et al., 2021). Chua and Shorey (2021) reported that inadequate systematic reviews had been conducted to synthesize evidence about end-of-life education interventions for nurses and nursing students. The following objectives guided their research synthesis: *"Therefore, this review aims to consolidate the available evidence on end-of-life educational interventions with respect to nurses and nursing students' attitude toward death and care of dying patients at immediate post-intervention (primary outcomes) and any follow-up timepoints (secondary outcomes)"* (Chua & Shorey, 2021, Introduction section).

Step 4: Was a Significant Clinical Question Developed to Direct the Research Synthesis?

A systemic review or meta-analysis is best directed by a relevant clinical question that focuses the review process and promotes the development of a quality synthesis of research evidence. Chua and Shorey (2021, Introduction section) stated the following clinical question that was essentially the same as their *aims:* "This review questions how effective end-of-life educational interventions are at improving nurses and nursing students' attitude toward death and care of dying patients at immediate post-intervention and follow-up timepoints."

The PICOS format (*p*articipants or population, *i*ntervention, *c*omparative interventions, *o*utcomes, and *s*tudy design) can be used to clarify the clinical question used to guide a systematic review or meta-analysis. The PICOS format (similar to the PICO format introduced earlier) is included in the PRISMA Statement (Page et al., 2021) and includes the elements presented in Box 13.3. The PICOS format can also be used to present the eligibility criteria that guide the search for relevant studies. Chua and Shorey (2021) used the original PRISMA guidelines

---

BOX 13.3 PICOS FORMAT FOR DIRECTING LITERATURE SEARCHES

P: *Population* or participants of interest (see Chapter 9, sampling)
I: *Intervention* needed for practice (see Chapter 8, discussion of interventions)
C: *Comparisons* of the intervention with control, placebo, standard care, variations of the same intervention, or different therapies (see Chapter 8, discussion of groups)
O: *Outcomes* needed for practice (see Chapter 14, outcomes research, and Chapter 10, measurement methods)
S: *Study design* (see Chapter 8, for study designs)

(Liberati et al., 2009) to guide their combined systematic review and meta-analysis, and the PICOS format to identify the eligibility criteria for their literature search.

Step 5: Were the Literature Search Criteria Clearly Identified?

Reports of systematic reviews and meta-analyses need to identify the inclusion and exclusion eligibility criteria used to direct the literature search (see Table 13.2). As discussed earlier, the PICOS format might be used to develop the search criteria with more detail for each of the elements. These search criteria might focus on the (1) type of research methods, quantitative, outcomes, or mixed methods; (2) population or type of study participants; (3) study designs, such as quasi-experimental and experimental; (4) sampling processes, such as probability or nonprobability sampling methods; (5) intervention and comparison interventions; and (6) specific outcomes measured. The search criteria also need to indicate the years for the review, language, and publication status of the studies to be included (Higgins & Thomas, 2020; Page et al., 2021). Chua and Shorey (2021) clearly, concisely presented their eligibility criteria in PICOS format to direct their literature search.

Population

Nursing students who studied in any educational institution and nurses who worked in any clinical setting, with no restrictions on the number of years of working experience, were included. Healthcare students and professionals of other disciplines were excluded.

Intervention

Any educational intervention with a set curriculum focused on training nurses and nursing students regarding end-of-life issues (bereavement, terminal care, death and dying, and palliative courses) were included.

Comparator

Studies with control groups which did not undergo any intervention, placebo control (undergo educational interventions on non-end-of-life issues), or waitlist control were included.

Outcomes

Included studies must measure either attitude toward death or attitude toward care of dying patients self-reported by participants at pre- and post-intervention. The immediate post-intervention values were of primary focus and follow-up measurements were of secondary interest.

Study Design

Only randomized controlled trials (RCTs), cluster RCTs and controlled clinical trials (CCTs) were included.

Language and Publication Status

Peer-reviewed journal articles and unpublished dissertations that were written in or translated to the English language were included.

(Chua & Shorey, 2020, Methods section)

Step 6: Were Information Sources Identified?

The key search terms, different databases searched, and search results should be recorded in the systematic review and meta-analysis publications. Sometimes authors provide a table that identifies the search terms and criteria. The PRISMA statement recommends presenting the full electronic search strategy used for at least one major database, such as CINAHL or MEDLINE (Jones et al., 2020; Page et al., 2021). The search strategy may be included as an appendix, supplementary file, or be available on request from the primary author.

Often, searches are limited to published sources in common databases, which excludes the grey literature from the research synthesis. Grey literature refers to sources that have limited distribution, such as theses and dissertations; articles in obscure journals; conference proceedings; government publications; and research reports for funding agencies, corporate organizations, and higher education (Woods et al., 2020). Most grey literature is not controlled by commercial publishers, making these sources difficult to access through database searches with limited referencing information. In the past, research syntheses often did not include grey literature that might have resulted in misleading biased results (Navarro et al., 2021; Pappas & Williams, 2011). In 2020, Woods et al. analyzed all citations ($n = 52,116$) from articles published in six of the top nursing journals and found that 10.4% of the citations were of grey literature. Government publications accounted for more than half of the grey literature cited. Thus nursing scholars are seeking out and citing grey literature in their publications.

Step 7: Was a Comprehensive, Systematic Search of the Literature Conducted?

Chua and Shorey (2021) detailed their search strategy for their research synthesis that included an extensive number of databases and other sources. They provided an example of the search strategy applied to Embase database in their supplementary file 1. In addition, they searched ProQuest Dissertations & Theses Global to identify relevant studies not published in journals or online (grey literature). The authors also conducted ancestry searches, which involves the use of citations from relevant studies to identify additional studies. The literature search strategy for this research synthesis is briefly presented in the following excerpt:

> Five electronic databases (PubMed, Embase, CINAHL, PsycINFO and ProQuest Dissertations & Theses Global) were searched from their respective inception dates to November 2020. Relevant reviews and included articles had their reference lists scrutinized and backward searching was conducted to find additional relevant studies. Authors of promising studies with unavailable full-texts were contacted to request full access to the articles. All search results were exported to Endnote Version X8, where they were sorted according to their databases and had their duplicates removed. Titles and abstracts of all studies were screened against the eligibility criteria. Next, full-texts of potential studies were perused to establish their relevance. Study selection was conducted by two independent reviewers who held discussions to resolve any discrepancies.
>
> (Chua & Shorey, 2021, Study selection section)

Step 8: Were the Selection Process for Studies and Collection of Data From the Sources Detailed?

The selection of studies for inclusion in a systematic review or meta-analysis is a complex process that initially involves the review and removal of duplicate sources. The abstracts of the remaining studies are reviewed by two or more authors and sometimes by an external reviewer to ensure that they meet the criteria identified in step 5 (see Table 13.2). The abstracts might be excluded based on the study participants, interventions, outcomes, or design not meeting the search criteria. The data abstracted from the studies also needs to be discussed and often presented in tables

(Page et al., 2021). Chau and Shorey (2021) provided a detailed description of the process they used to select studies and the data obtained from these studies:

> *Characteristics related to the study's sample, design, outcomes measured, intervention content, duration and method of delivery were extracted using a data extraction form. The mean and standard deviation values of the review's outcomes were extracted. When these specific values were not provided, relevant formulas were used to transform the data to obtain the values (Higgins & Green, 2011). Any discrepancies that arose between the two independent reviewers were discussed until consensus was reached.*
>
> *(Chua & Shorey, 2021, Data extraction section)*

Step 9: Were Publication and Reporting Biases Addressed?

Even with rigorous literature searches, authors of meta-analyses and systematic reviews are often limited to mainly published studies. The nature of the sources can lead to biases and inaccurate conclusions in the research synthesis. The common publication biases that can occur in conducting and reporting research syntheses include time lag bias, location bias, duplicate publication bias, citation bias, and language bias. Publication bias occurs because studies with positive results are more likely to be published than studies with negative or inconclusive results. Higgins and Thomas (2020) found that the odds were four times greater that positive study results would be published versus negative results. Time lag bias of studies, a type of publication bias, occurs because studies with negative results are usually published later, sometimes 2 to 3 years later, than studies with positive results. Sometimes, studies with negative results are not published at all, whereas studies with positive results might be published more than once (duplicate publication bias). Location bias of studies can occur if studies are published in lower impact journals and indexed in less searched databases. A citation bias occurs when certain studies are cited more often than others and are more likely to be identified in database searches. Language bias can occur if searches focus just on studies in English when important studies also exist in other languages. Reporting bias might occur if certain results are missing from the synthesis. Chua and Shorey (2021) reduced location, citation, and timeframe biases by searching a variety of databases from their inception dates to November 2020, identifying 17,142 records or possible sources. These sources were reviewed, and 6120 duplicate records (abstracts or articles) were removed. The nine studies selected for synthesis were from six different countries, but only the studies in English were included in the review (language bias). The outcomes (attitude toward death and attitude toward care of dying patients) measurement methods were not described, resulting in reporting bias (Page et al., 2021).

Step 10: Were the Synthesis Methods Detailed?

Authors of systematic reviews provide details of the methods used to synthesize relevant sources. Chua and Shorey (2021, Data synthesis section) reported: "Characteristics of the included studies and the interventions were summarized narratively. Meta-analyses were conducted to pool data for the outcomes."

Step 11: Was the Study Selection Documented?

The Results section of a systematic review identifies the studies that are excluded and the specific number of studies included in the final review. The study selection process is best documented using a flow diagram. Chua and Shorey (2021) documented their selection of studies for their review in Fig. 13.1 and also in the narrative. The flow diagram included the four phases identified in the 2009 PRISMA Statement (Liberati et al., 2009): (1) *identification* of the sources, (2) *screening* of the source, (3) *eligibility* requirements met, and (4) *included* studies. As indicated in Fig. 13.1, nine studies were included in the systematic review. Fig. 13.2 presents the new flow diagram format

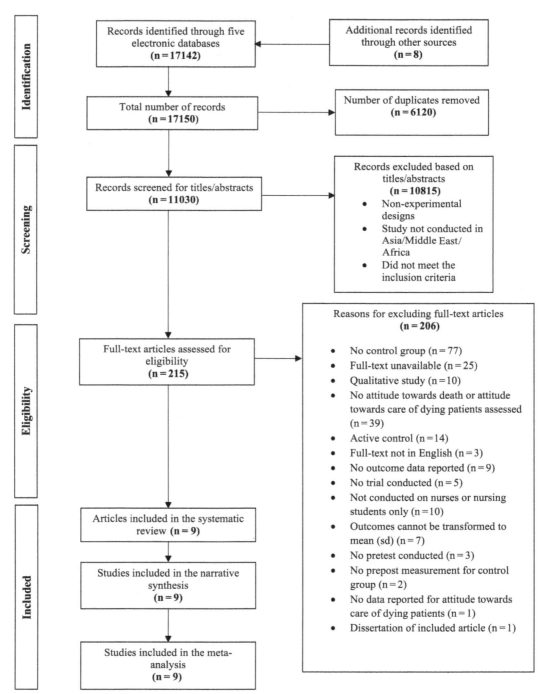

FIG. 13.1 PRISMA Flow Diagram. (From Chua, J. Y. X., & Shorey, S. [2021]. Effectiveness of end-of-life educational interventions at improving nurses and nursing students' attitude toward death and care of dying patients: A systematic review and meta-analysis. *Nurse Education Today, 101,* 104892. https://doi. org/10.1016/j.nedt.2021.104892.)

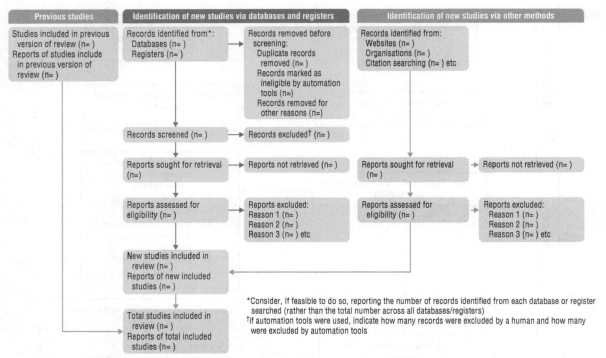

FIG. 13.2 PRISMA 2020 Flow Diagram for Updated Systematic Reviews that Include Searches of Databases, Registers, and Other Sources. (From Page, M. J., McKenzie, J. E., Bossuyt, P. M., Boutron, I., Hoffmann, T. C., Mulrow, C. D.,...Moher, D. [2021]. The PRISMA 2020 statement: An updated guideline for reporting systematic reviews. *Systematic Reviews, 10*, 89. https://doi.org/10.1186/s13643-021-01626-4.)

for systematic reviews included in the Page et al. (2021) article on the PRISMA 2020 statement. You can expect to see this format in future systematic reviews and meta-analyses publications.

Step 12: Were Key Elements of the Studies Presented?

Key elements of studies in systematic reviews and meta-analyses are best identified by constructing a table describing the characteristics of the included studies, such as the purposes of the studies, populations, sampling processes, interventions, outcomes, and results (Cooper, 2017; Page et al., 2021). Chua and Shorey (2021) developed a table to document key information from the nine studies they reviewed. The table summarized the study characteristics, such as authors, year of publication, country where the study was published, research design, number of participants and their age, intervention duration, and review of outcomes. Five of the studies were RCTs, and three studies were controlled clinical trials.

Step 13: Were the Studies Critically Appraised and the Risks for Biases Described?

Two or more experts need to review the studies independently and make judgments about their quality. The critical appraisal of the studies is often difficult because of the differences in types of participant, design, sampling method, intervention, outcome variable and measurement method, and presentation of result. The studies are examined for risks of methodological and outcome reporting biases. Methodological bias is often related to design and data analysis problems in studies. For example, studies might have limitations related to the sample, intervention, outcome measurements, and analysis techniques that result in methodological bias. Outcome reporting bias occurs when study results are not reported clearly and with complete accuracy. For example, reporting bias occurs when researchers selectively report positive results and not negative results, or positive results might be addressed in detail, with limited discussion of negative results. Following critical appraisal, the studies are often rank ordered based on their quality and contribution to the development of the review (Page et al., 2021). Chua and Shorey (2021) provided a clear, concise discussion of the quality appraisal conducted on the studies in their synthesis. The appraisal tools used were described, and the risks for methodological and outcomes reporting biases were identified.

> The Cochrane Risk of Bias tool was used to assess five types of biases for all studies: selection bias, performance bias, detection bias, attrition bias, and reporting bias (Higgins & Green, 2011). Each study's overall bias rating was determined by the worst score it received for any domain. …

> Quality appraisal of the body of evidence at the outcome level was determined by the Grades of Recommendation, Assessment, Development, and Evaluation (GRADE) approach. Each outcome was initially accorded high quality and this rating was dropped to moderate, low or very low. … The online GRADEpro software was used to rate each review's outcome separately. … Any discrepancies were resolved by holding discussions between the reviewers. … Inter-rater agreement between both reviewers was approximately 98% and the Cohen's kappa value was 0.96. … Both outcomes, attitude toward death and attitude toward care of dying patients, were rated as very low quality.
>
> (Chua & Shorey, 2021, Quality appraisal section)

Step 14: Was a Meta-Analysis Conducted as Part of the Systematic Review?

Some authors conduct a meta-analysis as a part of the synthesis of sources for their systematic review (Page et al., 2021). Because a meta-analysis involves the use of statistics to summarize results of different studies, it usually provides strong, objective information about the effectiveness of an intervention or solid knowledge about a clinical problem (Bertolaccini & Spaggiari, 2020; Ruppar, 2020). Chua and Shorey (2021) did include a meta-analysis as part of their synthesis report that is discussed in the following Critically Appraising Meta-analyses section.

Step 15: Were the Results of the Review Clearly Presented?

The results of a systematic review and meta-analysis should include a description of the study participants, types of intervention implemented in the studies, outcomes measured, and measurement methods. The results of the different types of interventions might be best summarized in a table that includes (1) study source; (2) structure of the intervention (stand-alone or multifaceted); (3) specific type of intervention (e.g., physiological treatment, education, counseling, behavioral therapy); (4) delivery method (e.g., demonstration and return demonstration, verbal, video, self-administered); (5) length of time the intervention is implemented; and (6) statistical differences between the intervention and control, standard care, placebo, or alternative intervention groups (Page et al., 2021).

The systematic review by Chua and Shorey (2021) focused on an end-of-life educational intervention. The duration of the interventions was presented in table format and varied greatly from one study to another. The educational sessions ranged from 50 to 90 minutes in length, and the number of sessions ranged from 5 to 13 per study over 3 to 16 weeks. The content of the educational interventions in the different studies was not addressed. The interventions were an area of methodological and reporting bias in this research synthesis.

In systematic reviews, the outcomes, including primary and secondary outcomes, are best summarized in a table. This table might include (1) the study source; (2) outcome variable(s), with an indication as to whether it was a primary or secondary outcome in the study; (3) measurement method used for each study outcome variable; and (4) quality of the measurement methods, such as the reliability and validity of a scale or the precision and accuracy of a physiological measure. The outcomes examined by Chua and Shorey (2021) were attitude toward death and attitude toward care of dying patients. Only one study measured both outcomes, and three studies included follow-up measurements of the outcomes. The instruments used to measure the two outcomes were not identified, and no discussion of reliability or validity was provided. As discussed earlier, the outcomes, attitude toward death and attitude toward care of dying patients, were rated very low quality by the GRADE approach. The varied educational interventions and questionable measurement methods caused the researchers to state "there is very little confidence in the effect estimated in this review" (Chua & Shorey, 2021, Limitations section).

Step 16: Did the Report Conclude With a Clear Discussion Section?

In a systematic review or meta-analysis, the discussion of the findings includes an overall evaluation of the interventions implemented and the outcomes measured. The limitations of the review also need to be addressed. Finally, the Discussion section needs to provide conclusions and recommendations for practice, policies, and future research (Higgins & Thomas, 2020; Page et al., 2021). Chua and Shorey (2021) provided a discussion of their findings, limitations, and implications for practice and further research. Overall, the end-of-life educational interventions did improve nurses and nursing students' attitudes toward death and caring for dying patients. However, the serious risks for methodological and outcomes reporting biases led the authors to make several recommendations for further research with few implications for practice. The following excerpt provides conclusions for the Chua and Shorey (2021) research synthesis.

Conclusion

This review showed that end-of-life educational interventions are able to improve nurses and nursing students' attitude toward death and care of dying patients at immediate post-intervention. Sustainability of this improvement at any follow-up timepoint could not be determined due [to] insufficient data and thus warrant future investigation. Improving nurses and nursing students' attitude toward death is challenging. [H]ence interventions are recommended to be longer than 2 months and include spiritual components. Future trials should promote combined learning sessions for nurses and nursing students, as well as group-based and online segments to improve participants' learning experience. Grief management is another critical topic that should be discussed. Moreover, future research would be required to examine how an improvement in attitude toward death and care of dying patients among nurses and nursing students is translated into clinical practice. Lastly, due to this review's limitations and uncertainties, future research is needed to corroborate current findings.

(Chua & Shorey, 2021, Conclusion section)

Step 17: Was a Clear, Concise Report Developed for Publication?

A systematic review report needs to include the content discussed previously using the PRISMA 2020 Statement (Page et al., 2021). When critically appraising a systematic review, you can use

Table 13.2 to indicate if the step is present, and comment about its quality with supporting rationale. In summary, Chua and Shorey (2021) conducted a quality systematic review following the PRISMA guidelines for publication. The title clearly indicated the type of synthesis conducted, and the PICOS format was used to present the eligibility search criteria. A knowledge gap was identified for nursing practice, and the aim of the review focused on this area. The selection of studies for the synthesis was clearly presented in a flow diagram and documented with rationale. The studies selected for the systematic review were critically appraised, and the results from these syntheses were presented in tables and narrative. The publication concluded with appropriate findings, limitations, and detailed recommendations for further research. However, the studies were of such poor quality, the systematic review provided limited knowledge for practice.

Step 18: Was Registration Information for the Review Provided?

The protocol and review should be registered with information about the registered name and number documented in the publication. Chua and Shorey (2021, Methods section) reported: "A protocol can be found on the PROSPERO website (CRD42021224121)."

Step 19: Were Funding and Competing Interests Addressed?

Chua and Shorey (2021) reported they received no funding from public, commercial, or not-for-profit agencies. They also declared they had no conflict of interest.

📄 **RESEARCH/EBP TIP**

A quality systematic review includes a transparent, complete, and accurate account of why the review was conducted, what was done, and what was found. Systematic reviews should follow the PRISMA 2020 statement guidelines (Page et al., 2021).

Critically Appraising Meta-Analyses

A meta-analysis is conducted to pool or combine statistically the results from previous studies into a single quantitative analysis that provides one of the highest levels of evidence (Cooper, 2017; Page et al., 2021; Ruppar, 2020). Meta-analyses are usually conducted with a small number of studies (5–15) to determine the effectiveness of particular interventions but are also conducted to determine the strength of relationships among study variables or concepts (Bertolaccini & Spaggiari, 2020). This objective analysis technique is conducted to determine the overall mean effect of an intervention while examining the influences of variations in the studies, such as design, intervention, outcomes, and measurement methods. Heterogeneity in the studies included in a meta-analysis can lead to different types of methodological and outcome reporting bias (previously discussed). Meta-analyses that include more homogeneous (similar) studies have less bias and usually provide more valid findings (Cooper, 2017). However, Ruppar (2020) provides direction for synthesizing studies with heterogeneity to improve the meta-analysis outcomes.

Statistically combining data from several studies results in a large sample size, with increased power to determine the true effect of an intervention. The ultimate goal of a meta-analysis is to determine whether an intervention (1) significantly improves outcomes, (2) has minimal or no effect on outcomes, or (3) increases the risk for adverse events. Meta-analysis is also an effective way to resolve conflicting study findings and controversies that have arisen related to a particular intervention (Higgins & Thomas, 2020).

Strong evidence for using an intervention in practice can be generated from a meta-analysis of quality studies, such as RCTs and other experimental studies. However, the conduct of a meta-analysis depends on the accuracy, clarity, and completeness of information presented in studies. Box 13.4 provides a list of information that needs to be included in a research report to facilitate the conduct of a meta-analysis (Ruppar, 2020). You might use this information as a checklist to determine whether the reports of RCTs and other interventional studies are complete.

The steps for critically appraising a meta-analysis are similar to those for critically appraising a systematic review (see Table 13.2). The PRISMA 2020 statement (Page et al., 2021), Cochrane Collaboration guidelines for meta-analysis (Higgins & Thomas, 2020), and other resources (Bertolaccini & Spaggiari, 2020; Cooper, 2017; Ruppar, 2020) were used in critically appraising the meta-analysis from the Chau and Shorey (2021) study. Many of the steps related to the meta-analysis were discussed previously in the systematic review section; thus only a brief discussion is presented here with emphasis on the statistical results and findings from the meta-analysis.

BOX 13.4   RECOMMENDED REPORTING BY RESEARCHERS TO FACILITATE THE CONDUCT OF META-ANALYSES

Demographic Variables Relevant to Population Studied
- Age
- Gender
- Marital status
- Ethnicity
- Education
- Socioeconomic status

Methodological Characteristics
- Sample size (experimental and control groups)
- Type of sampling method
- Sampling refusal rate and attrition rate
- Sample characteristics
- Research design
- Groups included in study—experimental, control, comparison, placebo groups
- Intervention protocol and fidelity discussion
- Data collection techniques
- Outcome measurements
  - Reliability and validity of instruments
  - Precision and accuracy of physiological measures

Data Analysis
- Names of statistical tests
- Sample size for each statistical test
- Degrees of freedom for each statistical test
- Exact value of each statistical test
- Exact p value for each test statistic
- One-tailed or two-tailed statistical test
- Measures of central tendency (mean, median, and mode)
- Measures of dispersion (range, standard deviation)
- Post hoc test values for ANOVA (analysis of variance) test of three or more groups

Clinical Question Directing a Meta-Analysis

The clinical question developed for a meta-analysis is usually clearly focused: "What is the effectiveness of a selected intervention?" The PICOS format discussed earlier might be used to generate the clinical question (see Box 13.3).

Objectives and Questions to Direct a Meta-Analysis

Researchers need to identify the specific objectives used to guide their meta-analysis.

Search Criteria and Strategies for Meta-Analyses

The search criteria are usually more narrowly focused for a meta-analysis than a systematic review to identify the specific studies examining the effect of a particular intervention. For example, Chua and Shorey (2021) selected five studies for conducting meta-analyses to examine the attitudes of nurses and students toward death and another five studies for attitude toward care of dying patients postintervention. Only one study was included in both meta-analyses because it measured both outcome variables.

Possible Biases for Meta-Analyses

Publication, methodological, and outcome reporting biases (discussed earlier) can weaken the validity of the findings from meta-analyses (Bertolaccini & Spaggiari, 2020; Higgins & Thomas, 2020; Ruppar, 2020). An analysis method termed the *funnel plot* can be used to assess for biases in a group of studies. This discussion of funnel plots is brief but will hopefully provide you with some understanding of the funnel plot diagrams included in most meta-analyses. Funnel plots provide graphic representations of possible effect sizes (ESs) for interventions in selected studies (see Chapter 9 for the calculation of ES; Kim et al., 2022). The ES, or strength of an intervention in a study, can be calculated by determining the difference between the experimental and control groups for the outcome variable. The mean difference between the experimental and control groups for several studies is easier to determine when the outcome variable is measured by the same scale or instrument in each study. However, the standardized mean difference (SMD) must be calculated in a meta-analysis when the same outcome, such as depression, is measured by different scales or methods. More details on SMD are provided later in this section.

Fig. 13.3 shows a hypothetical funnel plot of the *SMDs* from 13 studies. The studies with small sample sizes are toward the bottom of the graph, and the studies with larger samples are toward the top. The *SMDs* from the studies are fairly symmetrical or are equally divided by the line through the middle of the funnel in the graph. A symmetrical funnel plot indicates limited publication bias. Asymmetry of the funnel plot is mainly the result of publication bias but also of methodological bias, outcome reporting bias, heterogeneity in the studies' sample sizes and interventions, and chance (Higgins & Thomas, 2020; Ruppar, 2020). Chua and Shorey (2020) did not provide a funnel plot in their research synthesis.

Results of Meta-Analysis

Many nursing studies examine continuous outcomes or outcomes that are measured by methods that produced interval- or ratio-level data. For example, physiological measures to examine blood pressure (BP) produce ratio-level data. Likert scales, such as the Center for Epidemiologic Studies Depression Scale, produce interval-level data (see Chapter 10 for a copy of the Center for Epidemiologic Studies Depression Scale). Therefore BP and depression are continuous outcomes. The effect of an intervention on a continuous outcome in a meta-analysis is determined by the mean difference between two groups. The mean difference is a standard statistic that identifies the

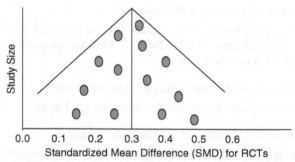

FIG. 13.3 Funnel Plot of Standardized Mean Differences for Hypothetical Randomized Controlled Trials (Rcts) With Limited Bias.

absolute difference between two groups. It is an estimate of the amount of change caused by the intervention (e.g., end-of-life education) on the outcomes (e.g., attitude toward death and toward care of dying patients), on average, compared with the control group. The mean difference is reported in a meta-analysis to identify the effect of an intervention but is appropriate only if the outcome is measured by the same scale in all of the studies (Higgins & Thomas, 2020).

A *SMD*, or *d*, is a summary statistic that is reported in a meta-analysis when the same outcome is measured by different scales or methods. The *SMD* is sometimes referred to as the standardized mean ES. Chua and Shorey (2021) provided no discussion of the scales used to measure the outcomes (attitudes toward death and care of dying patients). Studies that have differences in means in the same proportion to the standard deviations have the same *SMD* (*d*), regardless of the scales used to measure the outcome variable. Statistical software can be used to calculate the *SMD*. The differences in the means and standard deviations in the studies in the meta-analysis are assumed to be the result of the measurement scales and not variability in the outcome (Cooper, 2017; Ruppar, 2020). The meta-analysis results for Chua and Shorey (2021) are presented in the following excerpt:

Attitude Toward Death

The meta-analysis conducted for the five studies that assessed attitude toward death at immediate post-intervention...showed a statistically non-significant small effect favoring the intervention group (SMD = 0.25, 95% CI [confidence interval]: −0.02 to 0.53, Z = 1.79, p = 0.07). ...

Attitude Toward Care of Dying Patients

The meta-analysis conducted for the five studies that assessed attitude toward care of dying patients at immediate post-intervention...showed a statistically significant small effect favoring the intervention group (SMD = 0.46, 95% CI: 0.09 to 0.83, Z = 2.41, p = 0.02).

(Chua & Shorey, 2021, Results section)

Discussion of Meta-Analysis Findings

The findings for the systematic review for Chau and Shorey (2021) were described previously, so the following excerpt focuses only on the findings from the two meta-analyses.

This meta-analysis examined the effectiveness of end-of-life educational interventions in improving nurses and nursing students' attitude toward death and care of dying patients and results suggest that they are effective in doing so. ... Current results suggest that end-of-life educational interventions are more effective in improving nurses and nursing students' attitude toward care of dying patients compared to their attitude toward death. The effect size of the attitude toward care of dying patients was greater than that of the attitude toward death and also showed statistical significance, unlike that of the attitude toward death.

(Chua & Shorey, 2021, Results section)

In summary, the studies included in the meta-analyses had increased risk of biases, varied interventions, and outcomes rated as very low quality. Therefore Chua and Shorey (2021) reported there was very limited confidence in the effects estimated by the meta-analyses. The findings from this synthesis are not ready for use in practice, and many areas were identified for further research (see the Discussion section of systematic review).

📄 **RESEARCH/EBP TIP**

A meta-analysis including an adequate number (5–10) of quality studies (e.g., RCTs) provides the strongest evidence for determining the effectiveness of a nursing intervention in practice. The conduct of meta-analyses is essential for generating evidence to build an EBP in nursing.

CRITICALLY APPRAISING META-SYNTHESES OF QUALITATIVE RESEARCH

Qualitative research synthesis is the process and product of systematically reviewing and formally interpreting and integrating the findings from qualitative studies (Bergdahl, 2019; France et al., 2019; Munn et al., 2019). Various synthesis methods for qualitative research have appeared in the literature, such as meta-synthesis, meta-ethnography, meta-aggregation, qualitative meta-summary, and qualitative systematic review (Bergdahl, 2019; Butler et al., 2016; France et al., 2019; Munn et al., 2019). Qualitative researchers disagree about the best method to use for synthesizing qualitative studies or whether a single synthesis method would suffice. Although the methodology is not standardized for qualitative research synthesis, researchers recognize the importance of summarizing qualitative findings to generate important knowledge for practice and policy development (Bergdahl, 2019; France et al., 2019). Within the Cochrane Collaboration, the Cochrane Qualitative Methods Group has been formed for the discussion and development of synthesis methodology in the area of qualitative research (Higgins & Thomas, 2020).

In the literature, many of the syntheses of qualitative research are identified as a meta-synthesis. Methodological articles have been published to describe the process for conducting a meta-synthesis, but this synthesis process is still evolving (Butler et al., 2016; France et al., 2019). However, meta-ethnography has growing acceptance as a quality methodology for promoting the completeness and clarity in the reporting of qualitative syntheses (France et al., 2019; Munn et al., 2019). The term meta-synthesis is used in this text and is defined as the systematic compilation, integration, and translation of qualitative study results using different conceptual views to consolidate knowledge of fundamental importance to nursing (Bergdahl, 2019). Therefore the focus is on interpretation rather than the combining of study results as with quantitative research synthesis. Meta-synthesis involves the breaking down of findings from different studies to discover essential features and then the combining of these ideas into a unique, transformed whole. According to Sandelowski and Barroso (2007), a meta-summary is a step in conducting meta-synthesis that involves summarizing findings across qualitative reports to identify knowledge in a selected area. Meta-summary is similar to meta-aggregation in summarizing qualitative research findings and is not comprehensive enough to use in synthesizing knowledge to advance nursing science

(Bergdahl, 2019). Tong et al. (2012) developed the Enhancing Transparency in Reporting the Synthesis of Qualitative Research (ENTREQ) Statement that has been appearing in the literature with selected meta-syntheses (Munn et al., 2019). Merging ideas from different sources, the questions in the following Critical Appraisal Guidelines box were developed to guide students and RNs in critically appraising meta-syntheses. Tanganhito and colleagues (2020) conducted a qualitative evidence synthesis focused on the breastfeeding experiences and perspectives of women with postnatal depression (PND). This synthesis was developed using ENTREQ and is presented as an example to guide you in critically appraising qualitative research syntheses. This meta-synthesis is available in the online Research Article Library.

？ CRITICAL APPRAISAL GUIDELINES

Critically Appraising Meta-Syntheses

A. **Introducing and Focusing the Meta-Synthesis**
1. Did the title of the report identify it as a meta-synthesis?
2. Did the abstract include the aim or clinical question addressed, literature search process, methodology for synthesizing qualitative studies, results, and conclusions?
3. Did the authors clearly identify the aim or objective of their meta-synthesis?
4. Was the meta-synthesis framed to clarify its focus and scope, making it manageable?
5. Did the authors provide a rational for conducting a meta-synthesis?

B. **Searching the Literature and Selecting Sources**
6. Did the authors conduct a systematic and comprehensive search for and retrieval of qualitative studies in the target area of the synthesis? Who conducted the search?
7. Was the process for selecting studies for the meta-synthesis detailed?

C. **Critical Appraisal of Studies and Results**
8. Was the process for critically appraising the studies described? Who conducted the critical appraisal of the qualitative studies?
9. Was the analysis of the qualitative studies' findings detailed and the results clearly presented?

D. **Discussion of Meta-Synthesis Findings and Conclusions**
10. Did the authors clearly discuss the interpretation of the findings from the qualitative studies?
11. Were the findings from the meta-synthesis clearly presented, including the themes identified and/or a model or map of the overall findings?
12. Were the conclusions from the meta-synthesis clearly and concisely presented?
13. Was the meta-synthesis report complete and concise? (Bergdahl, 2019; Butler et al., 2016; France et al., 2019; Higgins & Thomas, 2020; Lewin et al., 2018; Munn et al., 2019; Tong et al., 2012)
14. Was the meta-synthesis registered through a national or international organization and documented in the report?

Introducing and Focusing the Meta-Synthesis

In their title, Tanganhito et al. (2020) reported a qualitative evidence synthesis was conducted but did not call it a meta-synthesis. The researchers provided a quality abstract of their synthesis that included Background, Aim, Method, Findings, and Conclusion sections. A qualitative research synthesis needs to be focused by a clearly stated aim. The aim of the qualitative research synthesis is usually an important area of interest for the individuals conducting it and a topic with an adequate body of qualitative studies. In addition, the aim should focus on the identified gap in the knowledge base. The scope of a meta-synthesis is an area of debate, with some qualitative researchers recommending a narrow, precise approach and others recommending a broader, more inclusive approach. However, researchers recognize that focusing is essential for making the synthesis process manageable and the findings meaningful and potentially transferable to practice. Most authors develop research questions or objectives to focus their qualitative research synthesis (Butler et al., 2016; France et al., 2017; Lewin et al., 2018). The background, aim, and review questions for the qualitative synthesis by Tanganhito et al. (2020) are presented in the following excerpt:

Background

Studies show that postnatal depression affects around 10–16% of women globally. It is associated with earlier cessation of breast feeding, which can negatively impact infants' long-term development. Mechanisms underpinning associations between mental health and women's decision to commence and continue to breastfeed are complex and poorly understood.

(Tanganhito et al., 2020, p. 231)

Aim

This review aimed to synthesize evidence from qualitative studies considering the breastfeeding experiences, perspectives, and support needs of women with PND. The review aimed to explore reasons for initiation, continuation, and early cessation of breastfeeding among these women. A search of Cochrane Library and PROSPERO found no current or planned reviews on this topic.

(Tanganhito et al., 2020, p. 231–232)

Method

The review was developed in line with "Enhancing transparency in reporting the synthesis of qualitative research (ENTREQ)" guidelines. It was registered on the PROSPERO international prospective register of systematic reviews (PROSPERO 2018 CRD42018090841). Two primary and one secondary review questions were developed to support identification of the available evidence.

Primary questions

What are the experiences and perspectives of breastfeeding among women with postnatal depression? What are the breastfeeding support and advice needs of women with postnatal depression?

Secondary question

What are the factors affecting decisions to initiate, continue or stop breastfeeding among women with postnatal depression?

(Tanganhito et al., 2020, p. 232)

Searching the Literature and Selecting Sources

Most authors agree that a rigorous search of the literature needs to be conducted. The search needs to include databases, books and book chapters, full reports of theses and dissertations, and conference reports. Researchers often document the specific search strategies they conducted to locate relevant qualitative studies for their synthesis. The search criteria need to be detailed in the synthesis report, and the years of the search, keywords searched, and language of the sources need to be discussed. Meta-syntheses are usually limited to qualitative studies only and do not include mixed methods studies. Also, qualitative findings that have not been analyzed or interpreted, such as unanalyzed quotes, field notes, case histories, stories, and poems, are usually excluded (Butler et al., 2016; France et al., 2019; Higgins & Thomas, 2020). The search process is usually very fluid, with the conduct of additional computerized and hand searches to identify more studies and grey literature (Navarro et al., 2021).

Tanganhito et al. (2020) detailed the eligibility criteria for the inclusion of qualitative studies and conducted an extensive literature search for relevant studies. An example of one of their electronic searches is included in their report. The authors Daniela Da Silva Tanganhito (DDST) and Yan-Shing Chang (Y-SC) collaborated to devise the search strategies and to check and revise them as needed. DDST and Y-SC also screened abstracts and full-text articles for the eligibility requirement and inclusion in the synthesis. The combined work of these two authors greatly strengthened this literature review. The following excerpt presented the search criteria, search strategies, and selection of studies for Tanganhito et al. (2020) synthesis.

Eligibility Criteria

Studies published in English from any settings were considered if they presented qualitative primary research centered on the experiences, perspectives, support and advice needs of breastfeeding among women with symptoms of PND. Adhering to the definition of PND provided in the introduction of this review, studies were considered if they included women who had onset of symptoms of depression within one year postpartum, who perceived or self-reported themselves as having postnatal depression, who completed screening tools which indicated they were likely to have symptoms of PND. ...Reviews, grey literature and publications such as policy documents, opinion papers and guidelines in which primary research data were not reported were excluded.

Search Strategy

Searches were conducted in six databases: CINAHL, Maternity and Infant Care, MEDLINE, PsycInfo, Scopus, and Web of Science on 21st January 2018. These searches were updated on 9th July 2018. Reference lists of three relevant reviews and included papers were hand searched for other relevant articles. Initial keywords and index terms included postnatal depression, postpartum depression, perinatal depression, breastfeeding, infant feeding, experience, perspective, view, and need were searched. The initial electronic searches were conducted by DDST who discussed with Y-SC. The results of searches were discussed. The searches were checked and revised by Y-SC. Final agreed searches were then completed on the selected databases by DDST. An example of an electronic search of one selected database is presented in Fig. 1 [see the article]. All publications identified by the search were initially assessed for relevance based on the title by DDST and verified by Y-SC. Following initial assessment, abstracts were screened against inclusion criteria by DDST and a random sample of 20% were independently screened by Y-SC. Papers which were considered to be relevant were retrieved for full texts and independently screened by DDST and Y-SC. Any disagreements were resolved through discussion. Papers were excluded if they did not meet the inclusion criteria described above or answer the review questions.

(Tanganhito et al., 2021, pp. 232–233)

Critical Appraisal of Studies and Results

The critical appraisal process for qualitative research varies among sources. Usually a table is developed as part of the appraisal process, but this is also an area of debate because tables of studies are more often included in syntheses of quantitative studies. The table headings might include (1) authors and year of source, (2) purpose or aim of the synthesis, (3) design, (4) methodological orientation, (5) participants, (6) key findings, and (7) other key content relevant for comparison. This table provides a display of relevant study elements so that a comparative appraisal might be conducted (France et al., 2019; Higgins & Thomas, 2020; Lewin et al., 2018; Munn et al., 2019). The comparative analysis of studies involves examining methodology and findings across studies for similarities and differences. The frequency of similar findings might be recorded. The differences or contradictions in studies need to be resolved, explained, or both. The critical appraisal results in the final selection of studies for inclusion in the meta-synthesis. The selection process is often presented in a flow diagram similar to the one presented in Fig. 13.1 in the discussion of systematic reviews. Varied analysis techniques often are used by the researchers to translate the findings of the different studies into a new or unique description.

Tanganhito et al. (2020) critically appraised their studies and presented their results with assessment scores in a table. They also included a flowchart that documented their selection process for determining the six studies to include in their synthesis. The characteristics of these studies were also concisely presented in a table. The following excerpt from the Tanganhito et al. (2020) study briefly presents the critical appraisal process and results.

Results

Following the initial systematic search, 11560 publications were identified. A total of 9179 remained after removing duplicates. After evaluation of titles, 136 abstracts were screened. Fifteen full texts were retrieved and assessed. ...Reference lists of relevant reviews and selected papers were searched, and one further paper was identified. Quality assessment was undertaken independently by DDST and Y-SC for six included papers. ...Quality assessment scores of these papers are presented in Table 1 [see article] which shows that two of the papers scored 10. The other papers were scored 8 or 9. One common reason for losing a mark was failure to discuss the relationship between the researchers and participants. No further papers were selected following the updated search in July 2018. All six papers were from high-income countries and presented qualitative data relevant to the review questions. ...A summary of study characteristics is shown in Table 2 [see article].

(Tanganhito et al., 2020, p. 233)

Discussion of Meta-Synthesis Findings and Conclusions

A meta-synthesis report includes findings presented in different formats based on the knowledge developed and the perspective of the authors. A synthesis of qualitative studies in one area might result in the discovery of unique or more refined themes explaining the area of synthesis. The findings from a meta-synthesis might be presented in narrative format or graphically presented in a model or map. Authors should also identify the limitations of the meta-synthesis. The report often concludes with recommendations for further research and implications for practice (France et al., 2019; Lewin et al., 2018; Munn et al., 2019).

Tanganhito et al. (2020) identified the themes that evolved from the synthesis and the relevant conclusions from their qualitative synthesis. They also included a discussion of limitations, implications for practice, and recommendations for further research. The findings and conclusions from this study are briefly presented in the following excerpt:

Findings

Five themes were identified: (1) desire to breastfeed and be a "good mother", (2) struggles with breastfeeding, (3) mixed experiences of support from healthcare professionals, (4) importance of practical and social support, (5) support for mental health and breastfeeding. Most women with postnatal depression expressed strong intentions to breastfeed, although some perceived "failure" to breastfeed triggered their mental health problems. Practical and non-judgmental support for their mental health needs and for successful breastfeeding from healthcare professionals, family and friends are needed.

Conclusion

Most women with postnatal depression desired to breastfeed but experienced breastfeeding difficulties that could impact on their mental health. By offering women with postnatal depression tailored and timely support, healthcare professionals could help women minimize breastfeeding problems, which could consequently impact on their mental well-being and ensure they and their infants have opportunity to benefit from the advantages that breastfeeding offers.

(Tanganhito et al., 2020, p. 231)

📄 RESEARCH/EBP TIP

A meta-synthesis is a way to reinterpret, compare, and translate qualitative studies into a consolidated body of knowledge with fundamental importance to nurses in practice.

CRITICALLY APPRAISING MIXED METHODS RESEARCH SYNTHESES

Nurse researchers have increased the conduct of mixed methods studies over the last 15 years, but the quality of these studies continues to be a concern (Beck & Harrison, 2016; Irvine et al., 2020). Many of the nursing mixed methods studies lack the integration of the data and the findings from the quantitative and qualitative components of the study (Irvine et al., 2020; McKenna et al., 2021). The lower quality of these studies makes it difficult for researchers to synthesize study findings to identify knowledge for education, practice, and policy development. The synthesis process for mixed methods studies is an evolving process. Initially, Harden and Thomas (2005) identified this process as mixed methods synthesis. Sandelowski et al. (2012) identified this process as mixed methods-mixed research synthesis that they defined as a form of a systematic review in which the findings from qualitative and quantitative studies are integrated. Higgins and Thomas (2020) referred to this synthesis of quantitative, qualitative, and mixed methods studies as a mixed methods systematic review.

The synthesis of mixed methods studies involves aggregation and configuration. "Research synthesis by aggregation depends on both qualitative and quantitative findings being conceived as potentially addressing the same factors or aspects of a target phenomenon" (Sandelowski et al., 2012, p. 323). Research synthesis by configuration occurs when diverse individual findings or sets of aggregated findings are arranged into a coherent theoretical framework or model. Heyvaert et al. (2013) termed the synthesis of qualitative, quantitative, and mixed methods studies as a mixed methods research synthesis (MMRS). MMRS is the term that is used frequently in the literature and is included in this text. MMRS might include various study designs, such as a variety of types of qualitative research (see Chapter 3; Creswell & Poth, 2018) and descriptive, correlational, and quasi-experimental quantitative studies (see Chapter 2; Creswell & Creswell, 2018; Higgins & Thomas, 2020; Kazdin, 2017).

Conducting MMRS involves implementing a complex synthesis process that includes expertise in synthesizing knowledge from quantitative, qualitative, and mixed methods studies. There are different approaches to synthesizing the findings from studies using different methods, such as separate synthesis and integrated synthesis. Separate synthesis involves synthesizing the findings from quantitative studies separately from qualitative studies and integrating the findings from these two syntheses in the final report. Integrated synthesis is used when quantitative and qualitative research findings are thought to extend, confirm, or refute each other (see Chapter 14; Beck & Harrison, 2016; Creswell & Plano Clark, 2018).

Further work is needed to develop the methodology for conducting MMRS. The steps seem to overlap with the systematic review process described previously, and some researchers use the PRISMA guideline when conducting an MMRS. The critical appraisal process for MMRS is not clearly developed. Therefore the guidelines for critical appraisal of MMRS in this text focuses on the quality of the following basic elements: abstract, aims, clinical question, literature search, critical appraisal of studies, results, findings, and conclusions. These appraisal guidelines are presented in the following box.

? CRITICAL APPRAISAL GUIDELINES
Mixed Methods Research Syntheses

A. **Introduction of the Mixed Methods Research Synthesis (MMRS)**
   1. Did the title identify the type of research synthesis conducted?
   2. Was a clear, concise abstract presented that included the aim of the review, data sources, study selection process, results, findings, and conclusions?
   3. Did the aim and/or clinical question guide the MMRS?

B. **Literature Search Methods and Selection of Sources**
   4. What were the search criteria for identifying quantitative, qualitative, and mixed methods studies?
   5. Were the search strategies detailed enough to identify relevant quantitative, qualitative, and mixed methods studies?
   6. Was a rigorous search of the literature conducted and detailed in the final report?
   7. Was the process for selecting relevant quantitative, qualitative, and mixed methods studies for the synthesis described?

C. **Critical Appraisal of Studies and Results**
   8. Did the authors of the review present a table and narrative that demonstrated a comparative appraisal of how the studies were conducted?
   9. Were critical appraisals of the studies summarized in the final report, and were the results provided?

D. **Findings, Conclusions, and Implications for Practice, Policy, and Research**
   10. Was a clear synthesis of study findings presented? Did this synthesis effectively integrate the findings from quantitative, qualitative, and mixed methods studies?
   11. Were the implications for practice, policy, and research identified and appropriate (Beck & Harrison, 2016; Creswell & Plano Clark, 2018; Heyvaert et al., 2013; Higgins & Thomas, 2020; Irvine et al., 2020)?

Introduction of the Mixed Methods Research Synthesis

An MMRS should include a clearly stated title that identifies the type of synthesis conducted and its focus. The abstract needs to include the aim, process for locating sources, selection of studies for the review, results, findings, and conclusions (Heyvaert et al., 2013; Irvine et al., 2020). The introduction section for an MMRS should include the problem, gap in knowledge, and aim of the synthesis.

The MMRS of Tatar and colleagues (2018, p. 40) is presented as an example and included the following title: "Factors Associated with Human Papillomavirus (HPV) Test Acceptability in Primary Screening for Cervical Cancer: A Mixed Methods Research Synthesis." This title clearly identifies the focus and type of synthesis conducted. The abstract included relevant information but would have been clearer to the reader with specific headings. The investigators thought it important to synthesize research in this area so healthcare providers and others might have the knowledge needed to encourage women to accept HPV testing for cervical cancer. The problem and objective for this MMRS are presented in the following excerpt:

Historically, the mainstay of cervical cancer screening was represented by cytology (i.e., Papanicolaou or Pap test) to screen for cervical cellular abnormalities. In recent years, HPV DNA tests (hereafter HPV test or testing) capable of identifying high-risk HPV types have been developed. Multiple studies have shown that HPV testing is more sensitive than cytology in detecting cervical intraepithelial neoplasia in primary cervical cancer screening (hereafter primary screening). ... Overwhelming evidence suggests that a negative HPV test provides more reassurance to a woman that she is at low-risk for cervical lesions than a Pap test. ... This evidence has led to new recommendations that incorporate HPV testing as a primary screen for cervical cancer in women aged between 30 and 65 years. ...

No synthesis has been carried out to examine what factors' impact (e.g. facilitators, barriers) on HPV test acceptability in primary screening. As new guidelines have been developed and are in the process of being implemented worldwide, we aimed to provide a comprehensive description of psychosocial factors related to HPV testing and to assess their influence on HPV testing acceptability in primary screening for cervical cancer with the ultimate goal to guide interventions to promote screening.

(Tatar et al., 2018, p. 41)

Tatar et al. (2018) identified a significant clinical problem that could be addressed by conducting an MMRS. No previous synthesis had been conducted to examine the factors that could affect HPV testing acceptability. The objective of this synthesis addressed the gap in knowledge to promote primary screening of women for cervical cancer.

Literature Search Methods and Selection of Sources

Tatar et al. (2018) conducted an MMRS using the PRISMA statement to guide the reporting of their synthesis (Moher et al., 2009). Therefore the critical appraisal is similar to the one conducted on the systematic review by Chua and Shorey (2021) with the guidelines presented in Table 13.2. Tatar et al. (2018) provided detailed, relevant literature search criteria and comprehensive search strategies. They also clearly presented the process for selecting relevant quantitative, qualitative, and mixed methods studies for their synthesis. These steps are briefly presented in the following study excerpt:

We searched MEDLINE, Embase, PsycINFO, CINAHL, Global Health and Web of Science for journal articles between January 1, 1980 and October 31, 2017. The search strategy was developed for MEDLINE by our team, validated by an experienced McGill librarian and then adapted for the other databases (Appendix A). The following eligibility criteria were applied: 1) Population: women of all ages for whom primary cervical cancer screening is recommended, 2) Outcome: psychosocial factors related to acceptability of HPV testing in primary screening for cervical cancer, 3) Study design: empirical studies, without restrictions of study methodology, 4) Languages: English or French or German. The selection of references was performed by two researchers (OT and AN).

(Tatar et al., 2018, p. 41)

The study selection flow diagram is presented in a figure [similar to Fig. 13.1 in Chua & Shorey, 2021 study]. *We retained 22 primary studies: 5 of qualitative methodology...15 of quantitative methodology…and 2 in which both methodologies were used. …Seventeen studies originate in high income countries (8-USA, 2-Canada, 5-Europe, and 2 in Australia) and five in low and middle income countries (1-Mexico, 1-El Salvador, 1-China, 1-India, and 1 in Nigeria). In 14 quantitative studies, statistical tests of significance to assess acceptability were reported; these studies were included in the integration phase.*

(Tatar et al., 2018, p. 42)

Critical Appraisal of Studies and Results

Mixed methods synthesis requires data extraction from the different types of studies, and the information is often presented in a comparative table. The headers in the table usually included author and year, objective, design, data collection methods, sampling, participants, data analysis, and results. Data extraction from qualitative studies needs to be addressed as well. The studies need to be critically appraised with a tool to determine potential biases. Tatar et al. (2018) detailed their data extraction process and their critical appraisal of the studies included in their synthesis. Four of the 22 studies selected for synthesis had high risk for bias and were of questionable quality, which could limit the confidence in the findings.

A data extraction sheet was developed in Excel and included author, title, publication date, country, objectives, study design, quantitative data collection and analysis methods, qualitative methodology, qualitative data collection methods and analysis, and number of participants. From qualitative studies, we extracted qualitative raw data without any interpretation or analysis (e.g., quotes). From quantitative studies, we extracted outcomes of acceptability (e.g. proportions, means, odds ratios). …

We performed deductive-inductive qualitative thematic analysis to identify factors related to HPV testing. Deductively, we identified themes based on two frameworks widely used in health behavior research: The Health Belief Model (HBM) (Champion & Skinner, 2008) and the Theory of Planned Behavior (TPB). …Inductively, we developed new themes (i.e., not covered by HBM and TPB) through an iterative process, which consisted of reading the studies (and new themes) multiple times, allowing researchers to assure accurate interpretation of study results. Themes (hereinafter called factors) were further grouped into categories to enable a structured reporting of the results of the qualitative phase. The factors and categories were developed independently by two researchers (OT and ET) and then validated by the research team.

(Tatar et al., 2018, p. 41)

Quality appraisal revealed low risk of bias in 18 studies and high risk of bias in 4 studies. … In the high risk of bias studies, theoretical frameworks were not used, the validity and reliability of the measurement methods were not assessed, no sample size calculations were provided…and few details were provided related to the recruitment procedure and research setting.

(Tatar et al., 2018, p. 42)

Findings, Conclusions, and Implications for Practice, Policy, and Research

Tatar et al. (2018) reported a quality discussion of their MMRS findings. The findings from this synthesis are summarized in Fig. 13.4, which included a framework of the influencing factors on HPV test acceptability. Tatar et al. (2018) also identified the limitations of their synthesis and the

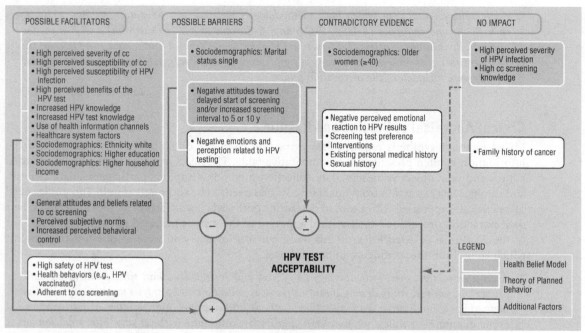

FIG 13.4 Influence of Factors on HPV Test Acceptability. *cc,* Cervical screening; *HPV,* human papillomavirus. (From Tatar, O., Thompson, E., Naz, A., Perez, S., Shapiro, G. K., Wade, K.,...Rosberger, Z. [2018]. Factors associated with human papillomavirus (HPV) test acceptability in primary screening for cervical cancer: A mixed methods research synthesis. *Preventative Medicine, 116*[1], 47.)

need for additional research in this area. They discussed their conclusions that included the implications for practice presented in the following excerpt:

Conclusions

By synthesizing findings of both qualitative and quantitative studies, our review provides a wide perspective related to factors of HPV testing in primary cervical cancer screening. Our results can inform designing interventions to increase primary HPV-based cervical cancer screening uptake in high income countries, but even more so in low and middle income countries where the incidence of cervical cancer is highest and where, as suggested by previous research...implementing a primary HPV testing program could be lifesaving.

(Tatar et al., 2018, p. 49)

📄 RESEARCH/EBP TIP

The MMRS enables findings from quantitative, qualitative, and mixed methods studies to be integrated to identify evidence useful in practice and to provide direction for future research.

MODELS TO PROMOTE EVIDENCE-BASED PRACTICE IN NURSING

EBP is a complex phenomenon that requires integration of the best research evidence with clinical expertise, patient needs, and patient values in the delivery of quality, safe, cost-effective care

(QSEN Institute, 2020; Straus et al., 2019). The two most common models used to facilitate EBP in nursing are the Stetler Model of EBP (Stetler, 2001, 2010) and the Iowa Model of Evidence-Based Practice to Promote Excellence in Healthcare (Cullen et al., 2018; Iowa Model Collaborative, 2017). This section introduces these two models, which might be used to implement evidence-based protocols, algorithms, and guidelines in clinical agencies.

Stetler Model of Research Utilization to Facilitate Evidence-Based Practice

An initial model for research utilization in nursing was developed by Stetler and Marram in 1976 and expanded and refined by Stetler in 1994 and 2001. The most current Stetler Model of Research Utilization to Facilitate Evidence-Based Practice provides a comprehensive framework to enhance the use of research evidence by nurses to facilitate EBP. Stetler published this model in 2010, and it is presented in Fig. 13.5. As indicated in the model, research evidence can be used at the institutional or individual level. At the institutional level, synthesized research knowledge is used to develop or update protocols, algorithms, policies, procedures, or other formal programs implemented in the institution. Individual nurses, such as RNs, APNs, educators, administrators, and policymakers, use this model to summarize research and use the knowledge to make decisions in practice, influence educational programs, and guide political decision making. The following sections briefly describe the five phases of the Stetler Model: preparation, validation, comparative evaluation/decision making, translation/application, and evaluation (Box 13.5). Anderson and Jenson (2019, p. 114) used the Stetler Model to conduct an "integrative review of the literature to identify violence risk-assessment screening tools that could be used in acute care mental health settings." This review is used as an example in the discussion of Phases I to III of the Stetler Model (see Box 13.5). Phases IV and V were not completed by Anderson and Jenson (2019) because implementation was not within the scope of their inquiry.

Phase I: Preparation

The intent of Stetler's model (Stetler, 2010) is to ensure critical thinking is initiated by nurses to use research evidence in practice. The first phase (preparation) involves selecting sources of research evidence; defining the issue, catalyst, or problem to be addressed; affirming the nature, degree, and priority of the problem; and defining the outcomes for the catalyst(s) (see Fig. 13.5). The agency's priorities and other external and internal factors that could be influenced by or could influence the proposed practice change must be examined. After the purpose of the evidence-based project has been identified and approved by the agency, a detailed search of the literature is conducted to determine the strength of the evidence available for use in practice. The research literature might be reviewed to solve a difficult clinical, managerial, or educational problem; to provide the basis for a policy, standard, algorithm, or protocol; or to prepare for an educational program or other type of professional presentation. As mentioned earlier, Anderson and Jenson (2019) used the Stetler Model of EBP to direct their literature review to identify a violence risk-assessment screening tool. The following excerpt briefly discusses Phase I:

Phase I: Preparation

Preparation consists of identifying the purpose, context, and sources of evidence (Grove et al., 2013). A detailed search was conducted to determine the strength of the evidence, leading to the recommendation within this article.

(Anderson & Jenson, 2019, p. 114)

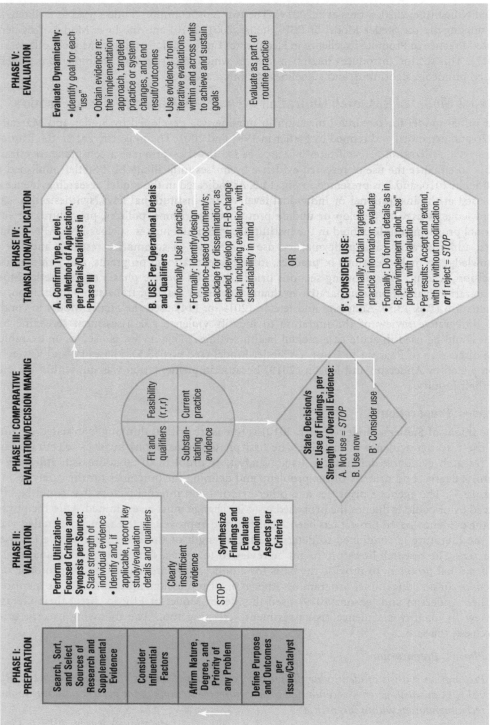

FIG. 13.5 Stetter Model, Part I: Steps of Research Utilization to Facilitate Evidence-Based Practice. (From Stetler, C. B. [2010]. Stetler model. In J. Rycroft-Malone & T. Bucknall [Eds.], *Models and frameworks for implementing evidence-based practice: Linking evidence to action* [pp. 53–55]. Wiley-Blackwell.)

PHASE I: PREPARATION	PHASE II: VALIDATION	PHASE III: COMPARATIVE EVALUATION/DECISION MAKING	PHASE IV: TRANSLATION/APPLICATION	PHASE V: EVALUATION

Purpose, Context, and Sources of Evidence:
 	
• **Potential Issues/Catalysts:** *= a problem, including unexplained variations; less-than-best practice; routine update of knowledge; validation/routine revision of procedures, etc; or innovative program goal*
• **Affirm/clarify perceived problem/s, with internal evidence re: current practice** *[baseline]*
• **Consider other influential internal and external factors,** e.g., timelines
• **Affirm and focus on high priority issues**
• **Decide if need to form a team, involve formal stakeholders, and/or assign project lead/facilitator**
• **Define desired, measurable outcome/s**
• **Seek out systematic reviews/guidelines first**
• **Determine need for an explicit type of research evidence,** if relevant
• **Select research sources with conceptual fit**
	Credibility of Evidence and Potential for/Detailed Qualifiers of Application:
	
	• **Critique and synopsize essential components, operational details, and other qualifying factors, per source**
	  ○ *See instructions for use of utilization-focused review tables,* with evaluative criteria, to facilitate this task; fill in the tables for group decision making or potential future synthesis
	• **Critique *systematic reviews and guidelines**
	• **Reassess fit of individual sources**
	• ***Rate the level and quality of each individual evidence source per a "table of evidence"**
	• **Differentiate statistical and clinical significance**
	• **Eliminate noncredible sources**
	• **End the process if there is clearly insufficient, credible external evidence that meets your need**
	
	*Stetler, Morsi, Rucki, et al. *Appl Nurs Res* 1998; 11(4):195–206 for noted tables, reviews, and synthesis process
		Synthesis and Decisions/Recommendations per Criteria of Applicability:
		
		• ***Synthesize the cumulative findings:**
		  ○ *Logically organize and display the similarities and differences across multiple findings, per common aspects or subelements of the topic under review*
		  ○ *Evaluate degree of substantiation of each aspect/subelement; reference any qualifying conditions for application*
		• **Evaluate degree and nature of other criteria:** *feasibility **(r,r,r = risk, resources, readiness);** pragmatic fit, including potential qualifying factors to application; and nature of **current practice, including the urgency/risk of current issues/needs
		• **Make a decision whether/what to use:**
		  ○ *Can be a personal practitioner-level decision or a recommendation to others
		  ○ *Judge strength of decision: indicate if primarily "research-based" (R-B) or, per high use of supplemental info, "E-B"; note level of strength of recommendation/s per related* table; note any qualifying factors that may influence individualized variations
		  ○ **If decision = "Not use" research findings:**
		    ○ *May conduct own research or delay use till additional research done by others*
		    ○ *If still decide to act now, e.g., on evidence of consensus or another basis for practice, consider need for similar planned change and evaluation.*
		  ○ **If decision = "Use/Consider Use," can mean a recommendation for or against a specific practice**
			Operational Definition of Use/Actions for Change:
			
			• **Types** = *cognitive/conceptual, symbolic and/or instrumental*
			• **Methods** = *informal or formal; direct or indirect*
			• **Levels** = *individual, group or department/organization*
			• **Direct instrumental use:** *change individual behavior (e.g., via assessment tool or Rx intervention options); or change policy, procedure, protocol, algorithm, program, etc.*
			• **Cognitive use:** *validate current practice; change personal way of thinking; increase awareness; better understand or appreciate condition/s or experience/s*
			• **Symbolic use:** *develop position paper or proposal for change; or persuade others regarding a way of thinking*
			• **Formal dissemination and change/implementation strategies should be planned per relevant research and local barriers:**
			  ○ *Passive education is usually not effective as an isolated strategy. Use Dx analysis** and an ***implementation framework to develop a plan. Consider multiple strategies: e.g., opinion leaders, interactive education, reminders and audits.*
			  ○ *Focus on context & to enhance sustainability of organization-related change*
			• **CAUTION: Assess whether translation/product or use goes beyond actual findings/evidence:**
			  ○ *Research evidence may or may not provide various details or a complete policy, procedure, etc.; indicate this fact to users, and note differential levels of evidence therein*
			• **Consider need for appropriate, reasoned variation**
			• **WITH B, where made a decision to *use* in the setting:**
			  ○ *With formal use, may need a dynamic evaluation to effectively implement and continuously improve/refine use of best available evidence across units and time*
			• **WITH B', where made a decision to *consider use* and thus obtain additional, pragmatic information before a final decision:**
			  ○ *With formal consideration, do a pilot project*
			  ○ *With a pilot project, must assess if need IRB review, per relevant institutional criteria*
				Alternative Evaluations:
				
				• **Evaluation per type, method, level: e.g., consider conceptual use at individual level****
				• **Consider cost-benefit of change + various evaluation efforts**
				• **Use RU-as-a-process to enhance credibility of evaluation data**
				• **For both dynamic and pilot evaluations, include:**
				  ○ ****formative, regarding actual implementation and goal progress*
				  ○ *summative, regarding identified end goal and end-point outcomes*
				
				NOTE: Model applies to all forms of practice, i.e., educational, clinical, managerial, or other; to use effectively, read 2001 and 1994 model papers.
				
				**Stetler et al, 2006 re: dx analysis
				
				***E.g.: Rogers' re: implications of attributes of a change; Rycroft-Malone et al, ᵅPARIHS (2002) and Green and Krueter's PRECEDE (1992) models re: implementation
				
				ᵅStetler, 2003 on context
				ᵅᵅStetler and Caramanica, 2007 on outcomes

FIG. 13.5, cont'd

BOX 13.5 FIVE PHASES OF THE STETLER MODEL FOR EVIDENCE-BASED PRACTICE

Phase I: Preparation
Phase II Validation
Phase III: Comparative Evaluation/Decision Making
Phase IV: Translation/Application
Phase V: Evaluation

Phase II: Validation

In the validation phase, research reports are critically appraised to determine their scientific soundness. If the studies are limited in number or are weak, or both, the findings and conclusions are usually considered inadequate or insufficient for use in practice, and the process stops. The quality of the research evidence is greatly strengthened if a systematic review or meta-analysis has been conducted in the area in which you want to make an evidence-based change (Cullen et al., 2018; Melnyk & Fineout-Overholt, 2019). If the research knowledge base is strong in the selected area, a decision needs to be made regarding the priority of using the evidence in practice by the clinical agency (see Fig. 13.5). Phase II from the Anderson and Jenson (2019) article is presented in the following excerpt:

Phase II: Validation

Validation outlines the need for a comprehensive literature search to determine the scientific soundness of current literature (Grove et al., 2013). The following section describes the primary literature review, which identified various violence risk–assessment screening tools used in acute care mental health settings.

Primary review. The aim of the primary literature review was to identify violence risk–assessment screening tools used in acute care mental health settings. A search of the EBSCO-host and CINAHL databases identified 60 articles. An additional search of PubMed, focusing on meta-analysis and systemic reviews, produced another 57 articles. Inclusion criteria for the literature search: written in English, peer-reviewed journals, and contained one or a combination of selected keywords (assessment, mental health, screening, tools, violence). Of the 117 articles identified, further review of the abstracts excluded studies within forensic mental health populations and publication dates before 2010. . . . Twenty articles were selected for further examination.

Fifteen violence risk–assessment screening tools were identified in the literature. Eight of the 15 tools were identified for evaluation. . . . Studies were excluded if they did not review validity and reliability of the tool and were published before 2010. Four of the 6 tools . . . warranted further exploration.

Secondary review. The aim of the secondary review was to further explore the literature identified as violence risk–assessment screening tools. Secondary review was conducted with searches in the CINAHL, PubMed, and PsycINFO databases, resulting in an additional 77 studies. . . . Of the 77 abstracts reviewed, 42 were selected for review and 32 were selected for further evaluation. Information from the primary and secondary searches [were provided in a figure].

(Anderson & Jenson, 2019, pp. 114–115)

Phase III: Comparative Evaluation/Decision Making

Comparative evaluation includes four parts: (1) fit and qualifiers of the evidence for the health-care setting, (2) feasibility of using the research findings, (3) substantiation of the evidence, and (4) concerns with current practice (see Fig. 13.5). To determine the fit of the evidence in the clinical agency, the characteristics of the setting are examined to determine the forces that would facilitate or inhibit the evidence-based change. Stetler (2010) believed the feasibility of using research evidence for making changes in practice necessitated examination of the three rs: (1) potential risks, (2) resources needed, and (3) readiness of the people involved (see Fig. 13.5).

Substantiating evidence is produced by replication, in which consistent, credible findings are obtained from several studies in similar practice settings. The studies generating the strongest research evidence are RCTs, meta-analyses of RCTs, and quasi-experimental studies. The final comparison involves determining whether the research information provides credible, empirical evidence for making changes in the current practice. The research evidence must document that an intervention increases the quality and safety in current practice by solving practice problems and improving patient outcomes. By conducting Phase III, the overall benefits and risks of using the research evidence in a practice setting can be assessed. If the benefits (improved patient, pro-vider, or agency outcomes) are much greater than the risks (complications, morbidity, mortality, or increased costs) for the organization, the individual nurse, or both, then using the research-based intervention in practice is feasible.

Three conclusions are possible during the decision-making phase: (1) not to use the research evidence, (2) to use the research evidence now, and (3) to consider using the evidence (see Fig. 13.5). The decision *not* to make a change in practice is usually due to the poor quality of the research evidence, costs, and other potential problems. The decision to use research knowledge in practice now is determined mainly by the strength of the evidence. Depending on the research knowledge to be used in practice, the individual nurse, hospital unit, or agency might make this decision. Another decision might be to consider using the available research evidence in practice, but not immediately. When a change is complex and involves multiple disciplines, the individuals involved often need additional time to determine how the evidence might be used and what mea-sures will be taken to coordinate the involvement of different health professionals in the change. The application of Phase III of Stetler's Model from Anderson and Jenson's (2019) integrative review is presented in the following excerpt:

> ### Phase III: Comprehensive Evaluation/Decision Making
>
> Phase III addresses evaluation of the literature and provides a recommendation for practice (Grove et al., 2013). … The recommendation for violence risk–assessment screening tools was based on predictive validity, calibration, discrimination, and reliability reported in the literature.
>
> **Comprehensive evaluation.** Over past decades, several violence risk–assessment screening tools have been studied to establish predictive validity (based on calibration and discrimination) for assessing the likelihood of violence. … Calibration of an assessment is defined as the ability of the tool to predict risk with actual observed risk. Discrimination of an assessment is defined as the ability of the tool to assess tendency toward violence.
>
> (Anderson & Jenson, 2019, p. 115)

Phase IV: Translation/Application

The translation and application phase involves planning for and using the research evidence in practice. The translation phase involves determining exactly what knowledge will be used and how that knowledge will be applied to practice. The use of the research evidence can be informal or formal and direct or indirect (see Fig. 13.5; Stetler, 2010). The application of research evidence includes direct instrumental use, cognitive use, and symbolic use. Instrumental use is the direct and formal application of research evidence to support the need for change in nursing interventions or practice protocols, algorithms, and guidelines. Cognitive use is a more informal, indirect use of the research knowledge to modify one's way of thinking or appreciation of an issue. Cognitive application may improve the nurse's understanding of a situation, allow analysis of practice dynamics, or improve problem-solving skills for clinical problems. Symbolic use occurs when position papers or proposals for change are developed to persuade others toward a new way of thinking (see Fig. 13.3).

The application phase includes the following steps for planned change: (1) assess the situation to be changed, (2) develop a plan for change, and (3) implement the plan. During the application phase, educational programs, protocols, policies, procedures, or algorithms are developed based on research evidence and implemented in practice (Stetler, 2001, 2010). A pilot project on a single hospital unit or in a specific healthcare clinic might be conducted to implement the change in practice, and the results of this project could be evaluated to determine whether the change should be extended throughout the healthcare agency or system.

Phase V: Evaluation

The final stage, evaluation, is to determine the effect of the research-based change on the patients, personnel, and healthcare agency. The evaluation process can include informal and formal activities conducted by administrators, nurse clinicians, and other health professionals (see Fig. 13.5). Informal evaluations include self-monitoring or discussions with patients, families, peers, and other health professionals. Formal evaluations might include case studies, audits, quality improvement projects, and translational or outcomes research projects.

An example of Phase IV and Phase V of the Stetler Model is presented using the study by Sher (2018). Sher (2018, p. 1) implemented an "educational program for parents of neonates on nasal continuous positive airway pressure [NCPAP]" that was guided by the Stetler Model (Stetler, 2010). The practice problem focused on the stress of parents with preterm infants on NCPAP, who worried about holding their infant and the possible complications of NCPAP.

A review of the literature suggested family-centered educational programs are able to decrease stress and increase parental confidence. The purpose of this project was to develop a family-centered education program focused on the education of parents of infants on NCPAP in the NICU [neonatal intensive care unit]. ...Stetler's evidence-based practice model was used to guide this project. ... Evidence was collected in a systematic review of published peer-reviewed journal articles. The Johns Hopkins Nursing evidence-based appraisal tool was used to evaluate relevant articles. ...The curriculum, supporting handouts for participants, and implementation and evaluation plans were developed and were provided to the institution as a complete solution to the practice problem [Phase IV of Stetler's Model]. The project may promote positive social change for caregivers, patients, and patients' families by enhancing outcomes such as improved infant behavior, increased parental emotional well-being, and increased caregiver satisfaction [Phase V of Stetler's Model].

(Sher, 2018, p. 1)

📄 **RESEARCH/EBP TIP**

The Stetler Model (2010) is a valuable resource that includes the steps to guide nurses in making appropriate evidence-based changes in their practice.

Iowa Model of Evidence-Based Practice

Nurses are actively involved in conducting research, synthesizing research evidence, and developing evidence-based guidelines for practice. The Iowa Model of Evidence-Based Practice (EBP) was developed as a practical process for promoting EBP (Titler et al., 1994, 2001). The most current revision and validation of the Iowa Model was conducted by the Iowa Model Collaborative (2017, p. 175): "The Iowa Model-Revised remains an application-oriented guide for the EBP process. Intended users are point of care clinicians who ask questions and seek a systematic, EBP approach to promote excellence in health care" (Fig. 13.6). In a healthcare agency, triggers, such as issues or opportunities, initiate the need for change. These triggers can include clinical or patient-identified issues; organization, state, or national initiative(s); new research evidence in a nursing area; accrediting agency requirements/regulations; and/or philosophy of care (Cullen et al., 2018). The triggers are evaluated and prioritized based on the needs of the patients, nurse providers, and clinical agency. The next step is the statement of the question or purpose of the EBP project. Is the topic of this question a priority for nurses and the healthcare agency? If the answer is no, consider another issue/opportunity for an EBP project (see Fig. 13.6). If the topic is a priority, a team is formed to assemble, appraise, and synthesize the body of evidence available (Cullen et al., 2019; Iowa Model Collaborative, 2017).

In some situations, the research evidence is inadequate to make changes in practice, and additional studies are needed to strengthen the knowledge base. Sometimes the research evidence can be combined with other sources of knowledge (theories, scientific principles, expert opinion, and case reports) to provide fairly strong evidence for developing research-based protocols for practice. The strongest evidence is generated from meta-analyses of several RCTs, systematic reviews that usually include meta-analyses, and individual experimental studies (Cochrane Collaboration, 2021). If the evidence is sufficient, the team then designs and pilots the practice change. The next question the EBP team must address: Is the change appropriate for adoption in practice? If the answer is no, then the practice change should be redesigned and pilot-tested again (see Fig. 13.6).

If the outcomes of the pilot test are favorable, the next step is to integrate and sustain the practice change by identifying and engaging key personnel and *hardwiring* the change into the system. The indicators of the practice change are monitored over time by quality improvement to determine its effect on patients, nurses, and/or agency in terms of quality, safety, and costs. The team and other nurses involved in the EBP change should take actions as needed to sustain the practice change (Iowa Model Collaborative, 2017). The final step is to disseminate results of the evaluations of the practice change's efficacy and expand the change to other appropriate areas (see Fig. 13.6).

📄 RESEARCH/EBP TIP

More than 90% of the nursing research leaders in Magnet-designated hospitals use an EBP model to implement research evidence into practice, and the Iowa Model was the most frequently used to promote EBP in healthcare agencies (Speroni et al., 2020).

Application of the Iowa Model of Evidence-Based Practice

Trentadue and colleagues (2020) implemented an EBP project to standardize infusion therapy practices in nonhospital outpatient ambulatory clinic settings. These authors reported that RNs in ambulatory care setting were not consistently following national evidence-based guidelines, which

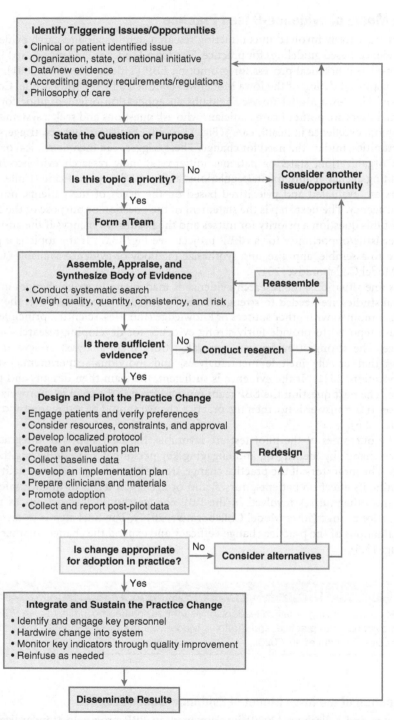

FIG. 13.6 The Iowa Model-Revised. (From Iowa Model Collaborative. [2017]. Iowa Model of Evidence-Based Practice: Revisions and validation. *Worldviews on Evidence-Based Nursing, 14*[3], 178. https://doi.org/10.1111/wvn.12223.)

resulted in practices that were highly variable and of unknown quality. They used the Iowa Model of EBP to implement their EBP change, which is briefly presented in the following excerpt.

Methods

The Iowa Model-Revised (2017) guided the project methodology. This model is endorsed by the organization's Nursing Research Innovation Council because of its pragmatic approach to achieving EBP change and its success in improving both process and outcomes across a variety of practice concerns. Following are the key components of the Iowa Model and a description of how use of this tool steered the organization's evidence-based infusion practices.

Identifying Triggering Issues/Opportunities

The Ambulatory Care Shared Governance Practice Council meets monthly to review and prioritize ambulatory care clinical issues. Each year the council selects 1 EBP improvement project. Nurses identified considerable variability in infusion therapy practices (e.g., types of medications administered intravenously, patient monitoring, and use of infusion pumps). In 2017, standardization of infusion practices was identified as a priority to provide safe, consistent, evidence-based patient care.

State the Question/Purpose

Using a PICO statement clarifies the project's aim by identifying: P–the specific patient population, I–the intervention, C–the comparison group, and O–the outcomes. The PICO question for this initiative was: What are the best practices for safe, effective infusion therapy in the non-hospital outpatient department (non-HOD) ambulatory care setting?

Obtain Administrative Support and Create a Team

An EBP team was formed specifically for this project with representatives from the Ambulatory Care Shared Governance Council…and nurses from a variety of clinics and urgent care. The Shared Governance Council members represent more than 121 non-HODs across a large geographic area in the Midwestern United States. Non-HODs are not covered under Joint Commission or similar accreditation programs as HODs. In this organization there are 73 single primary care provider clinics, 48 large multispecialty clinics, and 37 urgent care sites (located in one of the aforementioned clinics). Nurses in non-HOD clinics provide a range of infusion therapy services, such as the administration of hydrating solutions, long-term intravenous (IV) antibiotic therapy for infectious diseases and diuretic therapy for heart failure….

Assemble, Appraise, and Synthesize the Evidence

An extensive appraisal of evidence regarding infusion therapy practices was conducted. This process was particularly helpful to identify potential barriers to implementing practice changes. The evaluation included:
- *A review of the infusion therapy in ambulatory care literature*
- *A review of the organization's infusion therapy policies and procedures*
- *A review of ambulatory care infusion incident reports*
- *An inventory of ambulatory care infusion pumps (conducted by biomedical engineering and information technology personnel who traced pumps by make, model, Wi-Fi capacity, availability, and functionality)*
- *A list of IV medications administered in the ambulatory care settings (obtained from the System Infusion Device Council)*

- *System infusion therapy educational offerings (both required and elective)*
- *A survey of ambulatory care RN current infusion practices.*

This multidimensional appraisal of system evidence revealed several strengths and limitations. A system librarian's literature search yielded 16 publications. Team members reviewed all the publications and found the Infusion Nurses Society's (INS) Infusion Therapy Standards of Practice (the Standards) most instructive. ... The team found no literature specifically testing the application of the Standards in non-HOD ambulatory care settings. ... Because this was the first attempt to standardize ambulatory care infusion practices, it was not surprising that the organization's current infusion therapy policies and procedures were focused on hospitalized patients. Several gaps/differences were identified, including differences in terminology, catheters and supplies, training requirements, use of topical anesthetics, and use of infusion pumps. The incident reporting process was complex and oriented more toward the hospital setting, which made it difficult to report and virtually impossible to identify infusion errors in the ambulatory care setting. ... A small number of nurses are the only RN in their clinic, and many nurses report to non-clinical managers, creating unique training and competency testing challenges.

(Trentadue et al., 2020, p. 352)

Design and Pilot the Practice Change

Based on the synthesis of evidence, the team identified 4 key areas to improve practice:

1. *Standardize the IV medication list. The EBP team asked the System Infusion Device Council to examine the types of solutions and medications administered intravenously, the frequency of administration, and the use of an infusion pump. ...*
2. *Update the organization's infusion therapy policy and procedures to be inclusive of ambulatory care. The Standards indicates that they can be applied across settings. There was organizational consensus that evidence-based procedures must be in place to support safe nursing practice, and those practices must be consistent across all settings. ... This time-consuming process took almost 1 year to complete and required the use of the same infusion therapy equipment/pumps and supplies across all sites of service.*
3. *Establish ambulatory care infusion therapy training and competency requirements. Not all ambulatory care clinic settings provided infusion therapy services. ... To improve patient satisfaction and enhance safety, a decision was made that patients would receive consistent infusion therapy services within the medical group. Infusion therapy competency training of staff was outlined. ... The inpatient and outpatient areas share the same electronic health record (EHR). The infusion therapy EHR template was revised and a tip sheet was developed to support consistent documentation of the types of catheter(s) placed and insertion dates.*
4. *Standardized use of pumps and Wi-Fi connectivity. Standardization of pump technology was necessary to ensure that staff had the competence, as well as supplies, for safe use. ...*

Evaluate Appropriateness of Change in Practice

The Ambulatory Care Shared Governance Practice Council and System Infusion Device Council wholeheartedly endorsed the practice changes outlined: (1) create standardized lists of high-risk patients and medications requiring an infusion pump; (2) develop a systemwide infusion therapy policy and procedure; (3) design standardized ambulatory care infusion competencies; and (4) standardize use of pumps with Wi-Fi connectivity. ...

Integrate and Sustain a Practice Change

The key to integrating and sustaining a practice change is standardization. ... Several approaches were required to ensure that best practices are implemented and followed. This increased the complexity of the project but also ensured that changes would be hardwired into practice and workflow.

Results

Significant progress was made in advancing the standardization of infusion therapy in some but not all areas. Having an organizational standard of high-alert medications and high-risk populations was greatly appreciated and embraced by nursing staff. A new EHR report allows the System Infusion Device Council to monitor the types and volumes of medications administered via IV routes, ensuring rapid follow-up on any deviations. ...

Conclusions and Implications

The primary aim of this project was to build the Ambulatory Care Shared Governance Practice Council's capacity for EBP. The application of the Iowa Model was valuable in providing the team with a solid framework. ... As health care continues to evolve from hospital to ambulatory care settings, we anticipate the need for more EBP interventions in ambulatory care nursing. ... An important step, as ambulatory nursing takes on this task, is to continue to disseminate successful strategies for building and testing EBPs to other nurses working in ambulatory care.

(Trentadue et al., 2020, pp. 353–354)

📄 **RESEARCH/EBP TIP**

EBP change requires a multifaceted approach that takes into consideration the evidence available, attitudes of the practicing nurses, the organization's philosophy, and national organizational standards and guidelines. Therefore EBP changes are best guided by frameworks such as the Iowa and Stetler models of EBP.

IMPLEMENTING EVIDENCE-BASED GUIDELINES IN PRACTICE

Research knowledge is generated every day and must be critically appraised and synthesized to determine the best evidence for use in practice (Bertolaccini & Spaggiari, 2020; Grainger, 2021). This evidence has been developed into numerous evidence-based guidelines by researchers, expert clinicians, educators, policy developers, and consumers. These guidelines are available on many national and international websites and in referred professional journals. This section focuses on the resources for evidence-based guidelines and provides an example of a guideline for the management of hypertension (HTN) in adults (Whelton et al., 2018).

Resources for Evidence-Based Guidelines

Since the 1980s, the Agency for Healthcare Research and Quality (AHRQ) has had a major role in identifying health-related topics and promoting the development of evidence-based guidelines in these areas (http://www.ahrq.gov). The first evidence-based guidelines sponsored by the AHRQ were developed by panels of nationally recognized researchers in the topic area, expert clinicians (e.g., physicians, nurses, pharmacists, social workers), healthcare administrators, policy developers, economists, government representatives, and consumers. The group members designated the scope of the guideline and conducted extensive reviews of the literature, including relevant systematic reviews, meta-analyses, meta-syntheses, mixed methods research syntheses, individual studies,

BOX 13.6   **WEBSITES FOR IDENTIFYING EVIDENCE-BASED GUIDELINES FOR NURSING PRACTICE**

- Association of Women's Health, Obstetric and Neonatal Nurses: https://awhonn.org
- Centers for Disease Control and Prevention: https//www.cdc.gov/
- Guidelines International Network: https://www.g-i-n.net/
- Complementary and Alternative Medicine: https://www.nccih.nih.gov/health/providers/clinicalpractice
- National Association of Neonatal Nurses: https://www.nann.org/
- National Institute for Clinical Excellence (NICE): https://www.nice.org.uk/
- Oncology Nursing Society: https://www.ons.org/
- Clinical Practice Guidelines: https://www.aafp.org/family-physician/patient-care/clinical-recommendations/clinical-practice-guidelines/clinical-practice-guidelines.html
- US Preventive Services Task Force: http://www.uspreventiveservicestaskforce.org

and theories (Moriarty, 2019). The evidence-based guidelines developed were examined by consultants, other researchers, and additional expert clinicians for their input. Based on the experts' critique, the AHRQ revised and packaged the guidelines for distribution to healthcare professionals. At present, standardized guideline development ranges from a structured process, such as the one just discussed, to a less structured process where a guideline is developed by a group of individuals or a healthcare organization.

The AHRQ initiated the National Guideline Clearinghouse (NGC) in 1998 to store EBP guidelines. The NGC included thousands of publicly available EBP guidelines and related documents. Regretfully, this site was closed in July 2018 when the funding for this project was discontinued. Currently, AHRQ is searching for organizations that might support the work of the NGC (2018). In addition, numerous government agencies, professional organizations, healthcare agencies, and universities provide evidence-based guidelines for practice. Box 13.6 includes resources for identifying current evidence-based guidelines for nursing practice.

Implementing an Evidence-Based Guideline for Managing Hypertension in Adults

Evidence-based guidelines have become the standards for providing care to patients in the United States and other countries. The 2017 evidence-based guideline for the prevention, detection, evaluation, and management of high BP in adults was sponsored by the American College of Cardiology and American Heart Association (Whelton et al., 2018). The guideline was developed and published without commercial support, and the members of the task force volunteered their time for writing and reviewing the guideline. This guideline provides clinicians with directions for (1) implementing lifestyle interventions; (2) setting BP goals; and (3) initiating BP-lowering medication based on age, diabetes, and chronic kidney disease (CKD). Nurses and other healthcare providers can use this guideline to select the most appropriate interventions for each individual patient diagnosed with HTN.

Nursing students and RNs need to assess the usefulness and quality of each evidence-based guideline before they implement it in their practice. Fig. 13.7 presents the Grove Model for Implementing Evidence-Based Guidelines in Practice. In this model, nurses identify a practice problem, search for the best research evidence to manage the problem in their practice, and identify an evidence-based guideline. These guidelines are often considered the national standard for managing a health problem (Gray & Grove, 2021; Moriarty et al., 2019). Assessing the quality and usefulness of the guideline involves examining (1) the authors of the guideline, (2) the significance of the healthcare problem, (3) the strength of the research evidence, (4) the link to national standards, and (5) the cost-effectiveness of using the guideline in practice. The quality of the 2017 guideline for managing HTN is discussed using these criteria (Whelton et al., 2018).

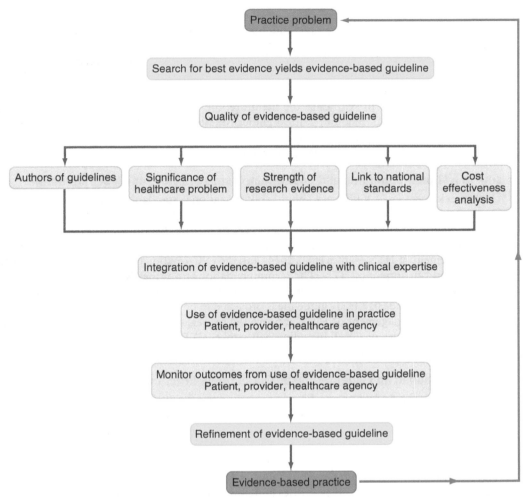

FIG. 13.7 Grove Model for Implementing Evidence-Based Guidelines in Practice.

Authors of the Guideline

The committee for the development of the 2017 HTN guideline included cardiologist, internist, geriatrician, nurse, nephrologist, pharmacist, physician assistant, and two lay/patient representatives. The clinicians were from several professional organizations (Whelton et al., 2018). These members were specifically selected based on their strong and varied expertise to develop an evidence-based guideline for the management of HTN.

Significance of Healthcare Problem

HTN continues to be the most common condition that is managed in primary care and can lead to myocardial infarction (MI), stroke, renal failure, and death if not detected and effectively managed. The 2017 HTN guideline provides evidence-based recommendations for patients with or at risk for CVD. The guideline was developed for healthcare practices in the United States but could have an effect globally (Todkar et al., 2021; Whelton et al., 2018).

Strength of Research Evidence

Whelton et al. (2018) detailed their methodology for reviewing relevant literature, selecting quality sources, and synthesizing these sources. The literature searches focused on RCTs but also includes systematic reviews, cohort studies, nonrandomized comparative and descriptive studies, and expert opinion. Additional studies that were published during the writing of this guideline were reviewed through June 2016. The studies selected for review were of high quality, which was documented in the review. To synthesize the literature, the task force members conducted a formal systematic review to address four critical clinical questions related to HTN. The results of the literature synthesis were presented in table and narrative format and made available to the readers in the article by Whelton et al. (2018) and online.

Link to National Standards and Cost-Effectiveness of Evidence-Based Guideline

Quality evidence-based guidelines should link to national standards and be cost-effective (see Fig. 13.7). The task force reviewed associated guidelines and statements and documented those that were pertinent to the writing of the 2017 HTN guideline. This guideline also built on the other national guidelines, such as the Joint National Committee (JNC) 8 evidence-based guideline for the management of HTN (James et al., 2014) and the JNC 7 national guideline for the assessment, diagnosis, and treatment of HTN. The recommendations from the JNC 7 were supported by the Department of Health and Human Services and disseminated through the NIH (Chobanian et al., 2003). The use of the 2017 HTN guideline is projected to be cost-effective because the recommendations for the management of HTN improve the management of high BP in adults, which decreases the incidences of CVD, including MI, stroke, CKD, heart failure, and related mortality (Todkar et al., 2021; Whelton et al., 2018).

Implementation of an Evidence-Based Guideline in Practice

The next step is for student nurses, RNs, and APNs to use the 2017 HTN evidence-based guideline in their practice. Student nurses and RNs need to accurately take and record patients' BPs in EHRs to ensure quality measurement of outcomes. The BP value should be based on an average of two or more careful readings on two or more occasions (Whelton et al., 2018). The designated BP categories for adults in the 2017 HTN national guideline include normal, elevated, and HTN (stages 1 and 2), which are presented in Table 13.3. Nurses are responsible for educating patients and their families about the BP categories and how to take and record their BP accurately at least

TABLE 13.3 CATEGORIES OF BLOOD PRESSURE IN ADULTS

BLOOD PRESSURE CATEGORY	SYSTOLIC BLOOD PRESSURE	AND/OR	DIASTOLIC BLOOD PRESSURE
Normal	<120 mm Hg	And	<80 mm Hg
Elevated	120–129 mm Hg	And	80–89 mm Hg
Hypertension stage 1	130–139 mm Hg	Or	80–89 mm Hg
Hypertension stage 2	≥140 mm Hg	Or	≥90 mm Hg

Blood pressure (BP) is based on an average of two careful readings obtained on two occasions. Individuals with systolic BP and diastolic BP in two categories should be designated to the higher BP category.
Data from Whelton, P. K., Carey, R. M., Aronow, W. S., Casey, D. E., Collins, K. J., Himmelfarb, C. D.,...Wright, J. W. (2018). 2017 Guideline for the prevention, detection, evaluation, and management of high blood pressure in adults: Executive summary: A report of the American College of Cardiology/American Heart Association task force on clinical practice guidelines. *Hypertension, 71*(6), 1269–1324. https://doi.org/10.1161/HYP.0000000000000066.

BOX 13.7   MODIFIABLE RISK FACTORS IN PATIENTS WITH HYPERTENSION

- Current cigarette smoking, secondhand smoking
- Diabetes mellitus
- Dyslipidemia/hypercholesterolemia
- Overweight/obesity
- Physical inactivity/low fitness
- Unhealthy diet

Modifiable risk factors are factors that can be changed and when changed may reduce cardiovascular disease risk.
Adapted from Whelton, P. K., Carey, R. M., Aronow, W. S., Casey, D. E., Collins, K. J., Himmelfarb, C. D.,...Wright, J. W. (2018). 2017 Guideline for the prevention, detection, evaluation, and management of high blood pressure in adults: Executive summary: A report of the American College of Cardiology/American Heart Association task force on clinical practice guidelines. *Hypertension, 71*(6), 1269–1324. https://doi.org/10.1161/HYP.0000000000000066.

once a day. If an elevated BP is noted, the values need to be reported to an APN or physician for management.

Adults' BPs are affected by modifiable risk factors and relatively fixed risk factors. The modifiable risk factors are presented in Box 13.7. The relatively fixed risk factors include CKD, family history of HTN, increased age, low socioeconomic status, low educational status, male gender, obstructive sleep apnea, and psychosocial stress (Whelton et al., 2018). RNs and nursing students need to educate patients and families about the modifiable and fixed HTN risk factors to increase their understanding of HTN. The major role of nurses in managing HTN involves educating patients and families about lifestyle modifications (LSMs), which focus on the modifiable risk factors, such as smoking, overweight, unhealthy diet, and physical inactivity (see Box 13.7). Table 13.4 includes the recommendations for the management and follow-up of adults with HTN for RNs, APNs, and physicians (Whelton et al., 2018). RNs and nursing students need to implement a variety of interventions to promote LSMs in patients (see Table 13.4) and provide them education about follow-up. Individuals with high BP readings consistent with stage 1 or stage 2 HTN should be reported to APNs and physicians. The APNs and physicians will initiate or revise HTN medication treatments based on the health circumstances and values of their patients (see Table 13.4).

The outcomes for the patient, provider, and healthcare agency for the management of HTN need to be examined. The outcomes should be recorded in the patients' EHRs and include (1) BP readings for patients; (2) patient education provided regarding LSMs; (3) current lifestyle behaviors of patients; (4) incidence of diagnoses of HTN based on the 2017 HTN guideline; (5) appropriateness of the pharmacological therapies implemented to manage HTN; and (6) incidence of stroke, MI, heart failure, CKD, and CVD and related mortality over a period of 1 to 20 years. The healthcare agency outcomes include access to care by patients with HTN, patient satisfaction with care, and costs related to diagnosis and management of HTN, in addition to the HTN complications previously mentioned. This EBP guideline is scheduled for review and revision every 6 years based on clinical outcomes, outcome studies, new RCTs, systematic reviews, and meta-analyses (Whelton et al., 2018).

📄 RESEARCH/EBP TIP

The review and implementation of evidence-based guidelines by nurses is essential for developing EBP for the nursing profession and healthcare agencies. You need to organize your evaluation and implementation of evidence-based guidelines in practice by use of a model, such as the Grove Model for Implementing Evidence-Based Guidelines in practice.

TABLE 13.4   RECOMMENDATIONS FOR MANAGEMENT AND FOLLOW-UP OF ADULTS WITH HYPERTENSION

CATEGORIES OF HTN IN ADULTS[a,c]	NURSING STUDENTS AND RNS INTERVENTIONS	APNS AND PHYSICIANS
	LSMS[b] AND FOLLOW-UP	PHARMACOLOGICAL MANAGEMENT OF HTN
Normal BP	LSMs and follow-up in 1 yr	
Elevated BP	LSMs and follow-up in 3–6 mo	Nonpharmacological therapy
Stage 1 HTN	LSMs and follow-up in 3–6 mo if BP goal is met and in 1 mo if not met	Pharmacological therapy (1–2 drugs)
Stage 2 HTN	LSMs and follow-up in 1 mo and then 3–6 mo based on BP values	Pharmacological therapy (usually more than one drug)

[a]Management is determined by the highest BP category.
[b]LSMs or nonpharmacological therapy include education and support in the following areas: balanced diet, regular exercise program, achieving normal weight, smoking cessation, and reduced dietary salt and alcohol. Emphasis on education and support should expand with elevated BP and stages 1 and 2 HTN.
[c]Patients with diabetes mellitus or chronic kidney disease need education about management of these diseases and the link with HTN.
APN, Advanced practice nurse; *BP*, blood pressure; *HTN*, hypertension; *LSM*, lifestyle modification; *RN*, registered nurse.
Adapted from Whelton, P. K., Carey, R. M., Aronow, W. S., Casey, D. E., Collins, K. J., Himmelfarb, C. D.,...Wright, J. W. (2018). 2017 Guideline for the prevention, detection, evaluation, and management of high blood pressure in adults: Executive summary: A report of the American College of Cardiology/American Heart Association task force on clinical practice guidelines. *Hypertension, 71*(6), 1269–1324. https://doi.org/10.1161/HYP.0000000000000066.

INTRODUCTION TO EVIDENCE-BASED PRACTICE CENTERS

In 1997 the AHRQ launched its initiative to promote EBP by establishing 12 evidence-based practice centers (EPCs) in the United States and Canada (AHRQ, 2021a). The functions of EPCs are described in the following excerpt:

> The **evidence-based practice centers** develop evidence reports and technology assessments on topics relevant to clinical, social science/behavioral, economic, and other healthcare organization and delivery issues—specifically those that are common, expensive, and/or significant for the Medicare and Medicaid populations. With this program, AHRQ became a "science partner" with private and public organizations in their efforts to improve the quality, effectiveness, and appropriateness of health care by synthesizing the evidence and facilitating the translation of evidence-based research findings. Topics are nominated by non-federal partners such as professional societies, health plans, insurers, employers, and patient groups.
>
> *(AHRQ, 2021a)*

Through the EPC Program, the AHRQ awards 5-year contracts to institutions to serve as EPCs. These centers review all relevant scientific literature on clinical, behavioral, organizational, and financial topics to produce evidence reports. These reports are used to inform and develop coverage decisions, quality measures, educational materials, tools, guidelines, and research agendas. The AHRQ developed the following criteria as the basis for selecting a topic to be managed by an EPC:

- *High incidence or prevalence in the general population and in special populations, including women, racial and ethnic minorities, pediatric and elderly populations, and those of low socioeconomic status.*
- *Significance for the needs of the Medicare, Medicaid, and other Federal health programs.*
- *High costs associated with a condition, procedure, treatment, or technology, whether due to the number of people needing care, high unit cost of care, or high indirect costs.*
- *Controversy or uncertainty about the effectiveness or relative effectiveness of available clinical strategies or technologies.*
- *Impact potential for informing and improving patient or provider decision making.*
- *Impact potential for reducing clinically significant variations in the prevention, diagnosis, or management of a disease or condition; in the use of a procedure or technology; or in the health outcomes achieved.*
- *Availability of scientific data to support the systematic review and analysis of the topic.*
- *Submission of the nominating organization's plan to incorporate the report into its managerial or policy decision making....*
- *Submission of the nominating organization's plan to disseminate derivative products to its members and plan to measure members' use of these products, and the resultant impact of such use on clinical practice.*

(AHRQ, 2021b)

The AHRQ (2021b) website provides names of the EPCs and the focus of each center. This site also provides a link to the evidence-based reports produced by these centers. These EPCs have had an important role in the development of evidence-based guidelines since the 1990s and will continue to make significant contributions to EBP in the future.

INTRODUCTION TO TRANSLATIONAL RESEARCH AND TRANSLATIONAL SCIENCE

Some of the challenges related to EBP have resulted from the application of research knowledge to practice. Therefore a research strategy called translational research was developed to facilitate the use of research evidence in practice. Originally, the conduct of translational research was part of the National Center for Research Resources (NIH, 2021a). However, in December 2011, the National Center for Advancing Translation Sciences (NCATS) was developed as part of the NIH Institutes and Centers (NIH, 2021b). Translational research is an evolving strategy that is defined by the NIH as the translation of basic scientific discoveries into practical applications. It is the "process of turning observations in the laboratory, clinic, and community into interventions that improve the health of individuals and the public — from diagnostics and therapeutics to medical procedures and behavioral changes" (NIH, 2021b).

Translation research is part of translational science, which is "the field of investigation focused on understanding the scientific and operational principles underlying each step of the translational process" (NCATS, 2021). Basic research discoveries from the laboratory setting should be tested in studies with humans before application is considered. In addition, the outcomes from human clinical trials should be adopted and maintained in clinical practice. Translational research is encouraged by nursing and medicine to increase the use of evidence-based interventions in practice and to determine whether these interventions are effective in producing the outcomes desired (NCATS, 2021b; Norris et al., 2019; Reed et al., 2018; Weiss et al., 2018).

NCATS (2021) developed a model of the translational science spectrum, which presents it focus and goals (Fig. 13.8). This model represents the concepts and their interaction in the translational science spectrum at each stage of research along the path from the biological basis of health and disease to interventions that improve the health of individuals and the public. The spectrum is not linear or unidirectional; each stage builds on and informs the others. At all stages of the spectrum, NCATS develops new approaches, demonstrates their usefulness, and disseminates the findings. Patient involvement is a critical feature of all stages in translation.

The NIH (2021a) wanted to encourage researchers to conduct translational research, so the Clinical and Translational Science Awards (CTSA) Consortium was implemented in October 2006. The consortium started with 12 centers located throughout the United States and expanded to 39 centers in April 2009. The program was fully implemented in 2012 with about 60 institutions involved in clinical and translational science. The details for the CTSA Program are available at the following website: https://ncats.nih.gov/ctsa.

Initially the CTSA Program was focused on expanding the translation of medical research to practice. Therefore Westra and colleagues (2015, p. 600) developed "a national action plan for sharable and comparable nursing data to support practice and translation research." This plan provides direction for the conduct and use of translation research to change nursing practice (Norris et al., 2019). Organizations, such as the American Association of Critical Care Nurses, have identified translational research as a priority (Deutschman et al., 2019). Weiss et al. (2018) aligned translational research with EBP in achieving and maintaining Magnet status in hospitals. Dang and Dearholt (2018) detailed the importance of translation in facilitating evidence-based nursing practice at Johns Hopkins.

As you search the literature for relevant research syntheses and studies, you will note that translation studies are appearing more frequently. Wand and colleagues (2019, p. 10) conducted a "multi-site translation research project to implement and evaluate an innovative model of mental health nursing care in three EDs [emergency departments] in Australia." The researchers reported the following results from their translational study:

> There is incontrovertible evidence that the burden of mental health, drug health and behavioral problems in EDs is increasing. This necessitates the development of new models of care to meet mounting demands and support ED staff. However, implementing models of care that necessitate a significant change in workplace thinking and culture is complex and often messy. This multi-site pre-implementation study conducted as part of a larger translational research project illustrates how difficult transforming health care becomes when individuals place professional self-interest above improving service provision and the best interests of the public. Even with the weight of a solid evidence base, extensive consultation and significant high-level support, cooperation of key stakeholders is never guaranteed.
>
> (Wand et al., 2019, p. 15)

RESEARCH/EBP TIP

Translational studies are needed to promote the use of research findings in nursing practice and to determine the outcomes of EBP. However, national funding must be expanded to increase the conduct of translational and relevant outcomes studies.

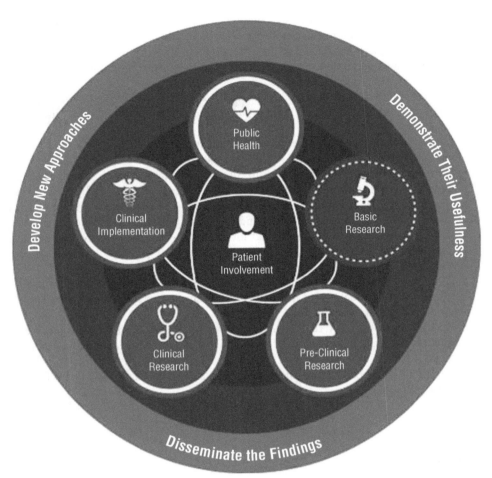

FIG. 13.8 National Science Spectrum. (From National Center for Advancing Translation Science. [2021]. *Translation Science Spectrum.* Retrieved from https://ncats.nih.gov/translation/spectrum.)

KEY POINTS

- EBP is the conscientious integration of best research evidence with clinical expertise and patient circumstances and values in the delivery of quality, safe, cost-effective health care.
- Best research evidence is produced by the conduct and synthesis of numerous high-quality studies in a health-related area.
- Nurses must be knowledgeable of the benefits and challenges associated with EBP.
- The PICO format is used to generate a clinical question to guide the use of current research evidence in practice.
- Guidelines are provided for critically appraising the research synthesis processes of systematic review, meta-analysis, meta-synthesis, and mixed methods research syntheses (MMRS).

- A systematic review is a structured comprehensive synthesis of the quantitative research literature to determine the best research evidence available to address a healthcare question.
- A meta-analysis is conducted to pool the results from previous quantitative studies statistically into a single quantitative analysis that provides one of the highest levels of evidence about the effectiveness of an intervention.
- A meta-synthesis is defined as the systematic compilation and integration of qualitative studies to expand understanding and develop a unique interpretation of study findings in a selected area.
- Reviews that include syntheses of various quantitative, qualitative, and mixed methods studies are often referred to as MMRS.
- The Stetler Model of Research Utilization to Facilitate Evidence-Based Practice provides a comprehensive framework to enhance the use of research evidence by nurses in practice.
- The Iowa Model of Evidence-Based Practice presents directions for implementing patient care based on the best research evidence and monitoring changes in practice to ensure quality care.
- Evidence-based guidelines developed for use in practice are described, and the guideline for the prevention, detection, evaluation, and management of high BP in adults is presented as an example.
- The Grove Model for Implementing Evidence-Based Guidelines in Practice is a series of steps nurses can use to determine the quality of evidence-based guidelines and to apply these guidelines in practice.
- EPCs, created by the AHRQ, have had an important role in the conduct of research, development of systematic reviews, and formulation of evidence-based guidelines in selected practice areas.
- Translational research is expanding in health care to translate basic scientific discoveries into practical applications.

REFERENCES

Agency for Healthcare Research and Quality. (2021a). *Research: Evidence-based practice centers (EPCs) program overview.* Retrieved from https://www.ahrq.gov/research/findings/evidence-based-reports/overview/index.html

Agency for Healthcare Research and Quality. (2021b). *Research: EPCs evidence-based reports.* Retrieved from https://www.ahrq.gov/research/findings/evidence-based-reports/index.html

American Nurses Credentialing Center. (2021a). *Find a Magnet organization.* Retrieved from https://www.nursingworld.org/organizational-programs/magnet/find-a-magnet-organization/

American Nurses Credentialing Center. (2021b). *Magnet model—creating a magnet culture.* Retrieved from https://www.nursingworld.org/organizational-programs/magnet/magnet-model/

Anderson, K. K., & Jenson, C. E. (2019). Violence risk-assessment screening tools for acute care mental health settings: Literature review. *Archives of Psychiatric Nursing, 33*(1), 112–119. https://doi.org/10.1016/j.apnu.2018.08.012

Beck, C. T., & Harrison, L. (2016). Mixed-methods research in the discipline of nursing. *Advances in Nursing Science, 39*(3), 224–234. https://doi.org/10.1097/ANS.0000000000000125

Bell, S. G. (2020). Evidence-based practice competencies for RNs and APNs: How are we doing? *Neonatal Network, 39*(5), 299–302. https://doi.org/10.1891/0730-0832.39.5.299

Beller, E. M., Glasziou, P. P., Altman, D. G., Hopewell, S., Bastian, H., Chalmers, I., ...PRISMA for Abstracts Group. (2013). PRISMA for abstracts: Reporting systematic reviews in journal and conference abstracts. *PLOS Medicine, 10*(4), e1001419. https://doi.org/10.1371/journal.pmed.1001419

Bergdahl, E. (2019). Is meta-synthesis turning rich descriptions into thin reductions? A criticism of meta-aggregation as a form of qualitative synthesis. *Nursing Inquiry, 26*, e12273. https://doi.org/10.1111/nin.12273

Bertolaccini, L., & Spaggiari, L. (2020). The synthesis of scientific shreds of evidence: A critical appraisal of systematic review and meta-analysis methodology. *Journal of Thoracic Disease, 12*(5), 3399–3403. https://doi.org/10.21037/jtd.2020.03.07

Butler, A., Hall, H., & Copnell, B. (2016). A guide to writing a qualitative systematic review protocol to enhance evidence-based practice in nursing and health care. *Worldviews on Evidence-Based Nursing, 13*(3), 241–249. https://doi.org/10.1111/wvn.12134

Champion, V. L., & Skinner, C. S. (2008). The health belief model. In K. Glanz, B. K. Rimer, & K. Viswanath (Eds.), *Health behavior and health education: Theory, research and practice* (4th ed., pp. 45–62). Jossey-Bass.

Chobanian, A. V., Bakris, G. L., Black, H. R., Cushman, W. C., Green, L. A., Izzo, J. L.,…National High Blood Pressure Education Program Coordinating Committee. (2003). Seventh report of the Joint National Committee on the prevention, detection, evaluation, and treatment of high blood pressure. *Hypertension, 42*, 1206–1252. https://doi.org/10.1161/01.HYP.0000107251.49515.c2

Chowdhury, S., Stephen, C., McInnes, S., & Halcomb, E. (2020). Nurse-led interventions to manage hypertension in general practice: A systematic review protocol. *Collegian, 27*, 340–343. https://doi.org/10.1016/j.colegn.2019.10.004

Chua, J. Y. X., & Shorey, S. (2021). Effectiveness of end-of-life educational interventions at improving nurses and nursing students' attitude toward death and care of dying patients: A systematic review and meta-analysis. *Nurse Education Today, 101*, 104892. https://doi.org/10.1016/j.nedt.2021.104892

Cochrane Collaboration. (2021). *Cochrane: Our evidence.* Retrieved from https://www.cochrane.org/evidence

Cochrane Nursing Care. (2021). *Cochrane Nursing: Resources.* Retrieved from https://www.nursing.cochrane.org/resources

Cocoman, A., & Murray, J. (2008). Intramuscular injections: A review of best practice for mental health nurses. *Journal of Psychiatric and Mental Health Nursing, 15*(5), 424–434. https://doi.org/10.1111/j.1365-2850.2007.01236.x

Cooper, H. (2017). *Research synthesis and meta-analysis: A step-by-step approach* (5th ed.). Sage.

Creswell, J. W., & Creswell, J. D. (2018). *Research design: Qualitative, quantitative, and mixed methods approaches* (5th ed.). Sage.

Creswell, J. W., & Plano Clark, V. L. (2018). *Designing and conducting mixed methods research* (3rd ed.). Sage.

Creswell, J. W., & Poth, C. N. (2018). *Qualitative inquiry & research design: Choosing among five approaches* (4th ed.). Sage.

Cullen, L., Hanrahan, K., Farrington, M., DeBerg, J., Tucker, S., & Kleiber, C. (2018). *Evidence-based practice in action: Comprehensive strategies, tools, and tips from the University of Iowa Hospitals and Clinics.* Sigma Theta Tau International.

Dang, D., & Dearholt, S. L. (2018). *Johns Hopkins nursing evidence-based practice: Model and guidelines* (3rd ed.). Sigma Theta Tau International.

Deutschman, C. S., Ahrens, T., Cairns, C. B., Sessler, C. N., Parsons, P. E., & Critical Care Societies Collaborative. (2019). Multisociety task force for critical care research: Key issues and recommendations. *American Journal of Critical Care, 21*(1), 15–23. https://doi.org/10.4037/ajcc2012632

Duncombe, D. C. (2018). A multi-institutional study of the perceived barriers and facilitators to implementing evidence-based practice. *Journal of Clinical Nursing, 27*(5–6), 1216–1226. https://doi.org/10.1111/jocn.14168

France, E. F., Cunningham, M., Ring, N., Uny, I., Duncan, E. A. S., Jepson, R. G.,…Noyes, J. (2019). Improving reporting of meta-ethnography: The eMERGe reporting guidance. *Psycho-Oncology, 28*(3), 447–458. https://doi.org/10.1002/pon.4915

Gallagher-Ford, L., Thomas, B. K., Connor, L., Sinott, L. T., & Melnyk, B. M. (2020). The effects of an intensive evidence-based educational and skills building program on EBP competency and attributes. *Worldviews on Evidence-Based Nursing, 17*(1), 71–81. https://doi.org/10.1111/wvn.12397

Gordon, C. (2021). COVID-19 vaccination: Intramuscular injection technique. *British Journal of Nursing, 30*(6), 350–353. https://doi.org/10.12968/bjon.2021.30.6.350

Gorsuch, P. F., Gallagher-Ford, L., Thomas, B. K., Melnyk, B. M., & Connor, L. (2020). Impact of a formal educational skill-building program based on the ARCC Model to enhance evidence-based practice competency in nurse teams. *Worldviews on Evidence-Based Nursing, 17*(4), 258–268. https://doi.org/10.1111/wvn.12463

Grainger, A. (2021). Critiquing a published healthcare research paper. *British Journal of Nursing, 30*(6), 354–358. https://doi.org/10.12968/bjon.2021.30.6.354

Gray, J. R., & Grove, S. K. (2021). *The practice of nursing research: Appraisal, synthesis, and generation of evidence* (9th ed.). Elsevier.

Grove, S. K., Burns, N., & Gray, J. R. (2013). *The practice of nursing research: Appraisal, synthesis, and generation of evidence* (7th ed.). Elsevier.

Harden, A., & Thomas, J. (2005). Methodological issues in combining diverse study types in systematic reviews. *International Journal of Social Research Methodology, 8*(3), 257–271. https://doi.org/10.1080/13645570500155078

Heyvaert, M., Maes, B., & Onghena, P. (2013). Mixed methods research synthesis: Definition, framework, and potential. *Quality & Quantity, 47*(2), 659–676. https://doi.org/10.1007/s11135-011-9538-6

Hickman, L. D., DiGiacomo, M., Phillips, J., Rao, A., Newton, P. J., Jackson, D., & Ferguson, C. (2018). Improving evidence based practice in postgraduate nursing programs: A systematic review. Bridging the evidence practice gap (BRIDGE project). *Nurse Education Today, 63*(1), 69–75. https://doi.org/10.1016/j.nedt.2018.01.015

Higgins, J. P., & Green, S. (Eds.) (2011). *Cochrane handbook for systematic reviews of interventions* (Version 5.1.0). The Cochrane Collaboration. Retrieved from https://training.cochrane.org/handbook/archive/v5.1/

Higgins, J. P. T., & Thomas, J. (2020). *Cochrane handbook for systematic reviews of interventions* (2nd ed.). Wiley Cochrane Series.

Iowa Model Collaborative. (2017). Iowa model of evidence-based practice: Revisions and validation. *Worldviews on Evidence-Based Nursing, 14*(3), 175–182. https://doi.org/10.1111/wvn.12223

Irvine, F. E., Clark, M. T., Efstathiou, N., Herber, O. R., Howroyd, F., Gratrix, L.,…Bradbury-Jones, C. (2020). The state of mixed methods research in nursing: A focused mapping review and synthesis. *Journal of Advanced Nursing, 76,* 2798–2809. https://doi.org/10.1111/jan.14479

Isseven, S. D., & Midilli, T. S. (2020). A comparison of the dorsogluteal and ventrogluteal sites regarding patients' levels of pain intensity and satisfaction following intramuscular injection. *International Journal of Caring Sciences, 13*(3), 2168–2179.

James, P. A., Oparil, S., Carter, B. L., Cushman, W. C., Denison-Himmelfard, C., Handler, J.,…Ortiz, E. (2014). 2014 evidence-based guidelines for the management of high blood pressure in adults: Report from the panel members appointed to the Eighth Joint National Committee (JNC 8). *Journal of the American Medical Association, 311*(5), 507–520. https://doi.org/10.1001/jama.2013.284427

Jiancheng, W., Jinhui, T., Lin, H., Yuxia, M., & Juxia, S. (2020). Has the reporting quality of systematic review abstracts in nursing improved since the release of PRISMA for abstracts? A survey of high-profile nursing journals. *Worldviews on Evidence-Based Nursing, 17*(2), 108–117. https://doi.org/10.1111/wvn.12414

Joanna Briggs Institute. (2021). *JBI EBP resources.* Retrieved from https://joannabriggs.org/ebp

Jones, E. P., Brennan, E. A., & Davis, A. (2020). Evaluation of literature searching and article selection skills of an evidence-based practice team. *Journal of the Medical Library Association, 108*(3), 487–493. https://doi.org/10.5195/jmla.2020.865

Kazdin, A. E. (2017). *Research design in clinical psychology* (5th ed.). Pearson.

Kim, M., Mallory, C., & Valerio, T. (2022). *Statistics for evidence-based practice in nursing* (3rd ed.). Jones & Barlett.

Lewin, S., Booth, A., Glenton, C., Manthe-Kaas, H., Rashidian, A., Wainwright, M.,…Nitesm J. (2018). Applying GRADE-CERQual to qualitative evidence synthesis findings: Introduction to the series. *Implementation Science, 13*(Suppl. 1), 2. https://doi.org/10.1186/s13012-017-0688-3

Liberati, A., Altman, D. G., Tetzlaff, J., Mulrow, C., Gotzsche, P. C., Ioannidis, J. P.,…Moher, D. (2009). The PRISMA Statement for reporting systematic reviews and meta-analyses of studies that evaluate healthcare interventions: Explanation and elaboration. *Annals of Internal Medicine, 151*(4), W-65–W-94. https://doi.org/10.7326/0003-4819-151-4-200908180-00136

Mackey, A., & Bassendowski, S. (2017). The history of evidence-based practice in nursing education and practice. *Journal of Professional Nursing, 33*(1), 51–55. https://doi.org/10.1016/j.profnurs.2016.05.009

McKenna, L., Copnell, B., & Smith, G. (2021). Getting the methods right: Challenges and appropriateness of mixed methods research in health related doctoral studies. *Journal of Clinical Nursing, 30,* 581–587. https://doi.org/10.1111/jocn.15534

MEDLINE (2021). *MEDLINE: Overview.* Retrieved from https://www.nlm.nih.gov/bsd/medline.html

Melnyk, B. M., & Fineout-Overholt, E. (2019). *Evidence-based practice in nursing & healthcare: A guide to best practice* (4th ed.). Wolters Kluwer.

Melnyk, B. A., Gallagher-Ford, L., Thomas, B. K., Troseth, M., Wyngarden, K., & Szalacha, L. (2016). A study of chief nurse executives indicates low prioritization of evidence-based practice and shortcomings in hospital performance metrics across the United States. *Worldview on Evidence-Based Nursing, 13*(1), 6–14. https://doi.org/10.1111/wvn.12133

Melnyk, B. M., Gallagher-Ford, L., Zellefrow, C., Tucker, S., Thomas, B., Sinnott, L. T., & Tan, A. (2018). The first U.S. study on nurses' evidence-based practice competencies indicates major deficits that threaten healthcare quality, safety, and patient outcomes. *Worldviews on Evidence-Based Nursing, 15*(1), 16–25. https://doi.org/10.1111/wvn.12269

Melnyk, B. M., Zellefrow, C., Tan, A., & Hsieh, A. P. (2020). Differences between Magnet and non-Magnet-designated hospitals in nurses' evidence-based practice knowledge, competencies, mentoring, and culture. *Worldviews on Evidence-Based Nursing, 17*(5), 337–347. https://doi.org/10.1111/wvn.12467

Moher, D., Liberati, A., Tetzlaff, J., Altman, D. G., & PRISMA Group. (2009*). Preferred reporting items for systematic reviews and meta-analyses: The PRISMA statement.* Retrieved from http://www.prisma-statement.org

Moore, F., & Tierney, S. (2019). What and how…but where does the why fit in? The disconnection between practice and research evidence from the perspective of UK nurses involved in a qualitative study. *Nurse Education in Practice, 34*(1), 90–96. https://doi.org/10.1016/j.nepr.2018.11.008

Moorhead, S., Swanson, E., Johnson, M., & Maas, M. L. (2018). *Nursing outcomes classification (NOC): Measurement of health outcomes* (6th ed.). Elsevier.

Moriarty, F., Pottie, I. K., Dolovich, L., McCarthy, L., Rojas-Fernandez, C., & Farrell, B. (2019). Describing recommendations: An essential consideration for clinical guideline developers. *Research in Social & Administrative Pharmacy, 15*(1), 806–810. https://doi.org/10.1016/j.sapharm.2018.08.014

Munn, Z., Dais, M., Tufanaru, C., Porritt, K., Stem, C., Jordon, Z.,…Pearson, A. (2019). Adherence of meta-aggregative systematic reviews to reporting standards and methodological guidance: A methodological review protocol. *JBI Database of Systematic Reviews and Implementation Reports, 17*(4), 444–450. https://doi.org/10.11124/JBISRIR-2017-003550

National Center for Advancing Translation Science (NCATS). (2021). *Translation science spectrum.* Retrieved from https://ncats.nih.gov/translation/spectrum

National Guideline Clearinghouse. (2018). *AHRQ: NGC to shut down July 16, 2018.* Retrieved from https://www.aafp.org/news/government-medicine/20180627guidelineclearinghouse.html

National Institute of Nursing Research. (2021). *About NINR: Mission & strategic plan.* Retrieved from https://ninr.nih.gov/aboutninr/ninr-mission-and-strategic-plan

National Institutes of Health. (2021a). *NIH: Clinical and translational research awards program.* Retrieved from https://ncats.nih.gov/ctsa

National Institutes of Health. (2021b). *NIH: National Center for Advancing Translational Scienc*e (NCATS). Retrieved from https://ncats.nih.gov/translation

Navarro, I., Soriano, J. M., & Laredo, S. (2021). Applying systematic review search methods to the grey literature: A review of education and training courses on breastfeeding support for health professionals. *International Breastfeeding Journal, 16*, 31. https://doi.org/10.1186/s13006-021-00373-5

Nicoll, L. H., & Hesby, A. (2002). Intramuscular injections: An integrative research review and guideline for evidence-based practice. *Applied Nursing Research, 16*(2), 149–162. https://doi.org/10.1053/apnr.2002.34142

Norris, A. E., Matsuda, Y., & Sarik, D. A. (2019). Implementing quality: Implications for intervention and translational science. *Journal of Nursing Scholarship, 51*(2), 205–213. https://doi.org/10.1111/jnu.12449

Ogston-Tuck, S. (2014). Intramuscular injection technique: An evidence-based approach. *Nursing Standard, 29*(4), 52–59. https://doi.org/10.7748/ns.29.4.52.e9183

Ost, K., Blalock, C., Fagan, M., Sweeney, K. M., & Miller-Hoover, S. R. (2020). Aligning organizational culture and infrastructure to support evidence-based practice. *Critical Care Nurse, 40*(3), 59–63. https://doi.org/10.4037/ccn2020963

Page, M. J., McKenzie, J. E., Bossuyt, P. M., Boutron, I., Hoffmann, T. C., Mulrow, C. D.,…Moher, D. (2021). The PRISMA 2020 statement: An updated guideline for reporting systematic reviews. *Systematic Reviews, 10*, 89. https://doi.org/10.1186/s13643-021-01626-4

Pappas, D., & Williams, I. (2011). Grey literature: Its emerging importance. *Journal of Hospital Librarianship, 11*(3), 228–234. https://doi.org/10.1080/15323269.2011.587100

Pintz, C., Zhou, Q., McLaughlin, M. K., Kelly, K. P., & Guzzetta, C. E. (2018). National study of nursing research characteristics at Magnet®-designated hospital. *Journal of Nursing Administration, 48*(5), 247–258. https://doi.org/10.1097/NNA.0000000000000609

Quality and Safety Education for Nurses (QSEN) Institute. (2020). *QSEN competencies: Definition* and pre-licensure knowledge, skills, and attitudes (KSAs). Retrieved from http://qsen.org/competencies/pre-licensure-ksas/

Reed, J. E., Howe, C., Doyle, C., & Bell, D. (2018). Simple rules for evidence translation in complex systems: A qualitative study. *BMC Medicine, 16*(1), 92. https://doi.org/10.1186/s12916-018-1076-9

Ruppar, T. (2020). Meta-analysis: How to quantify and explain heterogeneity? *Journal of Cardiovascular Nursing, 19*(7), 646–652. https://doi.org/10.1177/1474515120944014

Sandelowski, M., & Barroso, J. (2007). *Handbook for synthesizing qualitative research.* Springer.

Sandelowski, M., Voils, C. I., Leeman, J., & Crandell, J. L. (2012). Mapping the mixed methods-mixed research synthesis terrain. *Journal of Mixed Methods Research, 6*(4), 317–331. https://doi.org/10.1177/1558689811427913

Schnyder, J. L., Garrido, H. M. G., De Pijper, C. A., Daams, J. G., Stijnis, C., Goorhuis, A., & Grobusch, M. P. (2021). Comparison of equivalent fractional vaccine doses delivered by intradermal and intramuscular or subcutaneous routes: A systematic review. *Travel Medicine and Infectious Disease, 41*, 102007. https://doi.org/10.1016/j.tmaid.2021.102007

Sher, I. (2018). *Educational program for parents of neonates on nasal continuous positive airway pressure. Walden Dissertations and Doctoral Studies.* 4757. https://scholarworks.waldenu.edu/dissertations/4757.

Sisson, H. (2015). Aspirating during the intramuscular injection procedure: A systematic literature review. *Journal of Clinical Nursing, 24*(17/18), 2368–2375. https://doi.org/10.1111/jocn.12824

Speroni, K. G., McLaughlin, M. K., & Friesen, M. A. (2020). Use of evidence-based practice models and research findings in Magnet-designated hospitals across the United States: National survey results. *Worldviews on Evidence-Based Nursing, 17*(2), 98–107. https://doi.org/10.1111/wvn.12428

Stetler, C. B. (1994). Refinement of the Stetler/Marram model for application of research findings to practice. *Nursing Outlook, 42*(1), 15–25. https://doi.org/10.1016/0029-6554(94)90067-1

Stetler, C. B. (2001). Updating the Stetler Model of research utilization to facilitate evidence-based practice. *Nursing Outlook, 49*(6), 272–279. https://doi.org/10.1067/mno.2001.120517

Stetler, C. B. (2010). Stetler model. In J. Rycroft-Malone & T. Bucknall (Eds.), *Models and frameworks for implementing evidence-based practice: Linking evidence to action* (pp. 51–81). Wiley-Blackwell.

Stetler, C. B., & Marram, G. (1976). Evaluating research findings for applicability in practice. *Nursing Outlook, 24*(9), 559–563.

Straus, S. E., Glasziou, P., Richardson, W. S., & Haynes, R. B. (2019). *Evidence-based medicine: How to practice and teach EBM* (5th ed.). Elsevier.

Strohfus, P. K., Kim, S. C., Palma, S., Duke, R. A., Remington, R., & Roberts, C. (2017). Immunizations challenge healthcare personnel and affects immunization rates. *Applied Nursing Research, 33*, 131–137. https://doi.org/10.1016/j.apnr.2016.11.055

Tanganhito, D. D. S., Bick, D., & Chang, Y. (2020). Breast-feeding experiences and perspectives among women with postnatal depression: A qualitative evidence synthesis. *Women and Birth, 33*, 231–239. https://doi.org/10.1016/j.wombi.2019.05.012

Tatar, O., Thompson, E., Naz, A., Perez, S., Shapiro, G. K., Wade, K.,…Rosberger, Z. (2018). Factors associated with human papillomavirus (HPV) test acceptability in primary screening for cervical cancer: A mixed methods research synthesis. *Preventative Medicine, 116*(1), 40–50. https://doi.org/10.1016/j.ypmed.2018.08.034

The Joint Commission. (2021). *About The Joint Commission.* Retrieved from https://www.jointcommission.org/about-us/

Thomas, C. M., Mraz, M., & Rajcan, L. (2016). Blood aspiration during IM injection. *Clinical Nursing Research, 25*(5), 549–559. https://doi.org/10.1177/1054773815575074

Titler, M. G., Kleiber, C., Steelman, V. J., Rakel, B. A., Budreau, G., Everett, L. Q.,…Good, C. J. (1994). Research-based practice to promote the quality of care. *Nursing Research, 43*(5), 307–313.

Titler, M. G., Kleiber, C., Steelman, V. J., Rakel, B. A., Budreau, G., Everett, L. Q.,…Goode, C. (2001). The Iowa model of evidence-based practice to promote quality care. *Critical Care Nursing Clinics of North America, 13*(4), 497–509.

Todkar, S., Padwal, R., Michaud, A., & Cloutier, L. (2021). Knowledge, perception, and practice of health professionals regarding blood pressure measurement methods: A scoping review. *Journal of Hypertension, 39*(3), 391–399. https://doi.org/10.1097/HJH.0000000000002663

Tong, A., Flemming, K., McInnes, E., Oliver, S., & Craig, J. (2012) Enhancing transparency in reporting the synthesis of qualitative research: ENTREQ. *BMC Medical Research Methodology, 12*, 181. https://doi.org/10.1186/1471-2288-12-181

Trentadue, M. B., Rafter, D., Weiss, S., & Phelan, C. H. (2020). Utilizing an evidence-based practice approach to examining infusion therapy practices in non-hospital outpatient ambulatory clinic settings. *Journal of Infusion Nursing, 43*(6), 351–356. https://doi.org/10.1097/NAN.0000000000000394

Wand, T., Crawford, C., Bell, N., Murphy, M., White, K., & Wood, E. (2019). Documenting the pre-implementation phase for multi-site translational research project to test a new model emergency department-based mental health nursing care. *International Emergency Nursing, 45*(1), 10–15. https://doi.org/10.1016/j.ienj.2019.04.001

Wang, M., Zhang, Y., & Guo, M. (2021). Development of a cadre of evidence-based practice mentors for nurses: What works? *Worldviews on Evidence-Based Nursing, 18*(1), 8–14. https://doi.org/10.1111/wvn.12482

Warren, J. I., McLaughin, M., Bardsley, J., Eich, J., Esche, C. A., Kropkowski, L., & Risch, S. (2016). The strengths and challenges of implementing EBP in healthcare systems. *Worldviews on Evidence-Based Nursing, 13*(1), 15–24. https://doi.org/10.1111/wvn.12149

Weiss, M. E., Bobay, K. L., Johantgen, M., & Shirey, M. R. (2018). Aligning evidence-based practice with translational research. *Journal of Nursing Administration, 48*(9), 425–431. https://doi.org/10.1097/nna.0000000000000644

Westra, B. L., Latimer, G. E., Matney, S. A., Park, J. I., Sensmeier, J., Simpson, R. L.,…Delaney, C. W. (2015). A national action plan for sharable and comparable nursing data to support practice and translation research for transforming health care. *Journal of American Medical Informatics Association, 22*(3), 600–607. https://doi.org/10.1093/jamia/ocu011

Whelton, P. K., Carey, R. M., Aronow, W. S., Casey, D. E., Collins, K. J., Himmelfarb, C. D.,…Wright, J. W. (2018). 2017 Guideline for the prevention, detection, evaluation, and management of high blood pressure in adults: Executive summary: A report of the American College of Cardiology/American Heart Association task force on clinical practice guidelines. *Hypertension, 71*(6), 1269–1324. https://doi.org/10.1161/HYP.0000000000000066

Woods, S., Pillips, K., & Dudash, A. (2020). Grey literature citations in top nursing journals: A bibliometric study. *Journal of the Medical Library Association, 108*(2), 262–269. https://doi.org/10.5195/jmla.2020.760

14

Introduction to Additional Research Methodologies in Nursing: Mixed Methods and Outcomes Research

Susan K. Grove and Jennifer R. Gray

CHAPTER OVERVIEW

LEARNING OUTCOMES

After completing this chapter, you should be able to:

1. Provide a rationale for using mixed methods designs to address a research problem.
2. Describe pragmatism as a philosophical foundation for mixed methods research.
3. Distinguish between the quantitative and qualitative methods in mixed methods studies.
4. Describe mixed methods designs, such as convergent concurrent, exploratory sequential, and explanatory sequential.
5. Identify strategies to integrate quantitative and qualitative data in mixed methods studies.
6. Describe the challenges of conducting mixed methods studies.
7. Critically appraise a mixed methods study.
8. Identify the theoretical basis of outcomes research.
9. Discuss the history of outcomes research in nursing.
10. Describe the nursing-sensitive patient outcomes examined in outcomes research.
11. Discuss the structure, process, and/or outcomes examined in nursing outcomes studies.
12. Describe the role of outcomes research in determining the effects of nursing interventions and health services on patient outcomes.
13. Identify the methodologies used in published health outcomes studies.
14. Critically appraise nursing outcomes studies.

This chapter was developed to introduce you to mixed methods and outcomes research methodologies. These types of research have been conducted and their reports published more frequently in nursing since 2010. The content in this chapter was developed to provide you with a background for critically appraising mixed methods and outcomes studies. The first part of the chapter focuses on mixed methods research, followed by a discussion of outcomes research.

MIXED METHODS RESEARCH AND DESIGN

Clinical problems and their related research questions are frequently complex and multidimensional. Some researchers have studied these complex research questions by using quantitative and qualitative methods in the same study, an approach that is called mixed methods research (Creswell & Creswell, 2018; Tashakkori et al., 2021). Mixed methods studies allow researchers to capitalize on the strengths of numbers and words to answer different components or stages of a research question (Tashakkori et al., 2021). In this portion of the chapter, we describe some of the reasons why researchers select mixed methods designs and how they frequently base their studies on pragmatism as a philosophical foundation. You will also learn about different designs used in mixed methods studies, strategies used to integrate quantitative and qualitative data, some of the challenges of mixed methods studies, and how to critically appraise these studies.

Rationale for Conducting Mixed Methods Studies

Research methods must be selected to address the research question (Tashakkori et al., 2021). The research questions identified by nurses frequently address complex multilevel problems. For example, the *Future of Nursing 2020-2030* report has a clear message that nurses are uniquely positioned to address health inequities and promote improved health outcomes (National Academies of Sciences, Engineering, and Medicine, 2021). Health inequities are complex problems created or influenced by personal, cultural, religious, political, and environmental forces. As nurses and other healthcare professionals identify research questions related to health inequities, they may realize neither quantitative nor qualitative methods alone may provide adequate answers.

Health inequities are not the only complex issues nurses must address. Consider hypertension (HTN) management (see Chapter 13 for national HTN management guidelines). Antihypertensive medications may improve patients' blood pressure when the prescriptions are filled and the medications are taken appropriately. The lack of income or insurance can affect whether a prescription is filled. Beliefs about medications and unresolved negative side effects may also affect medication adherence. A research team developing a nurse-led intervention related to HTN may develop a mixed methods study to capture quantitative data about the number of pills taken and qualitative data about individual and contextual factors affecting those behaviors. Combining the two types of data provides answers that uniquely address both individual and contextual aspects of complex research questions.

📄 RESEARCH/EBP TIP

Mixed methods research is well suited to address complex clinical and policy problems. Collecting two types of data may generate deeper and richer findings for potential use in practice.

Philosophical Foundations of Mixed Methods Designs

Researchers who implement mixed methods studies base their research on values that are neither purely the objective post-positivistic view of quantitative researchers nor the subjective constructivist view of qualitative researchers. Researchers who use mixed methods designs have exchanged the dichotomy of objective and subjective approaches for the middle ground of pragmatism (Tashakkori et al., 2021). For our purposes, pragmatism is a philosophy that focuses on solving

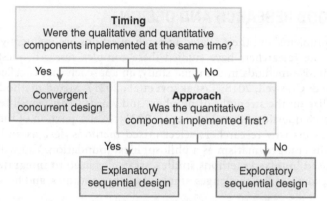

FIG. 14.1 Algorithm for Identifying Mixed Methods Designs.

problems by whatever methods fit the problem or question (Im, 2021). Pragmatists want to obtain the information that they believe they need to resolve an issue. With mixed methods designs, the researcher can allow the strengths of one method to compensate for the possible limitations of the other (Creswell & Poth, 2018). Stated in a more positive way, mixed methods research allows the strengths of each method to interact in a complementary way with the strengths of the other method. As an example, Browne and Braden (2020) conducted a mixed methods study to describe and quantify environmental turbulence in nursing practice, described as the interaction of unexpected changes and overlapping priorities of caring for multiple patients. Turbulence was identified as a confounding factor in measuring nursing workload, which is a necessary step in determining appropriate staffing levels and recognizing nurses' contributions to patient outcomes. Browne and Braden (2020) integrated the richness of nurses' descriptions (qualitative) and the objectivity of patient acuity, nurse/patient ratio, transfers, admission, and other quantifiable indicators to develop a comprehensive measurement method for environmental turbulence.

Overview of Mixed Methods Designs

When you read an article about a mixed methods study, notice whether the authors identified a specific design for the study. If they do not, your responses to the three questions in Fig. 14.1 will allow you to determine the design. The answers to these questions can result in a wide range of mixed methods designs. Mixed methods designs have been described and categorized in multiple ways. We focus in this chapter on three core designs commonly used in nursing and health research: (1) convergent concurrent design, (2) exploratory sequential design, and (3) explanatory sequential design (Creswell & Creswell, 2018; Tashakkori et al., 2021). Descriptions, diagrams, and example studies of these designs are provided to expand your understanding of mixed methods research. These core designs are frequently adapted to a study's research question or unique population.

Convergent Concurrent Design

The convergent concurrent design is selected when a researcher wishes to use quantitative and qualitative methods to confirm, cross-validate, or corroborate findings using a single sample or two samples from the same population (Creswell & Creswell, 2018). This design may also be called a *parallel design* because quantitative and qualitative data collection occur at or near the same time.

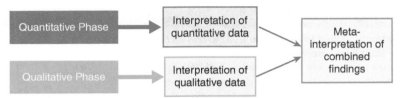

FIG. 14.2 Convergent Concurrent Mixed Methods.

The quantitative and qualitative data are analyzed separately and integrated during the interpretation phase. In Fig. 14.2, the rectangles on the top level represent the quantitative data collection and analysis processes, with the rectangles on the bottom representing the qualitative data collection and analysis processes. Notice that the results of the analysis are interpreted together. When the findings from the qualitative and quantitative methods yield the same findings, we call this *convergence*, which strengthens the evidence. When the findings from the two parts of the study are different, the researchers may be able to use the different findings to provide a broader description of the problem.

LoGiudice and Bartos (2021) recognized that the fears of infection, always-changing protocols, and repeated confrontations with death that nurses experienced in the first months of the coronavirus disease 2019 (COVID-19) pandemic were forces threatening the well-being of these nurses. The researchers recognized that multiple perspectives might more effectively describe the nurses' experiences, and they chose to use mixed methods. They selected a convergent concurrent design and used an online survey to explore nurses' resilience as they worked in critical care areas. Participants were recruited through websites and social media platforms for professional organizations. The American Association of Critical-Care Nurses posted a link to the online survey on their website (LoGiudice & Bartos, 2021). Research Example 14.1 includes excerpts from the study. The appraisal of the study's strengths and limitations follows the example.

RESEARCH EXAMPLE 14.1

After providing electronic informed consent, the participants completed a demographic form and then the 4-item BRCS [Brief Resiliency Coping Scale; Sinclair & Wallston, 2004] (quantitative data). ...They were asked to provide a written narrative in response to the request, 'As an acute care nurse working during the COVID-19 pandemic, please describe your experience of caring for your patients and for yourself. ...' Participants shared their experiences by typing their response in a free-text box (qualitative data). (LoGiudice & Bartos, 2021, p. 17)

Results

The final sample comprised 43 RNs. ...Participants had a mean age of 40.9 years (range, 23-64 years). ... Most nurses (n = 29) reported that patients with COVID-19 had died in their unit. (LoGiudice & Bartos, 2021, p. 18)

Discussion

In this study, we used narratives from nurses caring for patients with COVID-19 and their scores from the BRCS to form a robust picture of their experience and how these caregivers have been coping during the pandemic. Nurses working during the COVID-19 pandemic demonstrated medium resilience scores on the BRCS (mean score, 14.4). The qualitative themes from this study reflect both uncertainty ('What's the protocol

Continued

RESEARCH EXAMPLE 14.1—cont'd

today?') and certainty ('Proud to be a nurse'). ...Despite all that was happening, they continued to take pride in being on the front lines, showing up each day to provide care during the pandemic. They were especially empowered by the teamwork in which they and their fellow nurses engaged. On the other hand, the fear and the anxiety caused by constantly changing protocols, lack of research...and reuse of PPE [personal protective equipment] are examples of low resilient coping during a stressful situation. The qualitative thematic findings elucidate the medium mean resilience score for this sample of nurses. (LoGiudice & Bartos, 2021, p. 23).

In addition to the two themes identified in the excerpt, another theme related to how nurses were attempting to bridge the gap between patients and families, because the family members could not be with the patients. Other themes included "The never-ending 'sanitize' cycle" and "Restorative self-care" (LoGiudice & Bartos, 2021, p. 19).

A major strength of the study was that it was conducted during the COVID pandemic while the nurses' stressors were still being experienced. LoGiudice and Bartos (2021) also cited the mixed methods design as a strength. The limitations were the lack of racial and gender diversity and the small sample size for the quantitative portion of the study. The researchers are to be commended for timely implementation of a study that provided a unique insight into the experience of being a hospital nurse during a pandemic.

RESEARCH/EBP TIP

Mixed methods studies by representing multiple perspectives facilitate comprehensive descriptions of complex situations. Mixed methods studies can increase nurses' understanding of patients and family perspectives, a key component of implementing EBP.

Exploratory Sequential Design

The sequential designs provide the opportunity for results from the first phase of the study to shape the methods of the second phase (Gray & Grove, 2021). The exploratory sequential design follows that pattern. Qualitative data are collected and analyzed, followed by the researchers refining the methods for the quantitative phase. This strategy may be selected when researchers are initiating work with an understudied population or subgroup (Creswell & Creswell, 2018), hence the name *exploratory*. The researchers want to better understand the needs of the group and develop an intervention to address these needs. In the quantitative phase the researchers conduct initial testing of the intervention. Other researchers have used this design when measurement methods, such as a scale or survey, are lacking for a specific group. These researchers will explore the topic to be measured with the group, develop the instrument based on the group's input, and do initial testing in the second phase.

Fig. 14.3 provides a diagram of the stages of an exploratory sequential design. The left side of the figure begins with qualitative data collection followed by data analysis. The researchers use the findings of the first phase to refine the methods for the second phase, quantitative data collection and analysis. Ayoubi et al. (2020) conducted a mixed methods study with an exploratory sequential design in Iran to develop and refine an instrument to measure women's

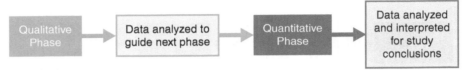

FIG. 14.3 Exploratory Sequential Mixed Methods.

perceptions of respectful maternity care (RMC). In some low-income countries, women may choose to give birth at home rather than endure possible disrespect and abuse from healthcare providers in hospitals. As part of an effort to improve maternal care, a reliable and valid instrument was needed to assess women's perceptions of the care they received (Research Example 14.2).

RESEARCH EXAMPLE 14.2

Literature review was followed by a qualitative study to elicit direct women's experiences of RMC. Three focus groups were conducted with 21 eligible women which were selected using purposeful sampling. The interview guide was created to facilitate the discussion, women were invited to talk about their actual and preferred labour and childbirth experiences. In this study the concept of RMC from the labouring women's perspectives was extracted in three main themes and seven sub-themes. (Ayoubi et al., 2020, Methods)

Review of the Women's Perspectives- Respectful Maternity Care [WP-RMCZ] by a panel of experts indicated very good content validity of the questionnaire. Evidence for construct validity of the questionnaire was obtained from exploratory factor analysis, which showed the stability of the three domains (Providing comfort, Participatory care, Mistreatment) and also demonstrated acceptable internal consistency. We therefore argue that this instrument is a useful tool for the assessment of subjective aspects of women's childbirth experiences and may be used for the evaluation of quality of childbirth care in maternity services. (Ayoubi et al., 2020, Discussion)

The WP-RMC questionnaire is a valid and reliable questionnaire for evaluating women's experiences of RMC that could assess subjective features of quality of childbirth care. This questionnaire can be used in maternity services trying to monitor and improve women's childbirth care experiences. (Ayoubi et al., 2020, Conclusion)

Ayoubi et al. (2020) achieved their goal of developing a measure of respectful maternal care. Another strength was the significant input of the women who comprised the target population. The researchers noted as a limitation that all testing was completed with women who had had normal vaginal deliveries. Future studies need to include women who had cesarean sections, complications, and other birthing challenges.

Explanatory Sequential Strategy

When using an explanatory sequential strategy, the researcher collects and analyzes quantitative data, and then collects and analyzes qualitative data to explain the quantitative findings (Fig. 14.4). The addition of qualitative data allows the quantitative findings to be expanded and put into context (Creswell & Clark, 2018). The nursing shortage continues to be a global problem, and little is

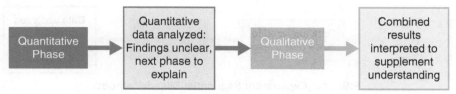

FIG. 14.4 Explanatory Sequential Mixed Methods.

known about why nurses leave the profession. In England, if a nurse does not work a specific number of hours each 3 years, he or she cannot renew their nursing registration (Garside et al., 2021). If the nurses decide to return to active practice, they are required to complete a return-to-practice (RtP) course. Garside et al. (2021) designed an explanatory sequential mixed methods study to understand the reasons the nurses in the RtP program left nursing and were now returning. Excerpts from the study are provided in Research Example 14.3.

RESEARCH EXAMPLE 14.3

A researcher-generated questionnaire was distributed to all students taking part in one of the RtP courses at the four collaborating institutions.... there were a total of 160 RtP participants.

The researchers administered a tool they developed to gather demographic and practice characteristics of the students. (Garside et al., 2021, p. 491)

A series of in-depth, semi-structured telephone interviews were conducted to explore the factors that influenced decisions to leave the profession (n = 20). Sampling for this phase was informed by phase 1 data, with selection from participants who had said in the questionnaire that they were prepared to be contacted for interview. (Garside et al., 2021, p. 492)

Two distinct categories of participants are apparent: those who left registered nursing practice for personal reasons through an unmanageable disequilibrium of their work/life balance; and those lacking the opportunity to advance in their career and maintain their nursing registration simultaneously. ... The finding of the current study that 83% of participants stay in employment during their vocational break raises the question of why so many participants felt forced to leave nursing, yet were adequately able to work in alternative employment during their absence from the profession. (Garside et al., 2021, p. 494)

Organisations and employers undoubtedly need to be more flexible and find creative solutions to demonstrate the valued contribution nurses make. ... This requires a greater understanding by policymakers and service managers of what motivates nurses to remain in practice. (Garside et al., 2021, p. 495)

The study conducted by Garside et al. (2021) described the unique perspectives of nurses who had left employment as a nurse. The researchers acknowledged, however, that the included nurses were likely different from nurses who had left but were not returning. Although a researcher-developed questionnaire is a limitation, Garside et al. (2021) minimized the limitation by seeking input from a statistician and an advisory group representing education, licensing bodies, and professional organizations. The identification of patterns of attrition and the effect of the type of setting on attrition were findings that can inform retention strategies of nurse employers.

> **RESEARCH/EBP TIP**
>
> Sequential mixed methods studies begin with the collection of either quantitative or qualitative data. These data are analyzed, and the results of the initial phase are used to refine the protocol and methods of the second phase. These studies generate evidence that may reflect patient values and perspectives more completely than either quantitative or qualitative studies.

Modification of a Core Design

Researchers often adapt the core mixed methods designs, previously introduced, to answer specific research questions. The study conducted by Browne and Braden (2020) that was mentioned earlier in this chapter was an example of a modified core design. Initially, Browne and Braden (2020) were interested in the workaround behaviors used by nurses related to safety technology. However, as they studied the effect of workarounds on workload, they found the current workload measures to be ineffective in capturing the unexpected events that increase work-related stress, such as troubleshooting broken equipment or assisting a new nurse with a combative patient. These unplanned, nonmeasured activities created what had been labeled by previous researchers as turbulence. The definition of turbulence, however, was unclear. Browne and Braden (2020) used an exploratory sequential design for their mixed methods study and then made modifications to achieve their goals.

After a thorough literature review, Browne and Braden (2020) collected qualitative data from key informants and local experts. The participants noted the need to collect additional examples of turbulence. As a result, the initial instrument was developed that included quantitative and qualitative questions. Instead of only quantitative data being collected in the second phase, Browne and Braden (2020) collected both and developed an initial instrument that was pilot tested with a small group of critical care nurses ($n = 19$). After revision, the survey was administered nationally with 296 respondents. Based on the analysis of the quantitative and qualitative data, the turbulence instrument was revised a second time. In the Conclusion of the study report, Browne and Braden (2020) proposed the next steps to be validity and reliability testing of the new instrument.

Challenges of Mixed Methods Designs

Teamwork

A team of researchers may be needed to develop and implement mixed methods studies. Ideally, the research team consists of health professionals who bring different perspectives, skills, and expertise (Creswell & Clark, 2018). However, a strong leader may be needed to balance these views and personalities into an effective team that produces rigorous studies. Additional time may be needed to develop the proposal and analyze qualitative data because of differing philosophical and conceptual beliefs.

Time Commitment

As you can surmise from the examples provided in this chapter, mixed methods studies require a longer time commitment than that required for single-method studies (Im, 2021). For example, the quantitative data collection for the Garside et al. (2021) study began in June 2015 and took 14 months. Once the quantitative data were analyzed, the interview prompts were developed and approved by an advisory group. Two researchers conducted the interviews, continuing until saturation was reached. To know they had reached saturation, the researchers must have been analyzing the qualitative data between interviews. The research report indicated it was accepted for publication by the journal in October 2020. Therefore the mixed methods study took at least 5 years to complete.

RESEARCH/EBP TIP

Mixed methods studies often require a team composed of researchers with expertise in collecting, analyzing, and integrating quantitative and qualitative data. Working with a team whose members have different views about research can be time-consuming, but the importance of the integrated evidence is worth the additional time and effort.

Funding

Complex research problems may require external funding to ensure the study is completed. Funding may provide salaries for the team leader and some members to dedicate most of their work time to a study. Even when that is not possible, funding may allow the research team to hire research assistants, statisticians, transcriptionists, and other personnel to complete some aspects of a study's work. When individual researchers conduct mixed methods studies, they may need additional funding to hire a consultant for the component of the study with which they are less familiar. Remember, however, that seeking funding is an additional step that adds more time to the research trajectory.

Combining Quantitative and Qualitative Data

Studies must be carefully designed to ensure congruence between the problem, purpose, questions, designs, data collection and analysis, and interpretation of the findings. Congruence of mixed methods studies can be especially challenging because quantitative and qualitative methods were founded within discrepant philosophies. Using pragmatism as an overriding philosophy, the motivation for the study and the desired outcome determine the best way to integrate the data of a mixed methods study (Tashakkori et al., 2021). Integration is the interface of the quantitative and qualitative data, which is what makes mixed methods designs unique (Creswell & Clark, 2018). Ideally, plans for integrating the data are part of the research proposal and may include building the second phase of the study on the findings of the first, expanding the view of a phenomenon, or strengthening support by interpreting the findings together.

Some researchers who use mixed methods designs advocate for converting the data from the qualitative phase to the same type of data that was generated by the quantitative phase, or vice versa (Cardoso et al., 2019). When this is done, qualitative codes may be counted and converted into quantitative data, or quantitative data may be converted to conceptual ideas or themes (Box 14.1). The capacity of mixed methods designs to answer the research questions depends on effective methods for integrating the data from each component.

Critically Appraising Mixed Methods Studies

Critically appraising mixed methods research begins with using the standards for quantitative and qualitative studies. The process also includes a component to assess the integration of the findings. The Mixed Methods Appraisal Tool (Hong et al., 2018) has become widely accepted. The mixed methods critical appraisal guidelines for this book reflect the criteria of the Mixed Methods Appraisal Tool, the qualitative critical appraisal guidelines in Chapter 3, and the quantitative critical appraisal guidelines in Chapter 8. The questions for the qualitative and quantitative phases of the study may be reversed to fit the study design. Building on your knowledge of quantitative and qualitative methods, learning how to critique mixed methods studies extends your capabilities as a scholar.

BOX 14.1 INTEGRATION STRATEGIES FOR MIXED METHODS DESIGNS

- Transform one type of data into the other
  - Count qualitative phrases that are the same
  - Count the number of qualitative participants who use the same phrase
  - Convert quantitative items to themes
- Contrast the results of the two phases
  - Side-by-side comparisons
  - Display jointly indicating similarities and differences
- Combine the results in a narrative
  - Present each quantitative result followed by related qualitative themes
  - Present the results of the two analyses followed by a paragraph with the combined meaning

? CRITICAL APPRAISAL GUIDELINES

Mixed Methods Studies

Introduction
1. Were the relevance and significance of the research question convincingly described?
2. Was an adequate rationale provided for using a mixed methods design (Hong et al., 2018)?
3. Was the specific mixed methods design identified?

Qualitative Phase
4. Was the qualitative approach appropriate for the research question?
5. How were the participants recruited for the qualitative phase?
6. How were the qualitative data collected and analyzed?
7. Did the researchers describe actions taken to ensure the accuracy of the data transcription and analysis?
8. Did the researchers provide participants' quotes to substantiate the themes or main ideas emerging from the analysis?
9. What were the strengths and weaknesses of the qualitative phase?

Quantitative Phase
10. Was the same sample used for both phases? If not, how were the participants for the quantitative phase selected?
11. Was there an intervention that was tested? If so, how was intervention fidelity maintained?
12. Were the measurement methods reliable and valid?
13. Were the appropriate statistical analyses used to answer the research questions?
14. What were the strengths and weaknesses of the quantitative phase?

Integration
15. If a sequential design was used, how were the results of the first phase analysis and its interpretation used to refine the methods of the second phase?
16. If a concurrent design was used, how were the results of the two phases integrated and interpreted to produce the findings?

Summary
17. What contributions to knowledge were made by conducting a mixed methods study, instead of two separate studies?
18. Summarize the strengths and weaknesses of the study.

Cardiovascular disease (CVD) is a major health problem in the United States and around the world. The prevalence of CVD is closely linked to diabetes and obesity, diseases whose prevalence continue to increase. A lack of self-care among persons with CVD can lead to poor health outcomes. However, initiating and maintaining self-care behaviors may be hindered by individual and work factors, because many persons with a CVD diagnosis continue to be employed, despite symptoms and limitations. Dickson et al. (2021) conducted a mixed methods study with persons, 50 years and older, who had been diagnosed with CVD and worked 35 hours or more per week for an employer (not self-employed). A sample of 108 participants completed seven quantitative instruments. In addition to sociodemographic variables, the researchers collected data to describe CVD self-care, organizational culture, job demands and security, supervisor and peer support, work-life balance, depression, anxiety, and physical functioning. From this sample, 40 persons were purposively selected who had a range of scores on the instruments. The researchers wanted to ensure that the qualitative sample had "maximum heterogeneity on specific attributes" that affected the study variables (Dickson et al., 2021, p. 448). Research Example 14.4 includes an excerpt from this mixed methods study followed by a critical appraisal.

RESEARCH EXAMPLE 14.4

Critical Appraisal of a Mixed Methods Study

Little is known about how older workers with CVD manage their conditions... within the context of employment. Thus, the purpose of this mixed methods study was to investigate the self-care practices of older workers with CVD and the relationship of organization of work...job-level factors...and self-care. ...Qualitative data about self-care within the context of work...were collected during tape-recorded interviews guided by a semi-structured interview guide. (Dickson et al., 2021, p. 447–448)

Data were integrated during the final stage of the analysis. In the first step of data integration, an informational matrix...was used to triangulate the qualitative data about self-care with the scores on the self-care instrument. ...Similarly, narratives of job-related characteristics elicited from the semi-structured interviews were compared with the JCQ [Job Content Questionnaire] results. ...Using these data integration techniques, results from the quantitative data were enhanced through the findings from the qualitative data to yield a broader perspective of the influences of self-care in this population. Methodological rigor...in this study was assured by using an audit trail, regular meetings with experts and member checking. (Dickson et al., 2021, p. 449)

This study uncovers the need for targeted self-care interventions that address the unique challenges of workers with CVD including balancing work, life and health demands. Our study results also suggest that there is an unmet workplace wellness need for older workers with CVD beyond current employer wellness programming that focuses on risk reduction. (Dickson et al., 2021, p. 453)

Critical Appraisal

Although the relevance and significance of CVD among older working adults was established, the rationale for using mixed methods was not clearly articulated. Dickson et al. (2021) described their study as being a convergent design. The participants for the quantitative sample were recruited from one urban area and from a website designed to nationally recruit research participants. The quantitative design did not include an intervention. The researchers reported satisfactory to high internal consistency coefficients in this sample for the instruments. There was no information provided about previous assessments of reliability and validity, which is a weakness of this phase (Waltz et al., 2017). With the number of instruments, the information may not have been included because of space limitations. Quantitative data were initially analyzed to ensure that assumptions for parametric analyses were met. Appropriate statistical analyses were used to answer the research questions (see Chapter 11; Grove & Cipher, 2020). The strength of the quantitative phase was the use of established instruments and the congruence of the conceptual and operational definitions.

For the qualitative data collection, the timing of the interviews was difficult to ascertain. However, because the methods of the qualitative phase were established before the study began, it is appropriate to call this a concurrent convergent design (see Fig. 14.2). The researchers clearly identified the methods of qualitative data collection, transcription, and analysis, including actions taken to ensure rigor. Participants' quotes were linked in a table to the qualitative themes of job control, workplace support, work-life balance, and organizational justice. The rigor of the qualitative phase was a strength. The only weakness identified was that most of the interviews were conducted by telephone and were relatively short (average of 42 minutes). However, the sample of 40 qualitative participants produced adequate data to address the narrow focus of the interview questions (Malterud et al., 2016).

In the integration matrix, additional quotes were included for each theme but differentiated in columns by whether the participant had adequate or inadequate self-care maintenance and adequate or inadequate self-care management. The participants' experiences captured in the interviews validated the quantitative findings and provided clarity for developing interventions to promote self-care in this population. Some details of the qualitative methods were missing, such as the timing of the interviews and who conducted them, but these might have been omitted because of the number of variables and three types of results (quantitative, qualitative, integration) to be reported in limited journal space. The strength of the study was the integration of the results of the two phases into a coherent whole.

📄 RESEARCH/EBP TIP

Mixed methods studies produce valuable, comprehensive, unique knowledge for understanding and managing patients and families with complex health problems. These studies provide nurses with expand perspectives in delivering EBP.

OUTCOMES RESEARCH

Outcomes research is a rigorous scientific method used to investigate the end results of health care. More specifically, health outcomes research is concerned with the effectiveness of healthcare interventions and health services (Barry et al., 2017; Kane & Radosevich, 2011). In the context of nursing, outcomes research focuses on how a patient's health status changes as a result of the nursing care received or the nursing services delivered (Moorhead et al., 2018). The outcomes of nursing care are the effects that people experience and desire, such as a change in their self-care ability or emotional status. For individuals with chronic conditions, for whom cure is not always possible, outcomes include quality of life, functioning, symptom management, depression, and mortality. The Agency for Healthcare Research and Quality (AHRQ, 2021) has a major role in promoting outcomes research to understand the end results of interventions and other healthcare practices. AHRQ supports the conduct and dissemination of outcomes research through the Patient-Centered Outcomes Research Institute (PCORI), which is discussed later in this chapter.

The momentum propelling outcomes research comes primarily from policymakers, insurers, and the public. They are basing payment for care on the economic efficiency of healthcare systems, especially the public health sector. As a result, there is a growing demand for data that document intervention effectiveness, justify the costs of care, and demonstrate improved patient outcomes. In that regard, nursing-sensitive outcomes have become an issue of increasing interest because of national concerns related to the quality of patient care (Moorhead et al., 2018). Because nurses are at the forefront of care delivery, the demand for professional accountability regarding patient outcomes dictates that we identify and document the outcomes influenced by nursing care.

The first part of this outcomes research section addresses the theoretical basis of outcomes research, provides a brief history of the emerging endeavors to examine outcomes, and explains the importance of outcomes research designed to examine nursing practice. The methodologies used in outcomes research are introduced to increase your understanding of these types of study and how the findings might be used in practice. This section on outcomes concludes with an introduction to guidelines that might be used to critically appraise outcomes studies. The movement to outcomes research and the approaches described in this chapter are a worldwide phenomenon (AHRQ, 2021; Barry et al., 2017; Kenner, 2017).

Outcomes research has similarities to quantitative research but is different in scope and design. Outcomes studies are more complex in design, populations, settings, and data analyses. The researchers engaged in outcomes studies are often from different disciplines, such as economics and public health, as well as from nursing and medicine. Health outcomes research is usually based on a theoretical framework by Donabedian (2005). This chapter provides only a brief introduction to the complex methodology of outcomes research so you might identify and critically appraise these studies focused on nursing care.

Theoretical Basis of Outcomes Research

The theorist Avedis Donabedian (1978, 1980, 1987) proposed a theory of quality healthcare and provided a process for evaluating it. This theory is still the dominating framework for outcomes research in healthcare disciplines. Other theories of outcomes have since been developed, but we will limit our discussion to Donabedian's theory. Although quality is the overriding construct of Donabedian's theory, his definition of quality was vague, "the balance of health benefits and harm" (Donabedian, 1980, p. 27). The Office of Disease Prevention and Health Promotion (ODPHP, 2020) and AHRQ (2018) expanded the definition of healthcare quality as the extent to which healthcare services provided to individuals and patient populations improve desired health outcomes. To achieve quality healthcare, the care must be safe, effective, patient-centered, timely, efficient, equitable, and consistent with current professional knowledge and practice.

Donabedian (1987) represented the key concepts and relationships in his theory using a cube. This cube, shown in Fig. 14.5, is used to explain the elements of quality healthcare. The three dimensions of the cube are health, the subjects of care, and the providers of care. The cube also incorporates three of the many aspects of health: physical-psychological function, psychological function, and social function. Donabedian (1987, p. 4) proposed that "the manner in which we conceive of health, and of our responsibility for it, makes a fundamental difference to the concept of quality and, as a result, to the methods that we use to assess and assure the quality of care."

Donabedian (1987, 2005) identified three foci of evaluation in appraising quality: structure (e.g., nursing units, hospitals, home health agencies, clinics), process (how care is provided, such as practice style or standard of care), and outcomes (end results of care). Each of these concepts is addressed in this chapter. A complete quality outcomes study requires the simultaneous inclusion of all three and an examination of the relationships among them. However, researchers have had little success in accomplishing this theoretical goal. Studies designed to examine all three concepts would require sufficiently large samples of various structures, each with the various processes being compared, and with large samples of study participants who have experienced the outcomes of those processes. The funding required and cooperation necessary to accomplish this goal have not yet been realized; however, there are examples of nursing research in which two or more

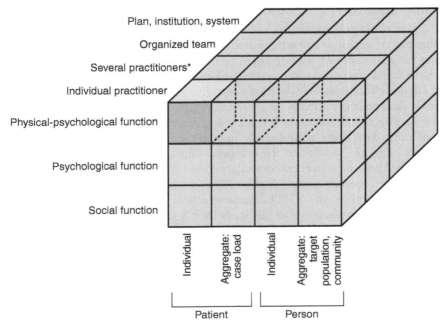

FIG. 14.5 **Level and Scope of Concern as Factors in the Definition of Quality.** *Of the same profession or of different professions.

aspects of structure, process, and/or outcomes have been examined. Numerous outcomes studies conducted by nurses in the United States (Wappel et al., 2021) and internationally (Chou et al., 2020) have explored the relationships among nursing services, nursing interventions, and patient outcomes. For example, Wappel and colleagues (2021) examined the effects of protein supplementation and mobility-based rehabilitation program on prolonged mechanical ventilation weaning success and increased discharge to home for patients with critical illnesses. These researchers reported that the program improved the prolonged mechanical ventilation weaning and discharge home rate. However, additional studies were recommended to examine the combined exercise and nutrition interventions.

Nursing services is a general concept referring to the organization and administration of nursing activities. Nursing service variables that have been studied include the skill mix and configuration of nursing personnel; staffing levels; assignment patterns; shift patterns; levels of nursing education, experience, and expertise; ratios of full-time to part-time nurses; level and type of nursing leadership available centrally and on units; cohesion and communication among the nursing staff and between nurses and physicians; implementation of clinical care maps; and the interrelationships of these factors (Lasater et al., 2021b; Moorhead et al., 2018). Lasater et al. (2021) studied hospital nurse-to-patient staffing ratios on patient outcomes. One of the coauthors of this study was Aiken, who is viewed as an expert and a leader in outcomes research.

📄 **RESEARCH/EBP TIP**

Nursing studies are focused on the effects of evidenced-based nursing interventions and services that improve health outcomes and promote the delivery of EBP.

Nursing-Sensitive Patient Outcomes

Nursing-sensitive patient outcomes (NSPOs) are considered sensitive because they are influenced by nursing care decisions and actions. It may not be caused by nursing but is associated with nursing. In various situations, *nursing* might be the individual nurse, nurses as a working group, the approach to nursing practice, the nursing unit or institution that determines the number of nurses, their salaries, educational levels of nurses, assignments of nurses, workload of nurses, management of nurses, and policies related to nurses and nursing practice. It might even include the architecture of the nursing unit. In whatever form, nursing actions have a role in the outcome, even though acts of other healthcare professionals, organizational factors, and patient characteristics and behaviors often are involved in the outcome. Think about the nursing interventions you have implemented and the influences they might have had on patient outcomes. Examples of NSPOs and their definitions are summarized in Table 14.1 (Doran, 2011; Moorhead et al., 2018). Chou et al. (2020) examined the NSPO adverse effects of using physical restraints with hospitalized older adults (see the discussion of this study later in this chapter).

The Nursing Role Effectiveness Model in Fig. 14.6 was developed to guide conceptualization and research related to nursing-sensitive outcomes. It also provided the theoretical basis for a systematic review of the "state of the science on nursing-sensitive outcomes measurement" (Doran, 2011, p. 15). Irvine et al. (1998) adapted Donabedian's (1987) theory of quality in their development of the Nursing Role Effectiveness Model. This model has three major components: structure, process (the nurses' roles), and patient and health outcomes.

Structure in outcomes research has three subcomponents: nurse, organization, and patient. Nurse variables that influence the quality of nursing care include factors such as experience level, knowledge, and skill level. Organizational components that can affect the quality of nursing care include staff mix, workload, and assignment patterns. Patient characteristics that can affect the quality of care and outcomes include health status, disease severity, and morbidity.

The process includes the nurse's role in outcomes, which has three subcomponents: nurse's independent role functions, nurse's dependent role functions, and nurse's interdependent role functions. The nurses' independent role functions include assessment, diagnosis, nurse-initiated interventions, and follow-up care. The patient and health outcomes of the independent role are clinical and symptom control, freedom from complications, functional status and self-care, knowledge of disease and its treatment, satisfaction, and costs (see Fig. 14.6). The nurses' dependent role functions include execution of medical orders and physician-initiated treatments. It is the dependent role functions that can lead to patient and health outcomes that are adverse events, such as infection, stroke, or kidney failure. Nurses' interdependent role functions include communication, case management, coordination and continuity of care, monitoring, and reporting. The interdependent role functions result in team functioning and affect the patient and health outcomes of the independent role. Patient and health outcomes are clearly interwoven into the entire care context (Irvine et al., 1998). This model can assist you in understanding the functions of nurses examined in outcomes studies.

Origins of Outcomes and Performance Monitoring

Florence Nightingale has been credited as being the first nurse to collect data to identify nursing's contribution to quality care by conducting research to examine patient outcomes (Magnello, 2010). However, efforts to collect data systematically to assess outcomes in more modern times did not gain widespread attention in the United States until the late 1970s. At that time, concerns about quality of care prompted the development of the Universal Minimum Health Data Set, which was followed shortly thereafter by the Uniform Hospital Discharge Data Set (Kleib et al., 2011). These

TABLE 14.1　NURSING-SENSITIVE PATIENT OUTCOMES AND DEFINITIONS

OUTCOME CONCEPT	DEFINITION
Functional status	Functional status is a multidimensional construct that consists of, at least, behavioral (e.g., performance of activities of daily living), psychological (e.g., mood), cognitive (e.g., attention, concentration), and social (e.g., activities associated with roles) components (Doran, 2011; Moorhead et al., 2018).
Self-care	Self-care behavior entails the practice of actions or activities that individuals initiate and perform, within time frames, on their own behalf in the interest of maintaining life, healthy functioning, continued personal development, and well-being (Moorhead et al., 2018; Orem, 2001; Sidani, 2011a).
Symptoms	"Symptoms refer to (a) sensations or experiences reflecting changes in a person's biopsychosocial functions, (b) a patient's perception of an abnormal physical, emotional, or cognitive state, (c) the perceived indicators of change in normal functioning, as experienced by patients, or (d) subjective experience reflecting changes in the biopsychosocial functioning, sensations, or cognition of an individual" (Sidani, 2011b, p. 132).
Pain	Pain has been defined as "the severity of observed or reported adverse cognitive and emotional response to physical pain" (Moorhead et al., 2018, p. 389).
Adverse outcome	An adverse outcome is defined as a consequence of injury caused by medical management or complication rather than by the underlying disease itself, and generally includes prolonged health care, a resulting disability, or death at the time of discharge (Doran, 2011).
Psychological distress	Psychological distress has been defined as "the emotional condition that one feels in response to having to cope with situations that are unsettling, frustrating, or perceived as harmful or threatening" (Lazarus & Folkman's work, as cited in Howell, 2011, p. 289).
Patient satisfaction with care	Patient "satisfaction with care outcomes describes an individual's perceptions of the quality and adequacy of health care provided" (Moorhead et al., 2018, p. 49).
Mortality rate	Mortality, in its simplest meaning, reflects death. "When examining death as a quality-of-care outcome, rates of death are examined for specific patient samples or populations" (Tourangeau, 2011, p. 411).
Healthcare utilization	"Healthcare utilization can be thought of as the sum or aggregate of services consumed by patients in their attempts to maintain or regain a level of health status, along with the costs of these services" (Clarke, 2011, p. 441).

data sets facilitated consistency in data collection among healthcare organizations by specifying the data elements to be gathered. The aggregated data were then used to perform an assessment of quality of care in hospitals and provide information on patients discharged from hospitals. However, those data sets did not include information about nursing care delivered to patients in the hospital. Without that information, the contribution of nursing care to patient, organizational, and system outcomes was rendered invisible. This major gap in information was addressed by the development of nursing minimum data sets in the United States and other countries worldwide (Werley & Lang, 1988).

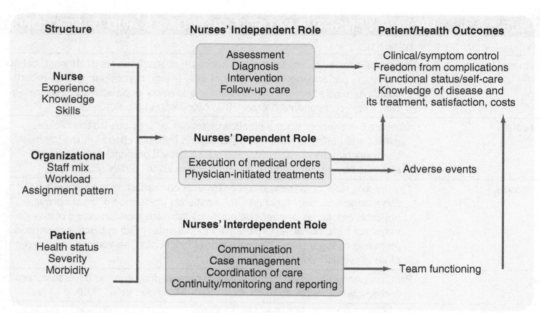

FIG. 14.6 Nursing Role Effectiveness Model. (From Donabedian, A. [1987]. Some basic issues in evaluating the quality of health care. In L. T. Rinke [Ed.], *Outcome measures in home care* [Vol. 1, pp. 3–28]. National League for Nursing; and Irvine, D. M., Sidani, S., & Hall, L. M. [1998]. Linking outcomes to nurses' roles in health care. *Nursing Economic$, 16*[2], 58–64, 87.)

National Initiatives in Outcomes Research

There are currently several outcomes' initiatives in the United States and internationally focused on the development of methods for measuring and reporting patient health outcomes. Some of the national outcome initiatives are briefly introduced, starting with the work of the AHRQ and followed by other examples of other nursing initiatives. These initiatives are paving the way for outcomes research by developing instruments and methodologies for examining patient outcomes and building large databases that are sources for outcomes research.

Agency for Healthcare Research and Quality

The AHRQ (2021), introduced earlier in this chapter, is one of the strongest supporters of research designed to improve the outcomes and quality of health care, reduce healthcare costs, address patient safety and medical errors, and broaden access to effective services. The AHRQ website (http://www.ahrq.gov) is a valuable source of information about outcomes research, funding opportunities, and results of recently completed research, including nursing studies.

An important AHRQ initiative is comparative effectiveness research that was initially funded by the American Recovery and Reinvestment Act (Recovery Act). This act allowed the AHRQ to expand its work in support of comparative effectiveness research, including enhancing the Effective Health Care Program. Grant money was designated for funding patient-centered outcomes research (PCOR) within the PCORI. PCORI (2021) "helps people make informed healthcare decisions, and improves healthcare delivery and outcomes, by producing and promoting high-integrity, evidence-based information that comes from research guided by patients, caregivers, and

---

BOX 14.2 AGENCY FOR HEALTHCARE RESEARCH AND QUALITY RESEARCH PORTFOLIO

- Clinical practice
- Outcomes and effectiveness of care
- Evidence-based practice
- Primary care and care for priority populations
- Healthcare quality
- Patient safety and medical errors
- Organization and delivery of care and use of healthcare resources
- Healthcare costs and financing
- Health information technology
- Knowledge transfer

---

the broader healthcare community." The number one funding priority for the AHRQ is improving healthcare quality by supporting the implementation of PCOR. PCORI (2021) has a broad research portfolio, outlined in Box 14.2, that includes almost every aspect of health care.

National Quality Forum

The National Quality Forum (NQF) was created in 1999 as a national standard-setting organization for healthcare performance measures. The NQF portfolio of voluntary consensus standards includes performance measures, serious reportable events, and preferred practices (i.e., safe practices). The NQF (2021) collection of measures, reports, and tools can be found online (http://www.qualityforum.org/Measures_Reports_Tools.aspx). Approximately one-third of the measures in NQF's portfolio are measures of patient outcomes, such as mortality, readmissions, health functioning, depression, and experience of care. The NQF includes several nursing-sensitive measures in its performance measurement portfolio. Those that were submitted by the American Nurses Association (ANA) under the National Database of Nursing Quality Indicators (NDNQI) are presented in Box 14.3. These indicators are the first nationally standardized performance measures of nursing-sensitive outcomes in acute care hospitals and have been designed to assess healthcare quality, patient safety, and a professional and safe work environment. Although most of the measures in use focus on the failure to meet expected standards, the NQF believes that quality is as

---

BOX 14.3 AMERICAN NURSES ASSOCIATION NATIONAL DATABASE OF QUALITY INDICATORS

- Nursing staff skill mix
- Nursing care hours per patient day
- Catheter-associated urinary tract infection rate
- Central line–associated bloodstream infection rate
- Fall and injury rates
- Hospital- and unit-acquired pressure ulcer rates
- Nurse turnover rate
- Registered nurse practice environment scale
- Ventilator-associated pneumonia rate

much about influencing positive outcomes as about avoiding negative outcomes. Therefore the NQF is currently developing national standards to evaluate the quality of health care based on how patients feel.

National Database of Nursing Quality Indicators

In 1994 the ANA, in collaboration with the American Academy of Nursing Expert Panel on Quality Health Care, launched a plan to identify indicators of quality nursing practice and to collect and analyze data using these indicators throughout the United States (Mitchell et al., 1998). The goal was to identify and/or develop nursing-sensitive quality measures. Donabedian's theory was used as the framework for the project. Together, these indicators were referred to as the ANA Nursing Care Report Card, which could facilitate benchmarking or setting a desired standard that would allow comparisons of hospitals in terms of their nursing care quality.

In 1998 the ANA provided funding to develop a national database to house data collected using nursing-sensitive quality indicators. This became the NDNQI (Montalvo, 2007). Participation in NDNQI meets requirements for the American Nurses Credentialing Center (ANCC, 2021) Magnet Recognition Program®, and more than 20% of database members participate for that reason. The data in the NDNQI have been transitioned and are now managed by Press Ganey (2021). Some of the NDNQI nursing-sensitive indicators and subindicators are summarized in Table 14.2; the measures are identified as structure, process, and/or outcomes. The relationships among the structure, process, and outcomes constructs are presented in Fig. 14.7.

The Collaborative Alliance for Nursing Outcomes California Database (CALNOC, 2021) was developed to house nurse-sensitive outcomes data. As with NDNQI, the CALNOC database was recently transitioned to Press Ganey (2021). The Centers for Medicare & Medicaid Services (CMS, 2021) Hospital Quality Initiative, American Hospital Association, Federation of American Hospitals, and The Joint Commission maintain databases that are also important resources for outcomes research.

Outcomes Research and Nursing Practice

Outcome studies provide rich opportunities to build a stronger scientific underpinning for nursing practice. More nurses are becoming involved in health outcomes research by collaborating with other healthcare professionals in conducting studies. Some universities focus on outcomes research, such as the University of Pennsylvania School of Nursing that has a Center for Health Outcomes and Policies. Ideally, we would like to understand the outcomes of nursing practice within a one-to-one nurse-patient relationship; however, in most cases, the nursing effect is shared because more than one nurse cares for a patient. In addition, nurse managers and nurse administrators have control over the nursing staff and the environment of nursing practice, and this control affects the autonomy of the nurse to implement practice. Consequently, outcomes research must first focus on how nursing care is organized rather than on what nurses do. Keep this in mind as you review outcomes studies in the nursing literature.

Evaluating Outcomes of Care

This section discusses approaches to examine structural variables, processes of care, and health outcomes. As introduced earlier, Fig. 14.7 demonstrates the relationship of structure and process that influences healthcare outcomes. Donabedian's (1987) theory requires that identified outcomes be clearly linked with the process that caused the outcome. Researchers need to define the process and justify the causal links with the selected outcomes in their studies. Desirable outcomes examined in outcomes studies need to address issues of concern to patients, such as long-term

TABLE 14.2 AMERICAN NURSES ASSOCIATION NATIONAL DATABASE OF NURSING QUALITY INDICATORS

INDICATOR	SUBINDICATOR	THEORY COMPONENT(S)
1. Nursing care hours per patient day[a,b]	a. RN b. LPN, LVN c. UAP	Structure
2. Patient falls with or without injury[a,b]	a. Injury level	Process and outcome
3. Pediatric pain assessment, intervention, reassessment cycle		Process
4. Pediatric peripheral intravenous infiltration rate		Outcome
5. Pressure ulcer prevalence	a. Community acquired b. Hospital acquired c. Unit acquired	Process and outcome
6. Psychiatric, physical, and sexual assault rate		Outcome
7. Restraint prevalence[b]		Outcome
8. RN education and certification		Structure
9. RN satisfaction survey options[a,c]	a. Job satisfaction scales: Full and short form versions b. Practice environment scale[b]	Process and outcome
10. Skill mix—percentage of total nursing hours[a,b]	a. RN b. LPN, LVN c. UAP d. Number of total nursing care hours supplied by agency staff (%)	Structure
11. Voluntary nurse turnover[b]		Structure
12. Nurse vacancy rate		Structure
13. Nosocomial infections	a. Urinary catheter–associated urinary tract infection[b] b. Central line catheter–associated bloodstream infection[a,b] c. Ventilator-associated pneumonia[b]	Outcome

[a]Original ANA nursing-sensitive indicator.
[b]NQF-endorsed nursing-sensitive indicator.
[c]The RN survey is annual, whereas the other indicators are quarterly.
ANA, American Nursing Association; *LPN*, licensed practical nurse; *LVN*, licensed vocational nurse; *NQF*, National Quality Forum; *RN*, registered nurse; *UAP*, unlicensed assistive personnel.

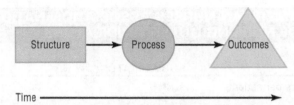

Time ————————————————————————————→

FIG. 14.7 Donabedian's Theory of Quality Focused on Structure, Process, and Outcomes. (Adapted from Donabedian, A. [2003]. *An introduction to quality assurance in health care.* Oxford University Press.)

symptoms or ability to conduct activities of daily living. In addition, the outcomes must be relevant to the goals of the health professionals, the healthcare system of which the professionals are a part, and society.

Outcomes are time dependent. Some outcomes may not be apparent for a long time after the process that is purported to have caused them, whereas others may be identified immediately. Some outcomes are temporary, and others are permanent. Did the researchers discuss these time elements in their study? Many factors other than health care may influence outcomes. For example, particular patient factors, such as the pathophysiology of the disease, treatment compliance, genetic predisposition to disease, age, propensity to use resources, high-risk behaviors (e.g., smoking, poor dietary habits, drug abuse), and lifestyle, must be considered. Environmental factors, such as air quality, public policies related to smoking, and occupational hazards, must be included. The responsibility for outcomes may be distributed among the providers, patients, employers, insurers, community, and governmental agencies. In critically appraising outcomes studies, you need to note any patient and environmental factors that might have influenced the study findings (Kane & Radosevich, 2011; Moorhead et al., 2018). For example, Binder et al. (2021) used Donabedian's model to guide the implementation of structure and process changes for the COVID-19 response in the emergency department (ED) of a suburban Westchester County hospital in New York. These changes were implemented to promote high-quality outcomes for the patients with COVID-19 and the safety of the ED staff. Binder et al. (2021) detailed the structure, process, and outcomes for their study in a model. Fig. 14.8 identifies the structures and processes of care implemented to promote quality outcomes for the patients and healthcare professionals in the ED.

Outcome studies include both proximal and distal outcomes. A proximal outcome is an outcome that is close to the delivery of care. An example of a proximal outcome is signs and symptoms of disease (Moorhead et al., 2018). A distal outcome is removed from proximity to the care or service received and is more influenced by external (nontreatment or nonintervention) factors than a proximal outcome. Quality of life is an example of a distal outcome. Moorhead and colleagues (2018) initially developed and continue to update the Nursing Outcomes Classification, an important source that identifies proximal and distal nurse-sensitive outcomes for research and practice.

Evaluating Structure of Care

The elements of organization and administration, as well as provider and patient characteristics that guide the processes of care, are referred to as the structures of care (see Fig. 14.7). You know that the organization of nursing care and nursing leadership influence nursing practice and, in turn, patient outcomes. These are called structural variables in Donabedian's (1987) Theory of Quality. For example, autonomy in clinical nursing practice is a structural variable, which is

Structure	Process	Outcome
Presence of waiting room nurse	Screening of patients, staff and visitors	Number of patients evaluated in emergency department
Presence of coronavirus hotline	Pre-arrival notification of PUIs	Number of patients tested for COVID
Presence of separate area of persons under investigation for COVID (PUIs)	Specific PPE guidelines for various care areas	Percentage of patients who left without being evaluated
Availability of UV-light pulsating robots	Environment cleaning	Number of daily sick calls
Capacity of infection-controlled care areas	Telehealth initiation and follow-up	Percentage of staff who are known to have contracted COVID
Use of negative pressure areas during high-risk aerosolizing procedures	Distribution of PPE	Return visits
Presence of outdoor screening tent	Daily communication to staff	Mortality
Availability of testing supplies	Provision of daily-use scrubs	Asymptomatic spread
Availability of personal protective equipment (PPE)	Testing criteria	Hospitalizations
Presence of critical airway team for intubation		Complications

FIG. 14.8 **Measures as Described Using the Donabedian Model.** COVID-19, coronavirus disease; PUI, person under investigation for COVID-19; UV, ultraviolet. (From Binder, C., Torres, R. E., & Elwell, D. [2021]. Use of the Donabedian Model as a framework for COVID-19 response at a hospital in suburban Westchester County, New York: A facility-level case report. *Journal of Emergency Nursing, 47*[2], 242. https://doi.org/10.1016/j.jen.2020.10.008.)

recognized as critically important to achieving positive patient outcomes. To achieve the Magnet hospital designation, the nurses in the facility must have autonomy, which empowers them to provide EBP to promote positive outcomes for patients and their families (ANCC, 2021).

In an outcomes study, researchers often discuss the administration and providers of care in their study setting. They might include leadership, organizational hierarchy, decision-making processes, distribution of power, financial management, and administrative decision-making processes. Nurse researchers investigating the influence of structural variables on quality of care and outcomes have studied factors such as nurse staffing, nursing education, nursing work environment, hospital characteristics, and organization of care delivery. For example, Lasater et al. (2021b) examined the effects of hospital nurse-to-patient staffing ratios and sepsis bundles on patient outcomes. Sepsis bundles are a set of evidence-based interventions implemented to prevent sepsis. The researchers noted that having a strong nurse-to-patient ratio resulted in lower within-hospital mortality, lower 60-day mortality, fewer 60-day readmissions, and reduced length of stay (LOS; see later in this chapter for a critical appraisal of this study).

In evaluating structures, the unit of measure is the structure. The evaluation requires access to a sufficiently large sample of *like* structures, with similar processes and outcomes, which can then be compared with a sample of another structure providing the same processes and examining the same outcomes. For example, nurse researchers have examined different structures for providing primary health care, such as the private physician office, community-oriented primary care clinic, rural clinics, and nurse-managed center. Alternatively, nurse researchers might examine nursing care provided in structures of private hospitals, county hospital, and teaching hospitals associated with a health science center. In each of these examples, the focus of research would be the effect of structure on the processes and outcomes of care. For example, Lasater et al. (2021a, p. 46) conducted an outcomes study to "compare surgical patient outcomes and costs in hospitals with better versus worse nursing resources and to determine if value differs across these hospitals for patients with different mortality risks." Nursing resources were defined as patient-to-nurse ratios, skill mix, proportions of nurses with bachelor's degrees, and nurses' work environment.

In the United States, nursing homes, home healthcare agencies, and hospitals are required to collect quality variables that have been defined precisely and measured in specific ways and to report them to the federal government. This mandate was established because of considerable variation in the quality of care in these structures. Various government agencies analyze the quality of these structures so they can adequately oversee the quality of care provided to the US public. These data are made available to the public so that individuals can make their own determination of the quality of care provided by various nursing homes, home healthcare agencies, and hospitals. Researchers can also access these data for studies of the quality of various structures. To access these data on the internet, you can search using the phrases "nursing home compare," "home health compare," and "hospital compare." In addition to being able to select a specific hospital, nursing home, or home healthcare agency, you can access considerable information about quality related to each of these structures of health care.

Evaluating Process of Care

Clinical management or the process of care implemented by nurses was more of an art than a science until EBP was emphasized (Melnyk & Fineout-Overholt, 2019; Melnyk et al., 2020). There are multiple components of clinical management, many of which have not yet been clearly defined or tested. Three components of process that are of interest are standards of care, practice styles, and costs of care. Standards of care and practice styles are included in the following subsections, but costs of care are discussed later in this chapter.

Standards of care. A standard of care is a norm on which quality of care is judged. Clinical guidelines, critical paths, care maps, and care bundles define standards of care for specific situations. In that regard, Donabedian (1982, 1987, 1988) and other researchers have recommended the development of specific criteria to be used as a basis for judging the quality of care. These criteria may take the form of clinical guidelines or care maps based on evidence that the care contributed to the desired outcomes. The clinical guidelines published by the AHRQ established norms or standards against which the validity of clinical management can be judged. These norms are now based on clinical practice guidelines available through a variety of professional organizations, such as the Oncology Nursing Society (2021), and governmental agencies, such as the Centers for Disease Control and Prevention (CDC, 2021) and the CMS (2020).

Practice styles, practice patterns, and evidence-based practice. The style of a nurse's practice is another dimension of the process of care that influences quality; however, judging what constitutes goodness in style and justifying the decisions made regarding it is very difficult. Practice pattern is a concept closely related to practice style. Practice style represents variations in how care is provided, whereas practice pattern represents variations in what care is provided. As discussed earlier, Chou et al. (2020) examined the adverse effects of using physical restraints (practice pattern) among older hospitalized adults.

📄 **RESEARCH/EBP TIP**

EBP is another dimension of the process of care that is considered a critical aspect of professional practice. The goal of EBP is the delivery of quality health care to improve patient outcomes that are documented through outcomes research.

Methodologies for Outcomes Studies

Outcomes research methodologies have been developed to link the care that people receive with the results they experience, thereby providing better ways to monitor and improve the quality of care (Donabedian, 2003, 2005). This section describes some of the current methodologies used in conducting outcomes research, including sampling methods, research strategies or designs, measurement processes, and statistical approaches. These descriptions were developed to provide a broad overview of the methodologies that you will see in outcomes studies. This knowledge will help you understand and critically appraise the methodologies used in these studies. For additional information, you can refer to the citations in each section and to other sources of outcomes research (Barry et al., 2017; Doran, 2011; Gray & Grove, 2021; Kane & Radosevich, 2011; Moorhead et al., 2018). Outcomes studies cross a variety of disciplines; therefore the emerging methodologies are being enriched by a cross-pollination of ideas, some of which are new to nursing research.

Samples and Sampling

The preferred methods of obtaining samples are different in outcomes studies. Random sampling is seldom used, with the exception of a randomized controlled trial (RCT), when a specific intervention or healthcare service is being evaluated. Usually, heterogeneous samples (with varied types of patients), rather than homogeneous samples (with similar patients), are obtained in outcomes research. Outcome researchers limit sampling criteria to obtain large, heterogeneous samples that reflect, as much as possible, all patients who would be receiving care in a real healthcare context. For example, samples need to include patients with various comorbidities and patients with varying levels of health status. In addition, individuals should be identified who do not receive nursing or medical treatment for their condition, because they may represent those who refuse treatment or who do not access the healthcare system.

Devising ways to evaluate the representativeness of such samples is problematic. For a sample to be representative, it must be as much like the target population as possible, particularly in relation to the variables being studied (see Chapter 9). Because the target population in outcomes research is often heterogeneous, there are many variables for which sample representativeness needs to be determined. Another challenge in outcomes research is to develop strategies for locating untreated individuals and including them in follow-up studies. The intent is to determine whether outcomes differ between those treated and those untreated. To address some of these challenges, outcomes researchers have used large databases as sample sources in observational research designs.

Large databases as sample sources. One source of samples for outcomes studies is large databases. As illustrated in Fig. 14.9, two broad categories of database emerge from patient care

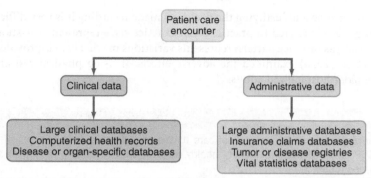

FIG. 14.9 Types of database emanating from patient care encounters. (Adapted from Gray, J. R., & Grove, S. K. [2021]. *The practice of nursing research: Appraisal, synthesis, and generation of evidence* [9th ed.]. Elsevier.)

encounters, clinical databases and administrative databases. Clinical databases are created by providers, such as hospitals, health maintenance organizations, accountable care organizations, and healthcare professionals. The clinical data are generated through routine documentation of care in the electronic health record or in relation to a research protocol. Some databases have been developed to gather data related to a specific disease, such as heart failure or breast cancer. With a clinical database, you can link observations made by many nurses over long periods to patient outcomes.

Administrative databases are created by insurance companies, government agencies, and others not directly involved in providing patient care. Administrative databases have standardized sets of data for enormous numbers of patients and providers. An example is the Medicare database managed by the CMS (2021). The administrative databases can be used to determine the incidence or prevalence of disease, geographical variations in medical care use, characteristics of medical care, and outcomes of care. Initiatives such as NQF, CALNOC, and NDNQI have made nursing data more accessible for large database research.

Common Study Designs Used in Outcomes Research

Although RCTs are considered the gold standard for clinical research, most outcomes studies use quasi-experimental or observational research designs, which are suitable for addressing questions of effectiveness and efficiency. Like RCTs, outcomes research sometimes seeks to provide evidence about which interventions work best for which types of patients and under what circumstances. However, the *intervention* being evaluated is not limited to medications or new clinical procedures but may also include the provision of social services and resources, or even the enforcing of specific policies and regulations by legislative and financial bodies. Outcomes researchers often consider additional parameters, such as cost, timeliness, convenience, geographical accessibility, and patient preferences. Outcomes studies frequently are not clearly identified in the research literature. Therefore common types of design used in outcomes research are briefly discussed to increase your ability to recognize and appraise these studies.

Prospective cohort studies. A prospective cohort study uses an epidemiological study design in which the researcher identifies a group of people who are at risk for experiencing a particular event and then follows the group over time to observe whether the event occurs. Sample sizes for these studies need to be extremely large, particularly if only a small portion of the at-risk group will experience the event. The entire group is followed over time to determine the point at which the event occurs (such as a fall), variables associated with the event, and outcomes for those who experienced the event in comparison with those who did not.

Liu (2021) implemented a prospective cohort design to determine the effects of simulation on nursing students' beliefs about prognosis and long-term outcomes for individuals with mental health conditions. The National League for Nursing (2020) and other nursing organizations have recommended expanding the focus on managing patients with mental illness in nursing curricula. In this study a virtual simulation mental health intervention, structured using videos and a protocol, was implemented to expand nursing students' knowledge in this area. The abstract from this study is presented in Research Example 14.5.

🔬 RESEARCH EXAMPLE 14.5

Prospective Cohort Study

Research/Study Excerpt
Abstract

Background: *Virtual simulation as an emerging technology is thought to be most amenable to mental health nursing education. This study aims to evaluate the effects of virtual simulation on undergraduate nursing students' beliefs about prognosis and long-term outcomes for people with depression and schizophrenia.*

Methods: *A prospective cohort design was used in this study. Students' responses were compared between the simulation cohort (n = 149) and the nonsimulation cohort (n = 150) at a school of nursing in the United States.*

Results: *Nursing students developed a greater insight into the prognosis of people with depression after receiving virtual simulation. Furthermore, virtual simulation increased nursing students' optimistic beliefs about the long-term outcomes for people with depression and decreased their pessimistic beliefs about the long-term outcomes for people with schizophrenia.*

Conclusions: *Virtual simulation can be used as an effective experiential learning tool to foster undergraduate nursing students' positive beliefs about and attitudes toward mental illness.* (Liu, 2021, p. 1)

Critical Appraisal
Liu (2021) clearly indicated that a prospective cohort design was used to conduct her study. This design was appropriate to address the aims identified in this outcomes study. The findings from this study were positive, but Liu (2021) reported delays in data collection that could have influenced the study results. Therefore she recommended that the findings not be generalized to other nursing students before additional studies are conducted in this area.

Retrospective cohort studies. A retrospective cohort study includes an epidemiological study design in which the researcher identifies a group of people who have experienced a particular event. This is a common research technique used in the field of epidemiology to study occupational exposure to chemicals. Events of interest to nursing that could be studied in this manner include a procedure, episode of care, nursing intervention, and/or diagnosis. Nurses might use a retrospective cohort study to examine the outcome of a cohort of women who had undergone a mastectomy for whom a urinary bladder catheter was placed during surgery. The cohort is evaluated after the event to determine the occurrence of changes in health status. Nurses are interested in the pattern of recovery after an event or, in the case of catheterization, the incidence of bladder infections in the months after surgery.

On the basis of the study findings, researchers calculate the relative risk of the identified change in health for the group. Relative risk is the probability of the outcome occurring in the exposed group versus the probability of the outcome in the unexposed (control) group. For example, if death were the occurrence of interest, the expected number of deaths would be determined. The observed number of deaths divided by the expected number of deaths and multiplied by 100 yields a standardized mortality ratio (SMR), which is regarded as a measure of the relative risk of the studied group to die of a specific condition (Grove & Cipher, 2020). In nursing studies, patients might be followed over time after discharge from a healthcare facility to determine complication rates and the SMR. An extensive number of outcomes studies have been conducted focused on exposure to COVID-19, incidence of the disease after exposure, and the SMR for those hospitalized with COVID-19.

In retrospective cohort studies, researchers commonly ask patients to recall information relevant to their previous health status. This information is often used to determine the amount of change occurring before and after an intervention. Recall can easily be distorted, thereby misleading researchers in determining outcomes. Some sources of recall distortion include (1) the question posed to the study participant may be conceived or expressed incorrectly; (2) the recall process may be in error; and (3) the measurement of recall may result in the recall appearing to be different from what occurred (Herrmann, 1995). You need to examine closely the data collection process in outcomes studies that include participant recall.

Chou and colleagues (2020) conducted an outcomes study to examine the adverse effects of restraint use among hospitalized elderly patients. The researchers provided a detailed definition of physical restraints to accurately determine what proportion of the patients met the criteria for being restrained. The abstract from this study is presented in Research Example 14.6.

RESEARCH EXAMPLE 14.6

Retrospective Cohort Study

Research/Study Excerpt

Abstract

Objectives: To evaluate the negative effect of physical restraint use on the hospital outcomes of older patients.

Design: A retrospective cohort study.

Setting: Internal medicine wards of a tertiary medical center in Taiwan.

Participants: Subjects aged 65 years and over who were admitted during April to Dec 2017 were recruited for study.

Measurements: Demographic data, geriatric assessments (polypharmacy, visual impairment, hearing impairment, activities of daily living before and after admission, risk of pressure ulcers, change in consciousness level, mood condition, history of falls in the previous year, risk of malnutrition and pain) and hospital conditions (admission route, department of admission, length of hospital stay and mortality) were collected for analysis.

Results: Overall, 4,352 participants (mean age 78.7 ± 8.7 years, 60.2% = male) were enrolled and 8.3% had physical restraint. Results of multivariate logistic regression showed that subjects with physical restraints were at greater risk of functional decline (adjusted odds ratio 2.136, 95% confidence interval 1.322-3.451, $p = 0.002$), longer hospital stays (adjusted odds ratio 5.360, 95% confidence interval 3.627-7.923, $p < 0.001$) and mortality (adjusted odds ratio 4.472, 95% confidence interval 2.794-7.160, $p < 0.001$) after adjustment for covariates.

Conclusion: The use of physical restraints during hospitalization increased the risk of adverse hospital outcomes, such as functional decline, longer length of hospital stay and mortality. (Chou et al., 2020, p. 160)

Critical Appraisal

Chou and colleagues (2020) reported they had conducted a hospital-based retrospective cohort study in the article title, abstract, and Methods section. The final sample size reported in the abstract ($N = 4352$) was inconsistent with the sample reported in the Results section ($n = 3460$). In addition, the physical restraint incidence was reported to be 8.3% in the abstract and 5.4% in the Results section. This inconsistent reporting of information decreases the confidence in the findings (Gray & Grove, 2021). The outcomes were LOS, functional decline, and mortality, which were appropriate for this study and precisely measured. The adverse outcomes were significantly affected when physical restraints were used, which supports reducing restraint use in hospitalized elderly patients. The limitations identified included (1) the incidence of restraint use was underestimated in the sample and (2) only patients in internal medicine were included in the study. Patients in intensive care units were not included in the study, so these findings cannot be generalized to patients in intensive care units or other areas not studied.

Population-based studies. Population-based studies are conducted within the context of the patient's community rather than the context of the medical system. With this method, all cases of a condition occurring in the defined population are included, not just the cases treated at a particular healthcare facility. The latter could introduce a selection bias. To avoid selection bias, the researcher might make efforts to include individuals with the condition who had not received treatment.

Community-based norms of tests and survey instruments obtained in this manner provide a clearer picture of the range of values than the limited spectrum of patients seen in specialty clinics. Estimates of instrument sensitivity and specificity are more accurate (see Chapter 10). This method enables researchers to understand the natural history of a condition or the long-term risks and benefits of a specific intervention (Doran, 2011; Kane & Radosevich, 2011).

Economic studies. Many of the problems studied in outcomes research address concerns related to the efficient use of scarce resources and thus to economics. Health economists are concerned with the costs and benefits of alternative treatments or ways of identifying the most efficient means of care. Economic evaluation has been defined as a "set of formal, quantitative methods used to compare two or more treatments, programs, or strategies with respect to their resource use and their expected outcomes" (Guyatt et al., 2015, p. 781). An economist defines the term *efficiency* as the least expensive method of achieving a desired end while obtaining the maximum benefit, or outcome, from available resources. If available resources must be shared with other programs or other types of patient, an economic study can determine whether changing the distribution of resources will increase the total benefit or welfare.

Measurement Methods

The selection of appropriate outcome variables is critical to the success of an outcomes study. As in any study, the researcher must evaluate the evidence of validity and reliability of the measurement methods. Outcomes selected for nursing studies should be those most consistent with nursing practice and theory (Moorhead et al., 2018). In some studies, rather than selecting the final outcome of care, which may not occur for months or years, researchers use measures of intermediate endpoints or proximal outcomes. Intermediate endpoints are events or markers that act as precursors to the final outcome. It is important, however, to document the validity of the intermediate endpoint in predicting the outcome. In early outcomes studies, researchers selected outcome measures that they could easily obtain, rather than those most desirable for an outcomes study. Later outcome studies selected outcome measures from secondary data sources. This selection involves secondary analysis, which is any reanalysis of data or information collected by other researchers, organizations, or agencies (see Chapter 10; Gray & Grove, 2021), which can be unreliable depending on the initial data collection.

As discussed earlier, most outcomes researchers obtain their study data from clinical and administrative databases. When critically appraising an outcomes study, you need to assess the quality of the databases used for data collection. For other measurement methods used in outcomes study, the reliability, validity, and sensitivity of the instruments should be appraised and summarized (see Chapter 10). Sensitivity to change is an important measurement property to consider in outcomes research because researchers are often interested in evaluating how outcomes change in response to healthcare interventions (Polit & Yang, 2016). As the sensitivity of a measure increases, statistical power increases, allowing smaller sample sizes to detect significant differences (Bandalos, 2018; Grove & Cipher, 2020; Waltz et al., 2017).

Statistical Methods for Outcomes Studies

Although outcomes researchers test for the statistical significance of their findings, that evaluation is not considered enough to judge the findings as important. Their focus is the clinical importance of study findings (see Chapter 11). In analyzing data, outcomes researchers have moved away from statistical analyses that use the mean to test for group differences. They now place greater importance on analyzing change scores and use exploratory methods for examining the data to identify outliers.

Analysis of Change

With the focus on outcomes studies has come a renewed interest in methods of analyzing change. Harris's (1967) text is the basis for most of the current approaches to analyzing change. However, some new ideas have emerged regarding the analysis of change (Polit & Yang, 2016). For some outcomes, the changes may be nonlinear or may go up and down, rather than always increasing. Therefore, it is as important to uncover patterns of change as it is to test for statistically significant differences at various time points. Some changes may occur in relation to stages of recovery or improvement. These changes may occur over weeks, months, or even years. A more complete picture of the process of recovery is obtained by examining the process in greater detail and over a broader range. In reading outcomes studies, you might note that the researchers developed a recovery curve, which provides a model of the recovery process.

Analysis of Improvement

In addition to reporting the mean improvement score for all patients treated, it is important to report what percentage of patients improved. Did all patients improve slightly, or is there a divergence among patients, with some improving greatly and others not improving at all? This divergence may best be illustrated by plotting the data. Researchers studying a specific treatment or approach to care might develop a standard or index of varying degrees of improvement that might occur. The index would allow for better comparisons of the effectiveness of various treatments. Characteristics of patients who experience varying degrees of improvement and outliers should be described in the research report. This step requires that the study design include baseline measures of patient status, such as demographic characteristics, functional status, and disease severity measures. An analysis of improvement allows for better judgments to be made about the appropriate use of various treatments (Polit & Yang, 2016).

📄 **RESEARCH/EBP TIP**

Outcomes studies usually include prospective and retrospective cohort designs, data from large databases, and analyses to examine patients' recovery in determining the effectiveness of evidence-based nursing care.

Critical Appraisal of Outcomes Studies

This section discusses approaches for critically appraising outcomes studies. Guyatt and colleagues (2015) outlined the methodology for critically appraising study designs, including those typically used in outcomes research. The guidelines might be used to address studies of economic analysis, retrospective cohort design, health-related quality of life, and prospective cohort design. An example of the types of questions to consider in critically appraising outcome studies is provided in the following box.

? CRITICAL APPRAISAL GUIDELINES

Outcomes Research

Critical appraisals of outcomes studies are organized by three broad questions: What are the results? Are the results valid? How can I apply the results to patient care? Exposure in these guidelines can refer to interventions, staffing models, and/or healthcare policy.

1. **What are the results?**
   a. How strong is the association between exposure and outcome?
   b. Were the results statistically significant? Were the results clinically important?
   c. How precise was the estimate of effect? Were the confidence intervals for the effect large or small? Small confidence intervals reflect greater precision in the estimate of effect.
2. **Are the results valid?**
   a. In a prospective cohort study, did the exposed (intervention) and unexposed (non-intervention) control groups start and finish with the same risk of outcome? How was exposure defined?
   b. Was the exposure related to nursing care or health policy? In nursing outcome studies, exposure could refer to a specific nursing intervention, staffing model, or even healthcare policy.
   c. In a retrospective cohort study, did the exposed and control groups have the same chance of being exposed in the past? In a retrospective cohort study, the researcher would be interested in determining whether outcomes differ for individuals exposed in the past to an identified health risk, health condition, or health service by following individuals longitudinally after the specific exposure?
3. **How can I apply the results to patient care and/or policy?**
   a. Were the study patients like the patients in my practice setting?
   b. Was follow-up sufficiently long to assess an effect on outcome?
   c. Is the exposure like what might occur in my practice setting?
   d. What is the magnitude of effect? This question requires you to consider whether the effect was clinically important to make it worthwhile to change practice.

As discussed earlier, Lasater and colleagues (2021b) conducted an outcomes study to examine whether patient-to-nurse staffing ratios are associated with clinical outcomes for patients admitted with sepsis in New York state hospitals. In addition, the effects hospital adherence to the severe sepsis/septic shock EBP sepsis bundles had on patient outcomes were examined and the extent improved staff ratios benefited these patients. Data were obtained from several large databases, with the final patient sample including 52,177 Medicare patients between the ages of 65 and 99 years who were discharged from one of 116 study hospitals. Research Example 14.7 includes the abstract from the Lasater et al. (2021b) study.

$ RESEARCH EXAMPLE 14.7

Critical Appraisal of an Outcomes Study

Research/Study Excerpt
Abstract

Background: Despite nurses' responsibilities in recognition and treatment of sepsis, little evidence documents whether patient-to-nurse staffing ratios are associated with clinical outcomes for patients with sepsis.

Methods: Using linked data sources from 2017 including MEDPAR [Medicare provider analysis and review] patient claims, Hospital Compare, American Hospital Association, and a large survey of nurses, we estimate the effect of hospital patient-to-nurse staffing ratios and adherence to the Early Management Bundle for patients with Severe Sepsis/Septic Shock [SEP-1] sepsis bundles on patients' odds of in-hospital and 60-day mortality, readmission, and length of stay. Logistic regression is used to estimate mortality and readmission, while zero-truncated negative binomial models are used for length of stay.

Continued

RESEARCH EXAMPLE 14.7—cont'd

Results: Each additional patient per nurse is associated with 12% higher odds of in-hospital mortality, 7% higher odds of 60-day mortality, 7% higher odds of 60-day readmission, and longer lengths of stay, even after accounting for patient and hospital covariates including hospital adherence to SEP-1 bundles. Adherence to SEP-1 bundles is associated with lower in-hospital mortality and shorter lengths of stay; however, the effects are markedly smaller than those observed for staffing.

Discussion: Improving hospital nurse staffing over and above implementing sepsis bundles holds promise for significant improvements in sepsis patient outcomes. (Lasater et al., 2021b, Abstract)

Critical Appraisal

Lasater et al. (2021b) conducted an extremely important outcomes study to address the critical healthcare problem of sepsis. The cross-sectional design of this study was strong, including an extremely large sample of patients from several hospitals. The sample was achieved by using a variety of relevant databases that included patients from 116 hospitals. Registered nurses (RNs) practicing in New York hospitals were surveyed about staffing levels and other aspects of their work environment. The response rate to the survey was 17% but included 13,000 RN responses, with an average of 24 RNs responding per hospital who were working in adult medical surgical units. The representativeness of the sample was strong because of the large number of RN responses obtained from numerous hospitals. However, the results are limited to adult medical surgical units in the hospitals.

The study outcome variables had precise, accurate operational definitions. These variables included initial hospital mortality (14.9%), 60-day mortality (28.6%), 60-day readmission (23.5%), and the average hospital LOS (8.5 days). The staffing effect was strongly associated with these outcome variables, resulting in statistical significance and clinical importance. The confidence intervals were small, reflecting greater precision in the estimate of the staffing effect. The SEP-1 bundle effect was not nearly as strongly associated with the outcome variables. This study focused on associations and therefore does not claim a causal relationship between nurse staffing and patient outcomes. In addition, the researchers had to rely on publicly available data from hospitals to determine the adherence to the SEP-1 bundle. This study has many strengths and few limitations, which support the validity of the results and the credibility of the findings.

The study findings clearly support increasing the patient-to-nurse staffing ratio to improve the outcomes of patients with sepsis. In addition, the patient-to-nurse staffing ratios were more important than adhering to the EBP sepsis bundles. The Lasater et al. (2021b) study provided support for the Safe Staffing for Quality Care Act that would require hospitals to comply with safe nurse staffing ratios. This study demonstrates the importance of outcomes research in determining quality, safe nursing practice to direct the implementation of essential health policies.

RESEARCH/EBP TIP

Outcomes studies are essential for examining the structures and processes of care that affect healthcare outcomes. The knowledge generated from outcomes research enables nurses to improve the quality, safety, and costs of care delivered in practice.

KEY POINTS

- Mixed methods research combines quantitative and qualitative research methods to answer a research question with a pragmatic focus.
- Data in mixed methods studies may be collected sequentially or concurrently.
- The three core mixed methods designs are (1) convergent concurrent designs, (2) exploratory sequential designs, and (3) explanatory sequential designs.

- Convergent concurrent designs include simultaneous quantitative and qualitative data collection, separate analysis of each set of data, and integration of the results to produce the findings.
- Exploratory sequential designs begin with qualitative methods to learn more about the research topic and refine the methods of the quantitative phase. The design is frequently used to explore the aspects of a phenomenon and generate potential questions or items for an instrument. The new instrument undergoes initial psychometric testing in the quantitative phase.
- Explanatory sequential designs begin with the collection, analysis, and interpretation of quantitative data, followed by a qualitative phase. These studies are most useful in providing answers to "why" and "how" questions that arise from quantitative findings.
- Mixed methods research strategies require a depth and breadth of research knowledge, as well as a significant commitment of time and resources.
- Experienced researchers plan the integration of the quantitative and qualitative data or the results of their analyses before the mixed methods study begins. Integration of the data can be displayed in tables, graphs, or matrices.
- Outcomes research examines the end results of patient care.
- Donabedian (1987, 2005) developed the theory on which many outcomes studies are based with quality as the overriding construct.
- Donabedian identified three components of evaluation in appraising quality: structure, process, and outcome.
- The goal of outcomes research is to evaluate outcomes that are clearly linked with the process that caused them.
- The focus of outcomes research in nursing is NSPOs that are *sensitive* because they are influenced by nursing.
- Some of the common outcome studies' methodologies include prospective and retrospective cohort studies, population-based studies, and economic analysis.
- Outcomes studies generally use large representative, heterogeneous samples rather than random samples. Most of the data for outcomes studies are obtained from large clinical and administrative databases.
- Critical appraisal of outcomes studies focuses on similarity of the exposed cohort and unexposed (control) cohort, adequacy and completeness of follow-up, reliability and validity of the outcome measure(s), and statistical and clinical significance of the study findings.

REFERENCES

Agency for Healthcare Research and Quality. (2018). *Six domains of health care quality.* Retrieved from https://www.ahrq.gov/talkingquality/measures/six-domains.html

Agency for Healthcare Research and Quality. (2021). *Mission and budget.* Retrieved from https://www.ahrq.gov/cpi/about/mission/index.html

American Nurses Credentialing Center. (2021). *ANCC Magnet Recognition Program™.* Retrieved from https://www.nursingworld.org/organizational-programs/magnet

Ayoubi, S., Pazandeh, F., Simbar, M., Moridi, M., Zare, E., & Potrata, B. (2020). A questionnaire to assess women's perception of respectful maternity care (WP-RMC); Development and psychometric properties. *Midwifery, 80,* 102573. https://doi.org/10.1016/j.midw.2019.102573

Bandalos, D. L. (2018). *Measurement theory and applications for the social sciences.* The Guilford Press.

Barry, R., Smith, A. C., & Brubaker, C. E. (2017). *High-reliability healthcare: Improving patient safety and outcomes with six sigma* (2nd ed.). Health Administration Press.

Binder, C., Torres, R. E., & Elwell, D. (2021). Use of the Donabedian Model as a framework for COVID-19 response at a hospital in suburban Westchester

County, New York: A facility-level case report. *Journal of Emergency Nursing, 47*(2), 239–255. https://doi.org/10.1016/j.jen.2020.10.008

Browne, J., & Braden, C. J. (2020). Nursing turbulence in critical care: Relationships with nursing workload and patient safety. *American Journal of Critical Care, 29*(3), 182–191. https://doi.org/10.4037/ajcc2020180

Cardoso, V., Trevisan, I., Cicolella, D. A., & Waterkemper, R. (2019). Systematic review of mixed methods: Method of research for the incorporation of evidence in nursing. *Texto Contexto Enferm, 28*, e20170279. https://dx.doi.org/10.1590/1980-265X-TCE-2017-0279

Centers for Disease Control and Prevention. (2021). *About CDC 24-7.* Retrieved from https://www.cdc.gov/about/default.htm

Centers for Medicare and Medicaid Services. (2021). *Explore & download Medicare provider data.* Retrieved from https://data.cms.gov/provider-data

Centers for Medicare and Medicaid Services. (2020). *Inpatient Rehabilitation Facility (IRF) Quality Reporting Program (QRP).* Retrieved from https://www.cms.gov/Medicare/Quality-Initiatives-Patient-Assessment-Instruments/IRF-Quality-Reporting

Chou, M. Y., Hsu, Y. H., Wang, Y. C., Chu, C. S., Liao, M. C., Liang, C. K.,…Lin, Y. T. (2020). The adverse effects of physical restraint use among older adult patients admitted to the internal medicine wards: A hospital-based retrospective cohort study. *Journal of Nutrition, Health, & Aging, 24*(2), 160–165. https://doi.org/10.1007/s12603-019-1306-7

Clarke, S. P. (2011). Health care utilization. In D. M. Doran (Ed.), *Nursing outcomes: The state of the science* (2nd ed., pp. 439–485). Jones & Bartlett.

Collaborative Alliance for Nursing Outcomes. (2021). *About us: Our history.* Retrieved from https://www.ahrq.gov/downloads/pub/advances2/vol1/advances-aydin_2.pdf

Creswell, J. W., & Clark, V. L. P. (2018). *Designing and conducting mixed methods research* (3rd ed.). Sage.

Creswell, J. W., & Creswell, J. D. (2018). *Research design: Qualitative, quantitative, and mixed methods approaches* (4th ed.). Sage.

Creswell, J. W., & Poth, C. N. (2018). *Qualitative inquiry & research design: Choosing among five approaches* (4th ed.). Sage.

Dickson, V., Jun, J., & Melkus, G. (2021). A mixed methods study describing the self-care practices in an older working population with cardiovascular disease (CVD): Balancing work, life and health. *Heart & Lung, 50*, 447–454. https://doi.org/10.1016/j.hrtlng.2021.02.001

Donabedian, A. (1978). *Needed research in quality assessment and monitoring.* U.S. Department of Health, Education, and Welfare, Public Health Service, National Center for Health Services Research.

Donabedian, A. (1980). *Explorations in quality assessment and monitoring.* Health Administration Press.

Donabedian, A. (1982). *The criteria and standards of quality.* Health Administration Press.

Donabedian, A. (1987). Some basic issues in evaluating the quality of health care. In L. T. Rinke (Ed.), *Outcome measures in home care* (Vol. I, p. 338). National League for Nursing. (Original work published in 1976.)

Donabedian, A. (1988). The quality of care: How can it be assessed? *Journal of the American Medical Association, 260*(12), 1743–1748. https://doi.org/10.1001/jama.260.12.1743

Donabedian, A. (2003). *An introduction to quality assurance in health care.* Oxford University Press.

Donabedian, A. (2005). Evaluating the quality of medical care. *Milbank Quarterly, 83*(4), 691–729. https://doi.org/10.1111/j.1468-0009.2005.00397.x

Doran, D. M. (Ed.). (2011). *Nursing outcomes: The state of the science* (2nd ed.). Jones & Bartlett.

Garside, J., Stephenson, J., Hayles, J., Barlow, N., & Ormrod, G. (2021). Explaining nursing attrition through the experiences of return-to-practice students: A mixed-methods study. *British Journal of Nursing, 30*(8), 490–496. https://doi.org/10.12968/bjon.2021.30.8.490

Gray, J. R., & Grove, S. K. (2021). *The practice of nursing research: Appraisal, synthesis, and generation of evidence* (9th ed.). Elsevier.

Grove, S. K., & Cipher, D. J. (2020). *Statistics for nursing research: A workbook for evidence-based practice* (3rd ed.). Elsevier.

Guyatt, G., Rennie, D., Meade, M. O., & Cook, D. J. (2015). *Users' guides to the medical literature: Essentials of evidence-based clinical practice* (3rd ed.). McGraw-Hill Medical.

Harris, C. W. (1967). *Problems in measuring change.* University of Wisconsin Press.

Herrmann, D. (1995). Reporting current, past, and changed health status: What we know about distortion. *Medical Care, 33*(Suppl. 4), AS89–AS94.

Hong, Q., Pluye, P., Fabregues, S., Bartlett, G., Boardman, F., Cargo, M.,…Vedel, I. (2018). *Mixed methods appraisal tool (MMAT) version 2018: User guide.* Retrieved from https://www.mcgill.ca/familymed/research/projects/mmat

Howell, D. (2011). Psychological distress as a nurse-sensitive outcome. In D. M. Doran (Ed.), *Nursing outcomes: The state of the science* (2nd ed., pp. 285–358). Jones & Bartlett.

Im, Y. (2021). Designing appropriate mixed methods nursing research. *Journal of Korean Academy of Nursing, 51*(2), 133–137. https://doi.org/10.4040/jkan.51201

Irvine, D. M., Sidani, S., & Hall, L. M. (1998). Linking outcomes to nurses' roles in health care. *Nursing Economic$, 16*(2), 58–64, 87.

Kane, R. L., & Radosevich, R. M. (2011). *Conducting health outcomes research.* Jones & Bartlett Learning.

Kenner, C. A. (2017). Trends in US nursing research: Links to global healthcare issues. *Journal of Korean Academic Nursing Administration, 23*(1), 1–7.

Kleib, M., Sales, A., Doran, D. M., Malette, C., & White, D. (2011). Nursing minimum data sets. In D. M. Doran (Ed.), *Nursing outcomes: The state of the science* (2nd ed., pp. 487–512). Jones & Bartlett.

Lasater, K. B., McHugh, M., Rosenbaum, P. R., Aiken, L. H., Smith, H., Reiter, J. G., ... Silber, J. H. (2021a). Valuing hospital investments in nursing: Multistate matched-cohort study of surgical patients. *BMJ Quality & Safety, 30*(1), 46–55. https://doi.org/10.1136/bmjqs-2019-010534

Lasater, K. B., Sloane, D. M., McHugh, M. D., Cimiotti, J. P., Riman, K. A., Martin, B., ... Aiken, L. H. (2021b). Evaluation of hospital nurse-to-patient staffing ratios and sepsis bundles on patient outcomes. *American Journal of Infection Control, 49*(7), 868–873. https://doi.org/10.1016/j.ajic.2020.12.002

Liu, W. (2021). The effects of virtual simulation on undergraduate nursing students' beliefs about prognosis and outcomes for people with mental disorders. *Clinical Simulation in Nursing, 50*, 1–9. https://doi.org/10.1016/j.ecns.2020.09.007

LoGiudice, J. A., & Bartos, S. (2021). Experiences of nurses during the COVID-19 pandemic: A mixed-methods study. *AACN Advanced Critical Care, 32*(1), 14–26. https://doi.org/10.4037/aacnacc2021816

Magnello, M. E. (2010). The passionate statistician. In S. Nelson, & A. M. Rafferty (Eds.), *Notes on Nightingale: The influence and legacy of a nursing icon* (pp. 115–129). Cornell University Press.

Malterud, K., Siersma, V., & Guassora. A. (2016). Sample size in qualitative interview studies: Guided by information power. *Qualitative Health Research, 26*(13), 1753–1760. https://doi.org/10.1177/1049732315617444

Melnyk, B. M., & Fineout-Overholt, E. (2019). *Evidence-based practice in nursing & healthcare: A guide to best practice* (4th ed.). Wolters Kluwer.

Melnyk, B. M., Zellefrow, C., Tan, A., & Hsieh, A. P. (2020). Differences between Magnet and non-Magnet-designated hospitals in nurses' evidence-based practice knowledge, competencies, mentoring, and culture. *Worldviews on Evidence-Based Nursing, 17*(5), 337–347. https://doi.org/10.1111/wvn.12467

Mitchell, P. H., Ferketich, S., & Jennings, B. M. (1998). American Academy of Nursing Expert Panel on Quality Health Care: 1998 Quality Health Outcomes Model. *Image—Journal of Nursing Scholarship, 30*(1), 43–46. https://doi.org/10.1111/j.1547-5069.1998.tb01234.x

Montalvo, I. (2007). *National Database of Nursing Quality Indicators (NDNQI).* Retrieved from http://ojin.nursingworld.org/MainMenuCategories/ANAMarketplace/ANAPeriodicals/OJIN/TableofContents/Volume122007/No3Sept07/NursingQualityIndicators.html

Moorhead, S., Swanson, E., Johnson, M., & Maas, M. L. (2018). *Nursing outcomes classification (NOC): Measurement of health outcomes* (6th ed.). Elsevier.

National Academies of Sciences, Engineering, and Medicine. (2021). *The future of nursing 2020-2030: Charting a path to achieve health equity.* The National Academies Press. https://doi.org/10.17226/25982

National League for Nursing. (2020). *vSim for nursing.* Retrieved from http://www.nln.org/centers-for-nursing-education/nln-center-for-innovation-in-education-excellence/institute-for-simulation-and-technology/vsim-for-nursing-medical-surgical

National Quality Forum. (2021). *Measures, reports, & tools.* Retrieved from https://www.qualityforum.org/Measures_Reports_Tools.aspx

Office of Disease Prevention and Health Promotion. (2020). *About ODPHP.* Retrieved from https://health.gov/about-odphp

Oncology Nursing Society. (2021). *About ONS.* Retrieved from http://www.ons.org/about

Orem, D. (2001). *Nursing concepts of practice* (6th ed.). Mosby.

Patient-Centered Outcomes Research Institute. (2021). *PCORI: About us.* Retrieved from http://www.pcori.org/about-us

Polit, D. F., & Yang, F. M. (2016). *Measurement and the measurement of change.* Wolters Kluwer.

Press Ganey. (2021). *Clinical excellence.* Retrieved from https://www.pressganey.com/solutions/clinical-excellence

Sidani, S. (2011a). Self-care. In D. M. Doran (Ed.), *Nursing outcomes: The state of the science.* (2nd ed., pp. 79–130). Jones & Bartlett.

Sidani, S. (2011b). Symptom management. In D. M. Doran (Ed.), *Nursing outcomes: The state of the science* (2nd ed., pp. 131–199). Jones & Bartlett.

Sinclair, V. G., & Wallston, K. A. (2004). The development and psychometric evaluation of the Brief Resilient Coping Scale. *Assessment, 11*(1), 94–101. http://doi.org/10.1177/1073191103258144

Tashakkori, A., Johnson, R., & Teddlie, C. (2021). *Foundations of mixed methods research: Integrating quantitative and qualitative approaches in social and behavioral sciences* (2nd ed.). Sage.

Tourangeau, A. E. (2011). Mortality rate: A nursing sensitive outcome. In D. M. Doran (Ed.), *Nursing outcomes: The state of the science* (2nd ed., pp. 409–437). Jones & Bartlett.

University of Pennsylvania School of Nursing. (2021). *Center for Health Outcomes and Policy Research (CHOPR).* Retrieved from https://www.nursing.upenn.edu/chopr/

Waltz, C. F., Strickland, O. L., & Lenz, E. R. (2017). *Measurement in nursing and health research* (5th ed.). Springer.

Wappel, S., Tran, D. H., Wells, C. L., & Verceles, A. C. (2021). The effect of high protein and mobility-based rehabilitation on clinical outcomes in survivors of critical illness. *Respiratory Care, 66*(1), 73–78. https://doi.org//10.4187/respcare.07840

Werley, H. H., & Lang, N. M. (1988). *Identification of the nursing minimum data set.* Springer Publishing Company.

A

Absolute zero value Value of zero indicates the absence of the property being measured.

Abstract (adjective) Idea focuses on a general view of a phenomenon.

Abstract (noun) Clear, concise summary of a study, usually limited to 100 to 250 words.

Academic journals Periodicals that include research reports and nonresearch articles related to a specific academic discipline and/or research methodology.

Acceptance rate The percentage of participants meeting sampling criteria who consent to be in a study.

Accessible population plans The term is Accessible population: The portion of the target population to which the research has reasonable access.

Accuracy Comparable with validity in that it addresses the extent to which the physiological instrument measures what it is supposed to measure in a study.

Accuracy of a screening test Screening tests that are evaluated in terms of ability to predict or confirm the presence or absence of a condition correctly as compared with the criterion or gold standard.

Administrative data Collected within clinical agencies; obtained by national, state, and local professional organizations; and maintained by federal, state, and local agencies.

Administrative database Databases that are created by insurance companies, government agencies, and others not directly involved in providing patient care.

Alternate or equivalent forms reliability Also referred to as *equivalent forms reliability*; comparison of two instruments or scales measuring the same concept.

Analysis of covariance (ANCOVA) Statistical technique that allows the researcher to examine the effect of a treatment apart from the effect of one or more potentially confounding variables.

Analysis of variance (ANOVA) A parametric statistical technique conducted to examine differences among three or more groups.

Analyzing a research report Critical thinking skill that involves determining the value of the report's content.

Ancestry search Involves the use of citations from relevant studies to identify additional studies.

Anonymity The researcher cannot link participant identities to their individual responses.

Applied research Scientific investigation conducted to generate knowledge that will directly influence or improve nursing practice.

Article Paper about a specific topic and may be published together with other articles on similar themes in journals (periodicals), encyclopedias, or edited books.

Artifacts Objects made by people that have meaning within a culture.

Assent to participate in research Agreement of a child or adult to participate in a study.

Associative hypothesis Statement of a proposed relationship among variables that occur or exist together in the real world so that when one variable changes, the other changes.

Assumption Statement taken for granted or considered true, even though it has not been scientifically tested.

Attrition rate of a sample Number and percentage of participants who drop out of a study before it is completed, creating a threat to the internal validity of the study. The attrition rate is calculated by dividing the number of participants dropping out of a study by the original sample size. For example, if the sample size was 200, and 20 participants dropped out of the study, then $(20 \div 200) \times 100\% = 10\%$.

Audit trail Documentation of how data were collected, analyzed, and interpreted.

Authority Person(s) with expertise and power who is (are) able to influence the opinions and behaviors of others.

Autonomy Freedom of individuals to conduct their lives as they choose, without external controls.

B

Background for a problem Part of the research problem that indicates what is known or identifies key research publications in the problem area.

Basic research Scientific investigation conducted to increase knowledge or understanding of the fundamental aspects of phenomena and of observable facts without emphasis on specific applications.

Belmont Report Provides a strong foundation for conducting ethical research by identifying ethical principles to guide selecting subjects, informing them of the risks and benefits of a study, and documenting their consent.

Benefit/risk ratio Comparison of the potential benefits (positive outcomes) and risks (negative outcomes) of a study that is used by researchers and reviewers to ensure the ethical conduct of research.

Best research evidence The empirical knowledge generated from the synthesis of quality health studies to address a clinical problem; produced by the conduct and synthesis of numerous high-quality studies in a selected health-related area.

Between-group variance Variation of the group means around the grand mean; determined by conducting analysis of variance statistical techniques.

Bias A slant or deviation from the true or expected.

Bibliographic database Electronically stored compilation of citations relevant to a specific discipline or a broad collection of citations from a variety of disciplines; searchable by authors, titles, journals, keywords, or topic.

Bimodal distribution Data sets that have two modes.

Biochemical measure Determines microchemical values, such as laboratory tests for determining cholesterol values.

Biophysical measures Devices, equipment, or methods used to measure physiological and pathological variables, such as the stethoscope and sphygmomanometer to measure blood pressure (BP). Biophysical measures can be acquired in a variety of ways from instruments within the body (in vivo), such as a reading from an arterial line, or from application of an instrument on the outside of an individual (in vitro), such as a BP cuff.

Bivariate correlation Measure of the extent of the relationship between two variables.

Blinded to group assignment Data collectors do not know who has received the intervention and who is in the control or placebo group.

Blinding Withholding group assignment or other study information from data collectors, participants, and their healthcare providers to reduce potential bias.

Borrowing Involves appropriating and using knowledge from other fields or disciplines to guide nursing practice.

Bracket or bracketing Qualitative research technique in which a researcher identifies personal preconceptions to describe the phenomenon as reported by the participants.

Breach of confidentiality Intentional or nonintentional action that allows an unauthorized person to gain access to the raw data of a study.

Broad consent Agreement whereby a study participant gives the researcher permission to store, manage, and use private information for other studies.

C

Case study In-depth analysis and systematic description of one patient or a group of similar patients to promote understanding of nursing interventions, problems, or situations. Case studies are one example of the practice-related research conducted in nursing.

Causal hypothesis Proposes a cause-and-effect interaction between two or more variables, referred to as independent and dependent variables.

Causality A way of knowing that one event leads to or causes another.

Chi-square (x^2) test of independence Statistical test conducted to determine whether two variables are independent or related; can be used with nominal or ordinal data.

Citation Act of quoting a source, paraphrasing content from a source, using it as an example, or presenting it as support for a position taken.

Citation bias Preference that occurs when certain studies are cited more often than others and that are more likely to be identified in database searches.

Clinical database Databases that are created by providers such as hospitals, health maintenance organizations, accountable care organizations, and healthcare professionals.

Clinical expertise Knowledge and skills of healthcare professionals providing care. In nursing, clinical expertise is influenced by years of clinical experience, current knowledge of the research and clinical literature, and educational preparation. Evidence-based practice is a combination of best research evidence, clinical expertise, and patient circumstances.

Clinical importance Practical relevance of a positive statistical finding in a study.

Clinical journal Periodical containing research reports and nonresearch articles about practice problems and professional issues in a specific discipline.

Cluster sampling Sampling method in which a sampling frame that includes a list of all the states, cities, institutions, or units with which elements of the identified population can be linked is developed.

Coding Process of reading the data, breaking text down into subparts, and giving a label to that part of the text.

Coefficient of multiple determination (R^2) Refers to a statistical technique conducted when a study includes multiple independent variables to predict one dependent variable. R^2 is the percentage of the total variation that can be explained by all the variables that the researcher includes in the final prediction equation.

Coercion Overt threat of harm or excessive reward intentionally presented by one person to another to obtain compliance.

Cognitive use Application of research evidence that is a more informal, indirect use of the research knowledge to modify one's way of thinking or appreciation of an issue.

Common Rule Name given to the similarities among federal departments' chapters in the Code of Federal Regulations; includes the contents of a consent document, processes of obtaining informed consent, maintaining an institutional review board (IRB), levels of IRB review, and protection of vulnerable populations.

Comparative descriptive design Design used to describe variables and examine differences in variables in two or more groups that occur naturally in a setting.

Comparative evaluation Includes four parts: (1) fit and qualifiers of the evidence for the healthcare setting, (2) feasibility of using the research findings, (3) substantiation of the evidence, and (4) concerns with current practice to determine the fit of the evidence in the clinical agency. The characteristics of the setting are examined to determine the forces that would facilitate or inhibit the evidence-based change.

Comparison group Group that is not exposed to the research intervention.

Complex hypothesis Hypothesis that predicts the relationship (associative or causal) among three or more variables.

Comprehending a research report Critical thinking process used in reading a research report in which the focus is on understanding the major concepts and logical flow of ideas in a study.

Comprehending a source Action that requires reading an entire study carefully, focused on understanding major concepts and the logical flow of ideas within the study.

Concept Term to which abstract meaning is attached; basic element of a theory or the building blocks of theories.

Conceptual definition Definition that provides the theoretical meaning of a variable and is often derived from a theorist's definition of a related concept.

Conceptual model Set of highly abstract, related constructs that broadly explain phenomena of interest; expresses assumptions; usually reflects a philosophical stance; early nurse scholars labeled as the most abstract theories.

Conclusion A statement about the state of knowledge in relation to the topic area, which includes what is known and not known about the area.

Concrete   Refers to the realities or actual instances that focus on a specific instance rather than a general idea.

Concurrent validity   Extent to which an individual's score on a scale can be used to estimate his or her present or concurrent performance on another variable or criterion.

Conference proceedings   Collection of papers presented at a conference, which are later published; include the findings of pilot studies and preliminary findings of ongoing studies.

Confidence interval   Probability of including the value of the population within an interval estimate.

Confidentiality   Safe management of information or data shared by a participant to ensure that the data are kept private from others.

Confirmability   Extent to which other researchers can review the audit trail and agree that the authors' conclusions are logical.

Confirmatory factor analysis (CFA)   Data analysis used to validate the number of factors or subcomponents in the instrument.

Confounding variables   Types of extraneous variable that are not recognized until the study is in process or are recognized before the study is initiated but cannot be controlled.

Consent form   Written document that includes the elements of informed consent required by the Common Rule.

Construct   A broader category or idea that may encompass several concepts.

Construct validity   Degree to which an instrument actually measures the theoretic construct that it purports to measure; this involves examining the fit between the conceptual and operational definitions of a study variable.

Content validity   Examines the extent to which the measurement method includes all the major elements or items relevant to the construct or concept being measured.

Continuous data   Also referred to as interval- and ratio-level data because the data can be added, subtracted, multiplied, and divided because of the equal intervals and continuum of values.

Control   The ability to write a prescription to produce the desired results; having the power to direct or manipulate factors to achieve a desired outcome.

Control group   Group of elements or subjects not exposed to the experimental treatment in a study.

Convenience sampling   Nonprobability sampling; also called *accidental sampling*, a relatively weak approach because it provides little opportunity to control for biases; participants are included in a study because they happen to be in the right place at the right time.

Correlational designs   Variety of study designs developed to examine relationships between or among two or more variables in a single group in a study.

Correlational research   Systematic investigation of relationships between (among) two or more variables.

Covert data collection   Information about research participants that is collected without their knowledge or awareness.

Criterion-related validity   Strengthened when a study participant's score on an instrument can be used to infer his or her performance or status on another variable or criterion.

Criterion standard   Most accurate means of currently predicting or diagnosing a particular condition or current best practice.

Critical appraisal   An examination of the quality of a study to determine the credibility, meaning, and relevance of the findings for nursing knowledge and practice.

Critical appraisal of research   Careful examination of all aspects of a study to judge its strengths, limitations, meaning, and significance.

Critical ethnography   Qualitative study that focuses on the sociological and political factors of a culture.

Cronbach's alpha coefficient   Most commonly calculated to determine the internal reliability for scales with multiple items.

Cross-sectional design   Noninterventional design that includes a time element and involves collecting data at one point in time; participants may be in various stages of development, levels of education, severity of illness, or stages of recovery to describe changes in a phenomenon across stages.

Current sources   References cited in a research report that have been published within 5 years of the date at which the manuscript of the report was accepted for publication.

D

Data analysis   Involves organization and statistical testing of data to determine prevalence, relationship, and cause.

Data analysis process   Involves the management of numerical data using statistical analyses to produce study results in quantitative and outcomes research.

Data collection   Process of acquiring study participants from whom essential data are gathered to address the research purpose; precise, systematic gathering of information (data) relevant to the research purpose or the specific objectives, questions, or hypotheses of a study.

Deception   Misinforming participants about the intent of a study or data collection for research purposes.

Decision theory   Theory that assumes that all of the groups in a study (e.g., experimental and comparison) used to test a particular hypothesis are components of the same population relative to the variables under study.

Declaration of Helsinki   Declaration that clarifies the differences between therapeutic research and nontherapeutic research.

Deductive reasoning   Reasoning from the general to the specific or from a general premise to a particular situation or conclusion.

Degrees of freedom (*df*)   Freedom of a score's value to vary, given the values of other existing scores and the established sum of these scores.

Demographic or sample characteristics   Characteristics determined by analyzing data collected from study participants for demographic variables.

Demographic variables   Specific attribute variables of study participants that are collected to describe the sample, such as age, education, gender, marital status, income, and medical diagnosis.

Dependability   Documentation of steps taken and decisions made during analysis.

Dependent variable   Outcome that the researcher wants to predict or explain in research.

Description Involves identifying and understanding the nature and attributes of nursing phenomena and sometimes the relationships among these phenomena.

Descriptive correlational design Type of design implemented to describe variables and examine relationships among these variables.

Descriptive design Type of quantitative study design that may be used to develop theories, identify problems with current practice, or identify trends in the health promotion and disease prevention actions of a specific group, such as uninsured young adults.

Descriptive phenomenological research Research study in which its purpose is to describe experiences as they are lived or, in phenomenological terms, to capture the "lived experience" of study participants. The researcher brackets personal perspectives and experiences.

Descriptive research Exploration and description of phenomena in real-life situations. Its purpose is to provide an accurate account of characteristics of particular individuals, situations, or groups using numbers.

Descriptive statistics Summary statistics that allow the researcher to organize data in ways that give meaning and facilitate insight.

Design The rules that are used to achieve control in research; the detailed plan for a study.

Design validity Probability that the study findings are an accurate reflection of reality; encompasses the strength and threats to the quality of a study design.

Determining strengths and weaknesses in studies Second step in the critical appraisal of studies to determine their quality. To complete this step, the researcher must have knowledge of what each step of the research process should be like based on expert sources, such as this textbook and other research sources.

Dichotomous Variables that include only two values.

Diminished autonomy Condition of subjects whose ability to give informed consent voluntarily is decreased because of medications, mental illness, or intellectual or cognitive capacity.

Directional hypothesis Statement that predicts the nature (positive or negative) of the interaction between two or more variables.

Direct measures Measures used to count and quantify the variable itself and are considered objective with limited influence from judgment issues; used for determining the value of objective variables, such as waist circumference, temperature, heart rate, and BP.

Discomfort and harm Degree of potential and actual risk experienced by a subject participating in a study; risks can be physical, psychological, economic, emotional, or a combination thereof.

Dissertation Extensive, usually original research project completed as the final requirement for a doctoral degree.

Distal outcome Outcome removed from proximity to the care or a service received and that is more influenced by external (nontreatment or nonintervention) factors than a proximal outcome.

Duplicate publication Occurs when multiple papers report the same results from the same study. Researchers may recycle text from previous articles without referencing the source, a practice called self-plagiarism.

Duplicate publication bias Studies with positive results that are published more than once.

Dwelling with the data Term in qualitative data analysis used to indicate that the researcher has spent considerable time reading, rereading, analyzing, and reflecting on the data, codes, and themes.

E

Economic evaluation A set of formal, quantitative methods used to compare two or more treatments, programs, or strategies with respect to their resource use and their expected outcomes.

Education Structured presentation of information, usually by a person identified to be the expert (teacher).

Effect size Extent to which the null or statistical hypothesis is false or, stated another way, the strength of the expected relationship between two variables or differences between two groups.

Elements Individual units of the population and sample examined in studies.

Emic approach Studying behaviors from within the culture that recognizes the uniqueness of the individual.

Empirical literature Relevant studies published in journals, books, and online, as well as unpublished studies, such as master's theses and doctoral dissertations; comprised of knowledge derived from research.

Encyclopedia Authoritative compilation of information on alphabetized topics that may provide background information and lead to other sources but is rarely cited in academic papers and publications.

Environmental variables Types of extraneous variables composing the setting in which a study is conducted.

Equivalence Comparison of two versions of an instrument or of two observers measuring the same behavior or event.

Error in physiological measures Inaccuracy of physiological instruments related to the environment, users, study participants, equipment, and interpretation.

Ethical principles Standards and laws that protect human participants.

Ethnographic research A methodology that examines how cultures develop and are maintained over time.

Ethnonursing research Type of research developed by Leininger, that focuses mainly on observing and documenting interactions with people and how these daily life conditions and patterns are influencing human care, health, and nursing care practices.

Etic approach Viewing a culture as a naive outsider and analyzing its elements as a researcher.

Evaluating the credibility and meaning of the study findings Determining the validity, trustworthiness, significance, and contributions of the study by examining the relationships among the steps of the study, study findings, and previous studies' findings.

Evaluation Final stage in Stetler model of Research Utilization to Facilitate Evidence-Based Practice that determines the effect of the research-based change on the patients, personnel, and healthcare agency.

Evidence-based guidelines Rigorous, explicit clinical guidelines that have been developed based on the best research evidence available in that area.

Evidence-based practice (EBP) Conscientious integration of best research evidence with nurses' clinical expertise and patients' circumstances and values in the delivery of quality, safe, cost-effective health care.

Evidence-based practice centers (EPCs) Universities and healthcare agencies identified by the Agency for Healthcare Research and Quality that develop evidence reports and technology assessments on topics relevant to clinical, social science/behavioral, economic, and other healthcare organization and delivery issues, specifically those that are common, expensive, and/or significant for the Medicare and Medicaid populations.

Evidence of validity from contrasting groups Tested by identifying groups that are expected (or known) to have contrasting scores on an instrument.

Evidence of validity from convergence Determined when a relatively new or revised instrument is compared with an existing instrument(s) that measures the same construct.

Evidence of validity from divergence Type of measurement validity obtained by using two instruments to measure opposite variables at the same time.

Exclusion sampling criteria Characteristics that excluded or eliminate potential participants from the target population for safety reasons or specific characteristics that might alter their responses.

Exempt from review Reviews that include anonymous completion of surveys, interviews with participants in a government projects, and analyzing de-identified data collected for another purpose.

Expedited review Institutional review process for studies that involve minimal risks to participate.

Experiment Study that typically includes randomizing subjects into groups, collecting data, and conducting statistical analyses.

Experimental designs Types of design that focus on examining the differences in dependent variables thought to be caused by independent variables or interventions; the study design with the highest level of control.

Experimental group Group of participants who received the study intervention, also called treatment group.

Experimental research Objective, systematic, and highly controlled investigation of cause-and-effect relationships.

Experimenter expectancy When a researcher knows which participants received the intervention and collects the data.

Explained variance Amount of variation in values explained by the relationship between the two variables.

Explanation Clarification of relationships among variables and identification of reasons why certain events occur.

Exploratory analysis Examining all of the data descriptively prior to study-specific statistical analysis.

Exploratory-descriptive qualitative research Studies that do not identify a specific method or philosophical approach; often motivated by a desire to solve a problem; occurs in naturalistic settings.

Exploratory factor analysis (EFA) Data analyzation used to examine relationships among the various items of the instrument.

External validity Concerned with the extent to which study findings can be generalized beyond the study's sample.

Extraneous variables Variables that are not the focus of a study but can make the independent variable appear more powerful or less powerful than it really is.

F

Fabrication When researchers add data to the research record that were not collected from participants and create results that did not occur.

Face validity Part of content validity that verifies if an instrument looks like it is valid or gives the appearance of measuring the construct for which it was developed.

Factor Closely related items are grouped together.

Factor analysis Examines the interrelationships among large numbers of items on a scale and disentangles those relationships to identify clusters of items that are most intricately linked.

False-negative (result) Outcome of a diagnostic or screening test indicating that a disease is not present when it is present.

False-positive (result) Outcome of a diagnostic or screening test indicating that a disease is present when it is not present.

Falsification When researchers manipulate equipment, alter statistical results, or omit results that do not support the study's hypotheses.

Feasibility of a study Determined by examining the time and money commitment, researcher's expertise, availability of study participants, facility, and equipment.

Field notes Notations recorded by qualitative researchers during or immediate after data collection.

Findings Translated and interpreted results from a study.

Focused ethnography Observation and description of a defined, organizational culture conducted in a shorter period than a traditional ethnography.

Focus group Group used to obtain participants' perceptions of a specific topic in a permissive and nonthreatening setting.

Framework Abstract, logical structure of meaning, such as a portion of a theory, that guides the development of the study, may be tested in the study, and enables the researcher to link the findings to nursing's body of knowledge.

Frequency distribution Statistical procedure that describes the occurrence of scores or categories in a study.

Full review Institutional review process that involves more than minimal risk. This allows the researcher to describe their study, including how they can minimize the risks of the study and ensure fair selection of participants.

Funnel plots Graphic representations of possible effect sizes (*ESs*) for interventions in selected studies; may be done during a meta-analysis.

G

Generalization Extension of the conclusions made based on the research findings from the sample studied to a larger population; the application of information that has been acquired from a specific instance to a general situation.

General proposition Broad and abstract statement that can be applied across many types of nursing care and settings.

Going native Complication of observation in which the researcher becomes a part of the culture and loses the ability to observe clearly.

Gold standard Accepted benchmark for currently assessing and diagnosing a particular patient problem; serves as a basis for comparison with newly developed diagnostic or screening tests; also, a gold standard or benchmark for managing patients' care that is linked to patient outcomes.

Grand nursing theory Abstract, broad-scope theory that encompasses nursing actions and patient responses in multiple settings.

Grey literature Sources that have limited distribution, such as theses and dissertations; articles in obscure journals; conference proceedings; government publications; and research reports for funding agencies, corporate organizations, and higher education.

Grounded theory research Inductive technique that emerged from the discipline of sociology, examines social processes, and may result in a tentative theory.

Grouped frequency distribution Visual presentation used when continuous variables are being examined. Many measures taken during data collection, including age, body temperature, weight, laboratory values, scale scores, and time, are measured using a continuous scale.

Grove Model for Implementing Evidence-Based Guidelines in Practice Model developed that helps nurses identify a practice problem, search for the best research evidence to manage the problem in their practice, and identify an evidence-based guideline.

H

Healthcare quality Extent to which healthcare services provided to individuals and patient populations improve desired health outcomes.

Health Insurance Portability and Accountability Act (HIPAA) Federal regulations that protect an individual's health information created during clinical care, electronically stored, and transferred from one entity to another.

Heterogeneous Sample in which study participants have a broad range of values or scores on the variables being studied.

Highly controlled setting Environment structured for the purpose of conducting research. Laboratories, research or experimental centers, and training units in hospitals or other healthcare facilities are examples of highly controlled environments.

Highly sensitive test Screening or diagnostic test that is accurate for identifying the disease or a condition in a patient.

Highly specific test Screening or diagnostic test that is accurate in identifying the patients without a disease or condition.

History Event that occurs during a study and may influence a participant's response to the intervention or alter how a participant answers the questions on a scale or survey.

Homogeneous Sample in which the researchers narrowly define the sampling criteria to make the sample as similar as possible to control for extraneous variables.

Hypothesis Formal statement of the proposed relationship between two or more variables in a specified population.

I

Identifiable private information Information for which the identity of the participant is or may be readily ascertained by the investigator or associated with the information.

Identifying the steps of the research process First step in a critical appraisal. It involves understanding the terms and concepts in the report, as well as identifying study steps and grasping the nature, significance, and meaning of these elements.

Immersed Being in a culture over time that allows the researcher to become increasingly familiar with the culture.

Implications for nursing Meaning of study findings and conclusions for nursing knowledge, theory, and practice.

Implicit framework Relationships among variables found in previous studies without fully developing the ideas as a framework; provide limited guidance for developing and implementing a study and limit the contribution of the study findings to nursing knowledge.

Inclusion sampling criteria Characteristics that the participant or element must possess to be part of the target population.

Independent groups Groups in which the selection of one study participant is unrelated to the selection of other participants.

Independent variable Intervention that is manipulated or varied by the researcher to create an effect on the dependent variable. In correlational research, independent variables are measured to predict a single dependent variable.

Indirect measures or indicators Measurements focusing on abstract ideas, such as pain, depression, or adherence; obtained to represent the quantity of a variable by measuring one or more characteristics or properties that are related to it.

Inductive reasoning Type of reasoning from the specific to the general, in which particular instances are observed and then combined into a larger whole or general statement.

Inference Conclusion or judgment based on research evidence.

Inferential statistics Designed to address objectives, questions, and hypotheses in studies to allow inference from the study sample to the target population.

Informed consent Providing information to a potential participant and giving the person the opportunity to volunteer for the study.

Institutional review board (IRB) Committee organized in universities and clinical agencies to examine the ethical aspects of studies before they are conducted.

Instrumental use Application of research evidence that is the direct and formal use of research evidence to support the need for change in nursing interventions or practice protocols, algorithms, and guidelines.

Integrated synthesis Used when quantitative and qualitative research findings are thought to extend, confirm, or refute each other.

Intellectual critical appraisal of a study Rigorous, complete examination of a study to judge its strengths and weaknesses and to determine the credibility and meaning of the findings.

Intermediate end points Events or markers that act as precursors to the final outcome.

Internal consistency Also known as homogeneity reliability testing; used primarily with multi-item scales, in which each item on a scale is correlated with all other items on the scale to determine consistency of measurement.

Interval-level measurement Measurement that exists when scales have equal numerical distances between the intervals.

Internal validity Degree to which the study findings are a true reflection of reality rather than the result of extraneous variables.

Interpretation Process whereby the researcher places the findings in a larger context; may link different themes or factors in the findings to each other and existing knowledge.

Interpretation of research outcomes Formal process whereby researchers consider the results from data analysis, form conclusions, explore the clinical importance of the findings, consider the implications for nursing knowledge and theory, generalize or transfer the findings, and suggest further studies.

Interpretative phenomenological research Analyzing the data and presenting a rich word picture of the phenomenon, as interpreted by the participants and the researcher.

Interpreting research outcomes Examining the entire research process for strengths and weaknesses, organizing the meaning of the results, and forecasting the usefulness of the findings for evidence-based nursing practice.

Interrater reliability Comparison of the ratings given by multiple observers or raters to determine their equivalence in making observations or rating situations.

Intervention Treatment or independent variable implemented during the conduct of a study to produce an effect on the dependent or outcome variables; may be physiological, psychosocial, educational, or a combination of these.

Interventional design See *Experimental designs.*

Intervention fidelity Accuracy, consistency (reliability), and thoroughness with which an intervention is standardized by a protocol and is applied consistently each time it is implemented in a study.

Intervention group See *Experimental group.*

Interview Verbal communication between the researcher and study participant during which information is provided to the researcher.

Intuition Insight or understanding of a situation or event as a whole that usually cannot be explained logically.

Iowa Model-Revised Framework for the implementation of evidence-based practice (EBP) that was revised and validated by the Iowa Model Collaborative in 2017 and remains an application-oriented guide for the EBP process.

k Size of the gap between participants or elements selected from a list of participants or elements.

Key informant Participant in an ethnographic study with extensive knowledge and influence in a culture.

Keywords Terms or labels used to identify studies; major concepts, variables, or research methodologies listed near the beginning of a research report; can be used to search bibliographic databases to find articles on a particular topic.

Knowledge Essential information that is acquired in a variety of ways, is expected to be an accurate reflection of reality, and can potentially be used to direct a person's actions.

Landmark studies Significant research projects that have generated knowledge that influences a discipline and sometimes society as a whole.

Language bias Occurs if searches for systematic reviews focus only on studies in English, while important studies also exist in other languages.

Level of statistical significance Probability level at which the statistical results for relationships or differences are judged to be significant.

Levels of measurement Organized set of rules for assigning numbers to objects so that a hierarchy in measurement from low to high is established. The levels of measurement are nominal, ordinal, interval, and ratio.

Likelihood ratios (LRs) Additional calculations that can help researchers determine the accuracy of diagnostic or screening tests, based on the sensitivity and specificity of results.

Likert scale Type of scale designed to determine the opinions, perceptions, or attitudes of study participants. It contains a number of declarative statements, with a scale after each statement.

Limitations Restrictions in a study methodology and/or framework that may decrease the credibility and generalizability of the findings.

Line of best fit Best reflection of the values on the scatterplot.

Literature All written sources relevant to the topic that the researcher has selected, including articles published in periodicals or journals, internet publications, monographs, encyclopedias, conference papers, theses, dissertations, clinical journals, textbooks, and other books.

Location bias Occurs when studies are published in lower impact journals and indexed in less searched databases.

Logical positivism The philosophy that knowledge is developed based on strict rules of logic, objective truth, and laws.

Logical reasoning Defined process of thinking to draw conclusions.

Logistic regression Testing a predictor (or set of predictors) with a dichotomous dependent variable.

Longitudinal design Noninterventional research that involves collecting data from the same study participants at multiple points in time; participants are recruited for initial data collection followed by subsequent data collection at predefined points.

Low statistical power Increases the probability of concluding that there is no significant relationship between variables or significant difference between groups when there is a relationship or difference.

Manipulation Changing the value or aspects of the independent variable to measure its effect on the dependent variable; form of control used in quasi-experimental and experimental studies during the implementation of the intervention and its characteristics as they exist in a natural environment or setting.

Maps or models Diagrams that visually represent research frameworks; visual way to display the concepts and relationships among them.

Mean   Sum of the scores divided by the number of scores being summed.

Mean difference   Standard statistic that is calculated to determine the absolute difference between the means of two groups.

Measurement   Process of assigning values to objects, events, or situations in accord with some rule.

Measurement error   Difference between the actual true measure and what is measured.

Measures of central tendency   Midpoint in the data or as an average of the data. These measures are the most concise statement of the nature of the data in a study.

Measures of dispersion   Measures of individual differences of the members of the sample.

Median   The midpoint or the score at the exact center of the ungrouped frequency distribution—the 50th percentile.

Member checking   Interview process where the researcher provides the participant with the interview transcript or initial analysis of the data to review.

Meta-analysis   Statistical technique conducted to combine or pool the results from previous quantitative studies into a single statistical analysis that provides strong evidence about an intervention's effectiveness.

Meta-summary   Step in conducting meta-synthesis that involves summarizing findings across qualitative research reports to identify knowledge in a selected area.

Meta-synthesis   Systematic compilation and integration of qualitative studies to expand understanding and develop a unique interpretation of the studies' findings in a selected area.

Methodological bias   Occurs when studies selected for a systematic review have weaknesses in their design and data analysis.

Methodology   General type of research, such as qualitative or quantitative research.

Middle range theories   Relatively concrete conceptual descriptions with a limited number of concepts and propositions that can be applied in practice, used to guide studies, or tested by research; less abstract and narrower in scope than grand nursing theories but are more abstract than theories that apply to only a specific situation.

Mixed methods research   Approach to addressing a research question that combines quantitative and qualitative research methods in a single study.

Mixed methods research synthesis   A review, evaluation, integration, and summation of findings of a variety of study designs.

Mixed results   Study results that are usually the most common outcomes of studies.

Mode   Numerical value or score that occurs with greatest frequency in a set of data; it does not necessarily indicate the center of the data set.

Moderator   Person who will identify the ground rules of the focus group, ask preselected questions, and guide the discussion.

Monograph   Book on a specific subject, a record of conference proceedings, or a pamphlet; is usually a one-time publication.

Mono-method bias   The potential for inaccurate measurement when only one type of measurement is used to assess a construct.

Mono-operation bias   The potential for incomplete measurement when only one tool, questionnaire, or assessment is used to measure a construct.

Multicausality   Presence of multiple causes for an effect.

Multiple regression   Statistical technique conducted to analyze study data; analysis of the effect of two or more independent variables on a dependent variable.

N

Natural or field setting   An uncontrolled, real-life situation or environment.

Negative likelihood ratio (LR)   The ratio of true-negative results to false-negative results; calculated as follows:

$$\text{Negative LR} = (100\% - \text{sensitivity}) \div \text{specificity}$$

Negative relationship   Association in which a high score on one variable is correlated with a low score on the other variable.

Network sampling   Nonprobability sampling technique that is sometimes referred to as snowball or chain sampling, it involves finding a few participants who meet the sampling criteria and asking them for their assistance in finding others with similar characteristics.

Nominal-level measurement   Lowest level of quantification used, and the values are names or labels; sometimes referred to as categorical data.

Nondirectional hypothesis   Type of hypothesis stating that a relationship exists but does not predict the exact nature (positive or negative or strength) of the relationship.

Nonexperimental design   Descriptive and correlational design that focuses on examining variables as they naturally occur in an environment, not on the implementation of a treatment by the researcher.

Noninterventional design   See *Nonexperimental design*.

Nonparametric analysis   Statistical technique conducted if the variables are measured at the nominal and ordinal levels.

Nonprobability sampling   Nonrandom sampling technique in which not every element of the population has an opportunity for selection; commonly used in nursing studies because a limited number of study participants are available.

Nonsignificant (or inconclusive) results   Results that are often referred to as "negative" results and may be a true reflection of reality.

Nontherapeutic research   Type of research conducted to generate knowledge for science.

Normal curve   Theoretical frequency distribution of all possible values in a population; however, no real distribution exactly fits the normal curve.

Null hypothesis (H_0)   Hypothesis that is used for statistical testing and interpretation of statistical results.

Nuremberg Code   The code that emphasizes voluntary consent and contains guidelines related to protecting subjects from harm and balancing the benefits and risks of a study.

Nurse's dependent role functions   Functions that include execution of medical orders and physician-initiated treatments.

Nurse's independent role functions   Functions that include assessment, diagnosis, nurse-initiated interventions, and follow-up care; evaluated by the patient outcomes of symptom control, freedom from complications, functional status and self-care, and knowledge of disease and its treatment, satisfaction, and costs.

Nurse's interdependent role functions   Functions that include communication, case management, coordination and continuity of care, monitoring, and reporting.

Nurse's role in outcomes   Nurse's role in outcomes of a study has three subcomponents: nurse's independent role functions, nurse's dependent role functions, and nurse's interdependent role functions.

Nursing Care Report Card   This report card could facilitate benchmarking or setting a desired standard that would allow comparisons of hospitals in terms of their nursing care quality.

Nursing process   Subset of the problem-solving process used by nurses to assess patients and implement a plan of care.

Nursing research   Scientific process of inquiry that may generate new knowledge or validate and refine existing knowledge; findings directly and indirectly influence the delivery of evidence-based nursing practice.

Nursing-sensitive outcome   Characteristic of the health of individuals or groups that are linked to the "quantity and quality of nursing care."

Nursing-sensitive patient outcome (NSPO)   Patient outcomes that are considered sensitive because they are influenced by nursing care decisions and actions.

Nursing services   General concept referring to the organization and administration of nursing activities.

O

Observation   Fundamental method of gathering data for qualitative studies, especially ethnographic studies.

Observational measurement   Measurement that involves an interaction in which the observer has the opportunity to watch the participant perform in a specific setting and rate the behavior on a numerical scale.

Odds ratio (OR)   The ratio of the odds of an event occurring in one group versus another group.

One-tailed test of significance   Analysis used in which the hypothesis is directional and extreme statistical values that occur in a single tail of the curve are of interest.

Open-ended interview   Type of interview in which the researcher may have only an initial question or statement to start the interview.

Operational definition   Description of how variables or concepts will be measured, manipulated, or controlled in a study.

Ordinal-level measurement   Method whereby data are assigned to categories that can logically be put in order.

Outcome reporting bias   Type of bias that occurs when study results are not reported clearly and with complete accuracy.

Outcomes research   Rigorous scientific method used to investigate the end results of health care; focused on examining the results of care and determining the changes in health status for the patient and family.

Outliers   Study data points that have extreme values (values that lie far from the other plotted points on a graph) that seem unlike the rest of the sample.

P

Paired groups   Participants or observations selected for data collection are related in some way to the selection of other participants or observations.

Parametric analyses   Statistical techniques conducted if variables are at the interval or ratio levels of measurement, and the values of the study participants for the variable are normally distributed.

Paraphrasing   Expressing existing ideas clearly in your own words.

Partially controlled setting   Environment that is manipulated or modified in some way by the researcher.

Participants   Individuals in nursing studies; previously called subjects.

Patient circumstances   Individual's physical condition, disease trajectory, family structure, economic resources, and educational level.

Pearson product-moment correlation (r)   Inferential analysis technique conducted to examine bivariate correlations in studies.

Peer reviewed   Primary source in which the authors submitted a manuscript to a publication editor, who identified scholars familiar with the topic to review and evaluate the manuscript.

Percentage distribution   Percentage of study participants in a sample whose scores fall into a specific group and the number of scores in that group; particularly useful for comparing the present data with findings from other studies that have different sample sizes.

Periodicals   Literature sources such as journals that are published over time and are numbered sequentially for the years published.

Permission to participate in research   Documentation that a parent(s) or guardian agrees for their child or guardian to be in a study.

Personal experience   Knowledge gained through participation in rather than observation of functions, including events, situations, or circumstances.

Phenomena   Events, processes, and situations experienced by human beings during their lives.

Phenomenology   Both a philosophy and a methodology congruent with the philosophy that guides the study of experiences or phenomena.

Philosophies   Rational, intellectual explorations of truths; principles of being, knowledge, or conduct.

Physiological measures   Instruments used to quantify the level of functioning of human beings.

PICOS or PICO format   Acronym for the population or participants of interest; intervention needed for practice; comparisons of interventions to determine the best intervention for your practice; outcomes needed for practice and ways to measure the outcomes in your practice. The "S" stands for study designs. The PICOS or PICO format is used to direct research syntheses.

Pilot study   A smaller version of a proposed study, and researchers frequently conduct these to refine the study sampling process, intervention, or measurement of variables.

Placebo group   Group of participants who receive an intervention that is like the intervention being tested.

Plagiarism   Using another person's work without citing the reference or otherwise giving that person credit.

Population All elements (individuals, objects, or situations) that meet certain criteria for inclusion in a study.

Population-based studies Studies conducted within the context of the patient's community rather than the context of the medical system.

Positive likelihood ratio (LR) Ratio used to determine the true-positive results to false-positive results. It is calculated by the following:

$$\text{Positive } LR = \text{sensitivity} \div (100\% - \text{specificity})$$

Positive relationship Numeric association in which a high score on one variable is correlated with a high score on another variable or a low score on one variable is correlated with a low score on another variable.

Post hoc analyses Three or more groups may be identified as being different than each other on a specific variable. The post-hoc analysis will determine which pairs of groups are significantly different.

Posttest-only design with a comparison group Quasi-experimental design used in situations in which a pretest is not possible.

Power Ability of the study to detect differences or relationships that actually exist in the population.

Power analysis Technique used to evaluate the adequacy of the sample size in quantitative and outcomes studies.

Practice pattern Represents variations in what care is provided.

Practice style Represents variations in how care is provided.

Precision Encompasses accuracy, detail, and order; degree of consistency or reproducibility of measurements made with physiological instruments.

Predatory journals Academic journals that bypass or minimize quality-control measures, including peer review.

Prediction Estimation of the probability of a specific outcome in a given situation that can be achieved through research.

Predictive correlational design Correlational design used to predict the value of one variable based on the values obtained for another variable or variables.

Predictive validity Extent to which an individual's score on a scale can be used to predict future performance or behavior on a criterion.

Primary data Data collected for a particular study.

Primary source Publication whose author originated or is responsible for generating the ideas published.

Principle of beneficence Ethical principle that encourages the researcher to do good instead of harm.

Principle of justice Ethical principle that states that human participants have a right to fair treatment.

Principle of respect for persons Ethical principle that indicates people should be treated as autonomous agents, with the right to choose whether to participate in research or withdraw from a study.

Privacy Freedom to determine the time, extent, and general circumstances under which private information will be shared with or withheld from others.

Probability Addresses the relative rather than the absolute causality of events.

Probability sampling Sampling method in which each person or element in a population has an opportunity to be selected for a sample.

Probability theory Explains the extent of a relationship, the probability that an event will occur in a given situation, or the probability that selected outcomes will occur in a study.

Probe Question or open-ended statement of a qualitative researcher during an interview to obtain more information from the participant about a specific interview question.

Problem statement Statement that indicates the gap in the knowledge needed for practice.

Process Structured, logical series of actions with a defined goal.

Professional practice Providing knowledgeable, skillful, and holistic care to patients, families, and communities as part of a healthcare team.

Proposition Relational statements in a study's framework that are tested through research.

Prospective Looking forward.

Prospective cohort study Uses an epidemiological study design in which the researcher identifies a group of people who are at risk for experiencing a particular event and then follows the group over time to observe whether the event occurs.

Protected health information Data generated and collected for research that can be linked to an individual.

Protocol Detailed plan for implementing an intervention and measuring its effects precisely and consistently.

Proximal outcome Outcome that is close to the delivery of care. An example of a proximal outcome is signs and symptoms of disease.

Publication bias Problems that can occur in conducting and reporting research syntheses including time lag bias, location bias, duplicate publication bias, citation bias, and language bias.

Purposive (or purposeful) sampling Referred to as judgmental or selective sampling; the researcher consciously selects certain participants or situations to include in the study.

Q

Qualitative research A systematic subjective approach used to describe life experiences and situations and give them meaning.

Qualitative research critical appraisal process Three-part process that consists of (1) identifying the components of the qualitative research process in studies; (2) determining study strengths and weaknesses; and (3) evaluating the trustworthiness, credibility, and meaning of study findings.

Qualitative research process Research process that involves identifying a researchable problem that can be addressed by collecting textual and observational data.

Qualitative research synthesis Process and product of systematically reviewing and formally integrating the findings from qualitative studies.

Quality and Safety Education for Nurses (QSEN) Initiative on identifying the requisite knowledge, skills, and attitude statements for each of the competencies for nurses and recommended strategies for incorporating the competencies into nursing education.

Quantitative research Formal, objective, systematic process in which numerical data are used to obtain information about the world.

Quantitative research critical appraisal process This process includes three basic steps: (1) identifying the steps of the research process in studies; (2) determining study strengths and weaknesses; and (3) evaluating the credibility and meaning of study findings; these steps occur in sequence, vary in depth, and presume accomplishment of the preceding steps.

Quantitative research process Involves conceptualizing a research project (gathering information, making observations, and identifying problems), planning and implementing that project, and communicating the findings.

Quasi-experimental design Plan for a study developed to facilitate the search for knowledge and examination of causality in situations in which complete control is not possible; determine the effectiveness of interventions when some aspect of an experiment cannot be implemented.

Quasi-experimental research Objective, systematic study of cause-and-effect relationships in settings with less control than experimental research.

Questionnaire Self-report form designed to elicit information through written, verbal, or electronic responses of the study participant.

Quota sampling Nonprobability convenience sampling technique with an added feature—a strategy to ensure the inclusion of participant types likely to be underrepresented in the convenience sample, such as minority groups, children, and those with limited access to health care.

R

Random measurement error Type of error in which the difference between the measured value and the true value is without pattern or direction (random).

Random sampling Sampling method in which everyone in the accessible population has an equal opportunity for selection.

Randomized controlled trial (RCT) Noted to be the strongest methodology for testing the effectiveness of an intervention because of the elements of the experimental design that limit the potential for bias and error.

Range Simplest measure of dispersion that is obtained by subtracting the lowest score from the highest score.

Rating scale A form of measurement involving scaling techniques; includes an ordered series of categories of a variable that are assumed to be based on an underlying continuum.

Ratio-level measurement Highest form of measurement meeting all the rules of other levels of measurement—mutually exclusive categories, exhaustive categories, ordered ranks, equally spaced intervals, and continuum of values.

Readability level Approximate educational level required to comprehend written information.

Reading a research report Method of reading that includes skimming, comprehending, and analyzing to facilitate an understanding of the study.

Reasoning Processing and organizing ideas to reach conclusions.

Recommendations for further research Including replications or repeating the design with a different or larger sample, using different measurement methods, or testing a modified or new intervention; may also include the formation of hypotheses to further test the framework in use.

Refereed journals Journals that have their articles critically appraised by expert peer reviewers.

Reference Documentation of the origin of a cited quote or paraphrased idea that provides enough information for the reader to locate the original material.

Reflexivity A researcher's acknowledgment of personal experiences and expectations that influence the study.

Refusal rate Percentage of potential subjects who declined to participate in the study and their reasons for not participating.

Regression analysis Statistical procedure used to predict the value of one variable when the value of one or more other variables is known.

Relational statement Explains the connection between two concepts.

Relevant studies Quality research with findings that have a direct bearing on the problem of concern.

Reliability Extent to which an instrument consistently measures a concept or phenomenon.

Reliability testing Method to determine the measurement error in an instrument used in a study.

Replication studies Reproductions or repetitions of a study that researchers conducted to determine whether the findings of the original study could be found consistently in different settings and with different study participants.

Reporting bias Occurs if certain results are missing from or inaccurately presented in a research report.

Representativeness Means that the sample, accessible population, and target population are alike in as many ways as possible.

Reputable journal Academic journal that uses peer review and other quality-control measures that are transparently described on their website.

Research Diligent, systematic inquiry or investigation to validate and refine existing knowledge and generate new knowledge.

Research concepts Ideas, experiences, situations, events, or cultures that are investigated in qualitative and mixed methods studies.

Research design Blueprint for conducting a study; maximizes control over factors that could interfere with the validity of the findings and guides the planning and implementation of a study in a way that is most likely to achieve the intended goal.

Researcher–participant relationship Involvement of the researcher with the participants of the study.

Research framework Abstract and logical structure of meaning that guides the development of a study and allows the researcher to link the findings back to the body of knowledge.

Research hypothesis Alternative hypothesis to the null hypothesis. It states that a relationship exists between two or more variables.

Research misconduct   The fabrication, falsification, or plagiarism in processing, performing, or reviewing research, or in reporting research results.

Research objective   Clear, concise, declarative statement that identifies the goals of a study.

Research problem   Area of concern in which there is a gap in the knowledge base needed for nursing practice. Research is conducted to generate essential knowledge to address the practice concern, with the ultimate goal of providing evidence-based practice. The research problem in a study needs to include significance, background, and problem statement.

Research process   Logical steps that involve rigorous application of a variety of research methods.

Research purpose   Statement generated from the problem that identifies a concise, clear statement of the specific focus or goal of the study.

Research question   Concise, clear interrogative statement that is worded in the present tense, includes one or more variables, and is expressed to guide the implementation of studies.

Research report   Written or verbal summary of the major elements of a study and identifies the contributions of that study to nursing knowledge.

Research setting   Site or location for conducting a study.

Research synthesis   Summary of relevant studies to determine the empirical knowledge in an area that is critical to the advancement of practice, research, and policy development.

Research synthesis by aggregation   Synthesis of mixed method study that depends on both qualitative and quantitative findings being conceived as potentially addressing the same factors or aspects of a target phenomenon.

Research synthesis by configuration   Synthesis of mixed method study that occurs when diverse individual findings or sets of aggregated findings are arranged into a coherent theoretical framework or model.

Research topics   Concept or broad issues that are important to nursing, such as chronic pain management, posttraumatic stress disorder assessment, prevention of the coronavirus (COVID-19) spread, and health promotion strategies for children.

Research variables   Qualities, properties, or characteristics identified in the research purpose and objectives, or questions that are observed or measured in a study.

Retrospective   Looking backward, usually in relation to time.

Retrospective cohort study   Epidemiological study in which the researcher identifies a group of people who have experienced a particular event.

Review of literature   Process of finding relevant research sources and theoretical sources, critically appraising these sources, synthesizing the results, and developing an accurate and complete reference list.

Review of relevant literature   Summary of current theoretical and empirical sources to generate a picture of what is known and not known about a particular problem and to document why a study needs to be conducted.

Rigor   Striving for excellence in research, which requires discipline, adherence to detail, precision, and accuracy.

S

Sample   Subset of the population that is selected for a study.

Sample attrition   The withdrawal or loss of participants from a study and can be expressed as either a number or a percentage.

Sample retention   Number of study participants remaining in and completing the study.

Sample size   Number of individuals participating in the study.

Sampling   Process of selecting participants who are representative of the population being studied.

Sampling criteria   List of the characteristics essential for inclusion or exclusion in the target population.

Sampling frame   List of every member of the target population using the sampling criteria to define eligibility.

Sampling method   Strategies used to obtain samples for studies.

Saturation   Point during a qualitative study when additional participants or data sources do not provide new information.

Scale   Self-report form of measurement composed of several items designed to measure a construct that is more precise than a questionnaire.

Scatterplot   Plot with two scales, horizontal and vertical, and is used to illustrate the dispersion of values on a variable.

Scientific theory   Framework for physiological studies; usually derived from physiology, genetics, pathophysiology, and physics.

Secondary analysis   Any reanalysis of data or information collected by other researchers, organizations, or agencies.

Secondary data   Data collected from previous research and stored in a database.

Secondary source   Publication whose author summarizes or quotes content from primary sources.

Seminal studies   The first studies on a particular topic that signaled the beginning of a new way of thinking on the topic and sometimes are referred to as classic studies.

Semistructured interview   Interaction between a researcher and participant guided by a fixed set of questions and no fixed responses.

Sensitivity   The proportion of patients with the condition or disease who have a positive test result, or true-positive rate.

Separate synthesis   Synthesizing the findings from quantitative studies separately from qualitative studies and integrating the findings from these two syntheses in the final report.

Setting   The location in which a study is conducted.

Significance of a research problem   Indicates the importance of the problem to nursing and health care and to the health of individuals, families, and communities.

Significant results   Results that agree with those predicted by the researcher and support the logical links developed by the researcher among the purpose, questions or hypotheses, variables, framework, and measurement tools.

Significant and unpredicted results   Results that are the opposite of those predicted by the researcher and indicate that flaws are present in the logic of the researcher and theory being tested.

Simple descriptive design   Used to examine variables in a single sample.

Simple hypothesis Statement of a relationship (associative or causal) between two variables.

Simple linear regression Conducted when one independent variable is used to predict one dependent variable.

Simple random sampling The most basic of the probability sampling plans that is achieved by randomly selecting elements from the sampling frame.

Situation-specific theory Theories that are more concrete than middle range theories and limited to a population and phenomenon or a nursing specialty; designed to propose approaches to specific nursing practice situations.

Skimming research reports Quickly reviewing a source to gain a broad overview of the content.

Social constructivism A shared reality that has been constructed through our interactions with individuals and groups.

Specificity The proportion of patients without the disease who have a negative test result, or true-negative rate.

Specific propositions Statements indicating a relationship between concepts that can be tested.

Stability reliability The reproducibility of scores with repeated measures of the same concept or attribute with a scale over time.

Standard deviation (*SD*) Measure of dispersion, which is the square root of the variance.

Standardized mean difference (*SMD*) Summary statistic that is reported in a meta-analysis when the same outcome is measured by different scales or methods.

Standardized mortality ratio (SMR) Observed number of deaths divided by the expected number of deaths and multiplied by 100. SMR is regarded as a measure of the relative risk of the studied group to die of a particular condition.

Standardized score Mechanism developed to transform raw scores using the means and standard deviations for a variable.

Standard of care Norm on which the quality of care is judged.

Statements Sentences that describe how concepts are connected to each other, usually in a theoretical framework.

Statistical analysis Techniques conducted to examine, reduce, and give meaning to a study's numeric data.

Statistical conclusion validity Concerned with whether the conclusions about relationships or differences drawn from statistical analyses are an accurate reflection of the real world.

Statistical hypothesis See *Null hypothesis*.

Stetler Model of Research Utilization to Facilitate Evidence-Based Practice Model developed by Stetler that provides a comprehensive framework to enhance the use of research evidence by nurses to facilitate evidence-based practice.

Stratified random sampling Method used when the researcher knows that some of the variables in the population are critical to achieving representativeness.

Structured interview Communication between the researcher and participant during which predetermined questions are asked in the same order for all interviews; can be used to collect quantitative data by assigning numbers to the answer options.

Structured observational measurement Measurement in which the researcher carefully defines what was observed, who conducted the observations, and how the observations were made, recorded, and coded as numbers.

Structure in outcomes Based on Donabedian's theory, structure of outcomes includes three subcomponents—nurse, organization, and patient.

Structures of care Elements of organization and administration, as well as provider and patient characteristics that guide the processes of care.

Subjects Individuals participating in a study (those being studied), who are sometimes referred to as participants.

Subject terms Standardized phrases, more formal than keywords that are used to identify studies on a topic during a literature review.

Substantive theory Conceptual structure of clearly identified concepts, definitions, and relational statements; can also be called *middle-range theories*; more commonly applied as frameworks in nursing studies.

Symbolic use Application of research evidence that occurs when position papers or proposals for change are developed to persuade others toward a new way of thinking.

Symmetrical Correlational analyses, which means that the variables are related to each other but the analysis gives no indication of the direction of the relationship.

Synthesis Clustering and interrelating ideas from several studies to promote a new understanding or provide a description of what is known and not known in an area.

Systematic measurement error Nonrandom measurement error in which the variation in measurement values from the calculated average is primarily in the same direction.

Systematic review A structured, comprehensive synthesis of the research literature to determine the best research evidence available to address a healthcare question.

Systematic sampling Conducted when an ordered list of all members of the population is available; involves selecting every *k*th individual on the list, using a starting point selected randomly.

T

Target population Entire set of individuals or elements who meet the sampling criteria.

Tentative theory Newly proposed conceptual structure that has had minimal exposure to critique by scholars and has undergone little testing.

Testable hypothesis A hypothesis that clearly predicts the relationships among variables and contains variables that are measurable or able to be manipulated in a study.

Test-retest reliability The determination of the stability of an instrument that measures variables that change minimally over time.

Textbook Monograph or book regarded as the standard for the study of a particular subject; may serve as a source of information for an academic course.

Theoretical literature Concept analyses, maps, theories, and conceptual frameworks that support a selected research problem and purpose.

Theoretical sampling Mainly implemented in grounded theory studies to explore the topic with different types of participants; method that is designed and implemented to develop a model, framework, or theory.

Theory Integrated set of defined concepts and statements that present a view of a phenomenon.

Therapeutic research Studies providing a patient with the opportunity for a potential benefit from an experimental treatment.

Thesis Report of a research project completed by a postgraduate student as part of the requirements for a master's degree.

Threats to validity Possible weaknesses in a study's design; organized into four categories—construct validity, internal validity, statistical conclusion validity, and external validity.

Time lag bias of studies Type of publication bias; occurs because studies with negative results are usually published later, sometimes 2 to 3 years later, than studies with positive results. Sometimes studies with negative results are not published at all.

Total variance Sum of within-group variance and between-group variance determined by an analysis of variance.

Traditions "Truths" or beliefs based on customs and habits.

Transcripts Typed records of audio recordings, video recordings, and notes made during observation.

Transferability Term used to describe the ability to transcend the sample and be applicable with similar participants.

Translation and application phase Stetler Model of Research Utilization to Facilitate Evidence-Based Practice phase that involves planning for and using the research evidence in practice.

Translational research An evolving strategy that is defined by the National Institutes of Health as the translation of basic scientific discoveries into practical applications.

Translational science The field of investigation focused on understanding the scientific and operational principles underlying each step of the translational process.

Translational science spectrum This model represents the concepts and their interaction in the translational science spectrum at each stage of research along the path from the biological basis of health and disease to interventions that improve the health of individuals and the public.

Treatment group Portion of a sample that receives the intervention being studied; group in which outcomes are expected to be different.

True measure or score Ideal or perfect measure.

True-negative (result) Diagnostic or screening test result that accurately indicates the absence of a disease.

True-positive (result) Diagnostic or screening test result that accurately indicates the presence of a disease.

Trustworthiness A determination that a qualitative study is rigorous and of high quality.

t-Test Statistical technique conducted to test for significant differences between two samples when variables are measured at the interval or ration level.

Two-tailed test of significance Analysis of a nondirectional hypothesis.

Type I error Occurs when the null hypothesis is rejected when it is true (e.g., when the results indicate there is a significant difference, when in reality there is not).

Type II error Occurs when the null hypothesis is regarded as true but is in fact false.

Unexpected results Results that are usually relationships found between variables that were not hypothesized and not predicted from the study framework.

Unexplained variance Variation between or among two or more variables that is the result of things other than the relationships.

Ungrouped frequency distribution Statistical distribution in which a table is developed to display all numerical values obtained for a particular variable; this approach is generally used on discrete rather than continuous data. Examples of data commonly organized in this manner are gender, ethnicity/race, and marital status, and values obtained from the measurement of selected research and dependent variables.

Unstructured interview Communication between the researcher and the participant that begins with a broad question. Participants are encouraged to elaborate on a topic, introduce new topics, and thereby control the content of the interview; commonly used to collect qualitative data.

Unstructured observation Spontaneously watching and recording what is seen in words.

Validation phase Stetler Model of Research Utilization to Facilitate Evidence-Based Practice phase wherein research reports are critically appraised to determine their scientific soundness.

Validity Extent to which an instrument indicates how well it measures the abstract concept it was developed to measure; the credibility of quantitative study findings due to the control and rigor of the study.

Validity from factor analysis A type of construct validity that involves the use of statistical techniques to determine the various dimensions or subcomponents of a construct of interest.

Variables Concepts at various levels of abstraction that are measured, manipulated, or controlled in a study.

Variance Measure of dispersion in which the scores in a study are calculated with a mathematical equation and indicate the spread or dispersion of the scores; the variance can be calculated on data only at the interval or ratio level of measurement.

Visual analog scale (VAS) Typically used to measure strength, magnitude, or intensity of individuals' subjective feelings, sensations, or attitudes about symptoms or situations.

Voluntary agreement Decision made by a prospective subject to participate in a study of his or her own volition, without coercion or any undue influence.

Vulnerable populations Potential research participants who are more susceptible to undue influence or coercion, such as children, prisoners, and those who are economically disadvantaged.

Websites Internet pages maintained by individuals, organizations, and companies to provide information, which must be evaluated for their accuracy, bias, and relevance prior to citation in a literature review.

Within-group variance Variation of individual scores in a group that will vary from the group mean; determined by conducting analysis of variance.

X

x-**Axis** Horizontal scale of a scatterplot; represents the possible values of the variable.

Y

y-**Axis** Vertical scale of a scatterplot; represents the number of times each value of the variable occurred in the sample.

Z

z-**Scores** Common standardized score; expresses deviations from the mean (difference scores) in terms of standard deviation units.

Note: Page numbers followed by "*f*" indicate figures, "*t*" indicate tables, and "*b*" indicate boxes.